Pharmacy In Bondage

Dr. Patrick Ojo

Pharmacy in Bondage
Copyright © 2021 Dr. Patrick Ojo

Library of Congress Control Number: 2021902160
ISBN-13: Paperback: 978-1-64749-350-9
Hardcover: 978-1-64749-351-6
ePub: 978-1-64749-352-3

All rights reserved. No part of this publication may be reproduced, distributed, or transmitted in any form or by any means, including photocopying, recording, or other electronic or mechanical methods, without the prior written permission of the publisher or author, except in the case of brief quotations embodied in critical reviews and certain other noncommercial uses permitted by copyright law.

Although every precaution has been taken to verify the accuracy of the information contained herein, the author and publisher assume no responsibility for any errors or omissions. No liability is assumed for damages that may result from the use of information contained within.

Printed in the United States of America

GoToPublish LLC
1-888-337-1724
www.gotopublish.com
info@gotopublish.com

BOOK ACCOLADES/REVIEWS/COMMENTS AND JUSTICE FOR PHARMACY.

1. HOLLYWOOD BOOK REVIEWS:

When it comes to the health profession, many people automatically associate the profession with that of a Doctor or Nurse. Yet there is another profession whose contributions have greatly added and aided the medical health career, and that is that of the Pharmacist. As scientist Tu You once said, "My choice of learning pharmacy was driven by my interests, curiosity, and a desire to seek new medicines for patients." In author Dr. Patrick Ojo's book "Pharmacy in Bondage", the author uses their expertise to fully explore the history of the world of Pharmacy. From the extensive knowledge and education pharmacists must undergo and their expertise with medicine to how undervalued and underutilized pharmacists are in the medical field and beyond, the author takes the time to perfectly outline this field in full. This is a lengthy, passionate and thorough read. The author really takes the time to delve into so much of the health profession and pharmacology in particular. From the history of the various branches of health and medicine to the history of pharmacy, comparing the curriculum of medical schools around the world to that of pharmacology, and the expertise pharmacists have with drugs and medicine overall, this book covers the topic in great detail, and yet never takes the time to assert itself as the dominate profession in the field of medicine. Instead the author encourages readers to seek a balance where all medical professionals work together for the good of the patient rather than themselves. This is a perfect book for those who enjoy reads involving medicine, health, and in particular pharmacology. In particular pharmacists and medical professionals will appreciate the detail and the insight into their field the book provides, and showcases the intense education that goes into the field. The author's expertise and knowledge shine through in every chapter, highlighting specific drug trials and cases and how pharmacology helps to bring the right medicine into the field. This was a detail-oriented, lengthy and educational read. Dr. Patrick Ojo's novel "Pharmacy in Bondage" is an enriching and thought-provoking read, and the author brilliantly focuses on the ins and outs of the pharmacological field in general that most average readers would not have been privy to. Be sure to grab your copy and see for yourself why pharmacists are not to be taken for granted.

A brief history of Pharmaceuticals: Medicine has come a long way from pure herbs and larvae and will likely continue to improve as time passes. Pharmaceuticals has always been an essential part of medical history as it maintains and improves the quality of human life by giving people easy access to medication and alternative treatments. This is done by studying the effects of different compounds on the human body when ingested. In Pharmacy in Bondage, the book published by author Patrick Ojo creates a detailed account of the history of pharmaceuticals consisting of its rise in popularity, its practices, and its repression into a forgotten medical science part. Society must recognize pharmacists are an essential part of the management of health. It is becoming more comfortable to ask for assistance at a pharmacy than to ask for help in more intricate medical facilities. "Pharmacists are critical to ensuring patient safety, optimal health outcomes, and controlling total healthcare spending." An informative point of view and one that is shared by many. Doctors are indeed the more well-known medical professionals, but pharmacists are Just as essential to human health and well-being. We have specialists who cater to every aspect of our lives except the poison that we pump into our bodies as drugs; all specialists are in control of their destiny except pharmacists who are treated as children in their area of jurisdiction; pharmacists are over-educated, under-utilized and marginalized medical practitioners. Copies of this informative work are available online at Amazon, BarnesandNoble, and GoToPublish. Read the hardships and criticisms the pharmaceutical branch of medicine must endure as well as read the history of such a traditional branch of medicine. This book addresses the challenges that pharmacists face in trying to make full use of in different health care settings.

Reviewed by: Tony Espinoza

2. 5 Star - 100% (5 out of 5) Book Review by D. Buffington, a Customer in Amazon.com: Buffington Reviewed Pharmacy In Bondage with the following caption -- Pharmacists make "The Difference" with regards to Medication Safety and Improved Health Outcomes. He tagged his review as Critical issue, noting that pharmacists are critical to ensuring patient safety, optimal health outcomes, and controlling total health care spend. This book addresses the challenges that pharmacists face in their attempt to be fully utilized across different health care settings. Like most of the reviewers in this section, Buffington is relatively unknown to the author and might not be a medical professional.

D. Buffington
Customer reviews, Amazon.com

3. United States of America Dept. of Health & Human Services through Secretary Kathleen Sebelius, 21st United States Secretary of Health and Human Services, 2009 — 2014 said via Associate Administrator Joyce G. Somsak, we certainly agree with "Pharmacy in Bondage" that clinical pharmacy services that are integrated into our healthcare system improve patient safety and patient outcomes. The Health Resources and Services Administration (HRSA), one of the agencies within the Department of Health and Human Services is at the forefront of this issue with a breakthrough effort to improve the quality of health care across America by integrating evidence-based clinical pharmacy services into the care and management of patients with chronic diseases. This initiative is called HRSA's Patient Safety and Clinical Pharmacy Collaborative (PSPC). To learn more about our efforts and to see the progress that the PSPC has made towards maximizing the value of clinical pharmacy services, please visit our Web site: http://www.hrsa.gov/patientsafety/default.htm. Teams of organizations that participate in this collaborative are implementing many of the principles contained in your book, Pharmacy in Bondage.

Secretary Kathleen Sebelius thru Joyce G.
Somsak, Associate Administrator.

4. Representative Bart Stupak in US Congress, Michigan (Democratic) - District 1, 103rd-111th (1993-2011): Rep Bart said as a member of the House Energy and Commerce Committee, I am familiar with the unique challenges involved in prescription drug regulation. I commend you for your knowledge of medicine, in particular pharmacology.

5. Representative Clifford "Cliff" Stearns in US Congress, Florida (Republican) – District 6, 101st-112th (1989-2012): Rep Clifford said "Pharmacy in Bondage" Couple my personal interest in our healthcare system and its escalating importance on a national level, I am sure to find your book very informative. Thanks for your thoughtfulness.

6. Representative Heather Wilson of New Mexico (Republican), in US Congress, New Mexico, District 1 105th -110th (1997-2009): Rep Heather did not only read the book, Pharmacy in Bondage twice or more but went ahead to introduce the Bill, H.R. 5780 — Medicare Clinical Pharmacist Practitioner Services Coverage Act of 2008 before the end of 110th Congress Session based on the message of the book. The Bill, H. R. 5780 was supported by cosponsors Rep. Marion Berry of Arkansa (Democratic) District 1 105th -111th (1997-2011), Rep David Price of North Carolina (Democratic) District 4 105th -116th (1997-Present), Rep Mike McIntyre of North Carolina (Democratic) District 7 105th -113th (1997-2015), Rep Bob Etheridge Of North Carolina (Democratic) District 2 105th -111th (1997-2011) and Rep Tom Udall of New Mexico (Democratic) District 3 106th -110th (1999-2009) and Senator of New Mexico 111th -116th (2009-Present). All of them read the book, Pharmacy in Bondage and supported pharmacy libration with the bill, H.R 5780.

7. **Lauren Arsonson on behalf of The Pharmacy Coalition comprising of Academy of Managed Care Pharmacy, American Association of Colleges of Pharmacy, American College of Clinical Pharmacy, American Pharmacists Association, American Society of Consultant Pharmacists, American Society of Health-System Pharmacists, Food Marketing Institute, National Alliance of State Pharmacy Association, National Association of Chain Drug Stores, National Community Pharmacists Association, Rite Aid Corporation and Walgreens Company** in a letter to Director Nancy-Ann Deparle of White House Office of Health Reform echoed many things from the book, Pharmacy in Bondage without direct quotations. Direct quotation from the letter reads "By promoting and utilizing the professional clinical skills and competencies of pharmacists, the goal of improve patient therapeutic outcomes will be more effectively realized. In addition, recognizing and relying on the clinical knowledge and expertise of pharmacists will help address the serious consequences of improper medication use which costs our nation close to $200 billion dollars a year in preventable medication-related errors. ----- It is time to optimize medication use by accessing the knowledge and skills of today's pharmacists — a highly trained and valuable, yet underutilized resource". The national organizations through the letter encouraged the incorporation of Pharmacy Principle For Health Care Reform in any US Health Care reform.

8. **Texas Pharmacy Association.** After book review of Pharmacy in Bondage by the Texas Pharmacy Association Editorial Board, the board requested that the book be described as a Prescription for Truth in order to better fit Texas Pharmacy Association's goals and member profile. Rx.perts, The official News Magazine of Texas Pharmacy Association.

> Rx.perts, 1624 East Anderson Lane, Austin,
> Texas 78752, 512-836-8350

9. **New York State Pharmacist Association** -- New York State Pharmacist: Century II, Official Publication of the Pharmacists Society of the State of New York (PSSNY) in its book review of Pharmacy in Slavery, twins publication of Pharmacy in Bondage highlighted in a caption **"Remember, we are fighting for the well being of our patients, not for power over other professionals."** The beginning of the review reads "Time brings advancement and growth to nearly every profession. Pharmacy is no exception to this phenomenon. As the future of pharmacy begins to evolve, we must look these changes

in the eye and welcome advancement of our profession. We must face the struggle for respect with strength and dignity. If we chose not to, we will be left behind while the rest of the medical community passes us by." The magazine reviewer, Dr. Bridget DuMont said It is our job as pharmacists, to embrace these changes with enthusiasm and confidence knowing that pharmacy is finally becoming what it has had the capability of being for centuries. She noted the comparison made in the book about many society's struggles with equality over time and how they overcome. Some of the struggles she cited from the book are Women's rights, the American Colonies versus Britain and Copernicus versus the Church. According to Dr. DuMont, The point being made was that pharmacists too can overcome the battle with society and the medical profession to become equal members of the health care profession if we are willing to fight for it. She said It is a proven fact that pharmacists take the most pharmacy courses of all medical professions and are therefore the drug experts. The proof is in the billions of dollars that pharmacists have saved patients and society by recommending more effective therapies and by detecting interactions before they occur. --- The book thoroughly refutes any accusation that pharmacists are not qualified to be medication experts with documented studies. Pharmacy in Slavery or Pharmacy in Bondage will inspire any pharmacist to utilize their degree to the fullest extent.---As we come together to demand respect let us remember Dr. Ojo's words, "The paramount interest in saving lives and unnecessary medical expenses/costs ought to be the utmost goal in using all available means and tools to strengthen pharmacists as drug specialists and enable pharmacy to overcome its deficiencies and stand on its feet---" then she repeated the above caption.

NY. Published bimonthly by PSSNY, 210 Washington Ave. Ext., Suite 101, Albany, NY 12203, 518-869-6595/800-632-8822.

10.   California Pharmacists Association — California Pharmacist, the official magazine of California Pharmacists Association advertised Pharmacy in Bondage with hints that elucidates 1 in 14 courses qualifies physician Assistants to prescribe drugs in just 1 year, 1 in 25 courses for Certified Nurse Practitioners, 1 in 17 courses for Optometrists and others but 7 in 10 courses do not qualify Clinical Pharmacists to prescribe drugs.

California Pharmacists Association, 4030 Lennane Drive, Sacramento, CA 95834. 916-779-1400, http://www.cpha.com.

11.   Long Island University Magazine tagged Pharmacy in Slavery, the twins publication of Pharmacy In Bondage as "A Prescription for

Truth" in its publication. The magazine noted that pharmacists have always taken a back seat to other health professionals, when in fact they provide life-saving services to patients each and every day. They acknowledges the Author's view that some changes have been made in the industry, but stressed that there still remains much to do to elevate the role of pharmacists and ensure that this specialty field becomes integrated at a different level in patient care.

        Long Island University Magazine, University Center, 700 Northern Blvd, Brookville, New York 11548-1327

12. **The Bloomsbury Review** reflected on the book, Pharmacy in Bondage and its twins publication Pharmacy in Slavery as a true professional reflection saying Pharmacy is branch of Medicine and not an errand boy of Medicine.

        The Bloomsbury Review, 1553 Platte Street, Suite 206, Denver, CO 80202-1167.

13. **12. The New York Times Book Review** of Pharmacy in Slavery, the twins publication of Pharmacy in Bondage showed how the book depicts an accurate account of pharmacy history, its slavery status, subservience, topsy-turvy fame, service to humanity, and awesome healthcare contribution. Pharmacists are overeducated, underutilized, and marginalized medical practitioners.

        The New York Times Book Review Company, 620 Eighth Avenue, New York, NY 10018. NYtimes.com/book, 800-NYTIMES (800-698-4637).

14. **Canada — Pharmacy Practice,** Professional Journal for Canada's Pharmacists. A Satirical Review of Pharmacy in Slavery, the twins publication of Pharmacy in Bondage by Professor Zubin Austin of Faculty of Pharmacy, University of Toronto showed a dogmatic view of a professor thoroughly schooled in an old system, belief in the old system and cannot break loose from it or come to terms with new pharmacy professional approach to medical practice and evolution in the medical field that has currently incorporated osteopathic medicine after much heresy, opposition and agitation, Dentistry — Optometry — Veterinary medicine — Physician Assistants —Certified Nurse Practitioners and others' prescribing acts after much heresy/opposition/agitation. The fact that pharmacy has been left out of this glorious fight because of our complacent, lack of willingness to fight for our rights in the medical field and indoctrination by the likes of Dr. Zubin is obvious in the book and other places. Dr. Zubin in his sarcastic review, said "The breathtaking scope of this subject, coupled with the almost inflammatory title of the book, suggests that readers may look forward to a provocative and insightful examination of interprofessional relationships. This was a self-serving review born out of envy with no specific interest for pharmacy profession and its projection in a challenging current/future medical field and the world. He ignored most of the studies and facts in the book that are worthy of intellectual investigations, analysis, deductions and publications (he as a University Professor, saddled with a lot of research work could have taking this as a research project and come up with his own results) for people to read and decide for themselves what is truth and fictions. He claimed that all the studies and facts in the book are the author's personalized account even though the author of Pharmacy in Bondage wasn't the publisher or originator of those studies and facts. In his words "Ojo provides a highly personalized account of the history of pharmacy, attempting to draw parallels between the professions of pharmacy and medicine and the history of colonial powers. While the metaphor is highly stretched, Ojo does make an important point — after years of "subjugation" to Physicians, most pharmacists, today simply do not know how to act as independent collaborative healthcare professionals." This last quotation from him is a clear indication of a profession in bondage or a profession incapable of operating as an independent specialty like other branches of medicine.

Pharmacy Practice, One Mount Pleasant Road, 7th Floor, Toronto, ON M4Y 2Y5, 416-764-3926.

15. Florida Pharmacy Association Vice President Michael Jackson: The book Pharmacy in Bondage is indeed an interesting analysis of our profession and its training modules in comparison with other health professions. Over the years our training has expanded both in scope and duration. Historically the first skillsets acquired by pharmacists were based upon an apprentice model. You demonstrate your knowledge and skills and "you're in". Today's pharmacy training is far beyond that and according to the author of Pharmacy in Bondage, is likely comparable or better than many other health professions. It is well known that the training of today's pharmacist candidates is developed for a practice that is only slowly beginning to emerge. There are many barriers in place including but not limited to regulatory restrictions, acceptance by some health care provider advocacy organizations and even from within our own profession. Pharmacy in Bondage peals back the mysterious environment we are in and suggests that tasks performed by other health care professionals can be better managed by pharmacists. This book is appropriate reading for not only those within pharmacy circles but also health care managers, administrators, policy makers and even other health care provider stakeholders. It will likely clear the air of misconception others may have about our industry and of capabilities.

Executive Vice President/CEO Michael A Jackson,
BPharm, CPh., Florida Pharmacy Association,
610 North Adams Street, Tallahassee, FL 32301.

16. **Former President of Florida Pharmacy Association and Member of Florida Board of Pharmacy,** Bob Parrado described Pharmacy in Bondage as Very interesting read. The book shows the difficult environment pharmacists are expected to practice in and still deliver quality healthcare. Patient safety has to be the most important factor when making business decisions.

Florida Pharmacy Association Ex-President Bob Parrado.

17. **Director of Information and Communication Technology (ICT - Retired) - Magnus Osagie Omoregie, The West African Examinations Council, Lagos, Nigeria:** The book, Pharmacy in Bondage is full of Historical, academic and journalistic analysis/quest. It gives an insight into the practice of medicine as a whole, revealing the inherent dilemma of Pharmacy profession, clinical pharmacists and pharmacists who are constantly faced with politicking, subjugation and other ills that are prevalent in traditional medicine practice through age-long 'Hippocratic Oath' and doctrines maintained over the years by medical doctors. In summary Pharmacy in Bondage acknowledges that, though medical doctors, dentists, optometrists, Veterinarians, and Pharmacists go through various rigorous inter/intradisciplinary course work that prepare them for their specialty/specialization but others except clinical pharmacist/pharmacist are allowed to be in charge of their destiny. The Pharmacist do not get the desired recognition in the medical field which is quite ironic and rather unfortunate. This creative, literary and academic presentation by Dr. Patrick Osarenren Ojo, whom I have been acquainted with his academic pursuits for several decades, has served as the needed instrument or tonic to question the norms in the practice of medicine and to liberate 'Pharmacy' as a medical profession for the benefit of mankind.

Magnus Osagie Omoregie, Director of Information and
Communication Technology (ICT) - Retired,
The West African Examinations Council, Lagos, Nigeria.

18. **Vice Mayor of the City of Miami Gardens — Dr. Erhabor Ighodaro:** More than ever and in an era of global health crisis, we need an approach to problem-solving that is holistic, integrated and based on

common sense. "Pharmacy in Bondage" is a cutting edge and out of the box view of medicine that allows solution based methodologies to take precedence over dogma

Hon Erhabor Ighodaro, PhD,
Vice Mayor, City of Miami Gardens

19.   18. Social Science Professor Edo Aikhionbare: PHARMACY IN BONDAGE, in this book, Dr. Patrick Ojo writes passionately with professional's depth of feelings about pharmacy in the medical field. His reflections in this area of healthcare are poignant, cogent, and eloquent. This brilliant work by an insider goes a long way to educate those of us that are laymen about the complementary interrelationships between all the various aspects of healthcare professionals, the relevance of pharmacy and pharmacists in the family of healthcare providers, and the need to liberate pharmacy from healthcare bondage. This book could not have been written at a better time than now for those who want to understand the role of pharmacy and pharmacists in modern world. Truly an intellectually rich book that develops an important thesis with verve. A great read indeed.

Dr. Edo-Aikhionbare, PhD,
Social science professor (Ret.),
Palm Beach State College, Palm Beach, Florida

20.   Engr Semi Ojo: The book "Pharmacy in Bondage" is easy, simple and interesting to read. The ease and Simplicity of the book lies in the fact that it is not just a book for medical professionals alone but everybody. People including High School Students, Dropouts, Self-educated and others can easily read and comprehend the book. The interesting part of the book lies in the overall message and that is thousands of human lives that will be saved in US and/or Millions of human lives that will be saved worldwide if specialists or pharmacists in this case are allowed to do what they do best in their area of specialization thereby controlling the poisons/drugs that we consume daily in a serious manner. This is a Nobel Prize winning book based on the message and practical implementation of the message in US and all over the World.

Semi Ojo, Electrical Engineer,
California State Dept of Transportation (Caltrans)
Intelligent Transportation System (ITS)/Communication Systems.

21.   Reviewed by: Dr. Felix o. Evbuomwan, Ph.D. In prehistoric time medicine, the doctor is the man or woman who develops and compounds herbal medicine (drugs) and administers the medicine through nurses or nurse midwives to the patients. Hierarchically, the person who develops the medicine leads the team of health care professionals. It is believed that diagnosing the ailment is only the first part of finding solution to health problems, the actual cure comes from the drug(s) that is given to the patient and so, whoever develops the drugs leads the team. In orthodox medicine on the other hand, over many generations the human society has gotten accustomed to or made believe that whoever makes the diagnosis of a sickness is considered to be the lead of the medical team, the doctor; which is quite a contrast to the prehistoric time medicine from which orthodox medicine evolved. As I began to read the book "Pharmacy in Bondage" written by Dr. Patrick Ojo, I saw it as a masterpiece that I believe, will hopefully correct the societal error of relegating pharmacist as subservient to medical doctors rather than co-laborers in the vineyard of health care professionals. The content of the book elucidates the need for societal reorientation in seeing Pharmacist as expert in drug manufacture, prescription and dispensing. Oftentimes, societies all over the world, pay more attention symbolically, to doctors and nurses in health care without giving equal credit to pharmacist. This in my view is an error, and it should be corrected.

The writing of this book should hopefully help to free "Pharmacy from the bondage' under which it has been for so many generations. It is a step in the right direction and I encourage everyone to get a copy and read it, our society will be better for it. Honest medical doctors will tell you that pharmacist deserves the same recognition and emoluments as they do, because of their unique training, if this is the case, the only thing that is needed for pharmacist and pharmacy to be delivered from its current bondage, is sufficient political clout as the medicals doctors currently have. Doctors should make the diagnosis of the sickness and refer the patients to the pharmacist who will prescribe the accurate medicine/drugs and the correct dosage that can effectively cure the sickness. The pharmacist by virtue of their training in pharmacology, pharmcognosy, Pharmaceutical chemistry, pharmaceutics etc, are better trained and better equipped to correctly prescribe medications and dosages, which will lead to lasting cures of the different sicknesses. I encourage all members of our societies all over the world both young and old, to buy the book "Pharmacy in Bondage" for further enlightenment on this topic and we as a people, will be better for it.

Dr. Felix o. Evbuomwan, Ph.D.
Senior AgroBioterrorism Operations Manager and Assistant Port Director, US Customs and Border Protection, Atlanta Field Office, Georgia. 1699 Phoenix Parkway, College Park, Georgia 30349, 678-284-5920.

JUSTICE FOR PHARMACY PROFESSION

As noted in the book, freedom and justice for unjust act is never given on a platter of Gold. The oppressed must be conscious of his status then let the oppressor know that it is unacceptable and he is willing and ready to fight for the freedom by any means necessary. This is the only time as portrayed in human history that the issue will be taking serious and the oppressed propinquity to freedom will be closer and closer until it is won. The big question for Pharmacy profession therefore is, are pharmacy professionals ready and willing to pay the price of freedom. It is a big question that demands big answer. Like many other similar situations noted in the book, situations such as the women liberation, Copernicus versus the Church and others, we are currently at the genesis of pharmacy professional liberation even though the oppression has been thousands of years old — older than other newer branches of medicine that gained their consciousness on time and subsequently strive for their specialty/liberation immediately afterwards thereby gaining their freedom/specialty/specialization.

Osteopathic physicians, Veterinarians, Optometrists, Dentists, Certified Nurse Pratitioners, Physician Assistants and others gained their consciousness on time through heresy, opposition and agitations; consequently, they gained freedom. With the exception of Physician Assistants who by the nature of their subtitle/discipline and modus operandi have to operate within the jurisdiction of Physicians, all others operate with their independence within their specialty. Certified Nurse Practitioners by their very nature are close in terms of subtitle/discipline and modus operandi to Physician Assistants but they have been able to wangle their way through the systems with mountainous strength and fight to defined their autonomy. Thus it is not unusual to see Certified Nurse Practitioners practicing on their own with separate clinics/offices run independently by them under the pretense of physicians' supervision. With all these in mind, how is it that pharmacy/pharmacy professionals abandoned the good fight or wait for others to fight the good fight for them and become complacent with the system. Is it that the system has thoroughly schooled them or the set of people that go into pharmacy profession/practice have different human composition from others, that is to say people as human beings will only see the light outside pharmacy but the moment they step into pharmacy they are blindfolded and can no longer see beyond their horizon. Alternatively, is pharmacy reward in terms of salary/remunerations so great that it blindfold them — if that be the case they are not the highest paid medical practitioners, as a matter of fact physicians and the above mentioned practitioners receives better salary/remuneration than them. The matter is further complicated by the fact that today's job market for pharmacist are constantly bombarded with the creation of auto-dispensing machines thereby eroding their once thought indispensable role of selling medications to the public/community as age long dispenser.

Today, competition with auto-dispensing machines coupled with numerous schools of pharmacy graduates pumped into the system years after years have resulted in supersaturated job market for pharmacy professionals. A decade or two ago, pharmacy professionals were inundated with sign-on bonus for job acceptance with thousands of dollars but today a good number of them are jobless with no salary or remuneration yet the graduates keep coming from the schools of pharmacy into already supersaturated job market. This condition, as bad as it appears is going to pave way for pharmacists to look for their niche through clinical services, awareness/consciousness and begin to fight for their rightful place in the medical field — something other branches of medicine have already done by taking advantage of the situation.

In this country, United States of America, one can conveniently trace the origin of pharmacy professional liberation/awareness/consciousness to Hepler and Strand. Hepler and Strand as noted in the book published their landmark research work in form of "Opportunities and Responsibilities in pharmaceutical care" in 1990 in American Journal of Hospital Pharmacy and the work became the major focus of attention for pharmacy evolution in medical field. Clinical pharmacy started earlier and underwent significant changes from 1960s to 1990s. Hepler and Strand work highlighted the significance of clinical pharmacy and the impact on the healthcare system. Consequently, the mantle of leadership and baton exchange to younger generation after Hepler and Strand degenerated into intellectual enhancement and clinical pharmacy training/practice with monetary reward. Monetary reward is good but the big problem is that there were no enough positions to absorb many graduating clinical pharmacists in the society. The end result was that this remuneration/monetary reward entice the attention of the lucky ones, those who because of their extreme academic excellence/clinical knowledge, parental influence and societal disposition in terms of race/religion/others gained the few jobs. Young clinical pharmacists with this kind of monetary reward see themselves as few lucky ones emerging into a privileged class among colleagues/classmates. This phenomenon in itself posed great danger to pharmacy profession because the young professionals became apathy to pharmacy professional plight and the faith of other unemployed colleagues. The young professionals that could have been pharmacy best hope were easily schooled into acceptances of pharmacy professional statusquo as an unchangeable phenomenon. They became docile and went with the flow. It is interesting to note that this same condition that catered to the needs of survival of the fittest is also going to galvanize the professional liberation because as noted above job market for clinical pharmacists/pharmacist is attenuating yearly while schools of pharmacy are pumping out graduates in astronomical manner into already supersaturated job market. Thus it is not unusual these days to see pharmacists accepting pharmacy technicians' salary for a starting pharmacist's position with the hope of moving up the ladder to their status or accepting real meager salary to go out of their home for daily job and other situations. The number of unemployed pharmacy graduates/pharmacists is already high enough and it is capable of igniting spontaneous revolution or liberation of movement provided the right ignition is in place.

The author of Pharmacy in Bondage has contributed enormously to pharmacy liberation movement. Besides the organized protests seen in the book, he has taking the fight to US elected officials. The first package along with a letter, this book — Pharmacy in Bondage, a flier, and some states pharmacy association publications with information about the book were sent to President George Bush, Vice President Dick Cheney, all senators and Representatives in 110th US Congress Session around June, 19, 2007. A sample of the letter is displayed below. As noted above the book Pharmacy in Bondage lead to the introduction of the Bill, H.R. 5780 by a Republican, Rep. Heather Wilson of New Mexico and it was cosponsor by Rep Marion Berry of Arkansa (Democratic), Rep. David Price of North Carolina (Democratic), Rep. Mike McIntyre of North Carolina (Democratic), Rep. Bob Etheridge Of North Carolina (Democratic) and Rep. Tom Udall of New Mexico (Democratic). Around February 10, 2009, a similar package was sent to President Barrack Obama, Vice President Joe Biden and letter to all Senators and Representatives in 111th Session of the US Congress. A sample of the letter to the 111th Congress is equally displayed below.

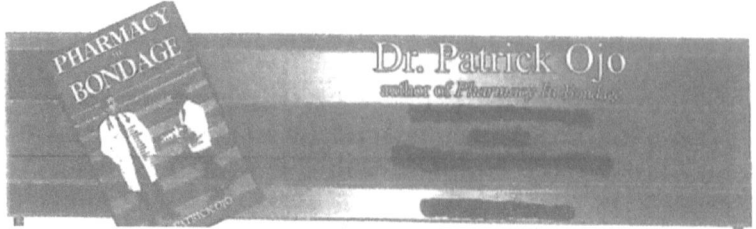

The Honorable
House of Representatives Washington, DC 20515
Dear Representative ----:

RE: PHARMACY IN BONDAGE

CAN YOU HELP TO LIBERATE THE PROFESSION?

There is no gainsay about the fact that pharmacists are overeducated, underutilized, and marginalized medical practitioners in the medical field. We as a nation are just beginning to grapple with the issue with the enactment of the Nursing Home Regulations in 1974, OBRA'90 in 1990, and, now, Medication Therapy Management (MTM), as part of the Medicare Prescription Drug and Modernization Act of 2003. Many will love to laugh away the above issue, but it is not funny. I decided to send you a copy of my newly published book Pharmacy in Bondage because of this issue. The book dives into the length and breadth of the medical field to excavate issues that have been swept under the rug, to buttress the plight of pharmacists and the pharmacy profession, and to highlight the need to liberate the profession for the benefit of mankind.

As reflected in the book, the plight of pharmacists and the pharmacy profession typifies the various human struggles against oppression Pharmacists are the downtrodden and oppressed group of medical practitioners in the medical field. If after reading the book, you have any doubt about any issues, especially the ones relating to course comparison, a committee can be set up to examine the authenticity of the issues.

This is not just an issue about the book or a trivial matter but something of vital national interest that has been echoed by Dr. David Kessler (an MD, attorney, and former FDA chairman), Dr. Cathy Worrall (a clinical pharmacist and certified nurse practitioners professor), Dr. Harris Gold (an MD and advocate for drug specialty), Dr. Raymond Woosley (an MD and an advocate for independent drug research -- CERT), Dr. Renal Cole (PharmD), Dr. David Flockhart (an MD), Dr. Kenneth Freeman (an MD) and others.

I have only taken the issue a step further with an investigation and a book. Today, specialization is the mainstay of society and with the aid of specialization, humanity is capable of achieving great heights or miracles of biblical proportion --- making the blind see, the deaf hear, separating conjoined twins, and others. However, pharmacy and drug treatment have been kept out of this specialization/miracle. There are specialists catering to every aspect of our lives, including life-threatening and non-life-threatening issues, except for the poison that is pumped into our bodies as drugs. All specialists are in control of their destiny, except pharmacists, who are treated like children in their supposed area of jurisdiction.

We are all living witnesses of the devastating effect of drugs, adverse drug reactions (ADR), and other drug problems in our nation today. Just in case we have any doubts about these drug problems, we might need to refresh our memories with these facts:

1. In 1990, the World Health Organization's (WHO) statistics showed that ADR cost us 1.6 million hospitalization and 160,000 deaths.

2. In 1992, the Fink study revealed 198,000 deaths and $76.5 billion costs because of drug-related morbidity and mortality.

3. In 1994, Lazaraous et al.'s meta-analysis study showed that hospital statistics alone revealed 106,000 deaths because of ADR. These statistics placed ADR as the 4th to 6th leading cause of death in our country, etc.

We now have a book on the issue and the title of the book is Drug-Induced Diseases --- Billion Dollar Patient Care Issue. Besides human tolls and the rising cost of health care because of drugs, drug treatment has grown out of proportion. We as a nation spent $2.7 billion on drugs in 1960; $12 billion in 1980; $60.8 billion in 1995; and $121.8 billion in 2000 (in sharp contrast, our quality of life and life expectancy did not improve by more than tenfold from 1980 to 2000). The number of prescription drugs dispensed rose from 400 million in 1950 to 1.5 billion in 1980 and 3 billion in 2000 for outpatient alone. The health care fraction of our Gross Domestic Product (GDP) rose from 5.2% in 1960 to 13.3% in 1992 and 14.4% in 2001. In 1992, we ranked 18th in the world in terms of life expectancy (75.6 years) despite our 13.3% GDP expenditure. Japan ranked first in the world the same year with 78.6 years and 6.8% GDP expenditure. In 1997, our average life expectancy was 76 years (an increase of 0.4 years compared to our huge financial expenditure in 6 years, from 1992 to 1997), while Hong Kong was on top of the world with 82.3 years. In spite of the fact that we outspent other nations on earth by 82% per person's health care, statistics revealed that by the year 2000, we ranked 37th in terms of quality of health or the fourth 10-best nations, along with Cuba, Chile, Denmark,

Dominica, Finland, Costa Rica, Slovenia, Brunei and Australia. France. along with Oman, Spain, Japan, Italy, Austria, San Marino, Andorra, Malta, and Singapore, were the first 10-best nations in the world the same year.

We are the world's largest producer and consumer of drugs, and we have no specialists catering to the poison we pump into our body as drugs in spite of our sophistication or advancement. Some will say that the reason why these other nations do better than us is not because their pharmacy profession operates differently from ours. That is true, but, in spite of the fact that there is no room for bondage in our modern-day society, it is important to know that the United States is number one in the world in many spheres of human endeavors. This is a great opportunity for us to champion the world's freedom again in another sphere of human endeavor before others take it from us. We can use the opportunity to improve our health care system, bridge the gap with these other nations, and move ahead of them before they start copying us. Some might say that life expectancy and quality of life are lagging indicators of our technological advancement, others view of our nation as the number one country in the world and our desire to remain on top of the world but the fact remains that these two parameters are key factors for measuring the greatness of any nation because a health nation is a wealthy nation. We cannot continue to assert our greatness if we cannot remain on top or in close proximity to the top (at least within first 10-best nations, like France and Japan) on these two vital issues.

Research studies discussed in the book, study upon study, and others vindicate clinical pharmacists as drug experts, or the most knowledgeable medical practitioner about drugs/medications, yet they have to obtain permission from other branches of medicine that do not know as much about the profession as the practitioners. In spite of the legal limitations, lack of professional autonomy, and the hindrances that prevent schools of pharmacy from teaching students how to prescribe drugs/medications, some of the studies showed that clinical pharmacists are ahead of other branches of medicine in terms of medication/drug treatment. For example:

- The course outline comparison presented in the book shows that pharmacists take more courses in school in pharmacy/drug treatment than other branches of medicine put together.

- The public opinion survey/study in the book, by Drug Topics and others, places pharmacists ahead of others in terms of drug knowledge (drug experts or medication specialists) in the medical field.

- The Carter et al., Thompson et al., Stimrnel et al., and other studies show that prescriptions written by clinical pharmacists are better than those written by other branches of medicine.

- The Schloemer and Zagogen study at Nicholas Hospital, Sheboygan, Wisconsin, shows clinical pharmacists' dexterity over others in terms of pharmacokinetics (other physicians did not know that the Aminoglycoside half-life in patients almost doubles with age more than 30 years). The Pharmacists armed themselves with this information to improve patients' health outcome and make some savings.

The Levin et al. study showed how clinical pharmacists at Good Samaritan Hospital, Baltimore, Maryland, reduced the number of Serum Drug Assay (SDA) for Digoxin alone from 95 to 57 in 5 months (unwanted SDA went down from 65 to 16). Prior to the program, a patient whose blood level was inappropriately drawn 2 to 3 hours after administration when the drug was in the distributive phase had the drug discontinued and was discharged home because of supposedly "toxic level." The patient was readmitted for the same reason, congestive heart failure (CHF), one week later. Digoxin ($10/month) is known to prevent or to reduce hospitalization for CHF patients.

Elenabaas et al.'s conducted a 12-month study at Truman Medical Center, Kansas City, Missouri, in 1979. The hospital, in January 1978, mandated that all drug blood level tests go through clinical pharmacist consultation and approval before the test. The study showed that the number of SDAs per month reduced from 151 ± 22 to 90 ± 15 (about 61 SDAs/month reduction) with some savings.

- The Bootman et al. study showed annual savings of 8,500 human lives and $3.6 billion in nursing home facilities across the country (this study alone did not only vindicate the Nursing Home Regulation Act of 1974 but proved that pharmacists are capable of being the master of their fate and the controller of their Destiny.

Bond et al.'s study showed savings of one human life and $244.88 every time the hospital spent $320 and $1, respectively, on clinical pharmacists' salaries --- this also amounts to 4.78 days/patient decrease in length of stay (LOS) in the hospital, etc.

The Ashville Project, a successful story (savings of $2,000/year/employee, reduced absenteeism, increased productivity, decreased sick days/leave etc) recently caught media attention. Talking about the achievement, an NBC newscaster said, on Saturday, February 24, 2007, that we all know that pharmacists dispense drugs and can also reduce health care costs when trained to do so. The general notion about pharmacists and dispensing, as portrayed by the newscaster, is such that no one needs specialized training for a dispensing role, and that is correct in the eyes of everybody both within and outside the pharmacy profession. The amazing thing about the Ashville Project is that one of the research studies showed that pharmacists need no further training in order to impact the health care system, reduce health care costs, and provide other benefits as noted above.

An engineer is an engineer because college work/courses lay emphasis on engineering. The same is true of accountants, optometrists, meteorologists, dentists, and others. Consequently, there is nothing unusual in pharmacy laying emphasis on drug treatment/pharmacy college work/courses. We just need to recognize pharmacy as a specialty. The truth is bitter, -- restricting the pharmacists' role to a mere dispensing function after 6 to 7 years of college work (this is bound to increase to 8 and more years in the near future with first-degree entry level and residency) is, in part, as good as:

*** Asking the electrical engineer to sell electric bulbs, wires, cables, gadgets, refrigerators, and generators after 4 years of college work.

***Asking the dentist to dispense (sell) toothpaste, toothbrushes, dentures, Fixodent, Seabond, oral gel, and prostheses after 8 years of college work.

* * *Asking the veterinarian to sell goats, cows, chickens, sheep, and eggs after 8 years of college work.

***Asking the agriculturalist to sell tomatoes, corn, potatoes, yams, broccoli, Spinach, and rice after 4 years of college work.

***Asking a lawyer to sell law books, court documents/orders, to be a process server after 7 years of college work.

***Asking a civil engineer to sell building materials, concrete, cement, shovels, and toilet bowls after 4 years of college work, etc.

It is interesting to note that pharmacists currently spend the same number of years in professional school training as many other professionals (e.g., dentists, veterinarians, optometrists, as well as other branches of medicine). This is not the era of autocracy (autocratic society) or authoritative medicine, but evidence-based society and medicine-based on empiricism. All that pharmacy is requesting is to apply the same evidence-based medicine to the issues at stake vis-a-vis, school course/curriculum comparison, drug expert/specialist study, etc.

The greatest insult anyone can pass on to humanity is to take humanity for granted. Besides that, the greatest insult the American Medical Association (AMA), American College of Physicians-American Society of Internal Medicine (ACP-ASIM), American Board of Medical Specialties (ABMS), and others, can pass on to pharmacy, pharmacists, and pharmacy organizations is to ignore these issues. The U.S. Congress, U.S. Senate, and the House of Representatives are greater than any individuals, organizations, and special interest groups in this country. Consequently, they can mandate the AMA, the ACP-ASIM, the ABMS, or other groups to conduct their own research or to duplicate ones mentioned in the book. Congress can conduct its own research on the issues through a special committee. If the results of the research/study are contrary to the ones in the book, the book will be pulled off the market.

The New York State Pharmacist Association publication, Long Island University Magazine, Laura Simonse of US Pharmacist and, recently, the Texas Pharmacy Association Editorial Board have reviewed the book and classified it as the basic truth or a prescription for truth. Others are in the making. The truth about pharmacy/pharmacists and the revelations contained in this book parallel those of Vice President Al Gore's book on global warming and the "Inconvenient Truth" documentary. Even though Mr. Gore was saying the right thing with the right message and reality as basic truth, it takes years for the country and the world to come to terms with the truth. The earlier we act to correct abnormalities or injustice of the past/present, the better we are, the greater society benefits. With regard to this bitter truth about pharmacy/medical community, the more lives we save, the greater health care costs are reduced, etc. Experience has shown that humanity strives well when experts/specialists put their ingenuity to practice, thereby minimizing risks and increasing benefits. No one can eliminate drug problems in the world; however, with the aid of internship, rotations, residency and fellowship, pharmacy liberation will reduce drug problems to the barest minimum in the country and the world.

Dear Representative, pharmacy liberation

- Is not a Republican or Democrat (partisan) issue but a human issue.

- Is not a rich American or a poor American issue, but an issue about improving and saving human lives.

- Is not a man's or a woman's issue but an issue about saving huge amounts of money for the health care system, employers, government, and the country.

- Is not a Black or a White issue but an issue of liberating one of the greatest professions in the history of mankind?

A journey of a thousand miles begins with one step. America, the envy of all nations, the shining city on the hill, as per President Reagan, and the pride of the world, can liberate pharmacy for the benefit of mankind. We on earth today have every tool within our reach to correct and to adjust the injustice of yesteryears, the same way the forefathers of our great nation fought until the last drop of their blood to liberate humanity from hereditary bondage. If the forefathers of our great nation were alive today, they would simply laugh and say this is what America is about --- freedom, not just for ourselves, but for others and for other spheres of human endeavors.

I look forward to Congress for pharmacy salvation, and I hope to follow up with a telephone and/or a visit in the future. I am enclosing, along with this package, a copy of Pharmacy in Bondage, a flyer, and some state pharmacy association publications with information about the book. The same package was sent to other Senators and Congressmen. A similar package has been sent to President Bush, and his staff has since replied to acknowledge the bookwork.

My passion for pharmacy freedom and the burning desire to bring attention to the plight of pharmacists/pharmacy in the medical field made me fall victim of an Internet Scam, and I lost about $250,000. With Western Union, Money Gram, and other receipts, the Federal Bureau of Investigation (FBI) empathized with me and was willing to bring the criminals to justice but referred me to the United States Secret Service Fraud Department (Miami Division), who just threw their hands up saying there was nothing they could do for me. Initially, the London Police were willing to help after personal contacts, but they were discouraged by the disposition of our Secret Service Fraud Department. They claimed it was too late for them to act at the time they received it, even though it was less than 6 months. At any rate, I have seen the light about pharmacy, and I will continue to pursue the just course until ------.

To crown it all, as a friend or acquaintance of pharmacy, Representative ---, can you help to liberate the profession for the benefit of mankind? I know you will, if only you can read the book, Pharmacy in Bondage. It is important to note that pharmacy liberation will not stop other branches of medicine from prescribing drugs just as the existence of dentistry, urology, pediatrics and others have not stopped other branches of medicine from attending to patients' oral problems, urinary tract infections/problems, children's health and others. Thanks for your time, understanding, and anticipated cooperation. I hope to hear from you. God bless you, and God Bless America.

Sincerely yours,
Dr. Patrick Ojo

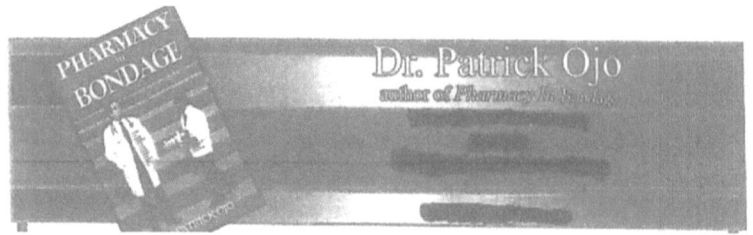

The Honorable
United States Senate
702 Hart Senate Office Building Washington, DC 20510

Dear Senator:

RE: PHARMACY IN BONDAGE

CAN YOU HELP TO LIBERATE THE PROFESSION?

Welcome to the 111th session of the U.S. Congress. I am sure that with a new president in office, you have much work ahead of you. This is a follow-up to the package that was mailed to you about the above issue around June 2007. The package included a letter addressed to you, a copy of Pharmacy in Bondage, a flier, and some state pharmacy association publications with information about the book, Pharmacy in Bondage. The book among other things reflects various research studies in Health care field, experimental views from people and others in the society as well as other issues that support pharmacy as an independent branch of medicine. Thank you for reviewing the package and the book if you have already done so.

I am delighted to acknowledge with appreciation the concerns and the responses from President George Bush, Vice President Dick Cheney, Senator Hillary Rodham Clinton, Senator Michael Enzi, Senator John Cornyn, Senator Chuck Nagel, Senator Jim Bunning, Senator Bob Corker, Rep. Robert Aderholt, Rep. Dutch Ruppersberger, Rep. Bart Stupak, Rep. Grace Napolitano, Rep. Cliff Sterns, and others before the end of 110th congress session. They took time from their busy schedules to reply to the package.

Special thanks to Rep. Heather Wilson of New Mexico not only for reading the book two or more times but also for introducing the Bill, H.R. 5780 --- Medicare Clinical Pharmacist Practitioner Services Coverage Act of 2008 before the end of 110th Congress session.. This act, supported by cosponsors Rep. Marion Berry of Arkansa, Rep. David

Price and Rep. Mike McIntyre of North Carolina, Rep. Bob Etheridge and Rep. Tom Udall of New Mexico in the 110th Congress, goes a long way to show our determination in liberating pharmacy from bondage. The cosponsors read the package and the book,

Pharmacy in Bondage and found the need to liberate the profession. Other members of Congress who initially could not read the book for one reason or the other subsequently found the time to do so.

As Americans, it is not our tradition to see the truth and the injustices and turn away. Rather, when we see the truth and the injustices we move swiftly to address them, like the human rights abuse in China, and that is what these honorable members of the House of Representatives, 110th Congress did. Unfortunately, the bill was overshadowed by the economic crisis before the end of 110th session. The need to reintroduce H.R. 5780 and see it through the House of Representatives and the Senate, or a similar bill through the Senate, cannot be overemphasized. If for any reason, you have doubts as to why H.R. 5780 was introduced into the House of Representatives, you can review and read the package or the book, Pharmacy in Bondage, once or twice. Similar package is sent along with this letter to all new senators and new members of the House of Representatives. Those who do not, or did not receive their packages (lost in transit) can order, free, a Congress's copy of the book, Pharmacy in Bondage or the package through 954 - 432 - 2794 or OTRICKOSA@CS.COM and it will be mailed to you at no cost.

The recent economic crisis, financial meltdown, and mortgage debacle reminds us of the need to rely more and more on specialists/experts because a "stitch on time saves nine." We could have avoided the problem if we had listen to the warning signs and advice given approximately two years earlier by Economists and Economic professors as well as the financial analysts who wrote about the issue. However, the fact that we listened to them eventually will help to avoid future calamity. We rely heavily on specialists and experts in all spheres of human endeavor. Pharmacy and pharmacists are no exception to the specialty rule. Clinical pharmacists and indeed, pharmacy reserve the right to decide their own destiny like all other branches of medicine, including Pharmacy's baby, anesthesiology, which is an integral part of pharmacy.

No special interest group or organization should be allowed to decide the fate of others however rich and powerful they may be. ABC world news recently revealed that the American medical association (AMA) is second after Chamber of Commerce in lobbying Congress and the public. ABC world news claims that AMA spent millions of dollars in lobbying the congress ($21.96 million in 2007 as per Lobbyists. Info). Certainly, pharmacy and pharmacists do not have such money to defend their interest and fight against injustices in medicine.

Nevertheless one thing is certain, and that is U.S. Congress (both the Senate and the House of Representative) as ombudsman of the masses, society, weak, voiceless, poor, and defenseless citizens and organizations can look directly at the AMA's eye and say "enough is a enough. We can no longer allow the injustices against pharmacy and pharmacists to continue because the evidence is overwhelming." Pharmacy deserves equal treatment and rights that are given to other branches of medicine e.g. dentistry, optometry, anesthesiology, pediatric, urology, dermatology, and others.

We do not need to look any further as to why pharmacy is in bondage; the answer is within our reach. For example, we are the world's largest producer and consumer of drugs. We have specialists catering to every aspect of our lives, except for drugs (poisons) that we pumped into our bodies every day. Anesthesiology (a baby) is a specialty of medicine, yet an infinitesimal part of pharmacy (the parent). In 1990, the World Health Organization's (WHO) statistics showed that adverse drug reactions (ADR) cost us 1.6 million hospitalizations and 160,000 deaths. J.L. Fink's study of ADR revealed 198,000 deaths and $76.5 billion in costs in 1992. Lazaraous et al.'s study showed 106,000 deaths from hospital statistics alone in 1994; these statistics placed ADR between fourth and sixth leading cause of deaths in our country. Many other statistics are listed in the book, Pharmacy in Bondage. Studies upon studies discussed in the book and in other sources show that clinical pharmacists and pharmacists save more human lives and money when allowed to display their ingenuity in their supposed area of jurisdiction (medication specialty) compared with others in the medical field.

Beside the above, we can best answer pharmacy liberation question by asking ourselves the following questions, "who is in charge of surgery?" I guess we will say surgeons; the same is true of anesthetics -- anesthesiologists, skin or dermatological conditions --- dermatologists, mouths/teeth or dental conditions --- dentists, eyes or ophthalmologic conditions --- optometrists/ophthalmologists, X-rays --- radiologists, animal health --- veterinarians, and others. The next question then is "who is in charge of drugs/medications or the poisons that we pumped into our bodies every day?" Are we right to say "all branches of medicine" including the above? This is a dangerous answer that deserves immediate attention in view of the human tolls resulting from adverse drug reaction, 4[h to 6s' leading cause of deaths in our country, U S. We cannot say that all branches of medicine are in charge of surgery, dentistry, anesthetics (pharmacy's baby), radiology, and other specialties so why pharmacy or medications/drugs? It is right to say that the existence of dentists, optometrists, dermatologists, radiologists and others have not stopped other branches of medicine from attending to mouths/teeth, eyes, skin, using X-rays in the case of radiology, and other human conditions so pharmacy liberation will not operate differently.

The reintroduction and passage of H.R. 5780, or a similar senate bill, will not only ensure the liberation of pharmacy, one of the greatest professions in the history of mankind, but also will reduce drug problems in this country and in other places to the barest minimum. Along with this letter, I have enclosed a sampled copy of my previous letter, Dr. Carla Frye' s introductory article about the profession, a flier and the book, Pharmacy in Bondage for new members of the Congress. In America, we do not need a Godfather to let the truth shine and for justice to reign. Rather the goodwill of the American people championed by congress and the president is enough to let the cat out of the bag by upholding the truth and letting justice reign supreme. We upheld the truth in the 18th century by standing up to the greatest power on Earth, the United Kingdom or British power. However intimidating and frustrating it may have been, we succeeded in fighting and declaring our independence in 1776. Today, however rich and powerful the American medical association may be, it is not greater than the British Authority of the 18th century, so we can stand by the truth and let justice reign supreme.

Health care reform without pharmacy's liberation is not only as good as tea without sugar or tantamount to mockery of our democracy but a slap in the face of the greatest civilization in the history of mankind. Health care reform without pharmacy liberation will amount to turning our back against injustices and oppression right under our noses, telling the world that injustice anywhere is not a threat to justice everywhere and epitomizing dictatorship in face of all evidence, facts, and figures. Anyway, health care reform or no health care reform, the Congress as well as the president of the United States can liberate pharmacy for the benefits of mankind. "Yes we can" if I may borrow the words of President Barrack Obama.

Dear Lawmakers (Senators and Representatives), the fate of pharmacy, as well as many innocent human lives (unnecessary deaths because of ADR), is in our hands and this is the moment of truth for us. We cannot afford to let humanity or pharmacy down through our inaction. Let us reintroduce and rally around H.R. 5780 and have it passed into law. Rep. Wilson's staff, especially Brad Runrou and Joe Mosei, were gracious in their cooperation with me before the end of 110th Congress session. Unfortunately, Rep.

Wilson, a Republican Congresswoman and an indomitable lion from New Mexico, lost her reelection bid. The fact that she is no longer in the Congress should not stop us from liberating pharmacy for the benefit of mankind. Any of the cosponsors or other goodwill members of the Congress can reintroduce H.R. 5780, or a similar bill into the senate.

Thanks for your precious time and cooperation. I look forward to hearing from you or seeing you to discuss the issues at stakes if you so desire. God bless you and God bless America,

Sincerely yours,
Dr. Patrick Ojo

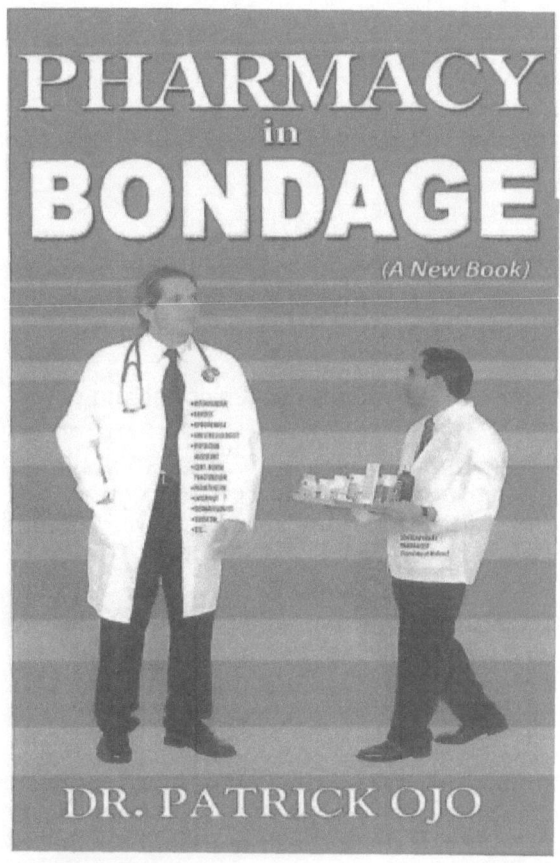

The book depicts an accurate historical account of pharmacy, its bondage, subservience, topsy-turvy fame, service to humanity and awesome contribution to the healthcare system of the US/ World.

Hints:
1 in every 14 courses qualifies Physician Assistant to prescribe drugs (in just 1yr)
1 in every 25 courses qualifies Cert. Nurse Pract. to prescribe drugs (no residency)
1 in every 11 courses qualifies Veterinarian to prescribe drugs (no residency)
1 in every 17 courses qualifies Optometrist to prescribe drugs (no residency)
1 in every 33 courses qualifies Dentist to prescribe drugs (no residency)
1 in every 17 courses qualifies other branches (Med) to prescribe drugs (With residency)

& 7 in every 10 courses do not qualify Clinical Pharmacist to prescribe drugs

Prescriptions written by Clinical Pharmacists are better than others in the Medical field.

PABULUM

*Is dispensing so great that pharmacists forget they went to school like every other professional?

*Which school of pharmacy teaches count and pour?

* If a dentist who does not know how penicillin kills bacteria can prescribe any drug from Pen VK to Percocet/Oxycontin, a pharmacist who knows and learns everything about the drug should be allowed to control his destiny.

* If a veterinarian who does not know how Xanax works to control animal anxiety can prescribe any drug from Amoxil to Percocet/Oxycontin, a pharmacist who studied the drug should be allowed to be the master of his fate.

* If an optometrist who does not know how Cosopt works to control eye pressure/glaucoma can prescribe any drug from Ciloxan to Diamox, a pharmacist who is vast about the drug should be allowed to champion his course/jurisdiction.

* If in the whole of their school life, maximum drug/pharmacy courses of 1½, For nurse practitioner and 2 for physician assistant make them prescribe most drugs then 42 should make pharmacist drug specialist according to specialization protocol.

The President, Vice President, all Senators, Congressmen and women have a copy of the book. Pharmacy is tired of being a medical and political football, played and won by those who know how to dribble and win the game in medicine.

Congressmen and women in Senate and House of Representative respond to pressure, people's yearnings and demands. Medical field is no exception, as a matter of fact the other branches of medicine namely Osteopathic medicine, Optometry, Veterinary medicine, Dentistry, and even Certified Nurse Practitioner as well as Physician Assistants gained their autonomy/specialty and/or prescription writing authority from the Congress by mounting series of pressure. It appears the apathy in pharmacy profession by the professionals is a monumental phenomenon that weighs heavily on the prospect of the profession. It wares on the various professional organizations, States and National body in form of American Pharmacists Association (APHA). Manners don't fall from heaven, the States Pharmacy Associations and APHA is as good as the professionals want it to be. Pharmacy professionals need to wake up and smell the coffee or face reality for themselves. APHA on the other hand is a so so organization in terms of agitating for pharmacy freedom, liberty and independence. To the credit of APHA they have been involved in numerous pharmacy issues including some successful and unsuccessful bills through the US Congress but their effort is like a drop of water in a bucket compared to the above professionals' organizations. I remembered vividly that I went to solicit APHA's assistance several times at the APHA office/building in Washington DC before and during the protest marches displayed in this book and the then Executive Vice President/CEO John Gan together with his Secretary refused to grant me audience as a member of APHA.

In the absence of APHA, I knew I have to do everything alone. No matter what happened, no matter the number of set back and failures, pharmacy liberation coupled with numerous lives to be saved from the dangers of medications usage is too great a price to let go so we must summoned enough courage to continue the fight by facing all obstacles/battles in a fearless manner. Pharmacy professionals' apathy in mobilizing forces to demand for their rightful place in medicine and influence others' impact in their professional practice is a big problem so any representative organization like APHA whose desire is to have a meaningful impact should have been on the lookout for every opportunity from anyone, members or nonmembers, professionals or nonprofessionals to encourage and not discourage efforts like this. Here and there efforts like this put enough pressure on law makers to do what is right for the people, professions (that was how others gained their independence/specialty) and others. Florida Pharmacy Association (FPA) and few other states did a better job in lending hand/assistance in this regard than APHA.

Besides the US Congress, the author of Pharmacy in Bondage equally visited various schools of pharmacy to promote pharmacy awareness/liberation as shown below with various Deans or Deans' office personnel including Dean Grossman of Long Island University, Brooklyn, New York

-- see pictures below:

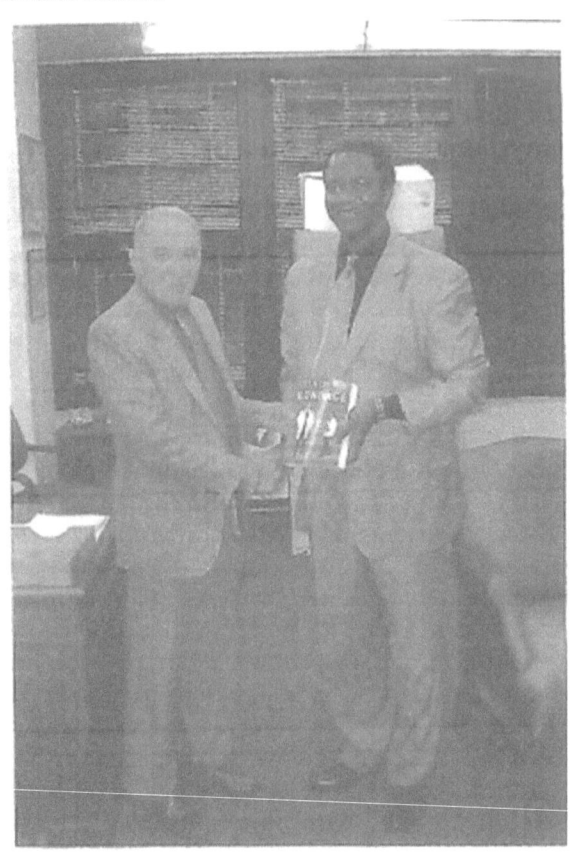

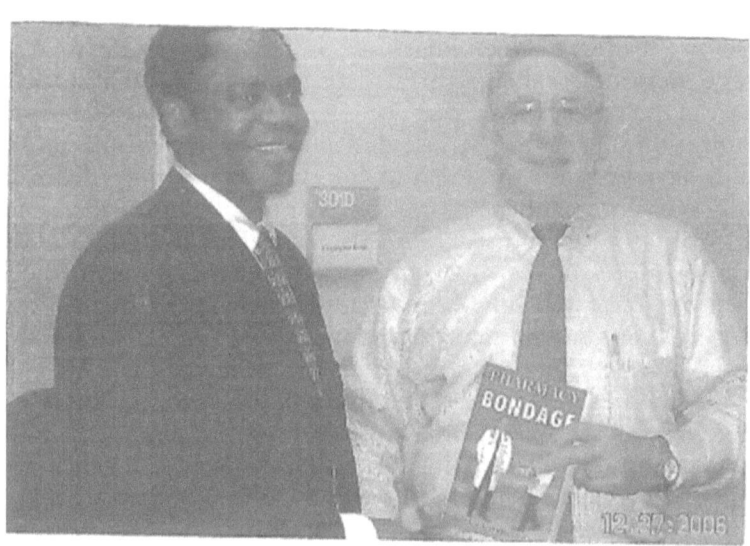

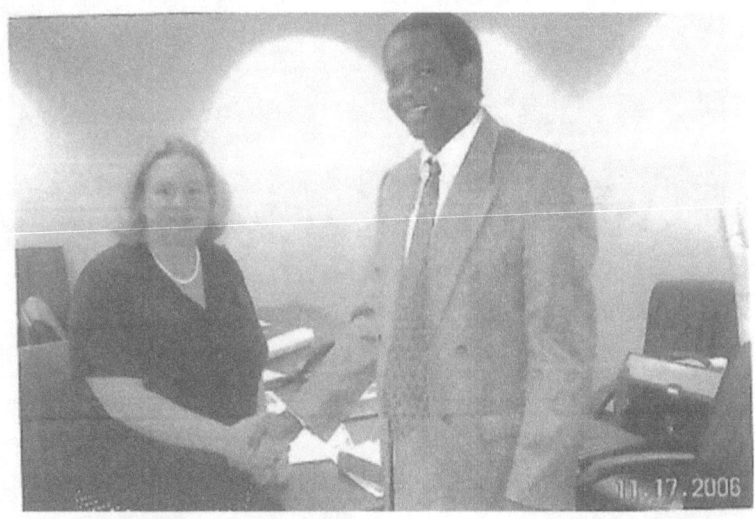

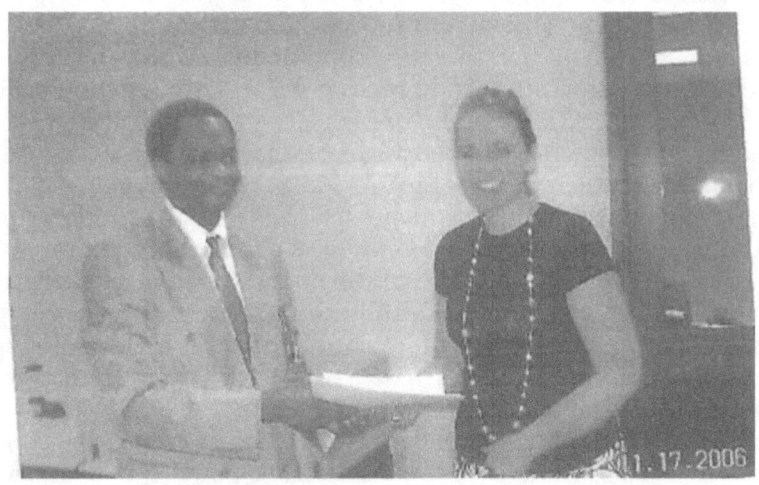

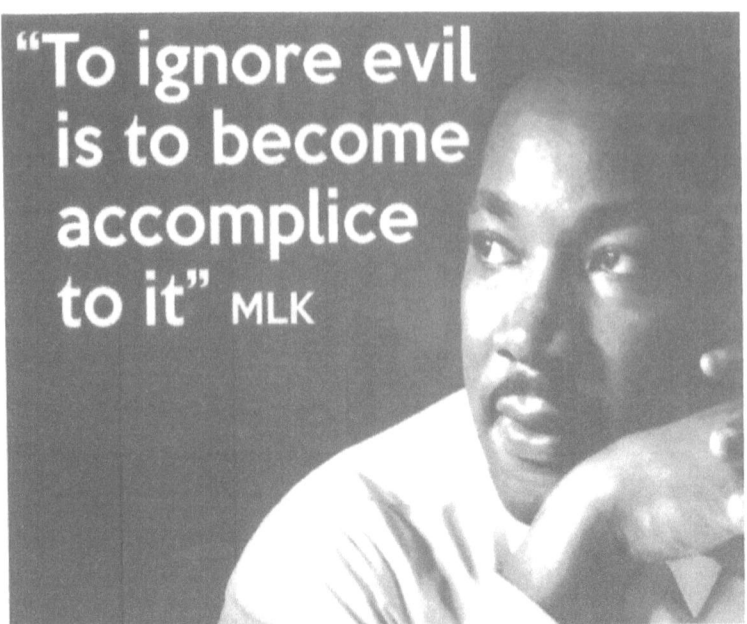

The last flyer with Martin Luther King quotation "To ignore evil is to become accomplice to it" signified a lot to humanity because it is a direct challenge to all human beings on the surface of this earth. This quotation coupled with late Congressman John Lewis saying "If you see something say something" indicate that we all have a responsibility to make humanity and the world a better place to live in or better than we found it. If anyone feels that the plight of pharmacy in the medical field is not an evil act then they are probably in a different world.

Simple human etiquette teaches us that you don't rub Peter to pay Paul or you don't take away food from the child to give to others. How will the Dentist feel if their role in the medical field is restricted to the selling of toothpaste, dentures, toothbrush and others after years of school work and in the same token others in the medical field are giving the authority to control them in their area of specialization/jurisdiction. The same is true of other specialties in medicine.

Giving other specialties prescriptive authority, even Certified Nurse Practitioners and Physician Assistants the same power over pharmacist in their supposed area of jurisdiction have the same ramification no matter how we look at it. Anyway undaunted by various obstacles, the Author of Pharmacy in Bondage went a little further in the quest for justice for pharmacy by taking American Medical Association (AMA) and American Board of Medical Specialties (ABMS) to UNITED STATES DISTRICT COURT, Southern District of Florida in Florida. He consulted various lawyers before going to the court as revealed below:

(Rev. 10/2002) General Document

UNITED STATES DISTRICT COURT
Southern District of Florida
Case Number: 07-61733
CIV-SEITZ
/ McALILEY

Dr. Patrick Ojo

Plaintiff

v.

American Medical Association (AMA)
&
American Board of Medical Specialties (ABMS)

Defendants

FILED by ___ D.C.
INTAKE
NOV 29 2007
CLARENCE MADDOX
CLERK U.S. DIST. CT.
S.D. OF FLA. - FT. LAUD.

MOTION TO GRANT PHARMACIST/PHARMACY EQUAL PROTECTION UNDER THE LAW

I, Patrick Ojo, plaintiff, in the above styled cause, wish to commence civil action for deprivation of constitutional rights, Civil Rights Act -- 42 U.S.C. §1983, under equal protection clause of U.S.C.A. Const. Amend. 14 against the above defendants. Equal protection guarantee anesthesiologist, dentist, veterinarian, optometrist, and other practitioners (branches) of medicine the right to put into practice their skills, knowledge, and technical know how acquired from years of school training but it is denied to me, other clinical pharmacists, and the entire pharmacy profession. No school of pharmacy teaches count and pour (dispensing), the norms for contemporary pharmacist including me that is compelled to abandon his skills/knowledge in place of dispensing functions only because of lack of equal protection. Nobody needs specialized training/ education for dispensing functions only. The defendants' failure to recognize Constitutional Amendment 14, equal protection under the law in relation to pharmacist/pharmacy amounts to keeping Pharmacy In Bondage.

The defendants deliberately refused to honor and recognize pharmacy as a specialty or an independent branch of medicine in spite of numerous studies and preponderance evidence that support the ideal. Ironically, such gesture has long been extended to anesthesiology, an integral/infinitesimal part of pharmacy, since June 1937. Besides recognizing anesthesiology as an independent branch of medicine, the defendants have gone further to recognize with prescriptive authority other less qualified branches and allied of medicine (dentists, veterinarians, optometrists, certified nurse practitioners, midwives, physician assistants etc) than pharmacy itself in it area of jurisdiction. Pharmacy In Bondage among other things discriminate against me, other clinical pharmacists/pharmacists and pharmacy profession in that we are made to take orders from physician assistants, certified nurse practitioners, dentists, veterinarians, optometrists and others (e.g. midwives etc) with infinitesimal/fragmented knowledge of drugs in our own area of jurisdiction. We cannot exercise the same rights as these healthcare practitioners even though we have greater knowledge of drugs and we are well acknowledged as drug specialists/medication experts in the medical community/world. In this motion, I, Patrick Ojo, the Plaintiff seeks among other things the need for the defendants to:

1. Define the term Specialty in Medical field, the application of such definition to drug treatment/therapy/management and the criteria for meeting such definition.

2. State why other branches of medicine including non-life threatening (e.g. nuclear medicine, ophthalmology, radiology, dermatology, dentistry etc.) deserves a specialty while life threatening poison that is pumped into our bodies as drugs do not. Today, drug treatment in our country, US is estimated to be 4th to 6th leading cause of death.

3. State why and how the school curriculum or course content of veterinary medicine, dentistry, optometry, physician assistant, certified nurse practitioner and other branches of medicine meet the requirements for prescribing authority while that of the school of Pharmacy does not. Veterinarian, dentist, and optometrist spend the same number of years in professional school training as the clinical pharmacist with no residency requirement. Residency is now part of all school of pharmacy curriculum in US and many pharmacy graduates are taking advantage of it.

4. State why school curriculum must be ignored in dealing with drug treatment/therapy/management or in defining therapeutician when the same curriculum is used to define other profession/professional (e.g. accountant, engineer, meteorologist, Physicist,

biologist, geologist etc). Pharmacy is known to offer more courses in drug treatment/therapy/management than any other discipline/profession in the country. All specialists or many professionals with less educational training (e.g. 4 years) are in control of their destiny, except pharmacists, who in spite of spending more years in school are treated like children in their supposed area of jurisdiction. School/professional training allow dentist to control dentistry, veterinarian to control animal health, ophthalmologist/optometrist to control ophthalmology, engineer to control engineering, biologist to control biology and many others but that is not the case with pharmacist/pharmacy. The existence of dentist has not stopped other branches of medicine from attending to patients' oral health neither has the existence of pediatrician stopped other branches of medicine from attending to children's health etc. Similarly, pharmacy autonomy as an independent branch of medicine will not stop other branches of medicine from prescribing drugs. In a nutshell specialization strengthen all professions including medicine and encourages interdependence/cooperation so why should I as a drug specialist/medication expert be treated differently from other professionals. What is good for the goose is good for the gander.

(Rev. 10/2002) General Document

5. State why they refused to acknowledge pharmacist/pharmacy as medication experts/drug specialists in the medical field or as an independent branch of medicine (like every other branch) in spite of numerous studies and preponderance evidence that support the profession/practitioners. Some of the studies showed that prescriptions written by clinical pharmacists are better than others in the medical field.

6. State why Americans or humanity must be deprived of the full benefits of pharmacy/pharmacists by keeping the profession in bondage contrary to popular views and overwhelming evidence.

7. State why other branches of medicine must continue to lord it over pharmacy/pharmacists in their supposed

area of jurisdiction (the well know drug experts/medication specialists).

8. State why anesthetic, an infinitesimal or integral part of pharmacy, is a branch of medicine while pharmacy itself, the parent of anesthetic is not.

Wherefore, I pray the court to examine critically the above issues and others as deem necessary, render justice and set Pharmacy free from bondage as an independent branch of medicine for the benefit of Americans/mankind. Pharmacy autonomy/freedom would not only enable me put into practice my prescriptions' writing skills, years of school training, and scholasticism like every other professionals but ensure that I am the master of my fate and controller of my destiny as a clinical pharmacist.

VERIFIED RETURN OF SERVICE

UNITED STATES DISTRICT COURT
THE SOUTHERN DISTRICT OF FLORIDA

CASE: 07-61733 CIV-SEITZ
CIVIL DIVISION

DR. PATRICK OJO

vs.

20 DAYS SUMMONS AND COMPLAINT
MOTION TO GRANT PHARMACIST/PHARMACY EQUAL
PROTECTION UNDER THE LAW

AMERICAN MEDICAL ASSOCIATION (AMA) AND
AMERICAN BOARD OF MEDICAL SPECIALTIES

ATTORNEY: DR. PATRICK OJO
3791 N.W. 78TH AVENUE UNIT #6
HOLLYWOOD, FL 33024

I received this writ on Date 12-1-07 at Time _____ and served same on AMERICAN MEDICAL ASSOCIATION at, 515 N. State, Chicago, IL on Date 12/4/07 Time 11:15am

[ ] **INDIVIDUAL:** By serving the within named defendant a copy to the above named document(s). F.S. 40.031

[ ] **SUBSTITUTE:** By serving a copy of the above named document(s) at the defendant usual place of abode on a person residing therein, to wit, _____ who is 15 years of age or older and informing the person of the contents.

[X] **CORPORATE SERVICE:** By serving a copy of the above named document(s) to Virginia Evans as Staff Assistant or any employee of defendant corporation in the absence of any superior officer, FS 48.081 when defendant corp. does not keep a registered agent present. FS 48.091

[ ] **SERVICE BY ACCEPTANCE:** By serving a copy of the above named document(s) to _____ as _____, as the person designated by the above named defendant to receive same on his/her behalf.

[ ] **MILITARY STATUS:** To my best knowledge, information and belief the said defendant at the time of service was not engaged to the military service of the United States. defendant to receive same on his/her behalf.

[ ] **NO SERVICE:** For the reason that diligent search and inquiry failed to locate above named defendant / witness in _____ County, State of _____.

COMMENTS: Assistant to Leonard Nelson

Under penalties of perjury, I declare that I have read the forgoing document and that the facts stated in it are true.
Date: 12-4-07

ATTORNEY SERVICES, INC.
3301 S.W. 137TH AVENUE
MIRAMAR, FL 33027
OFFICE (305) 829-2993

Susan Milby
Notary Public Seal State of Indiana
Lake County
My Commission Expires 11/14/2015

INDEX 166711

(Rev. 10/2002) Complaint

UNITED STATES DISTRICT COURT
Southern District of Florida

07-61733

Case Number: —————————— CIV - SEITZ

/McALILEY

Dr. Patrick Ojo

Plaintiff

v.

American Medical Association (AMA)
&
American Board of Medical Specialties (ABMS)

Defendants

FILED by _____ D.C.
INTAKE
NOV 29 2007
CLARENCE MADDOX
CLERK U.S. DIST. CT.
S.D. OF FLA.

COMPLAINT

I, Patrick Ojo, plaintiff, in the above styled cause, sues Defendants; American Medical Association (AMA) and American Board of Medical Specialties (ABMS). This action is filed under: Civil Rights Act -- 42 U.S.C. §1983 and equal protection clause of U.S.C.A. Const. Amend. 14 against the above defendants. Equal protection guarantee anesthesiologist, dentist, veterinarian, optometrist, and other practitioners (branches) of medicine the right to put into practice their skills, knowledge, and technical know how acquired from years of school training but it is denied to me, other clinical pharmacists, and the entire pharmacy profession. No school of pharmacy teaches count and pour (dispensing), the norms for contemporary pharmacist including me that is compelled to abandon his skills/knowledge in place of dispensing functions only because of lack of equal protection. Nobody needs specialized training/education for dispensing functions only. The defendants' failure to recognize Constitutional Amendment 14, equal protection under the law in relation to pharmacist/pharmacy amounts to keeping Pharmacy In Bondage.

The defendants deliberately refused to honor and recognize pharmacy as a specialty or an independent branch of medicine in spite of numerous studies and preponderance evidence that support the ideal. Ironically, such gesture has long been extended to anesthesiology, an integral/infinitesimal part of pharmacy, since June 1937. Besides recognizing anesthesiology as an independent branch of medicine, the defendants have gone further to recognize with prescriptive authority other less qualified branches and allied of medicine (dentists, veterinarians, optometrists, certified nurse practitioners, midwives, physician assistants etc) than pharmacy itself in it area of jurisdiction. Pharmacy In Bondage among other things discriminate against me, other clinical pharmacists/pharmacists and pharmacy profession in that we are made to take orders from physician assistants, certified nurse practitioners, dentists, veterinarians, optometrists and others (e.g. midwives etc) with infinitesimal/fragmented knowledge of drugs in our own area of jurisdiction. We cannot exercise the same rights as these healthcare practitioners even though we have greater knowledge of drugs and we are well acknowledged as drug specialists/medication experts in the medical community/world. In this motion, I, Patrick Ojo, the Plaintiff seeks among other things the need for the defendants to:

1. Define the term Specialty in Medical field, the application of such definition to drug treatment/therapy/management and the criteria for meeting such definition.

2. State why other branches of medicine including non-life threatening (e.g. nuclear medicine, ophthalmology, radiology, dermatology, dentistry etc.) deserves a specialty while life threatening poisons that is pumped into our bodies as drugs do not. Today, drug treatment in our country, US is estimated to be 4th to 6th leading cause of death.

3. State why and how the school curriculum or course content of veterinary medicine, dentistry, optometry, physician assistant, certified nurse practitioner and other branches of medicine meet the requirements for prescribing authority while that of the school of Pharmacy does not. Veterinarian, dentist, and optometrist spend the same number of years in professional school training as the clinical pharmacist with no residency requirement. Residency is now part of all school of pharmacy curriculum in US and many pharmacy graduates are taking advantage of it.

4. State why school curriculum must be ignored in dealing with drug treatment/therapy/management or in defining therapeutician when the same curriculum is used to define other profession/professional (e.g. accountant, engineer, meteorologist, Physicist, biologist, geologist etc). Pharmacy is known to offer more courses in drug treatment/therapy/management than any other discipline/profession in

the country. All specialists or many professionals with less educational training (e.g. 4 years) are in control of their destiny except pharmacists who in spite of spending more years in school training are treated like children in their supposed area of jurisdiction. School/professional training allow dentist to control dentistry, veterinarian to control animal health, ophthalmologist/optometrist to control ophthalmology, engineer to control engineering, biologist to control biology and many others but that is not the case with pharmacist/pharmacy. The existence of dentist has not stopped other branches of medicine from attending to patients' oral health neither has the existence of pediatrician stopped other branches of medicine from attending to children's health etc. Similarly, pharmacy autonomy as an independent branch of medicine will not stop other branches of medicine from prescribing drugs. In a nutshell specialization strengthen all professions including medicine and encourages interdependence/cooperation so why should I as a drug specialist/medication expert be treated differently from other professionals. What is good for the goose is good for the gander

5. State why they refused to acknowledge pharmacist/pharmacy as medication experts/drug specialists in the medical field or as an independent branch of medicine (like every other branch) in spite of numerous studies and preponderance evidence that support the profession/practitioners. Some of the studies showed that prescriptions written by clinical pharmacists are better than others in the medical field.

6. State why Americans or humanity must be deprived of the full benefits of pharmacy/pharmacists by keeping the profession in bondage contrary to popular views and overwhelming evidence.

7. State why other branches of medicine must continue to lord it over pharmacy/pharmacists in their supposed area of jurisdiction (the well know drug experts/medication specialists).

8. State why anesthetic, an infinitesimal or integral part of pharmacy, is a branch of medicine while pharmacy itself, the parent of anesthetic is not.

Wherefore, I pray the court to examine critically the above issues and others as deem necessary, render justice and set Pharmacy free from bondage as an independent branch of medicine for the benefit of Americans/mankind. Pharmacy autonomy/freedom would not only enable me put into practice my prescriptions' writing skills, years of school training, and scholasticism like every other professionals but ensure that I am the master of my fate and controller of my destiny as a clinical pharmacist.

AO 440 (Rev. 10/2002) Summons in a Civil Case

UNITED STATES DISTRICT COURT

Southern District of Florida

Case Number: 07-CV61733 SEITZ

———————————————————— X

Dr. Patrick Ojo

      Plaintiff

v.

American Medical Association (AMA)
&
American Board of Medical Specialties (ABMS)

      Defendants   X

SUMMONS IN A CIVIL CASE

TO: American Medical Association
515 N. State Street
Chicago, IL 60610

&

American Board of Medical Specialties (ABMS)
1007 Church Street, Suite 404
Evanston, IL 60201 - 5913

YOU ARE HEREBY SUMMONED and required to serve upon PLAINTIFF

Dr. Patrick Ojo
3791 NW 78th Avenue, Unit #6
Hollywood, FL 33024 - 8371.

An answer to the complaint which is herewith served upon you, within 20 days after service of this summons upon you, exclusive of the day of service. If you fail to do so, judgment by default will be taken against you for the relief demanded in the complaint. You must also file your answer with the clerk of this court within a reasonable period of time after service.

Clarence Maddox
CLERK OF COURT

NOV 29 2007

DATE

(BY) DEPUTY CLERK

AO 440 (Rev. 10/2002) Summons in a Civil Case (Reverse)

RETURN OF SERVICE

Service of the Summons and Complaint was made by me [1]	DATE: 12-4-07
NAME OF SERVER (PRINT): Lisa M Everett	TITLE: Process Server

Check one box below to indicate appropriate method of service

- ☐ Served personally upon the defendant. Place where served: _____

- ☒ Left copies thereof at the defendant's dwelling house or usual place of abode with a person of suitable age and discretion then residing therein.
  Name of person with whom the summons and complaint were left: Virginia Evans, Staff Assistant to Leonard Nelson. 515 N. State, Chicago, IL

- ☐ Returned unexecuted: _____

- ☐ Other (specify): _____

STATEMENT OF SERVICE FEES

TRAVEL	SERVICES	TOTAL $0.00

DECLARATION OF SERVER

I declare under penalty of perjury under the laws of the United States of America that the foregoing information contained in the Return of Service and Statement of Service Fees is true and correct.

Executed on 12-4-07
Date

Signature of Server

Address of Server: 202 E Ohio St. 372 Chicago, IL

Susan Milby
Notary Public Seal State of Indiana
Lake County
My Commission Expires 11/14/2013

(1) As to who may serve a summons see Rule 4 of the Federal Rules of Civil Procedure.

VERIFIED RETURN OF SERVICE

UNITED STATES DISTRICT COURT
THE SOUTHERN DISTRICT OF FLORIDA

CASE: 07-61733 CIV-SEITZ
CIVIL DIVISION

DR. PATRICK OJO

vs.

20 DAYS SUMMONS AND COMPLAINT
MOTION TO GRANT PHARMACIST/PHARMACY EQUAL
PROTECTION UNDER THE LAW

AMERICAN MEDICAL ASSOCIATION (AMA) AND
AMERICAN BOARD OF MEDICAL SPECIALTIES

ATTORNEY: DR. PATRICK OJO
3791 N.W. 78TH AVENUE UNIT #6
HOLLYWOOD, FL 33024

I received this writ on Date 12-1-07 at Time _____ and served same on AMERICAN MEDICAL ASSOCIATION at, 5151 N. State, Chicago, IL on Date 12/4/07 Time 11:15am

[ ] **INDIVIDUAL:** By serving the within named defendant a copy to the above named document(s). F.S. 40.031

[ ] **SUBSTITUTE:** By serving a copy of the above named document(s) at the defendant usual place of abode on a person residing therein, to wit, _____ who is 15 years of age or older and informing the person of the contents.

[X] **CORPORATE SERVICE:** By serving a copy of the above named document(s) to Virginia Evans as Staff Assistant or any employee of defendant corporation in the absence of any superior officer, FS 48.081 when defendant corp. does not keep a registered agent present. FS 48.091

[ ] **SERVICE BY ACCEPTANCE:** By serving a copy of the above named document(s) to _____ as _____, as the person designated by the above named defendant to receive same on his/her behalf.

[ ] **MILITARY STATUS:** To my best knowledge, information and belief the said defendant at the time of service was not engaged to the military service of the United States. defendant to receive same on his/her behalf.

[ ] **NO SERVICE:** For the reason that diligent search and inquiry failed to locate above named defendant / witness in _____ County, State of _____.

COMMENTS: Assistant to Leonard Nelson

Under penalties of perjury, I declare that I have read the forgoing document and that the facts stated in it are true.
Date: 12-4-07

ATTORNEY SERVICES, INC.
3301 S.W. 137TH AVENUE
MIRAMAR, FL 33027
OFFICE (305) 829-2993

Susan Milby
Notary Public Seal State of Indiana
Lake County
My Commission Expires 11/14/2015

INDEX 166711

AO 440 (Rev. 10/2002) Summons in a Civil Case (Reverse)

RETURN OF SERVICE

Service of the Summons and Complaint was made by me	DATE 12-4-07
NAME OF SERVER (PRINT) Lisa Everett	TITLE Process Server

Check one box below to indicate appropriate method of service

☐ Served personally upon the defendant. Place where served: _____

☒ Left copies thereof at the defendant's dwelling house or usual place of abode with a person of suitable age and discretion then residing therein.
Name of person with whom the summons and complaint were left: Susan O'Connell, Dr of Finance + Admin, 1007 Church St Ste 404 Evanston, IL

☐ Returned unexecuted: _____

☐ Other (specify): _____

STATEMENT OF SERVICE FEES

TRAVEL	SERVICES	TOTAL $0.00

DECLARATION OF SERVER

I declare under penalty of perjury under the laws of the United States of America that the foregoing information contained in the Return of Service and Statement of Service Fees is true and correct.

Executed on 12-4-07
Date

Signature of Server

807 S. Ohio Ste 372
Chicago, IL
Address of Server

Susan Milby
Notary Public Seal State of Indiana
Lake County
My Commission Expires 11/14/2015

(1) As to who may serve a summons see Rule 4 of the Federal Rules of Civil Procedure.

UNITED STATES DISTRICT COURT SOUTHERN
DISTRICT OF FLORIDA
Case No.: 07-CV-61733-SEITZ

Dr. Patrick Ojo
Plaintiff,
VS.
American Medical Association and American Board of Medical Specialties

Defendant.

MOTION FOR LIMITED APPEARANCE, CONSENT TO DESIGNATION AND REQUEST TO ELECTRONICALLY RECEIVE NOTICES OF ELECTRONIC FILING

In accordance with Local Rules 4.B of the Special Rules Governing the Admission and Practice of Attorneys of the United States District Court for the Southern District of Florida, the undersigned respectfully moves for the admission of William K. McVisk of the law firm of Johnson & Bell, Ltd., 55 East monroe Street, 41st Floor, Chicago, IL 60603 (313) 948-0229, for purposes of limited appearance as co-counsel on behalf of American Board of Medical Specialists, herein, in the above-styled case only, and pursuant to Rule 2B, Southern District of Florida, CM/ECF Administrative Procedures, to permit William K. McVisk to receive electronic filings in this case, and in support thereof states as follows:

1. William K. McVisk is not admitted to practice in the Southern District of Florida and is a member in good standing of the Illinois State Bar, the United States District Court Northern District of Illinois, the United States District Court for the Northern District of Indiana, and the United States District Court for the Southern District of Indiana, United States District Court for the Central District of Illinois.

2. Movant, Michael L. Elkins, Esquire, of the law firm of Fowler, White, Burnett, P.A., 1395 Brickell Ave., 14th Floor, Miami, Florida 33131 (305) 789-9213, is a member in good standing of the The Florida Bar and the United States District Court for the Southern District of Florida, maintains an office in this State for the practice of law, and is authorized to file through the

Court's electronic filing system. Movant consents to be designated as a member of the Bar of this Court with whom the Court and opposing counsel may readily communicate regarding the conduct of the case, upon whom filings shall be served, who shall be required to electronically file all documents and things that may be filed electronically, and who shall be responsible for filing documents in compliance with the CM/ECF Administrative Procedures. See Section 2B of the CM/ECF Administrative Procedures.

3. In accordance with the local rules of this Court, William K. McVisk has made payment of this Court's $75 admission fee. A certification in accordance with Rule 4B is attached hereto.

4. William K. MeVisk, by and through designated counsel and pursuant to Section 2B,

Southern District of Florida, CM/ECF Administrative Procedures, hereby requests the Court to provide Notice of Electronic Filings to William K. McVisk at email address:mcviskw@jbltd.com.

WHEREFORE, Michael L. Elkins, moves this Court to enter an Order William K. McVisk, to appear before this Court on behalf of American Board of Medical Specialists, for all purposes relating to the proceedings in the above-styled matter and directing the Clerk to provide notice of electronic filings to William K. McVisk.

Date: 01/24/2008

Respectfully submitted,

Michael L. Elkins
523781
Mle@fowler-white. com
Fowler, White, Burnett, P.A., 1395 Brickell Ave., 14th Floor,
Miami, Florida 33131 (305) 789-9213
(305) 789-9213
(305) 728-7513
Attorneys for American Board of Medical Specialties

CERTIFICATE OF SERVICE

I HEREBY CERTIFY that a true and correct copy of the foregoing Motion for Limited Appearance, Consent to Designation and Request to Electronically Receive Notices of Electronic Filings was served by U.S. Mail, on 01/24/2008, to Dr. Patrick Ojo, 3791 NW 78th Avenue, Unit 6, Hollywood, FL 33024-8371.

Michael L. Elkins

UNITED STATES DISTRICT COURT SOUTHERN DISTRICT OF FLORIDA

Case No.: 07-CV-61733-SEITZ

Dr. Patrick Ojo
Plaintiff,
VS.
American Medical Association and American Board of Medical Specialties
Defendant.

CERTIFICATION OF William K. McVisk

William K. McVisk, Esquire, pursuant to Rule 4B of the Special Rules Governing the Admission and Practice of Attorneys, hereby certifies that (1) I have studied the Local Rules of the United States District Court for the Southern District of Florida; and (2) I am a member in good standing of Illinois State Bar, United States District Court Northern District of Illinois.

William K. McVisk

UNITED STATES DISTRICT COURT SOUTHERN DISTRICT OF FLORIDA

Case No.: 07-CV-61733-SEITZ

Dr. Patrick Ojo
Plaintiff,
vs.
American Medical Association and American Board of Medical Specialties
Defendant.

ORDER GRANTING MOTION FOR LIMITED APPEARANCE OF WILLIAM MCVISK, CONSENT TO DESIGNATION AND REQUEST TO ELECTRONICALLY RECEIVE NOTICES OF ELECTRONIC FILING

THIS CAUSE having come before the Court on the Motion for Limited Appearance of William K. McVisk, and Consent to Designation, requesting, pursuant to Rule 4B of the Special Rules Governing the Admission and Practice of Attorneys in the United States District Court for the Southern District of Florida, permission for a limited appearance of William K. McVisk, in this matter and request to electronically receive notice of electronic filings. This Court having considered the motion and all other relevant factors, it is hereby

ORDERED AND ADJUDGED that:

The motion for Limited Appearance, Consent to Designation and Request to Electronically Receive Notices of Electronic Filings is GRANTED. William K. McVisk, is granted to appear and participate in this action on behalf of American Board of Medical Specialties. The Clerk shall provide electronic notification of all electronic filings to William K. McVisk, at mcviskw@jbltd.com.

UNITED STALES DISTRICT COURT SOUTHERN DISTRICT OF FLORIDA

CASE NO. 07-CV-61733-SEITZ

DR. PATRICK OJO,
Plaintiff,
V.
AMERICAN MEDICAL ASSOCIATION (AMA) and AMERICAN BOARD OF MEDICAL SPECIALTIES (ABMS),
Defendants.

NOTICE OF APPEARANCE

The law firm of FOWLER WHITE BURNETT P.A., notifies the Court and all interested parties of its appearance on behalf of the Defendant, AMERICAN BOARD OF MEDICAL SPECIALTIES (ABMS).

Respectfully submitted,
s/Michael L. Elkins
Michael L. Elkins
Florida Bar No. 523781
melkins fowler-white.com
Counsel for Defendant American Board of Medical Specialties (ABMS)
FOWLER WHITE BURNETT P.A.
Espirito Santo Plaza, 14th Floor
1395 Brickell Avenue
Miami, Florida
33131-3302
Telephone: (305) 789-9200
Facsimile: (305) 789-9201

CASE NO. 07-CV-61733-SEITZ

CERTIFICATE OF SERVICE

I hereby certify that on the 16th day of January, 2008, the foregoing document was electronically filed with the Clerk of the Court using CM/ECF. I also certify that the foregoing document is being served this day on all counsel of record on the attached Service List in the manner specified, either via transmission of Notices of Electronic Filing generated by CM/ECF or in some other authorized manner for those counsel or parties who are not authorized to receive electronically Notices of Electronic Filing.

s/ Michael L. Elkins
Michael L. Elkins
Florida Bar No. 523781

SERVICE LIST

DR, PATRICK OJO v.
AMERICAN MEDICAL ASSOCIATION (AMA) and
AMERICAN BOARD OF MEDICAL SPECIALTIES (ABMS)
CASE NO. 07-CV-61733-SEITZ

Dr. Patrick Ojo
3791 NW 78th Avenue Unit 6
Hollywood, FL 33024-8371
Service via Regular mail
[ecd] W:\74490\NOTAPP73.MLE (1/1618-12:28)

Case: 0:07-cv-61733-PAS Document #: 5 Entered on FLSD Docket: 12/14/2007 Page 1 of 7

UNITED STATES DISTRICT COURT

SOUTHERN DISTRICT OF FLORIDA

CASE NO. 07-61733-CIV-SEITZ/MCAL1LEY

DR. PATRICK OJO,
Plaintiff,
VS.
AMERICAN MEDICAL ASSOCIATION, et al.,
Defendant.

ORDER REQUIRING JOINT SCHEDULING REPORT

THIS MATTER came before the Court upon the filing of the Complaint. The Court has reviewed the Complaint and is otherwise fully advised. It is

ORDERED:

1. Plaintiff(s), through counsel, or if unrepresented, personally, shall provide copies of this order to all counsel and any unrepresented parties when they file an appearance in the case.

2. **Joint Scheduling Report (JSR)**. Pursuant to Fed.R.Civ.P 26(f) and Local Rule 16.1B, the parties are jointly responsible for conferring to develop a Joint Scheduling Report that sets out a proposed case management and discovery plan. By **February 26, 2008**, the parties must jointly file with the Court a scheduling report that includes a complete service list containing the names, addresses, phone, facsimile and bar numbers of each counsel. Parties need not submit a proposed scheduling order with the Report. **If Plaintiff has not effectuated service on all defendants at least forty (40) days from the date of this Order,** Plaintiff must file a motion to extend the time to file the JSR, specifying the date on which service will be completed and the JSR will be filed.

3. The **Joint Scheduling Report must include** the following:

A. A short, plain statement of the nature of the claim, any counterclaims, cross-claims or third-party claims with a good faith estimate of the specific dollar valuation of damages claimed and any other relief sought.

B. A brief summary of the facts that are uncontested or which can be stipulated to without discovery.

C. A list of the legal elements of each claim and defense asserted. Consult the Eleventh Circuit or applicable state standard jury instructions for such. This list will be used to help resolve relevance issues in discovery.

D. Whether discovery should be conducted in phases or limited to certain issues.

E. A detailed schedule of discovery for each party.

F. Proposed dates and/or deadlines for: Trial; to join other parties; to amend pleadings; to file motions (i.e., Class Certification, Summary Judgment, Daubert, Markman); to complete fact and expert discovery; to exchange Fed. R. Civ. P. 26(a) (3) disclosures; to complete mediation; and to hold any status, specialized hearings (i.e., Markman), and pretrial conferences. **All Fed. R. Civ. P. 26(a)(3)(A) disclosures must be made at least forty (40) days before the agreed fact discovery cutoff.** Fifteen (15) weeks must be scheduled between the Summary Judgment Motion deadline and the pretrial conference to complete briefing and ruling prior to the pretrial stipulation deadline. Pretrial Conferences are set a month before trial. **Attachment A to this order is a case management deadline worksheet for the parties' convenience.**

G. Estimated length of trial and whether it is jury or non-jury.

H. A list of all pending motions, whether each is "ripe" for review, the date each became ripe and a summary of the parties' respective positions with respect to each ripe motion.

I. Any unique legal or factual aspect of the case requiring the Court's special consideration,

J. A statement as to the need (or agreement) to refer matters, including motions to dismiss, motions for summary judgment and discovery to the Magistrate Judge or special master. As part of the Joint Scheduling Report, the parties shall jointly complete and file with the Court the **Magistrate Judge jurisdiction election form fur motions appended to this Order as Attachment B.** The Court will not accept unilateral submissions in this regard; thus, a "Yes" should be checked only if all parties agree. If all parties consent to a full disposition of the case by the Magistrate Judge, including trial and entry of final judgment, Attachment C is an election form which all parties must sign and tile.

K. The status and likelihood of settlement.

L. Any other matters that Local Rule 16.1B requires, or that may aid in the fair, expeditious and efficient management and/or disposition of this action.

4. Disclosures required under Fed. R. Civ. P. 26(a)(1)-(2) must be made at or before the time the parties confer to develop their case management and discovery plan. The parties must certify in the Joint

Scheduling Report that such disclosures have been made unless a party objects that the required disclosure(s) is not appropriate under the circumstances, and files an objection to the specific disclosure(s). Such filed objection must include a full explanation of the basis for the objection.

5. If after receipt of the parties' Joint Scheduling Report the Court determines that a

Rule I 6(b) Fed, R. Civ. P. scheduling and planning conference is necessary, it shall set a hearing. The parties should be prepared to argue all motions pending at the time of such hearing.

DONE AND ORDERED in Miami, Florida, this 13th day of December, 2007.

PATRICIA A. SEITZ
UNITED STATES DISTRICT JUDGE
cc: All counsel of record

IN THE UNITED STATES DISTRICT COURT FOR THE SOUTHERN DISTRICT OF FLORIDA

PATRICK OJO, M.D.,
Plaintiff,
v.
AMERICAN MEDICAL ASSOCIATION and AMERICAN BOARD OF MEDICAL SPECIALTIES,

Defendants.

DEFENDANT AMERICAN MEDICAL ASSOCIATION'S MOTION TO DISMISS PLAINTIFF'S COMPLAINT WITH INCORPORATED MEMORANDUM OF LAW

Defendant American Medical Association (the "AMA"), by and through its undersigned counsel, hereby files its Motion to Dismiss Plaintiffs Complaint With Incorporated Memorandum of Law. In support of said pleading, the AMA states as follows:

BACKGROUND

The American Medical Association ("AMA"), an Illinois non-profit corporation, is an association of approximately 250,000 physicians, residents, and medical students. Its members practice in every state, including Florida. The AMA was founded in 1847 to promote the science and art of medicine and the betterment of public health, and these remain its core purposes. Its members practice in all fields of medical specialization, and it is the largest medical society in the United States. The AMA is in, no way, a state actor or related to any arm of government.

Although difficult to discern, the pro se Complaint filed by Dr. Patrick Ojo ("Plaintiff") appears to attempt to assert a 42 U.S.C. § 1983 statutory and equal protection claim against the AMA (and Defendant American Board of Medical Specialties) asking that the pharmacy profession somehow be set free "from bondage." As discussed below, even if Plaintiff's Complaint actually asserted the elements of a § 1983 claim, it must still be dismissed for lack of subject matter jurisdiction as the case law is clear that the AMA is not any kind of "state actor" under that statute. Plaintiff's Complaint would also have to be dismissed, in the end, for failure to assert any of the elements of a § 1983 claim in his Complaint.

LEGAL ANALYSIS

Rule 12(b)(6) of the Federal Rules of Civil Procedure provides that a court must dismiss a plaintiff's complaint for failure to state a claim if it appears beyond doubt that the plaintiff can prove no set of facts which would entitle him to relief. See Hodges v. Buzzeo, 193 F. Supp. 1279, 1281 (M.D. Fla. 2002) citing Conley v. Gibson, 355 U.S. 41 (1957). In this case, Plaintiffs Complaint must be dismissed because Plaintiff can assert no set of facts that would entitle him to judgment against the AMA.

I. The AMA's Actions Do Not Violate the Fourteenth Amendment
A. The AMA Is Not A State Actor Under § 1983.

Although Plaintiff's Complaint never explains how the AMA has aggrieved him or his pharmacy profession or how the AMA's alleged actions somehow fall under the color of state law, there is simply no way that the AMA's conduct (whatever Plaintiff thinks happened) can violate the Fourteenth Amendment. It is well-settled that in order to state a claim under § 1983, a plaintiff must allege that he was deprived of a federal right by a person [or group] acting under color of state law. See Griffin v. City of Opa-Locka, 261 F.3d 1295, 1303 (11th Cir. 2001)(citing Almand v. DeKalb County, 103 F.3d 1510, 1513 (11th Cir. 1997). As Explained by the Eleventh Circuit, the "dispositive issue is whether the official was acting pursuant to the power he/she possessed by state authority or acting only as a private individual." Edwards v. Wallace Community College, 49 F.3d 1517, 1523 (11th) Cir. 1995). In other words, the defendant charged with the civil rights violation under § 1983 must be a person or association who may be fairly said to be a "state actor." Harvey v. Harvey, 949 F.2d 1127, 1130 (11th Cir. 1992). Moreover, where "the institution accused of a constitutional violation is private, the plaintiff will bear a heavier burden of showing that the questioned conduct is really tantamount to that of the State." Bailey v. McCann, 55o F.2d 1016, 1018 (5th Cir. 1977)(private association that licensed drivers and tracks in harness racing not a "state actor").

The AMA is a voluntary, non-profit association of physicians dedicated to advancing the medical profession. The AMA has no power to issue, suspend, revoke, or otherwise affect the licensing of doctors— or pharmacists-- practicing in Florida. Such authority rests entirely with the government, as it does in every other state. Indeed, the issue is so clear that case law has already determined voluntary medical associations not to be "state actors" under § 1983. See Ford v. Harris County Medical Society,

535 F.2d 321 (5th Cur, 1976)(voluntary medical association affiliated with the AMA not a "state actor). Moreover, in Brown v. Federation of State Medical Boards of the United States, 1985 WL 1659 (N.D. 111. 1985), the United States District Court held that the state medical board association was not a state agency as it did not license physicians and did little more than provide a testing service utilized by some of the states. The same result is demanded here.

Thus, Plaintiff's claim that the AMA is somehow keeping his pharmacy profession "in bondage" must fail for lack of subject matter jurisdiction because no state action or acts under color of state law occurred or could possibly occur. It is important to note that Plaintiff has not even alleged in his Complaint that the AMA acted under color of state law or was otherwise any kind of state actor, and it should be dismissed on this ground alone. Plaintiff simply can never make a case that a voluntary, national medical association, such as the AMA, acts under color of state law and, therefore, any dismissal of Plaintiff's § 1983 or constitutional claim must be with prejudice.

IL Plaintiff Has Not Complied With the Federal Pleading Rules

The Federal Rules of Civil Procedure contain pleading requirements for documents filed in federal court. Rule 8(a)(2) of the Federal Rules of Civil Procedure requires a complaint to contain "a short and plain statement of the claim showing that the pleader is entitled to relief." Rule 8(e)(2) requires that "[e]ach averment of a pleading shall be simple, concise, and direct." One important purpose of Rule 8 is so that the Court and the opposing parties can determine what is being claimed. A failure to comply with Rule 8 "makes it difficult to determine upon what authority and facts [the plaintiff] has relied." Washington v. Bauer, 149 Fed.Appx. 867, 871 (11th Cir. 2005).

Although pro se complaints like Plaintiff's should be liberally construed, such complaints must still comply with the procedural rules governing the proper form of pleadings. McNeil v. United States, 508 U.S. 106, 113 (1993). Plaintiff's prayer that this Court "render justice and set Pharmacy free from bondage as an independent branch of medicine for the benefit of Americans/mankind" simply is not an appropriate request for relief. The rest of his Complaint speaks in similar hyperbole. Moreover, under Rule 12(b)(6), Plaintiff's Complaint must be wholly dismissed for failure to state a claim as he has not even alleged any of the constitutional or statutory elements necessary to assert a § 1983 or equal protection claim.

CONCLUSION

WHEREFORE, for all the foregoing reasons, Defendant American Medical Association requests that: 1) Plaintiffs Complaint which appears to attempt to assert some kind of § 1983 and equal protection claim be dismissed with prejudice as the AMA is not a "state actor" and, thus, this Court lacks subject matter jurisdiction over such a claim: 2) Plaintiffs Complaint also be dismissed for failure to state a claim as he has alleged none of the statutory elements required of a § 1983 claim; 3) the Court consider awarding fees and costs; and, 4) the Court award any farther relief deemed just and proper.

January 24, 2007.

TRIPP SCOTT, P.A.
Attorneys for Defendant
AMA 110 S.E. 6th Street,
15th Floor Ft. Lauderdale, Florida 33301
(954) 525-7500
(954) 761-8475 facsimile
/s/ Stephanie Alexander. Esq.
STEPHANIE ALEXANDER
Florida Bar #: 0081078

CERTIFICATE OF SERVICE

I hereby certify that on January 24, 2007, I electronically filed the foregoing with the Clerk of the Court by using the CM/ECF system. A copy was also sent via U.S. Mail to Dr. Patrick Ojo, 3791 N.W. 78th Avenue, Hollywood, FL 33024.

By: /s/ Stephanie Alexander
Stephanie Alexander
Fla. Bar No. 00810178

UNITED STATES DISTRICT COURT SOUTHERN DISTRICT OF FLORIDA

CASE NO. 07-CV-61733-SEITZ

DR. PATRICK OJO,
Plaintiff,
v.

AMERICAN MEDICAL ASSOCIATION (AMA) and
AMERICAN BOARD OF MEDICAL SPECIALTIES (ABMS),

Defendants.

DEFENDANT'S MOTION TO DISMISS PLAINTIFF'S COMPLAINT AND INCORPORATED MEMORANDUM OF LAW

The Defendant, American Board of Medical Specialties ("ABMS"), by and through its attorneys, and pursuant to Federal Rule of Civil Procedure 12 (b)(2) and 12(b)(6), moves this honorable Court to dismiss plaintiff's Complaint, and in support of said motion states as follows:

I. INTRODUCTION

On November 29, 2007, Plaintiff, Dr. Patrick Ojo, filed this action, under 42 U.S.C. §1983, against ABMS and the American Medical Association. (See Plaintiff's Complaint). Plaintiff's general assertion is that Defendants, by refusing to recognize pharmacy as an independent branch of medicine, are in violation of the equal protection clause of the 14th Amendment.   (See Plaintiff's Complaint).

II. SUMMARY OF ARGUMENT

Plaintiff has failed to allege any facts linking the ABMS with the state of Florida and, therefore, has failed to establish a basis for personal jurisdiction over ABMS. Moreover, as set forth in the affidavit of Amy Horowitz, ABMS Vice President, ABMS has no substantial contacts with

Florida. In addition, because Plaintiff has failed to allege the deprivation of a federal right by a state actor, he has failed to allege facts sufficient to give rise to an equal protection claim.

III. ARGUMENT

A. This Court has no Personal Jurisdiction as ABMS Does Not Carry on Business in Florida and Does Not Have Any Contacts in Florida.

A plaintiff bears the burden of proving personal jurisdiction over nonresident defendants. Umbach v. Mercator Momentum Fund, L.P., 2007 U.S. Dist. LEXIS 74635, at *11-12 (S.D. Fla. 2007); Smolinski & Assocs. v. Continental Airlines, Inc., 2000 U.S. Dist. LEXIS 14685, at*3 (S.D. Fla. 2000). Plaintiff has not and cannot establish that ABMS carries on business or has any presence whatsoever in Florida.

ABMS is a not-for-profit corporation organized under the laws of Illinois, and its only office is in Illinois. To establish personal jurisdiction over a nonresident defendant, plaintiff must first show that Florida's long-arm statute provides a basis for jurisdiction. Sculptchair, Inc. v. Century Arts, Ltd., 94 F.3d 623, 626 (11th Cir. 1996). If a jurisdictional basis exists under the long arm statute, a plaintiff must also show that a defendant has sufficient minimum contacts with Florida as to satisfy traditional notions of fair play and substantial justice pursuant to the Due Process Clause of the 14th Amendment. Id. "Only if both prongs of the analysis are satisfied may a federal or state court exercise personal jurisdiction over a non-resident defendant." Umbach, 2007 U.S. Dist. LEXIS 74635, at *11; Robinson v. Giarniarco & Bill, P.C., 74 F.3d 253, 256 (11th Cir. 1996). Plaintiff has not satisfied either criterion.

The Florida long-arm statute has two sections. The first lists various acts by which a defendant submits to personal jurisdiction in Florida. Fla. Stat. §48.193(1). These acts include:

1. Operating or carrying on a business within Florida;
2. Committing a tortious act within Florida;

***

6. Causing injury to persons or property within Florida arising out of acts outside of Florida if the defendant was "engaged in solicitation or service activities within" Florida or "[p]roducts, materials, or things processed, serviced, or manufactured by the defendant anywhere were used or consumed within this state in the ordinary course of commerce, trade, or use";

ABMS does not operate or carry on a business in Florida. Horowitz Affidavit, ¶5. The plaintiff has not alleged that ABMS has committed any tortious acts in Florida. And while plaintiff alleges that his rights were violated, and plaintiff appears to be a Florida resident (plaintiff's state of residence is not alleged in the Complaint), there is no allegation that his alleged injuries arose out of any solicitation or service activities ABMS engaged in within Florida or that the injuries arose out of any products or materials processed, serviced or manufactured within Florida. None of the other bases for jurisdiction under §1(a) provide any conceivable basis for personal jurisdiction.

The second part of the long-arm statute provides for personal jurisdiction over a "defendant who is engaged in substantial and not isolated activity within this state, whether such activity is wholly interstate, intrastate, or otherwise." Fla.Stat. 48.193 (2). Florida courts have recognized that this requirement is the "functional equivalent of the continuous and systematic contact requirement for general jurisdiction under the Fourteenth Amendment Due Process Clause." American Color Graphics, Inc. v. Brooks Pharmacy, Inc., 2007 U.S. Dist. LEXIS 80093, *9 (M.D.Fla. 2007), citing Meier v. Sun International Hotels, 288 F.3d 1264, 1269 (11th Cir. 2002). As the court noted in Meier, the "due process requirements for general personal jurisdiction are more stringent than for specific personal jurisdiction, and require a showing of continuous and systematic general business contacts between the defendant and the forum state." 288 F.3d at 1269. Jurisdiction under §48.193(2) is only proper where a nonresident defendant procures business in Florida or solicits business through continued or sustained efforts. Price v. Point Marine, 610 So. 2d 1339, 1341 (Fla. Dist. Ct. App. 1992). It is insufficient for plaintiff to make only bare allegations of defendant's contacts without providing adequate factual details regarding defendant's contacts. Bond v. Ivy Tech State College, 167 Fed. Appx. 103, 106, 2006 U.S. App. LEXIS 3258, at *5-6 (11th Cir. 2006).

Here, plaintiff has made no allegations concerning ABMS' contacts, and indeed ABMS does not have any continuous or systematic general business contacts with Florida. ABMS does not have an office in Florida. Horowitz Aff. ¶5. It has no officers or employees in Florida. Id., ¶6. It does not maintain any bank account, telephone listing, yellow pages ads or other ads in Florida. Id., ¶5. ABMS does not engage in any public relations, publicity, charitable solicitations, or any business activities in Florida. Id. ABMS is not subject to taxes, regulation or licensing by Florida. Id. It derives no revenue from goods used or consumed in Florida or from services rendered in Florida. Id.

Accordingly, this Court should dismiss the Complaint pursuant to Fed.R.Civ.P. 12(b)(2) on the basis that the Court lacks personal jurisdiction over ABMS.

B. Plaintiff Has Failed to Allege Facts Sufficient to Give Rise to a 42 U.S.C. § 1983 Claim.

Under Federal Rule 8(a)(2), a plaintiff's complaint must provide the defendant with fair notice of the claim presented and the grounds upon which the claim rests. Bell Atlantic Corp. v. Twombly, 127 S.Ct. 1955, 1959 (2007); see also FED.R.CW.P. 8(a)(2). To avoid being dismissed under Rule 12(b)(6), the complaint must "raise a right to relief above the speculative level on the assumption that all of the complaint's allegations are true." Promark Engineered Systems, Inc.
v. Tyco Healthcare Group LP, 2007 U.S. Dist. LEXIS 47217, at *4 (S.D. Fla. 2007) (quoting Bell Atlantic Corp. v. Twombly, 127 S. Ct. 1955, 1964-65 (2007). Even though plaintiff is not required plead specific facts, plaintiff "must set forth enough facts to state a claim to relief that is plausible on its face." Pfeil v. Sprint Nextel Corp., 504 F. Supp. 2d 1273, 1275 (N.D. Fla. 2007).

1. Plaintiff Has Failed to Allege Facts Sufficient to Give Rise to Relief Under 42 U.S.C. §1983 Because No State Action Is Alleged.

Section 1983 provides for civil actions against anyone who, "under color of any statute, ordinance, regulation, custom, or usage, of any State ..., subjects, or causes to be subjected, any ... person within the jurisdiction thereof to the deprivation of any rights, privileges, or immunities secured by the Constitution and laws." 42 U.S.C. §1983. Here, the plaintiff appears to allege a Fourteenth Amendment equal protection violation. To set forth a cause of action under §1983, the complaint must allege: (1) the plaintiff's constitutional rights were deprived; and (2) the alleged conduct must have been committed by a person acting under color of state law. Shortz v. United Parcel Service, 179 Fed. Appx. 644, 645 (11th Cir. 2006); Focus on the Family v. Pinellas Suncoast Transit Auth., 344 F.3d 1263, 1276-77 (11th Cir. 2003).

Merely private conduct is excluded under the state action element of §1983, "no matter how discriminatory or wrongful." Focus on the Family v. Pinellas Suncoast Transit Auth., 344 F.3d 1263, 1 2 7 7 (11th Cir. 2003). Furthermore, the actions of a private entity are only considered state action in the following three situations: (1) where private actors perform a function traditionally the exclusive prerogative of the state; (2) where the government "has coerced or at least significantly encouraged the action alleged to violate the Constitution"; or (3) where "the state has so far insinuated itself into a position of interdependence with the [private party] that it was a joint participant in the enterprise."

Id. (quoting Willis v. Univ. Health Servs., Inc., 993 F.2d 837, 840 (11th Cir. 1993); Shortz, 179 Fed. Appx. at 645.

The plaintiff's complaint does not assert that the alleged constitutional violation was carried out by a state actor or that ABMS is a state entity (which it is not). Plaintiff also failed to assert any facts establishing that ABMS was performing a traditional government function, that the government coerced ABMS' conduct, or that the alleged conduct constituted joint action by ABMS and a state entity.

In addition to plaintiff's failure to allege state action on the part of ABMS, the fact remains that ABMS is not a government entity and does not perform any government functions. ABMS is a nonprofit organization, established in 1933, and serves to coordinate the activities of its member boards and to provide information to the public, the government, the profession and its members concerning specialization and certification in medicine. (Horowitz Aff., ¶2.) ABMS' mission is to maintain and improve the quality of medical care in the United States by assisting the member boards in their efforts to develop and utilize professional and educational standards for the evaluation and certification of physician specialists. Id. The purpose of certification is to assure the public that physicians certified in a specialty have the education and training needed by a specialist in that field of medicine and that they have demonstrated that they possess the necessary knowledge and skills of the specialty. Id., ¶3. Certification by an ABMS member board is voluntary. Id., ¶4. Board certification is not necessary for a physician to practice medicine in any state. Id. Nor is board certification by an ABMS member board required to prescribe drugs. Id.

> The Supreme Court described ABMS:
>
> Board certification of specialists in various branches of medicine, handled by the 23 member boards of the American Board of Medical Specialties, is based on various requirements of education, residency, examinations and evaluations. American Board of Medical Specialties, Board Evaluation Procedures: Developing a Research Agenda, Conference Proceedings 7-11 (1981). The average member of the public does not know or necessarily understand these requirements, but board certification nevertheless has "come to be regarded as evidence of the skill and proficiency of those to whom they [have] been issued." American Board of Medical Specialties, Evaluating the Skills of Medical Specialists 1 (7. Lloyd and D. Langsley eds. 1983).

Peel v, Attorney Registration & Disciplinary commission, 496 U.S. 91, 103, n.11 (1990). As certification by an ABMS member board is not required to practice medicine, and no state or governmental agency has any involvement in physician certification by ABMS member boards, there is no state action.

As such, Plaintiff's vaguely plead allegations clearly do not establish the alleged conduct was committed by a person acting under the color of state law.

2. Plaintiff Has Failed to Allege Facts Sufficient to Give Rise To Relief Under the Equal Protection Clause of the Fourteenth Amendment.

Even if plaintiff's vague allegations suggest that ABMS is a state actor, plaintiff has failed to allege facts giving rise to a valid equal protection claim. Where the challenged classification alleged in an equal protection claim does not burden a fundamental right or a suspect class, the Equal Protection Clause requires only that the classification be rationally related to a legitimate state interest. Whitaker v. Lee Memorial Health System, 177 Fed. Appx. 892, 894, 2006 U.S. App. LEXIS 10150 (11th Cir. 2006).

In the instant case, plaintiff's claim does not involve a fundamental right as certification of his medical specialty is not a fundamental right guaranteed by the Federal Constitution, and plaintiff, as a pharmacist, is not a member of a protected class. E.g., Gonzalez v. City of New York, 135 F. Supp. 2d 385 (E.D.N.Y. 2001)(discrimination against non-board certified physicians does not fall within fundamental right or suspect class, so rational basis test is applied.) Moreover, the classification against which plaintiff complains, that pharmacists are treated differently than physicians, is at least rational since the training and education of physicians and pharmacists is different. As the Supreme Court has stated, a "classification does not fail rational-basis review because it is not made with mathematical nicety or because in practice it results in some inequality." Heller v. Doe, 509 U.S. 312, 321 (1993)(internal quotations omitted). Whatever the similarities between the ability of physicians and pharmacists with respect to the use of drugs, ABMS is not obligated to treat them the same in determining whether to certify them within medical specialties.

The intent of physician certification performed by ARMS is to provide assurance to the public that physicians certified by an ABMS Member Board have successfully completed an approved training program and an evaluation process assessing their ability to provide quality patient care in the specialty. (Horowitz Aff., 11 3). ABMS member boards certify those physicians who have completed either allopathic or osteopathic medical school or an approved residency training program in their specialty. The certification procedures utilized by ABMS in certifying qualified medical specialties is completely rational and related to the legitimate purpose of ensuring quality healthcare to the public. As plaintiff has failed to allege facts sufficient to establish an equal protection claim, this Court should dismiss the Complaint against ABMS pursuant to Fed.R.Civ.P. 12(b)(6).

WHEREFORE, the Defendant, American Board of Medical Specialties, respectfully requests that this honorable Court dismiss Plaintiffs' Complaint against ABMS for lack of personal jurisdiction. In the alternative, ABMS requests that the Court dismiss the Complaint against ABMS for plaintiff's failure to state a claim upon which relief can be granted.

Respectfully submitted,
s/Michael L. Elkins
Counsel for Defendant American Board of Medical Specialties (ABMS)
FOWLER WHITE BURNETT P.A.
Espirito Santo Plaza, 14th Floor
1395 Brickell Avenue
Miami, Florida 33131-3302
Telephone: (305) 789-9200
Facsimile: (305) 789-9201

Human laws are human laws and they are indeed human in nature because they were made by man and for man. The Court system is the custodian of the laws and embodiment of it. Legal technicalities is not foreign to the court, thus a worst case scenario could find itself in the court today and end up being tossed out. That same case could resurface again and end up been the best case the court has witnessed on the ground of legal technicalities. Judges and Lawyers are human and very human in their approach to law and the court system. You could present the best case scenario with evidence, if a judge says or made up his mind to look the other way there is nothing you can do about it. You can equally present the worst case scenario with very little evidence, if the judge chose to stick with that little or one evidence in neglect of other multitude for his judgment then that is what it is and what you get. American President Richard Nixon once said whatever history has to say of me dependence on who write the history. He claimed that if any historian focus their attention on his "Impeachment" only then that is the only thing the readers is going to know about him; alternatively, if the same historian focus on everything about him except the "Impeachment" that is limited to just one page then the readers will get to know about him from the historian's perspective.

The court system is the best hope for humanity justice and in most cases or in many places around the world the system vindicates the just. Roe V Wade and Brown V Board of Education are two landmark justices in the history of US today, but the architect of these justices will tell you the degree of pessimism and obstacles that befall them before they see the light of the day. Recently, Miami-Dade County Mayor Carlos Gimenez said anyone or citizen has the right to go to court if he sees something wrong in the system or feels his own constitutional right has been violated one way and the other. This is exactly what made the author to go to the court to seek redress about pharmacy and pharmacy professionals' under-treatment in the medical field. The preponderance of evidence layout against the America Medical Association (AMA) and American Board of Medical Specialty (ABMS) in the above named case was overwhelming but the best defenses offered by the defendants through their lawyers are that the two organizations do not operate in Florida, they are not part of government (indirectly refereeing to the US Congress) and do not grant prescriptive authority even though they are directly involved in coordinating medical activities in all states throughout the country, US.

American Civil Liberties Union (ACLU) and few other organizations sympathized with the author but back off when they discovered the enormity of the financial involvement with no much support. The lawyers on the other hand were greatly concerned about the enormous task of taking up these two powerful organizations. By and large, after careful analysis and in conjunction with some of the lawyers' advice, the author decided in the spirit of he who fights and retreats lives to fight another day, to temporarily withdraw the case from the court as shown. As far as Pharmacy is concerned, all roads lead to heaven and it doesn't matter whichever means justice/victory/liberty comes whether through the government/elected officers (Congress), the court, awareness of professionals/people and others it is worthwhile. As indicated in the book, Pharmacy victory/justice/liberty is as sure as tomorrow's sun it is only question of time, Aluta Continua! Victoria Acerta!

UNITED STATES DISTRICT COURT

Southern District of Florida
Case Number: 07-61733-CIV-SEITZ

---------------------------------------X

Dr. Patrick Ojo

       Plaintiff,

v.

American Medical Association (AMA)
&
American Board of Medical Specialties (ABMS)

       Defendants.
---------------------------------------X

PLAINTIFF'S NOTICE OF VOLUNTARY DISMISSAL WITHOUT PREJUDICE

COMES NOW, Plaintiff Dr. Patrick Ojo, discontinues the above-styled action and hereby dismisses same without prejudice.

CERTIFICATE OF SERVICE

I HEREBY CERTIFY that a true and correct copy of the foregoing was served by U. S. Mail to: Michael L. Elkins, FOWLER WHITE BURNETT P.A. Espirito Santo Plaza, 14th Floor, 1395 Brickell Avenue, Miami, Florida 33131-3302 and Tripp Scott, 110 S.E. 6th Street, 15th Floor, Ft. Lauderdale, Florida 33301 on 02/04/2008.

/s/ Dr. Patrick Ojo
_____
Dr. Patrick Ojo

                              Plaintiff

               3791 NW 78th Avenue,
   Unit #6 Hollywood, FL 33024 - 8371
               Telephone: 954-432-2794
               E-Mail:Otrickosa@cs.com

DEDICATION

This book is dedicated to those who have worked relentlessly to bridge the gap between rich and poor, men and women, and blacks and whites.

Table of Contents

Dedication	v
Preface	ix
Acknowledgements	xvii

Chapter One	Introduction	1
Chapter Two	History of the Various Branches of Medicine	47
Chapter Three	History of Pharmacy	85
Chapter Four	Doctor of Pharmacy (PharmD) Degree	137
Chapter Five	Curriculum of Various Branches of Medicine in Comparism to Pharmacy	205
Chapter Six	Worldwide Study of Medical Schools' Curricula in Comparism to Schools of Pharmacy	359
Chapter Seven	Drug Specialists/Experts and the Medical Field	445
Chapter Eight	Pharmacy as a Life/Money-Saving Profession for Humanity: United States of America as a Case Example for the World	463
Chapter Nine	Medical Profession, Handwriting, and Errors	527
Chapter Ten	Epilogue	545

Appendix	561
Index	583

Preface

This book posits, to a large extent, an accurate historical account of pharmacy, its bondage, subservience, topsy-turvy fame, service to humanity, and awesome contributions to the health care system of the U.S. and the world. It also elaborates on the history and shortcomings of other branches of medicine, with or without pharmacy, and the need to liberate pharmacy for the benefit of mankind. My primary goal in writing this book stems from a personal encounter at the Long Island University, College of Pharmacy, Brooklyn, New York. On Thursday, May 11, 1995, I was on my way to the university library to study for one of my clinical pharmacy courses' examination, when I suddenly realized that something must be wrong with the health care system and its dealings with pharmacy profession. There were three clinical pharmacy courses in the first-degree program, and all students were required to pass them before graduating. These courses, among other things, demanded your knowledge of patients' SOAP (Subjective, Objective, Assessment, and Plan), and part of this SOAP has to do with your knowledge of patients' health/disease history, physical assessment data, laboratory values (e.g., sodium, potassium, red and white blood cells, bands or immature neutrophils, blood urea nitrogen, and other values—normal and abnormal levels, together with the consequences), drug treatment (e.g., drug choice, adverse drug reaction, drug/drug—drug/food interactions, and others), questions, answers, and others. It suddenly dawned on me on that fateful day that if I have to know all these and end up as a dispenser (throwing pills from bottle to bottle) then the essence of the education is defeated. What good does it serve to have all this great knowledge about pharmacy from a pharmacy school without an avenue to disseminate it to patients, or what good is it for me to acquire the knowledge if I can't use it? This was a millionaire question to which I sought to find an answer. As a chemist (graduate of chemistry), I had an avenue to use the knowledge I acquired from the University of Ife, Ile-Ife, Nigeria, by teaching students chemistry in high schools or secondary schools, but I noticed that that was not the case with pharmacy.

The answer to this question took me far and wide. I began by jotting notes, keeping all relevant documents, reading pharmacy journals and books, searching for facts and historical information about pharmacy, paying attention to speakers and clues during symposiums such as the Pharmacy Associations' conferences, in classrooms and elsewhere. The more I searched for facts from classrooms; first-degree pharmacy rotations at Maimonides Hospital, Brooklyn, New York; community pharmacies; and other places (e.g., during my tour of the six habitable continents of the world), the more the truth about pharmacy and the world of pharmacy unveiled itself and revealed the truth to me. Most of these facts are in the book. Some of the initial statements, views, and expressions that spurred me on include Jerry Seinfeld's views that the pharmacist needs no degree to perform his societal functions; a judge's view that the pharmacist is like a law book seller that does not know the contents of the books he is selling; Flexner's panel recommendations that declared pharmacy a non-profession and proscribed others such as osteopathic, chiropractic, etc., in 1910; Long Island University Dean of the School of Pharmacy, Dean Grossman's assertion during an entry-level PharmD symposium (around 1996) that the pharmacist knows more about drugs and medications than any other health care practitioner; Dr. Strand's mission, which was similar to but a little bit different from my vision (Dr. Strand, as a Doctor of Pharmacy degree student, was enigmatised by the question of pharmacy finality—where does it begin and end—and in a bid to find answer to the question she came across a British anthropologist who told her that pharmacy has no niche; she refused to accept that as an answer and forged ahead until she came across Dr. Hepler, with whom she formulated the pharmaceutical care experiment, and pharmaceutical care became the rallying point for modern pharmacy); and study upon study that justifies pharmacists' knowledge and others.

My inquisitiveness drove me to research the entire medical world and to be sensitive to the difference between pharmacy and other branches of medicine especially during rotations. The more I dove into the medical world, the more apparent was, on one hand, the inadequacy of other branches of medicine in dealing with drugs, drug problems, and treatment, while on the other hand was a greater demand for clinical pharmacy (to be the shepherd for sheep without a shepherd, pilot for an airplane without a pilot, and captain of a ship without a captain) for resolution. This explains why clinical pharmacy became my ultimate goal, so I decided to go back to school of pharmacy for my Doctor of Pharmacy degree shortly after graduating from the first-degree program. Clinical pharmacy has been and will be my ultimate goal in pharmacy; certain personal factors have prevented me from achieving my aim totally, but it will remain the major focus of my attention. Needless to say, there were obstacles all along the way, and the greater the huddles/obstacles the more resilient I became, because all huddles/obstacles merely betray weakness of the system and status quo that keep pharmacy in bondage. Few people may have intuitively felt what was going on around me at any given time, but many laughed and considered me a joke or jeered each time I highlighted some of the issues without disclosing my intention or goal. I looked at them, shook my head in disbelief at times, and forged ahead.

Shortly after graduating with a Doctor of Pharmacy degree from Nova Southeastern University, College of Pharmacy, Florida, in 1999, the final phase in writing this book began. I visited the Hollywood City, Florida, Town Hall Library several times for the history of various branches of medicine before I found the Marquis Who's Who. Except for the history of optometry and veterinary medicine, several searches at Nova Southeastern University health division/general library through Medline, IOWA abstract, shelves, subject and title headings, and others yielded nothing about the history of various branches of medicine. This was why I turned to the city hall local library for a solution. Marquis Who's Who, together with some other collections I acquired from other places, finalized my chapter two inquiry. I personally went to some schools such as the universities of Ife and Benin in Nigeria; Cambridge University in the UK; University de Paris in France; International University in Beijing, China; University of Sydney, Australia; and University of Rio de Janeiro, Brazil, to obtain the school curriculum of various branches of medicine and pharmacy. All other school curricula from Indian, Japan, Oxford University, Ashford University, schools in U.S., and others were obtained through phone calls, mail, and Internet services. I knew I had to do comparative analysis of schools' curricula of various branches of medicine and schools of pharmacy in order to prove my case to the whole world. Just as it was necessary to do school curriculum comparison, so it was important to conduct a drug specialist survey (to ascertain public opinion about pharmacists and drugs) and use numerous selected studies (about clinical pharmacists' activities and achievements in the U.S.) to justify the indispensable role of clinical pharmacists as drug experts/trained therapeutic physicians. Clinical pharmacists, and indeed other pharmacists, are able-bodied men and women who are capable of shaping their destiny and controlling their fate. These are men and women who, outside the pharmacy profession, are great leaders in their home and other places, so why must they be treated like children so much in the profession they revere? The harmful effect of bad handwriting in the medical community was highlighted to show the degree of pressure on medicine and how an independent/liberated pharmacy can help to reduce the pressure. I accept full responsibility for all views, perceptions, expressions, analysis, interpretations, and unseen/unintentional shortcomings of the book.

Clinical pharmacy supported by Doctor of Pharmacy degree and pharmaceutical care has emerged as a driving force to propel pharmacy profession to its final destination. Clinical pharmacy started in the U.S. in the 1930s by some first-degree-holder pharmacists who decided to go to the hospital for residence. It has taken firm hold of the profession in the United States; however, most pharmacists in the country have not yet turned to it. The major problem confronting clinical pharmacy in the U.S. today is professional autonomy; yet clinical pharmacists across the nation have proven critics of pharmacy wrong and showed that pharmacy practitioners are capable of being the master of their fate. As shown in the book, clinical pharmacists have greater knowledge of drugs than any other health care practitioners including traditional medical doctors; yet they are told to obtain permission or instruction from other branches of medicine, recall collaborative practice with other physicians, or prescriptions for legal drugs from optometrists, dentists, veterinary medical doctors, physicians assistants, and certified nurse practitioners. These health care practitioners' knowledge of drugs from the whole of their school life is no more than that of the first or second-year (at most) school life activity of the clinical pharmacists.

PABULUM FOR THE PHARMACY AND MEDICAL COMMUNITY

- Pharmacy/pharmacist is a branch of medicine and not an errand boy of medicine (EBOM).
- Treatment is to pharmacy as diagnosis is to other branches of medicine. Most physicians are trained diagnosticians, while clinical pharmacists are trained therapeuticians or therapeutic physicians.
- Except in pharmacy/medical community, there are no other places in the world where specialists are asked to take the back seat, warm up the bench, and watch while others do their job for them.
- Specialists are needed to cater to every aspect of our lives including auto repairs; house construction; and non-life-threatening cases such as dermatology, dentistry, and others, but when it comes to the poison (pills) we pump into our bodies every day, we exhibit a cavalier attitude.
- The pills (medications) you pump into your body through the mouth at dawn can send you to your grave at dusk instead of ameliorating your condition. Drugs are chemicals, and chemicals are poisons.

- Kings are kings only where there are slaves; slaves are slaves only where there are kings. Where there are no slaves, there are no kings and where there are no kings, there are no slaves. Similarly, traditional medical doctors have maintained their kingship position by keeping pharmacy in bondage while resisting any attempts to liberate the profession.
- Pharmacy was the first branch of medicine to be conceived as a specialty, yet it is the last to be liberated and nurtured to maturity.
- Freedom is a right and not a privilege; freedom is demandable and not negotiable. Each time a man goes around begging another man for freedom, he must realize that all he strived for is pseudo-freedom, otherwise considered second-class citizenship status. That is to say, each time a man negotiates freedom he compromises freedom. If the medical profession must do everything within its reach/power to deny pharmacy its inalienable rights and freedom, it must realize that it does not deserve the rights and freedom for itself.
- Except in pharmacy/medical community, there are no other places in the world where people are held responsible for other people's mistakes because of collective responsibility rule/law.
- Pharmacy, like every other profession, reserves the right to decide its fate, shape and control its destiny rather than leave it in the hands of others who do not know as much as the practitioners about the profession. Recent events and clinical pharmacists' professional activities in the U.S. have shown that the profession is capable of controlling and shaping its own destiny.
- Pharmacy is enslaved to other branches of medicine.

DO YOU KNOW?

- Do you know that 106,000 people died (taken from hospital data only) every year in the U.S. because of drug-related problems; this three-decade stable statistic placed drug-related mortality as the 4th to 6th leading cause of death in the country in 1994 (below stroke—150,108, and above pulmonary disease—101,077, accidents—90,523, and diabetes—53,894)?
- Do you know that five out every of 1,000 hospital admissions in the U.S. (i.e., 5,000 out of every one million) are due to drug therapy problems (next to cancer and above heart disease/diabetes)?
- Do you know that in 1995, ambulatory care patients alone spent well over 76 billion dollars on drug-related morbidity or illness, and that for every dollar we spend on drug treatment in this country we create drug-related problems that cost $1.33 in nursing homes?
- Do you know that in 1992, the U.S. spent 13.3% of its Gross Domestic Product (GDP) on health care, but ranked 18th in the world in terms of

life expectancy? In 1998, the same expenditure was 14.2% (14.4% by the year 2001) of the GDP, but ranked 37th in terms of health quality.

• Do you know that we as a nation spent $2.7 billion on drugs in 1960, $60.5 billion in 1995, and $121.8 billion in 2000, and that the number of prescription drugs dispensed rose from 400 million in 1950 to 1.5 billion in 1980 and 3 billion in 2000?

• Do you know that we are the world's greatest producer and consumer of drugs, and we have no experts/specialists in America catering to drug needs like other branches of medicine, consequently drugs are killing us?

• Do you know that Dr. Kessler, an MD, attorney, and former FDA chairman, blamed drug problems in this country on medical schools' inadequate training in drug therapy and clinical pharmacology (a few hours of study in the early years of student training as per Dr. Kessler)?

• Do you know that all aspects of medicine (including many non-life-threatening specialties such as dentistry, radiology, podiatry, rheumatology, dermatology, optometry, etc.) have specialists catering to them except the management of poisons we pump into our bodies in the name of drugs/pills?

• Do you know that if any aspect of medicine deserves a specialty, it is the management of the poisons we pump into our bodies? Such specialties ought to be the first consideration in medicine.

• Do you know that the early 20th century public outcry/uproar about physicians' inadequate training resulted in the establishment of Flexner's panel in 1908, the subsequent medical school reforms, and specializations? Today humanity is able to achieve miracles of biblical proportions (e.g., making the deaf hear with cochlea implant, blind see with retinal implants, and the separating of conjoined twins) with the aid of specializations, but pharmacy and drug treatment have been left out of this specialization and these miracles.

• Do you know that pharmacy was the first branch of medicine to be conceived as a specialty, yet it is the last to be liberated?

• Do you know that pharmacy/pharmacist is a branch of medicine and not an errand boy of medicine (EBOM)?

• Do you know that pharmacy is in bondage to other branches of medicine?

• Do you know that anesthesiology is an integral part of pharmacy, yet is a separate branch of medicine? It is all right for underage child to be free while the parent remain in bondage.

• Do you know that almost all physicians are trained diagnosticians, while clinical pharmacists are trained therapeutic physicians or therapeuticians (drug experts/specialists)?

• Do you know that at graduation, clinical pharmacists have greater knowledge of drugs than all other medical practitioners put together, but professional practices cause the former to lose almost everything while the latter begin to gain everything about drugs?

• Do you know that a survey of drug manufacturing company executives shows that pharmacists have greater knowledge of drugs (51%) than any other health care practitioners (physicians – 39%, nurses 4%, and others 6%), and that a similar survey of public opinion places pharmacists ahead of other branches of medicine?

• Do you know that without residency requirement, the dentists, optometrists, and veterinary medical doctors spend the same number of years in school training as the clinical pharmacists, yet the former can prescribe any drugs (except optometrists that are limited because of DEA registration) for the latter to dispense, and the later cannot do the same even though they have greater knowledge of drugs?

• Do you know that anywhere physician assistants (PA) and certified nurse practitioners (CNP) operate in offices they act like independent practitioners under the meaningless, theoretical phrase "supervision" with little or no drug knowledge? CNPs in some cases have separate offices from physicians, and physicians in most of the cohabitating offices have become administrative heads or colleagues. Little wonder why drugs are thrown at patients like candy bars, and people are dying from drugs like no man's business. More people die from prescribed legal drugs every year than from the terrorist attack on the World Trade Center.

• Do you know that approximately one pharmacy/drug-treatment course out of every 14 courses, maximum of 2 in just one year, qualifies a PA to write a wide range of prescriptions for the pharmacist to dispense to patients, while approximately one pharmacy/drug-treatment course out of every 25 courses, maximum of one and a half courses in two years, qualifies a CNP to prescribe a wide range of drugs for the pharmacist to dispense to patients?

• Do you know that prescriptions written by PAs and nurses account for 46.2% of physicians' office visits because of adverse drug reactions (ADRs), while those written by primary care physicians account for 55.98% (NCHS—1995 statistics)?

• Do you know that approximately one pharmacy/drug-treatment course out of every 17 courses, maximum of 4 courses in 3 years, qualifies the optometrist (limited by DEA registration) to write any prescription for the pharmacist to dispense to patients?

• Do you know that approximately one pharmacy/drug treatment course out of every 11 courses, maximum of 6 courses in 3 years, qualifies the veterinary medical doctor to prescribe any drug for the pharmacist to dispense to animals?

- Do you know that approximately one pharmacy/drug treatment course out of every 33 courses, maximum of 3 courses in 3 years, qualifies the dentist to write any prescription for the pharmacist to dispense to patients?
- Do you know that approximately one pharmacy/drug treatment course out of every 17 courses, maximum of 4 courses in 2 years of didactic classroom work (without rotations/residency), qualifies other branches of medicine (including osteopathic physicians) to prescribe any drug for the pharmacists to dispense to anybody?
- Do you know that approximately 8 out of every 10 courses (about 13.6 out of every 17) are diagnosis related in other branches of medicine, while about 2 out of every 10 courses are diagnosis related in schools of pharmacy?
- Do you know that clinical pharmacists/pharmacists take more diagnosis-related courses than medical doctors take pharmacy or drug treatment-related courses?
- Do you know that approximately 7 pharmacy/drug related courses out of every 10 courses, maximum of 42 courses in 3 years of didactic class work (without rotations), does not qualify clinical pharmacists to prescribe drugs for animals or people?
- Do you know that life experiences have shown that nothing can replace classroom didactic work; so no one expects the medical doctors to do a better job than the engineers in the engineering field (e.g., constructing bridges, electricity dams, roads, etc.) no matter how many years they spend in engineering rotations/residency?
- Do you know that studies have shown that prescriptions written by a clinical pharmacist are better than any other health care practitioner in spite of the fact that the law does not allow schools of pharmacy to teach the act of prescribing or permit pharmacists to prescribe freely?
- Do you know that studies upon studies have shown that clinical pharmacists can save lives and a large amount of money for the health care system if allowed to function as independent practitioners or trained therapeutic physicians/therapeuticians (drug specialists)? Two of these studies are the Bootman et al. study that showed savings of about 8,500 (0.5% of 1.7 million) human lives and $3.6 billion in nursing home facilities, annually; and the Bond et al. study that showed savings of one human life and $244.88 every time the hospital spent $320 and $1 respectively on a clinical pharmacist's salary—this also amounts to 4.78 days/patient decrease in length of stay (LOS) in the hospital.

For more information/facts, read the entire book.

Acknowledgements

God almighty, the creator of the universe, heaven, and Earth, and the overseer of all lives, human ambition, and goals and achievements, deserves the special grace and greatest acknowledgement for materialization of this work (book). Special thanks to my parents, Mr. and Mrs. Igbinehi Ojo, not only for the joy of my life but also their dedicated hard work in ensuring the success of their children. My late father sacrificed everything to the best of his ability to ensure that his children were educated at least to high school (secondary school) level as soon as he realized the importance of education. My mother, Mrs. Arumwunde Ojo, the youngest daughter of the late Madam Iduowonze Oviawe, supported my father fervently to ensure our educational success. Glory be to my grandmother Madam Enadeghe Oviawe, for her personal sacrifices in raising all her children and the children that grew under her tutelage. Enadeghe, the eldest daughter of Iduowonze, had no children of her own, and sleeping behind her on same bed as a child enabled me to listen to her yearnings, aspirations, and sobbing soul over the predicament. We both related to each other as mother and child like my other siblings (even my natural mother called her mum), and I couldn't understand why her sobbing soul couldn't accept me as her natural child. As a matter of fact, I didn't even know the difference between her and my natural mother until I grew to maturity. She was the only mother I knew for a good numbers of years in my childhood. At any rate, little did I know that she was merely responding to society's ignorance and perversion that derogates sterility. In a heredity-conscious society, having no children of your own is as good as not coming to life at all. The predicament alone is enough to galvanize the sympathy and empathy of others, but that is not always the case especially in a heredity-conscious society. Some people can be so sarcastic as to sing directly in your face that you have no purpose in life because you are working for the benefit of your fellow human beings, or remind you of your predicament at your most memorable/happy moment. She made me vow not to raise my hand against any woman on the surface of this Earth.

My great-grandmother Madam Iduowonze equally deserves commendations for her dedication to her children, endurance, and ability to starve at any given moment so that the children around her could feed. Madam Iduowonze Oviawe is the point of reference in the book; she is the granddaughter of Ezomo and her husband, Oviawe, is the son of Oloton, both of Benin City. I extend kudos to my late uncle Pa Aivehenyor Oviawe, for fervently supporting his mother and two sisters through life's peril after their father's death; and my late brother, Solomon Iyekoretin Ojo, for his commitment to our goals and family. His death in Nashville, Tennessee, in 1988 brought death closer to me and made me realize the fact that if death doesn't strike close to you, you don't know how cold the snatching hands are. The only thing that can be greater than Solomon's death in my entire life is my death, of which I will not be alive to experience it.

I acknowledge with great pride the role the following institutions played in shaping my life: Benin Baptist Model Primary School, Benin City, Evbuoneka Grammar School, Benin City, and the University of Ife, Ile-Ife (the greatest institution I ever attended in the world) all in Nigeria; and New York City Technical College, Brooklyn, Long Island University, Brooklyn, and Nova Southeastern University, Fort Lauderdale, Florida, all in the United States. My regards to Dr. Leanne Lai of Nova Southeastern University for her advice on the drug specialist study; Dr. G. E. Erhabor, head of the Department of Medicine, University of Ife, Ile-Ife, Nigeria; Dr. Allen Prince of Clinical Pharmacology (a department in the medical school), Oxford University, UK; Dr. Suzanne Manness of the Community College of Philadelphia and Anthony Brewer of Author House for their editing services; Dan Heise and Sarah Roscoe of Author House; Barbara Huang for Chinese translation of the questionnaire; Tatiana Guimaraes for Portuguese translation of the questionnaire and school curriculum; Fabia of PhD Pharmacy, Copacabana, Brazil, for her interview and pharmacy insight views in Brazil; the staff, especially Mr. George, of Apralido Hotel, Copacabana, Brazil; Leanne of Health Sense Pharmacy, Bernard Chan of Haymarket Pharmacy, Louis and Thole of Redmond—Fuss Chemists—all in Sydney, Australia; the staff of Blue Sky Mansion Hotel, Beijing (an affiliate of Beijing International Airport); the staff of the Hollywood City Hall Library, Florida; the students (especially for their hospitality—unlike the racist government officers at Sydney International Airport) and the admissions office staff of the University of Sydney (viz medical school, schools of pharmacy, veterinary medicine, and dental medicine), Australia; the admissions office staff of Cambridge University, UK; the admissions office staff of University de Paris, Paris, France; the faculty office staff of University of Ife (viz faculty of health science and pharmacy), Ile-Ife, and the University of Benin (viz faculty of health science and pharmacy), Benin City—all in Nigeria; the admissions office staff of Federal University of Rio de Janeiro (Universida de Federal do Rio de Janeiro—Center of Health Sciences and Pharmacy); admissions office staff of Beijing University, China; Rose Ojo of University of Benin Teaching Hospital, Nigeria; and Semi Ojo, Felix Oviawe, Owie Oviawe, Johnbull Agbonze, Dr. Bayo Shittu, Dr. Felix Evbuomwan and others for their contributions.

In an era when pharmacists' role in the health care delivery system has been trivialized by the count and pour system and it is extremely difficult to convince pharmacy staff (especially technicians) and pharmacists themselves that pharmacy is a branch of medicine and not an errand boy of medicine, the following technicians deserve a lot of commendations for exalting pharmacy/pharmacist: Mary Dean (a pillar), Monica Santana, Carmen Rosado, Winsome Johnson, Marie Brilliant, Maggie Neyra, Dulce Abrew, and a few others. According pharmacists with a Doctor of Pharmacy degree their due respect in pharmacy like the dentists, optometrists, veterinary medical doctors (all three specialists spent the same number of years in school training as the clinical pharmacists without a residency requirement), and other branches of medicine in their respective offices is not just a matter of "I don't care" or "It doesn't make any difference to me," but a matter of professional respect. This will go a long way toward changing the profession and people's perception of it from a pharmacist-customer (product-oriented services) to a pharmacist-patient (cognitive services) relationship. This gesture will not only enhance the profession, but also ensure that pharmacists take their proper role in medicine as therapeutic physicians or therapeuticians, drug experts/specialists, and perform their duties to patients as trained medical practitioners. If you don't care about your precious gift, personal property, or anything around you, others will consider it garbage and sweep it in the dustbin.

My special thanks to the United States of America for affording me the singular opportunity to see the world in its microscopic form rather than as a diverse, endless entity. It is difficult to imagine any other country on the surface of this Earth that would have given me a similar opportunity. I believe in the fact that the U.S., having provided me with the necessary tools to achieve my aim so far, will one day pave the way for me to accomplish my final life goal/vision of going to the moon. If I am not able to achieve this goal before my death, my spirit will be hovering in the country until one of my descendants is able to fulfill the dream. If, on the other hand, I am able to fulfill the dream then America will be sending a powerful message to the whole world that you can be born with great ambition anywhere in the world, and as long as you remain steadfast and committed to your dreams/goals you can achieve them. **GOD BLESS AMERICA.**

CHAPTER ONE

INTRODUCTION

Kings are kings only where there are slaves, and slaves are slaves only where there are kings. Where there are no kings, there are no slaves and where there are no slaves, there are no kings. Traditional medical doctors have maintained their kingship position by keeping pharmacy in bondage to them. The world as we now know it is a sophisticated world brimming with a tremendous amount of knowledge to be learned. In this world where there is so much information to be learned, pharmacy has had to become the determiner of its own fate. This decision will inevitably determine whether the profession sinks or swims. The medical profession as a branch of science has yet to grapple with the need to recognize pharmacy as an independent specialty. However, contemporary issues dictate that the medical profession can no longer ignore pharmacy and continue to deny pharmacy its rightful place in the medical world.

Throughout history, the plight of pharmacy has been comparable in magnitude to the following scenes: women versus men; Copernicus and Galileo versus the church; ANC, Mandela, Biko, and others versus apartheid South Africa; David versus Goliath; and the American Colonies versus the British Empire (American War of Independence). A brief description of these scenarios will help to explain the commonalities of these human events.

WOMEN VERSUS MEN

For centuries, men relegated women to the background, treating them like chattel (a piece of property). They used every tool within their reach including the Bible and established authority (e.g., government) to subjugate women. Many men claimed that women's place was home, and while at home their authorities were restricted to the kitchen. This deplorable situation permeated all human societies for millennia until various women's organizations such as the Women's Institute in Canada (1897) and Britain (1915) began to agitate for women's right to work outside the home. Politically, women suffered the same fate because they were repressed in various ways such as the unfortunate incident of the 1929 Aba riot in Nigeria (Abiola 1984). Generally, men thought that having women as mothers, wives, sisters, and daughters was enough to know everything about women; consequently, represent their views and interests politically outside the home. They later learned the bitter truth that no one can represent women better than women themselves. This notion is much more evident in the preaching of such great voices as Susan B. Anthony, an American political reformer. She paved the way for the enactment of 19th Amendment, which eventually granted women's right to vote in the U.S. by 1920. Today, women's contribution to the U.S. economy alone is generally immeasurable, but dollar-wise one can conveniently say billions if not trillions of dollars every year. By the year 2000, women's contribution to the U.S. economy was $877 billion per year (*Good Morning America* (*GMA*), April 4, 2001). This awesome contribution to the U.S. economy is one of the by-products of the women's liberation movement and it is enough to finance the annual budget of up to 50 poor nations or third world countries in the world today. Besides this, it is worthwhile to say that the personal assets of each of the following great women—Carly Fiorina, Betsy Holden, Meg Whitman, Indra Nooyi, Andrea Jung, Anne Mulcahy, Karen Katen, Pat Woertz, Abigail Johnson, Oprah Winfrey, Ann Moore, Judy McGrath, Collen Barrett, Shelly Lazarus, and others in U.S. (*Fortune* October 2002)—alone can conveniently finance some of the third world countries' annual budget. As at October 2003, women with assets over $3 million were said to outnumber men with over $3 million in assets in America. It is unimaginable to think of the Dark Ages and what the world would look like today without these women's wealth.

COPERNICUS AND GALILEO VERSUS THE CHURCH

The Earth was once thought to be the center of the universe on a flat platform. This view was held and propagated by the Ptolemy theory, Aristotelian physics, and the church for thousands of years. Any contrary views were considered blasphemy against God, the state, and the church; as a result there were severe consequences for such intransigent acts. It was under this atmosphere that Copernicus summoned the courage to brave the consequences and made his fearless proposal that the Earth and other planets orbit around the sun. He claimed that the sun and not the Earth was the center of the universe.

Unfortunately, Copernicus died in 1543, the year of his famous publication *On the Revolutions of the Heavenly Spheres*. Copernicus may have escaped the wrath of the state and church by virtue of his death; however, Galileo and few others of his supporters paid the price (Craig et al. 1990). Galileo was jailed and forced to recant the idea by the Inquisition in 1633. Today, an idea that was thought to be blasphemous or an abomination is the order of the day, the source of present-day scientific revolution (Webster 1990).

ANC, Mandela, Biko, and others versus Apartheid South Africa

The whites in South Africa used apartheid policy of segregation against nonwhites to secure and maintain political power in the country. The policy kept white minority in power to the detriment of blacks and others who were in the majority in South Africa. The blacks and others were subjugated, disenfranchised, and banned from entering certain areas in the country. The resultant back clash was such that the African National Congress (ANC) under the leadership of Nelson Mandela and others such as Steve Biko through various organizations fought back gallantly to regain the country from the hands of evil men. The battle was nurtured by bloody clashes such as the Sharpsville Massacre of 1961, a life sentence in jail for Mandela, the death of Steve Biko, and the killing and maiming of innocent souls that eventually resulted in international sanctions, pressure, and abandonment of the apartheid regime. Finally, Nelson Mandela was freed from jail after twenty-seven years in 1990 and the road to freedom was secured with free elections for South Africans. Today there is no more bloodshed and all citizens live not only in peace and tranquility but also in a nation where all blacks or whites have equal opportunities to contribute to the development of the country. The dismantling of the apartheid regime in South Africa has generally led to the uplift of humanity, blacks or whites, in the country, continent, and world at large.

David versus Goliath

The Bible says that the Philistines had gathered their war forces against Israel on the hill and the battle line was drawn. Goliath, a Philistine, a giant man over 9 feet tall and an experienced war veteran, dressed in dreadful war coat and armed with sword, spear, and javelin, came out from the Philistines to chastise the Israelites. He defied the Israelites and challenged them to choose a man to come forth and fight him, and whoever won the fight gained the upper hand in the battle. The Israelites and King Saul were disenchanted and terrified by Goliath's threat. They didn't know what to do for forty days about Goliath's threat. David, a boy and the youngest son of Jesse, was sent by his father to take some food to his brothers in the battlefield. He went to the battlefield and found the giant Goliath with his endless threats against Israelites. He was angered by the threats and wondered why this uncircumcised Philistine could defy the armies of the chosen people of God, the Israelites. He volunteered to counter the threat based on his experience as a shepherd boy who rescued sheep from the lion or bear's mouth. He faced Goliath with God on his side, his sling, and common stones from the stream. He slung the stone, which struck Goliath's forehead and killed him. The Philistines were paralyzed by Goliath's death; hence, the Israelites overran their army and conquered them. This brave act of courage on the part of David serves not only as a sermon for various churches today but also as encouragement for anyone to brave the unknown whenever it is necessary.

American Colonies versus Britain (American War of Independence)

The thirteen colonies of America were under the colonial rule of Britain. The British government had levied various forms of tax laws such as Sugar Act (1764), Stamp Act (1765) and Revenue Act (1767) on the American colonies. These taxes were to enhance the British government's financial status in order to maintain a standing army and expand its colonial territory in North America. The American colonies under George Washington revolted in 1775. They claimed that revenue collection without representation in the parliament was unjust; as a result they declared their independence in 1776. The writings of Thomas Paine, Patrick Henry, Thomas Jefferson, and other well-meaning great patriots helped to galvanize the public into action. The Revolution started with the Declaration of Independence in 1776 and continued till the British forces under Cornwallis were defeated at Yorktown in 1781 (Craig, Graham, and Kagan 1990). Today the United States is the greatest country on the surface of the Earth. The country is not only the envy of other nations but also a role model for democracy and a champion of the oppressed/human rights around the world. It is difficult to imagine the world without America today, but many do not know the price paid by the Founding Fathers.

Other issues are the Rosa Parks incident, Dr. Wigand versus the big tobacco companies (anti-smoking lawsuit), and many more. It is interesting to note that the challengers against authority figures have much in common with pharmacy. Some of these characteristics are that they were all considered inferior to the power in authority at that time; they all constituted the oppressed and downtrodden groups; and they all suffered various forms of humiliation, deprivation, and degradation. At one time or the other during the struggles, the challengers were considered toothless bull dogs, the vocal minority, arrogant fellows, intransigent beings, lawless people, and boisterous citizens who were doing nothing but making noise in the course of advancing their struggles. The powers that be used everything within their reach (government, law enforcement agents, mass media, enormous wealth, sophisticated weapons, legislatures, judiciary, etc.) to subjugate the challengers and educate the silent majority. They undermined and downplayed the effects of the challengers. The challengers, on the other hand, had nothing to lose except the struggle. The worst that could happen would be that the status quo remain the same. To begin with, the challengers had no power, no sophisticated weapons, no mass media, no legislature, no judiciary, no government, no law enforcement agents, and no wealth (in short, they were poor in comparison to the powers that be) on their side. They braved the unknown because they had the courage, willingness, determination, and the truth.

Besides professional humiliation, pharmacy has gone through series of vilifications, slanderous remarks, and attempts aimed at bringing it into disrepute. Three examples will perhaps serve as best examples of these remarks and put things in a generalized perspective. The first was the declaration made by Abraham Flexner, the medical school education reformer, who in 1910 claimed that pharmacy was not a profession. The second was a remark made by a judge in challenging pharmacy as a profession. He said:

"A pharmacist is nothing more than a bookseller in charge of selling law books to lawyers, students in law schools, and others."

He went further to say that selling these books does not guarantee him any status as a professional. In a nutshell, he was trying to indicate that selling these law books is not a guarantee that the bookseller knows the content of the books; hence, he cannot claim himself to be a lawyer, a surrogate, or an allied professional. The third and last one came from a number-one *New York Times* best-seller list. It was a book written by Jerry Seinfeld. Jerry in his satirical remarks in the mid-1990s wrote the following about pharmacists:

"And why does the pharmacist have to be two and a half feet up above everybody else? Who the hell is he? He's a stock boy with pills as far as I can tell. Why can't he be down there on the floor with you and me? Brain surgeons, airline pilots, nuclear physicists, we're all on the same level. But not him. He's gotta be two and a half feet up. "Look out, everybody, I'm working with pills up here. Spread out, 'gimme some room. I'm taking them from this bottle,' and I'm putting them in this little bottle. The only hard part of his whole job that I can see is typing everything onto that little, tiny label. He has to get a lot of words on there plus keep that small paper in the roller of the typewriter. That impresses me. But putting pills in a bottle with a white jacket on, I don't know why you need a diploma for that." (Bantam publication copyright 1993)

As bad as it sounds, many will argue that the truth is bitter, and Mr. Seinfeld has spoken the truth about the profession and a typical pharmacist that fits the expression. One can reasonably trace the validity of the views in the quotation as a portrayal of a profession in bondage. Like women; Copernicus and Galileo; ANC, Mandela, and Biko; David; blacks; the Founding Fathers of United States of America; Rosa Parks; Wigand; and others who were at one point considered inferior, unequal, second-class citizens, subhuman, and impotent, the pharmacy profession is suffering the same fate. At best it is logical to say that these views are an expression of absolute ignorance about the profession. Mr. Seinfeld probably might not be conscious of the fact that the pharmacist is operating within boundary of the laws that limit his knowledge output in terms of drugs, prescribing habits, and patient's education.

The term *profession* as defined by *Webster's Dictionary* means "one of a limited number of occupations or vocations involving special learning and carrying a certain social prestige e.g., law, medicine, and the church." Dr. McCarthy, in his book titled *Healthcare Delivery* (1998), defines profession in the health care field in terms of three criteria.

"Professionals provide, directly or indirectly, a vast range of services to the patient; possess specialized technical knowledge gained in particular schools or educational programs; are licensed to practice by an accepted credentialing body."

Although Flexner failed to recognize pharmacy as a profession and the first branch of medicine to be initiated out of necessity for specialty, it is pertinent to note that he also failed to define the term profession in the health care field. He, however, proposed the need for medical schools to produce clinicians and specialists in such areas as obstetrics, surgery, and cardiology. Instead of strengthening pharmacy along with other areas of specializations, Flexner's desire was to strangulate one of the longest-enduring professions in the history of mankind. Strengthening pharmacy, along with other areas of specializations, would have catalyzed its development and subsequent wish to take its proper place in medicine.

Medical education was formalized in United States of America in the early 17th century. This formal education was based purely on apprenticeship until the mid-19th century when several medical schools opened and operated without scientific basis/curriculum. Around 1860, the American Civil War, coupled with numerous deaths from infectious diseases, exposed the inadequacy of these medical schools and their lack of preparedness to deal with medical problems in a scientific manner. There was huge public outcry that eventually led to two sets of reforms. The first reform was modeled after the German pattern, which was more scientific by then. The second reform was sponsored by the Carnegie Foundation and undertaken by Abraham Flexner in 1908. The American Medical Association urged Abraham Flexner to conduct the study of medical schools in United States and Canada and publish his report. Flexner's panel conducted the study and published his report in 1910. The following was part of the findings/proposals:

- Change the basis of medical education by making allopathic medicine the only sanctioned form of practice.
- Abandon the apprenticeship mode of medical education.
- Close two thirds of medical schools, especially the weaker ones, and decrease the number of graduates through the graduation of fewer students.
- Increase the duration of training and mandate a baccalaureate degree as the criterion for admission.
- Improve quality with internships or and residence requirements.
- States' acceptance of national accreditation of medical schools under the American Medical Association.
- Base diagnosis and treatment of diseases on scientific method (e.g., formulation of hypotheses, experiment, and conclusion).
- Production of trained clinicians and specialists.

Most of the panel's proposals, including all of the above, were adopted and implemented throughout the country by 1930.

Contemporary pharmacy was conceived and left in the womb of medicine in Baghdad around the 9th century AD. The need for specialists to prepare sophisticated medicine (compounding) drove the Islamic physician Rhazes to create pharmacy as a branch of medicine. Like medicine, pharmacy education was based purely on the apprenticeship mode until the late 1800s. New York State passed a law in 1905 requiring all new pharmacists to have a diploma from a school of pharmacy, and various schools of pharmacy operated two, three, and four-year programs. Four of these schools had five-years Master of Science (MSc) degree programs in pharmacy. Many pharmacists opposed the idea of having a diploma or degree initially, but after Flexner's humiliation or utmost disregard for the profession and the U.S. War Department's subsequent refusal to commission pharmacists because of their low level of education, the situation changed for good. The changes that occurred led the American Association of Colleges of Pharmacy (AACP) to adopt the four-year minimum course of study in sciences in 1928. The AACP changed the four-year Bachelor of Science degree to five years in the late 1940s and the six-year Doctor of Pharmacy (PharmD) degree in 1992. A PharmD degree is now the adopted entry level for pharmacy practice in the country, and all schools are expected to be in full compliance by the year 2005.

Flexner and others may have cast aspersions on pharmacy but the fact remains that nothing can take away the truth from the profession and the society. Whatever yardstick anyone uses to judge or define a profession, pharmacy is not a pushover and the ideals behind its conception cannot be killed. Truth takes time in the form of minutes, hours, days, months, years, decades, or even centuries to materialize, and once it does, it is crystal clear, vivid, and plausible to all and sundry. As far as pharmacy is concerned, the truth is only a question of time and the day of reckoning is around the corner. Flexner advocated the replacement of apprenticeship with a scientifically based curriculum followed by residence in medical school/hospital. The idea was sound, but did Flexner consider the following?

1. The scientific curriculum of medical schools emphasizes diagnosis at the expense of every other thing. That is to say, the bulk of the didactic work (classroom work and internship) in medical school is centered on diagnosis, and a fragmented portion of it is assigned to drug knowledge, which eventually lays the basic foundation for drug treatment. The end result is such that at graduation, after four years in medical school (i.e., prior to residence) the graduate can conveniently call himself a diagnostician or diagnosis specialist and not a therapeutician or a drug specialist. Drug knowledge from medical school studies is so minimal that it does not give room for a well-rounded student in diagnosis and drug treatment. There is nothing wrong with emphasizing diagnosis in medical schools because of the specialty, but drug treatment/knowledge deserves equal treatment, and the only place where that can be given thoroughly is in schools of pharmacy. By the very nature of medical schools and their hectic curriculum/programs in diagnosis, it is virtually impossible to expand drug treatment/knowledge the same way diagnosis is treated.

Diagnosis and treatment are the two centerpieces in human ailment, and they both deserve equal treatment; one cannot be given greater priority over the other.

2. The apprenticeship was reintroduced as residence (housemanship or internship in a few cases; in most cases internship is a student learning exposure that occurs during the four-year didactic coursework as seen in many programs such as medicine, pharmacy, dentistry, optometry, veterinary medicine, engineering, architect, law, chemistry, etc.) as far as drug treatment is concerned. In a nutshell, the residence, which commences after four years of didactic work in medical school, was supposed to emphasize or build on what was learned in the classroom; but it turns out to be where drug knowledge is expected to be intensified as a way of bridging the discrepancy in classroom work. The intensity of drug knowledge does not surpass diagnosis during the internship. As a matter of fact, both programs—diagnosis and drug treatment—have the same status in terms of percentage allocation in classroom work and during internship/residency. The preceptor/trainer knows fully well that this is the last chance to imbibe drug knowledge, so greater effort is made to complete the training in both programs. This is the reason why drug knowledge gets a little more attention during internship/residency than in the classroom. The take-home lesson from internship/residency is such that the internship/residency is no different from apprenticeship in terms of drug knowledge because the preceptor/trainer's drug knowledge, views, preferences or favoritism, and bias are passed on to the intern/trainee.

3. The aim of introducing trained clinicians and specialists in medicine was to advance medicine for the benefit of mankind and prevent production of old- fashioned medical doctors who in most cases were jacks-of-all-trades (one physician is a dentist, dermatologist, optometrist/ophthalmologist, internist, cardiologist, veterinarian, allergist, neurologist, surgeon, pathologist, etc.), masters of none. Flexner failed to recognize the fact that diagnosis is to other branches of medicine as drug treatment is to pharmacy. This crucial view would have separated pharmacy as a branch/specialty of medicine and would have enhanced the profession to serve humanity better, because drugs are not just drugs, but poisons that we pump into our body daily. If any branch of medicine deserves specialty because of human advancement, pharmacy ought to be the first consideration.

In sharp contrast to what happens in medical school training, the pharmacist goes to school for three, four, or more years in the future to learn everything about drugs including scientific research. At graduation, he/she leaves school to start practicing the profession. That is to say, while graduates from medical school go into residence, graduates from a school of pharmacy (pharmacists) go to work. The pharmacist faces a downhill task as he/she continues to perform his/her daily job, while the medical school graduates faces an uphill task with his training and subsequent job performance after the training. A pharmacist's drug knowledge begins to deteriorate because of law limitations, job restriction, and the non-challenging job environment. He/she readily burns out and finds him/herself fitting the shoes of "Seinfeld pharmacist." At graduation, the least-knowledgeable pharmacist knows more about drugs than the average medical school graduate does, prior to residence. The medical doctor, on the other hand, continues to increase their drug knowledge in the absence of a solid background or foundation. The resultant consequence is such that doctors spend hours diagnosing real, complex cases, and the moment they unravel the mystery of diagnosis there is a sigh of relief. Complex cases that take hours to diagnose take a few minutes for them to recommend drugs on the basis of pharmacodynamics without due regard to other aspects of drug therapy (e.g., pharmacokinectics—absorption—distribution—metabolism—elimination, side effects, adverse drug reaction, drug/drug interactions, drug/food interactions, drug/disease interactions, and others) because they are not therapeuticians or drug specialists. What is even more disheartening is the fact that dentists, veterinary medical doctors, and optometrists go through the same number of years in school training in their respective fields as the pharmacists with even less drug knowledge than the medical doctors and without any residence requirement whatsoever, yet they can prescribe any drug (optometrists are limited to some extent) for the pharmacist to dispense.

All professionals go through prolonged specialized training in an abstract body of knowledge, and at graduation the fresh graduates go into their area of specialization to enhance their growth and knowledge. Here are some examples of how those designated as professionals are trained:

- A teacher goes through four years of college work in any field. At graduation he/she gains a job as a teacher, and as part of his/her responsibility he/she writes lesson plans for teaching the students, deciding how and what type of assignment to give the student. The profession aids him by building on what he has learned in school.
- An engineer goes through four or five years of college didactic work. After graduation, he starts working in one of many options:

1. Mechanical engineer: A profession that enables him/her to draw his/her plans in designing, constructing, fixing, repairing, and maintaining an engine. He/she learns and grows in the profession because college work has laid the foundation.
2. Electrical engineer: A profession that enables him/her to do the same thing with electrical equipments.
3. Civil engineer: A profession that enables him to do the same thing with roads and bridges.

- An architect goes through four years of college work. After graduation, he/she starts working. He/she draws up his plan on how to design a building and ensures that the plan is followed. He/she learns and grows in the profession because college work has laid the foundation for him/her.
- An accountant goes through four years college work. After graduation, he/she starts working. He/she learns and grows in the profession by planning his/her clients' accounts, audits, finances, and balance sheets. The college work laid the foundation for him/her to do the job.
- A meteorologist goes through four years of college study. After graduation, he/she starts working. He/she learns and grows in the profession by studying the weather. The college work laid the foundation for him/her to do the job.
- A lawyer goes through three years (after the bachelor's degree) of college work in law. After graduation, he/she starts working. He/she learns and grows in the profession by planning his/her clients' cases, mapping out strategies, and executing his/her plans in the court. He/she is able to do all this because college work has laid the foundation for him/her.

Ironically, the pharmacist goes through three or four years (five or six years with diploma entering level). After graduation, he/she goes to practice pharmacy, and he/she is meant to understand that he/she cannot write in a patient's chart about drugs, cannot prescribe legal drugs, cannot talk to patients about drugs without permission (especially prior to 1969), cannot plan a patient's regimen without permission, and cannot say anything about drug disease, direction, or the administration of drugs without permission. All he/she can do is to pour pills from bigger bottles into smaller bottles and dispense them to patients. The general practitioner, podiatrist, dermatologist, dentist, veterinarian, optometrist, physician assistant, and nurse practitioner can do most of the above or all of the above without any problems. The fate of pharmacy has been in the hands of the public right from its conception. At the beginning, the need for a specialist to prepare sophisticated medicine encouraged the growth of the profession, and shortly afterwards the specialists became dexterous in the act of compounding for all forms of ailments with or without prescriptions from physicians. The act of compounding placed pharmacy at the doorstep of the public, and people began to see the new specialists as magnanimous caregivers to whom they could turn with a prescription from a physician for complex cases and without a prescription for every simple ailment such as a cold or headache. The pharmacists' only charged for the compounded products they supplied and not for the service or advice they rendered to the patrons. They earned enough income from the compounded products to sustain their families and lifestyles; hence, they saw their free services, consultations, and advice as a magnet to bring members of the public to their locations. Pharmacy has metamorphosed through the ages from the era of compounding to apothecary, industrial drug manufacturing by pharmaceutical companies, and the contemporary quest for pharmaceutical care. They have been credited as the most accessible health care professionals in the community because of their dedication to human welfare and free health care services to people. The public has acknowledged and shows tremendous appreciation for the pharmacist's magnanimity. The most recent good gesture came from the Gallup poll in which pharmacy was rated as the most trusted profession in the country for more than a decade from 1988 to 1998 (11 years). That is to say, for more than a decade, pharmacy was rated the number-one trusted profession above clergymen, general practitioners, lawyers, dentists, and other professionals in the country. By the year 2002 and 2003, pharmacists' rating was 67%, and this placed them in fourth position. Pharmacists' average rating has been 65% since their inclusion in the annual CNN/*USA Today*/Gallup poll of professional honesty and ethics in 1981. In 2003, 1004 adults were randomly surveyed with a confidence interval of 3%, and the results showed that nurses had 83%; medical doctors/veterinarians had 68%; pharmacists had 67%; dentists had 61%; college teachers/engineers/policemen had 59%; clergy had 56%; psychiatrists had 38%; bankers had 35%; chiropractors had 31%; state governors had 26%; journalists had 25%; senators had 20%; business executives had 18%; congressmen had 17%; lawyers had 16%; stock brokers had 15%; advertising practitioners had 12 percent; insurance salesmen had 12%; HMO managers had 11%; and car salesmen had 7%. Pharmacy services, reputations, and public image have been the tools that kept the profession alive and viable in spite of the ridicule, derogatory remarks, and numerous perils aimed at subjugating and eliminating the profession. Pharmacy liberation is as sure as tomorrow's sun in spite of the above.

Pharmacy has revamped itself by setting pharmaceutical care in motion, an ideal aimed at liberating the profession from the era of count and pour or throwing pills from bottle to bottle. Pharmaceutical care has been defined as the responsible provision of drug therapy with the aim of reducing adverse drug reactions, maximizing efficacy and outcome, and improving quality of life. Numerous studies have revealed the tremendous impact of the pharmacist on health care system with the aid of pharmaceutical care. Some of these impacts are reflected in

a. decreased morbidity and mortality rates across the U.S.;
b. enormous savings of about $143.95 to $293.93 per patient per month for the U.S. health care system;
c. reduction in rates of hospitalization, emergency room visits, urgent care, and unscheduled clinic visits;
d. improved quality of life experiences by patients in internal medicine, oncology, bone marrow transplants, obstetric/gynecology, ophthalmology, HIV/AIDS condition, dermatology, nursing homes, and long-term care facilities;
e. the fact that prescriptions written by clinical pharmacists are better than those written by physicians and other health care providers put together. This high credit rating was based on drug choices, dosages, dosing intervals, clarity of instructions, benefits, and monitoring (Carter et al., *Pharmacothera* 17 (1997): 1275–84);
f. greater care for rural inhabitants, where physicians' absences have created a vacuum that has been filled by pharmacists' free access to the community;
g. the fact that pharmacists are better than physicians in improving patient compliance, making changes in physicians' drug regimens for patients, documenting allergies, nonprescription drug use, and medication histories.

Pharmaceutical care represents a paradigm shift in the health delivery system of the U.S. Many traditional medical doctors especially those in hospitals have now recognized the powerful knowledge of pharmacists as drug specialists; hence, they are now prepared to deal with them as colleagues and as another group of specialists within the medical field. Numerous factors such as human evolution, rising costs of health care, adverse drug reaction (ADR), and increased rate of hospitalization because of drug-related morbidity and mortality culminated in the advent of this pharmaceutical care. A brief discussion of these factors will provide an insight about the origin of pharmaceutical care.

♦ Human evolution and advancement entails change, and change is the prerequisite for progress. Generally people like to change for good, and some of these changes have resulted in increased life expectancy that precipitated chronic diseases as a major killer. Acute infectious diseases used to be a major killer in the world, and the biomedical model approach was sufficient for the world to deal with the problem. Human advancement helped to bring infectious diseases under control, but chronic diseases emerged with increased life expectancy and became a dominant factor. Unlike acute infectious diseases, the biomedical model was discovered to be inadequate in dealing with chronic diseases because of the involvement of lifestyle changes and multiple drug treatments. The inadequacy of the biomedical model led to the evolution of biopsychosocial model, which incorporated lifestyle changes and multiple drug regimens into the management of chronic diseases. This biopsychosocial model demands the attention of experts in drug treatment.

Additionally, media coverage of physicians' inaccurate predictions, inadequate treatment, inability to detect adverse drug reactions, malpractice/liability lawsuits, and other factors helped to educate the public and thus produced sophisticated consumers. These sophisticated consumers began to challenge physicians' authority and sought alternative means to their health care problems. They resisted the parent-child model relationship approach that was the standard of practice in most physicians' offices (clinic or hospital). The parent-child model entails the idea of a physician taking the role of a parent and the patient taking the role of a child. Some of the outcomes of the consumers' rebellion were the evolution of the consumer model of care (physicians and consumers assumed the role of coequals) and frequent visits to the pharmacy for greater knowledge about their drug regimen, therapy, adverse drug reaction, homeopathic remedies, etc. Consumers took advantage of pharmacists' free access to the community to solve their health problems. Their frequent visits led to greater confidence in the pharmacists' abilities and thus produced renowned, trusted professionals. As noted above, consumers' confidence continued to rate pharmacy as one of the most trusted professions in the country. Traditional medical doctors, on the other hand, have labored all their life to achieved their status; hence, none of them wants to lose their license or end up making payments for life to insurance companies because of a malpractice/liability suit. They all acknowledge the fact that it is better to be safe than to be sorry; consequently, they feel the onus to refer patients to specialists like dentists, dermatologists, clinical pharmacists, ophthalmologists, and others within the medical community whenever the need arises.

> Specialists in various fields of endeavor have proved that humanity is capable of achieving tremendous success and miracles of biblical proportions (e.g., making the blind to see, the lame to walk, the deaf to hear, the dumb to speak, etc.). This is particularly

true of the ophthalmologist/optometrist who can now use retinal transplant and/or laser beam treatment to aid the blind or repair human eye ailments. Dermatologists/Plastic Surgeons can now use plastic surgery to rejuvenate old faces. Gene scientists can replicate life through cloning. Dentists can now bleach and replace human teeth with no problems. Surgeons can now separate conjoined twins. Besides these highlighted benefits and human advancements, these experts/specialists have shown that they are capable of enhancing prevention that is better than cure, reducing the workload for the general practitioner and thus enhancing productivity/professional output, and minimizing or avoiding mistakes that can precipitate liability lawsuit and increased insurance premiums.

General practitioners and other medical practitioners have recognized the indispensable role of clinical pharmacists as therapeuticians/drug specialists. The vast body of knowledge available in the medical field dealing with human life makes it impossible for anyone to claim a monopoly over wisdom or conveniently assert himself as alpha and omega in solving human health problems; consequently, interdependence in medical fields as in other spheres of human life is now the order of the day. Today, we have discovered that a clinical pharmacists' position in hospitals is now more challenging than ever. Many hospitals now rely on pharmacy for their pharmacokinetics consultations; drug choices, drug monitoring, adverse drug reactions, and other treatment-related issues in intensive care units, cardiac units, ambulatory units, geriatric units, etc. Most doctors in these hospitals write their recommendations in the form of drug choice (e.g., vancomycin) for various ailments and request the pharmacy to follow up with dosages and monitoring. In some cases, the pharmacy is requested to come up with a drug of choice or ask for an opinion.

♦ The rising cost of health care has been a major source of concern for the government, employers, and consumers for the past three to four decades. For example, the country spent $2.7 billion dollars on drugs in 1960, $12 billion dollars in 1980, $60.8 billion dollars in 1995, $75.7 billion in 1997, $87.2 billion dollars in 1998, $103.9 billion in 1999, and $121.8 billion dollars in 2000 (Wallace Marsh, PhD, Nova Southeastern University—April 4, 2002). A breakdown of the 2000 expenses showed private payment of $95 billion ($39 billion out of pocket and $56 billion by insurance) and public payment of $26.5 billion (Medicare paid $2.3 billion and Medicaid paid $20.9 billion) for drugs. Some sources of health care cost increase have been attributed to inflation (22-33%), increased utilization (35-50%) and drug mix (27-33%). Prescription drug retail prices rose from an average of $2 in 1950 to $15 in 1990 and $50 in 2001. The number of prescription drugs dispensed by pharmacists rose from 400 million in 1950 to 1.5 billion in 1980 and 3 billion in 2000 for outpatients (*Journal of the American Pharmaceutical Association* 42 (2002). The Agency for Healthcare Research and Quality showed that in the year 2002, we spent $68 billion for heart condition, $58 billion for trauma, $48 billion for cancer and mental illness respectively, $45 billion for respiratory ailments (COPD and asthma), $32.5 billion for hypertension, $32 billion for arthritis and joint disorder, $28 billion for diabetes, $23 billion for back problems, etc. (Forbes 2005).

In addition, improper use of drugs is known to drain more than $76 billion from the nation's economy annually. Numerous studies have been conducted on the rising cost of health care in terms of drugs, and it has been shown that pharmacists, especially the clinical pharmacists, are well positioned through effective management (now with the aid of pharmaceutical care) to bring down the cost of drug expenditure and improper drug use. Clinical pharmacists are known to have better knowledge about drug efficacy, cost minimization, cost benefits, cost utilization, cost effectiveness, pharmacoeconomics, drug selection, dosages, and others than any other health care professionals.

♦ Adverse drug reaction (ADR) and increased rate of hospitalization because of drug-related morbidity and mortality: pharmaceutical care had its direct root from these concepts in the hospital. In 1974, Talley and Laventurier's study estimated that adverse drug reaction resulted in 140,000 deaths and one million patient hospitalizations. In 1976, McKenney and Harrison's study revealed that out of 216 admissions to a general medical/surgical unit, 59 (27%) were due to drug problems, which are mainly ADR 24 (11%) and others such as noncompliance, over dosage, or inadequate therapy 35 (16%). A study by Stewart et al. of psychiatric wards showed that 20% of psychiatry service admissions were due to drug toxicity, side effects, and noncompliance. In 1984, Lakshmanan et al. studied 834 hospital admissions in Ohio between July and August and found that 35 (4.2 %) were due to drug-related problems. In 1987, the Food and Drug Administration reported that ADR claimed 12,000 lives and resulted in 15,000 hospitalizations. These figures were reported to the FDA, and it is known that a small percentage, probably less than 10%, of cases is reported to FDA. In late 1980s, Dubois and Brook's study of preventable deaths in 12 hospitals found that 24% of 50 cerebrovascular accident deaths were due to inadequate fluid or sepsis management, nine deaths were deemed preventable; 16% of the 23 myocardial infarction preventable deaths were due to inadequate fluids management, 10% of them were due to inadequate arrhythmias control, and 5% of them were due inadequate sepsis control; and 50% of 70 pneumonia deaths were due to improper antibiotics or inadequate fluid management, and 17 deaths were preventable. In 1995, Bootman and Johnson projected that ADR cost the

U.S. economy about $76.6 billion, and 30% of the admitted hospital patients died, and 50% are deemed preventable deaths annually. In 1998, the *Journal of American Medical Association* (*JAMA*) reported that ADR claims 100,000 lives and results in one million hospitalizations and two million serious side effects annually. In 1999, the Institute of Medicine (IOM) reported that about 98,000 Americans died annually from medical mistakes, and 7,000 of these deaths are due to prescription drug errors. In 2002, Dr. Hepler cited a recent research study that claimed that in the U.S., the rate of drug-related preventable hospital admission problems was 5 out of every 1,000 admissions (i.e., 5,000 out of every 1 million admissions), and this statistic placed ADR behind all cancer admissions and above heart disease and diabetes mellitus admissions. *JAMA* and IOM reports placed ADR and medical mistakes as the 4th and 8th leading cause of death, respectively, in the U.S. The majority of these unimaginable numbers of causalities resulting from ADR have been blamed on bad handwriting, redundant names in medicine, errors in dosages, addition of drug(s) in treating ADR of previous regimens, increased workload, third-party pressure, patients' nagging, etc.

Knapp et al. studied the cost of drug-related morbidity and mortality and found that for pyelonephritis, patients with appropriate antibiotic therapy had on average a two-day shorter hospital length of stay (LOS) than those whose antibiotic therapy did not meet appropriate criteria ($P<0.05$); for pneumoccal pneumonia, patients with appropriate antibiotic therapy had a 2.2-day shorter LOS than those who did not meet the appropriate criteria ($P<0.05$). Eisenberg et al. studied the cost of drug toxicity by reviewing medical records of 1,756 patients who received aminoglycosides. They found that 7.3% of the patients developed nephrotoxicity with an additional cost of $2,501 or $183 per patient. Other studies have shown the impact of pharmacists on preventable drug-related morbidity and mortality. Kelly et al. conducted a randomized, clinical, controlled study of the impact of clinical pharmacist on intravenous fluid and medication administration. They showed a statistically significant difference of an average of 2.4 days in LOS. The pharmacist study group had an average of a 2.4-day shorter LOS than the control group (without pharmacist) had. Clapham et al. did a comparative controlled study of LOS and total cost per admission (TCA). The pharmacists were involved in patients' care in two major ways. The first method involved drug therapy review as part of cart check in a unit-dose system, and the second method involved drug use control (DUC) system with pharmacists rendering their services in patient care unit. The DUC systems patients had an average TCA of $1,300 and a 1.5-day shorter LOS than with the unit-dose system. Cumming et al. evaluated the effect of clinic pharmacy on ambulatory patients in a one-year retrospective case control study. They found that pharmaceutical services can significantly reduce rates of hospitalization and LOS in a sample of 129 patients. McKenney and Wasserman reviewed the findings of a Boston collaboration drug surveillance program and reported that nurses collected LOS and observed ADR in two bed study units over three thirty-day periods (October 1973, February and September 1974). During the first period, drugs were given to inpatients as per procedure with limited floor stock without any pharmacists; the second period had same procedure and four pharmacists to review drug therapy and consult to resolve any detected problems; and the third period was similar to the second period except that drugs were distributed in a unit-dose system. Statistics showed that LOS and ADR, respectively, for each group were: Period 1 (n = 77) 12 (8.7) and 21%; Period 2 (n = 64) 7.6 (5.9) and 16%; and Period 3 (n = 73) 8.3 (7.0) and 8%. The results revealed that patients who experience ADR were 50 to 80% likely to stay longer in a hospital than those who did not. In 1999, Pabis, Still, and Saklad conducted a study at the San Antonio State Hospital, a mental health institution, for one year and recorded 1,822 recommendations with a palm computer for 347 patients. The recommendations ranged from drug or dosage level changes, patient counseling, and monitoring, to no change advisable. The results revealed that a health care team with a pharmacist made an average of 5.4 interventions per patient and recorded a 6.3-day shorter LOS than those without pharmacists. The pharmacist cost avoidance was found to be $5.47 for every dollar investment, and physicians' approval of the pharmacists' interventions including residents was 97%. The state agency audited the hospital's clinical pharmacy internally and reported $4.09, compared to $5.47, for every dollar investment.

Thompson et al. studied the outcome of a trial with clinical pharmacists prescribing drugs in a geriatric setting or pharmacist management of long-term patients in a California nursing facility. The experimental group consisted of two pharmacists managing 67 patients' drug regimens with variations from new medication, dosage adjustment, and drug discontinuation to assessment and problem identification. The control group patients were managed by an internist in a private practice setting from February 1981 to January 1982. Results revealed that patients in the pharmacists' experimental group had significantly fewer deaths, fewer drugs, fewer hospitalization rates ($P = 0.06$), more discharges, and a greater savings ($7,000 per patient) than the internist's control group.

The project Impact started in March 1997 in Asheville, North Carolina. The pharmacists in the city decided to prove the worth of pharmaceutical care in improving a patient's health outcome and reducing total heath care costs for the city's employed diabetic patients. In the first year, the total savings of $20,000 for 40 employees was recorded, and their health status improved dramatically beyond the expectation of American Diabetic Association. For instance, the patients' average glycosylated hemoglobin $A1_c$ attenuated by 1.4% from 7.6 to 6.2%; total cholesterol level went down by 12mg/dl from 210 to 198mg/dl; and the average LDL (bad cholesterol) level decreased by 20mg/dl from 118 to 98mg/dl. The second year showed a 78% reduction in inpatient medical cost; 30% in outpatient medical costs; 62 % increase in prescription drugs; and 90% patients' satisfaction compared to 59 to 70% baseline with physicians. The project started with diabetic patients, and as at early 2001, about 365 employees were already receiving disease-state management in asthma, hyperlipidemia, diabetics, and hypertension in 32 communities. A projected economic benefit of the program revealed initial costs of $192,000, gross savings of $287,872 per 100 people in one year, reduced absenteeism and improved productivity, decreased sick leave by 50%, and a 28% decrease in per-patient overall health care cost. The most astonishing part of this project came from the findings of later studies, which showed that the pharmacist needs no additional training after the first degree (BSc) in order to impact patients' health care or outcome.

In France, two studies were conducted by Trunet et al. to determine the impact of drug-induced illness in intensive care unit admissions, mostly from acute care. In 1980, the first study revealed that out of 325 admissions, 4.3% were due to error in therapy and preventable ADR. In 1986, the second study revealed that out of 1,651 admissions, 2.6% were due to a preventable drug problem. Porter and Jick conducted a study on drug-related deaths among inpatients in 7 countries and found that a conservative estimate of approximately 1% of hospital admissions resulted in drug-related deaths, and 25% of these were preventable. They found that the drug-related death rate was largest in the U.S., with 1.2 deaths per 1,000 hospital admissions, and New Zealand was in a close second position.

Hepler and Strand's landmark research study heralded the genesis of pharmaceutical care. It changed the practice of pharmacy for many and how others viewed it. The research work was based on mental analysis/review of past studies that detailed the impact of pharmacists in the health care system. They highlighted past traditional roles that restricted pharmacists' activities in the medical field and defined drug-related morbidity and mortality in the following sense:

- Inappropriate prescription that is due to
    a. Inappropriate regime (drug, dosage form, route, interval, duration);
    b. Unnecessary regimen: for instance, prescribing antibiotics without a warranted medical condition. Dowell, Schwartz, and Phillips' study showed that about fifty million unnecessary antimicrobial prescriptions are written annually in the U.S. and

traditional medical practitioners have blamed the problem of antibiotic resistance on too many prescriptions being written (*GMA*—December 1998);
- Inappropriate delivery that is due to unavailable drugs because of economic barriers (pharmacy/patient), biopharmaceutical formulation problems, sociological barriers (failure to give drug by caretaker or institutional personnel), and dispensing error (incorrect prescription label, advice, and patient information);
- Inappropriate patient behavior due to compliance with inappropriate regimen or noncompliance with appropriate regimen;
- Inappropriate monitoring due to failure to recognize inappropriate therapeutic decision and /or effects of treatment on patient;
- Patient having medical problem that is the by-product of too much incorrect drug (toxicity), too little correct drug (sub-therapeutic treatment), drug/drug interaction, drug/laboratory interaction, and drug/food interaction.

In light of enormous evidence and a preponderance of medical problems facing the medical community, one would have expected leniency, sympathy, empathy, agitation, clamoring, and aggressive demand for specialists to take control of prescribing authority, be it the liberation and self-determination (autonomy) of pharmacy or the creation of a specialty within the medical field. Instead, the world has experienced greater delegation of power and prescribing authority to subordinates such as certified nurse practitioners (CNP), nurses, and physician assistants (PA) in medical offices/hospitals and psychologists in some states (e.g., New Mexico). Social workers, caseworkers, medical office managers, and secretaries in medical offices/hospitals are probably next in line to be considered on the basis of years of experience in this horrific delegation of prescribing authority. The nation and many states in the union have recognized the prescribing authority of these subordinates with an incredible list of drugs/formulary to be prescribed by them with or without physicians' permission. It is now known that majority of the cases that require supervision go unchecked, and many of these subordinates act independently. For instance, no physicians check CNP and PA diagnoses and prescribed drugs to make sure that everything is all right for the patients. Ironically, the pharmacists or drug specialists in most of the states are relegated to the background with little or no prescribing authority or are meant to fit the role of the "Seinfeld/Robot practicing pharmacist." Later chapters will reveal the fact that pharmacists received far greater knowledge/training in drugs than physicians.

Human experiences have shown that there are greater consequences each time we rob Peter to pay Paul, because we paid the price. Simple human etiquette tells us that we don't impoverish or enrich one profession at the expense of another because of tradition or ideology. The paramount interest in saving lives and unnecessary medical expenses/costs ought to be the utmost goal in using all available means and tools to strengthen pharmacists as drug specialists and enable pharmacy to overcome its deficiencies and stand on its feet through residence programs like most other specialties in the medical field. Instead, all effort was aimed at making pharmacy subservient to other branches of medicine. This subservience role can be traced to the following factors:

- Woman's job: In sharp contrast to reality, facts, and figures, the pharmacy profession has been seen by the male-dominated society as a woman's job because of its bondage. Many men considered the job of throwing pills from a big bottle to a smaller bottle as an undemanding and less strenuous job that requires little or no energy; as a result it is less deserving of men's attention in a male-dominated world. Like every other thing associated with women in the past, the profession is considered less important, low quality, and educationally inferior. This probably explains why a good number of traditional medical doctors get offended at a pharmacist's suggestion/advice about drug regimen. They treat pharmacists' suggestions/advice the same way they consider their patients' opinion, by rebuffing the good gesture; consequently, most pharmacists avoid the ego problem rather than go through any hassle. Like every other job, including medicine, that has opened its doors to women, pharmacy has a lot to show for it records and credits about gender balance. The Ya-chen study revealed how the number of women in the pharmacy profession rose from 5.8% in 1968-70 to greater than 25% in 1980 and 33% in 1994-96. The Fox study showed a greater proportion of women in pharmacy school: 51.9% of pharmacy students in 1982 and 30% of pharmacy graduates in 1976. In 1993, the American Association of Colleges of Pharmacy (AACP) revealed figures of pharmacy students' enrollment, which showed 63.2 percent (20,821) women and 36.8 percent (12,117) men (men are now reacting to pharmacy's strangulation, bondage, and greater encouragement of adding two more years to their educational career for a brighter future in other branches of medicine).

- Non-Western origin of the profession: This factor cannot be ruled out, because if pharmacy had originated from any of the Western nations, there would have been much interest in pursing its course to a logical end. Baghdad, Iraq, is the home origin of pharmacy in the world. The conception of pharmacy in the 9th century appears to be much easier than driving home its message and liberating the profession for the benefits of mankind 11 centuries later. Today, the origin of pharmacy is no longer the bone of contention, but rather the millions of lives and millions of health care dollars/costs the profession can save worldwide by being allowed to do what it does best.
- Drug treatment is one of the backbones of medicine, and relinquishing it to specialists is a problem for other branches of medicine. Generally human ailments have two major components: diagnosis and treatment. When people are sick they want to know the reason(s) why they are sick, and that in nutshell puts diagnosis at the forefront as one of the major backbones of medicine. Once diagnosed, the issue of treatment of a human ailment comes up as the second major backbone of medicine. Treatment of human ailments comes in various forms: drugs treatment, surgery, hypnotics (without drugs), body manipulations (chiropractics), acupuncture, and others. The most popular form of treatment involves the usage of drugs, and these drugs are either prescription drugs, over-the-counter (OTC) medications, homeopathic preparations, herbal products, or vitamins. Pharmacy is a general term for drugs/drug treatment. As noted earlier, medicine at the beginning of human history was an all-embracing term incorporating all branches of medicine including pharmacy until specialization and subsequent branches of medicine came into being. Specialization did not end general practice of medicine but witnessed the intermingling of specialization and general practice. Thus, the general practitioner retains their traditional role as patient gatekeeper attending to simple specialists' cases and referring complex cases to specialists. Specialists such as dentists, optometrists/ophthalmologists, surgeons, and others, on the other hand, seldom engage in general practice except when specialization is a by-product of general practice such as a hematologist. By and large, prescriptive authority is something many general practitioners and other branches of medicine view as one of the major backbones of medicine or their exclusive rights, and relinquishing or sharing it with specialists is tantamount to medical demise. They see it as an attempt to denigrate their personality,

professional image, and authority. Suffice it to say that this is not a new phenomenon to general practitioners, because they vehemently and passionately opposed the creation of all branches of medicine when specialization came into being at the beginning. Their bone of contention by then was that they would be left with nothing to do when you take away dentistry, optometry/ophthalmology, podiatry, dermatology, surgery, cardiology, and others from general practice. Today specialization is the rule and not the exception. Posterity has vindicated specialization and proven general practitioners wrong because they are still in practice alongside the specialists and their dignity remains intact. There is an element of truth in the fact that specialization might phase out general practice through a gradual process in the future, but this might not happen in our lifetime. The American Medical Association (AMA) is presently divided over the issue of granting prescribing authority to "nonphysicians," specifically pharmacists, the trained therapeutic physicians or therapeuticians/drug specialists. According to Joseph Breu's news brief in late 1999, the AMA House of Delegates interim meeting in San Diego finally took a stand against it. Sometime in June 1999, the AMA council submitted its report that stated "many nonphysicians had gained some level of prescribing authority in most states and that, given the current environment, the council felt there was little purpose in having the AMA establish additional policy opposing it" (*Drug Topics* January 2000).

- Complacency on the part of pharmacists and pharmacy organizations: Martin Luther King Jr. once said the reason why civil rights didn't come earlier was because of the salience of good people. In addition, it is worthwhile to say that no king in the course of human history has voluntarily relinquished his privileges even when such privileges involved enslavement of others for his benefit. If pharmacists do not want to be seen as 21st century slaves running around as medicine errand boys with their enormous drug knowledge that will be made redundant by Robot and other branches of medicine, they must be willing and ready to demand their rightful place in the medical community. Freedom is a right and not a privilege, and throughout the history of mankind it has never been given on a platter of gold. Relinquishing freedom on the part of the benefactor (king) and gaining freedom on the part of beneficiary (slave) entails a bitter struggle, however simple it may be. The mere realization of it by the beneficiary is something that brews bitter acrimony on both sides. However, the first phase of the struggle is self-realization of the bondage by the enslaved or slave. The second phase is characterized by demand for freedom by the slave, while the third or final phase is marked by a struggle crown with success or the granting of freedom at the end. For years, many pharmacists and pharmacy organizations have remained aloof and complacent of whatever position that was dictated to them by others. Some at one point or another saw the light and wanted to break loose of the shackles that bound them in bondage, but were brought down by other forces or hacked down by the powers that be. If a slave does not recognize his bondage and let those responsible for his condition know that his condition is unacceptable to him, and the king is happy with the status quo, then the situation remains perpetually unchallenged; as a result there will be no change.

In view of this, on August 30, 2004, Dr. Patrick Ojo organized a peaceful protest on Capitol Hill and in front of American Medical Association (AMA) building/office in Washington, D.C., to let the lawmakers and those responsible for pharmacists' professional bondage know that the pharmacists are aware of their condition and it is totally unacceptable to them. Dr. Patrick Ojo intends to continue with the campaign/event as an annual/regular occurring ritual until Americans and the whole world hear about the plight of pharmacy and do something about it.

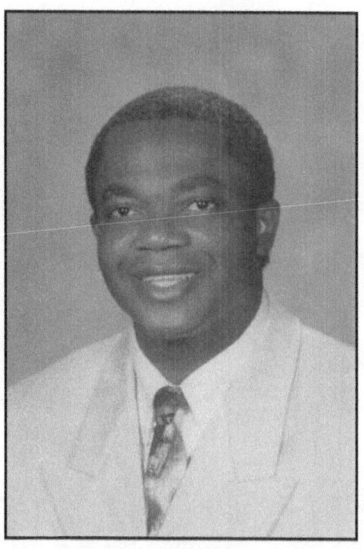

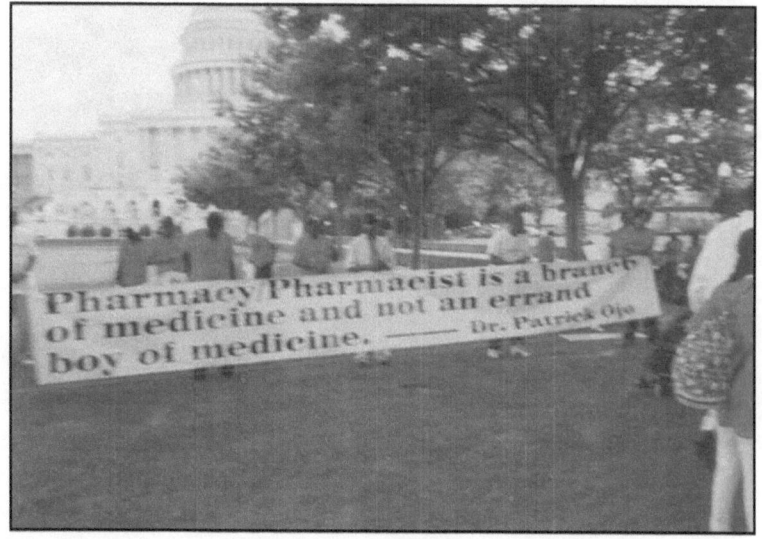

Above: Dr. Patrick Ojo at the beginning of the protest; *Below:* protesters with a banner in front of the Capitol Hill building, Washington, D.C.

Pharmacy was the first branch of medicine to be conceived as a specialty, yet the last to be liberated.
— Dr. Patrick Ojo

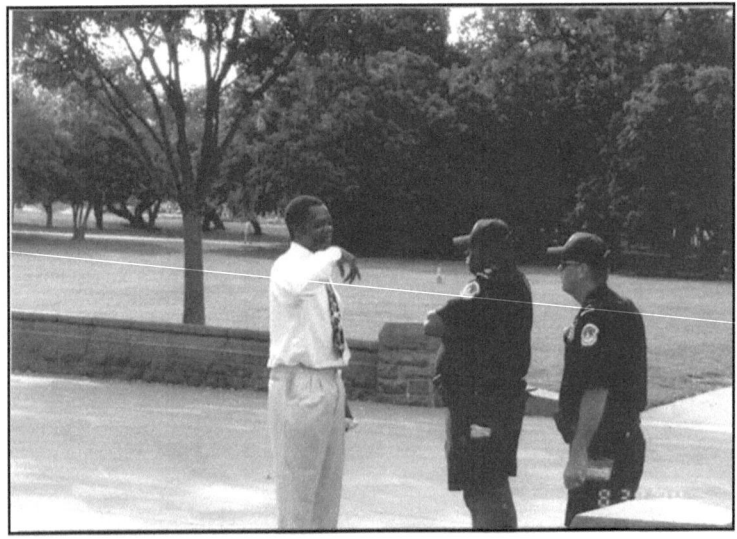

Top: One of the banners carried by a protester;
bottom: Ojo explaining to Capitol Hill police the nature of the protest, permission, and composition of the protest.

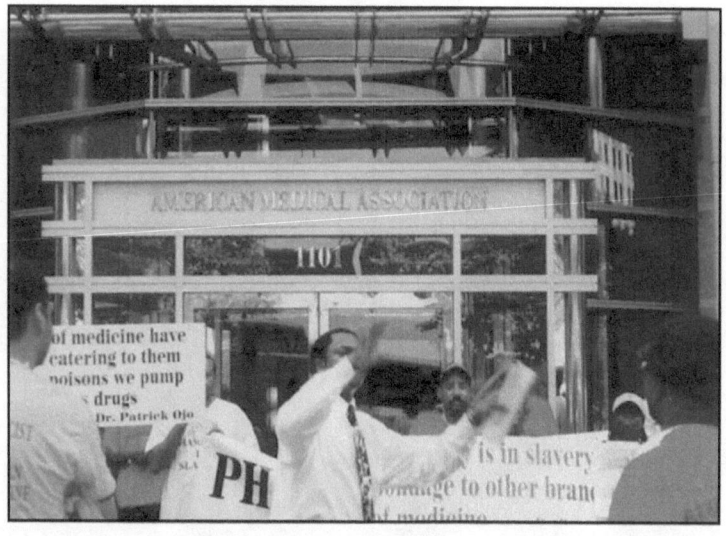

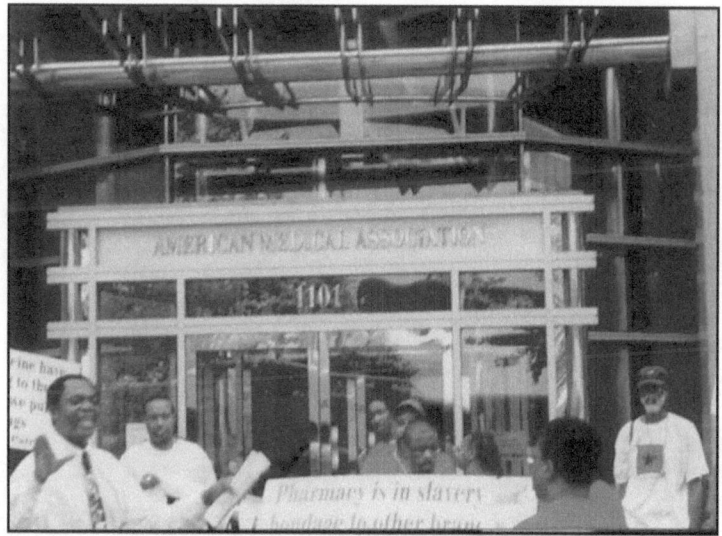

Top: Ojo trying to calm the protesters;
bottom: Ojo delivering a speech about the protest in front of the American Medical Association building, Washington, D.C.

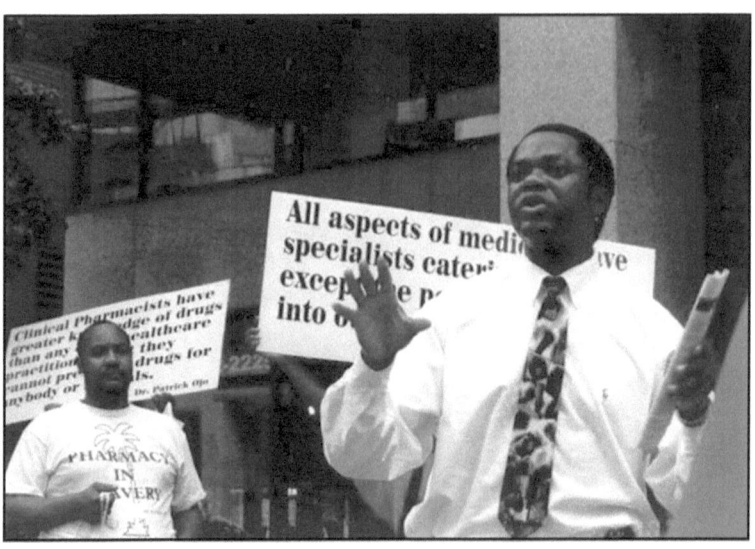

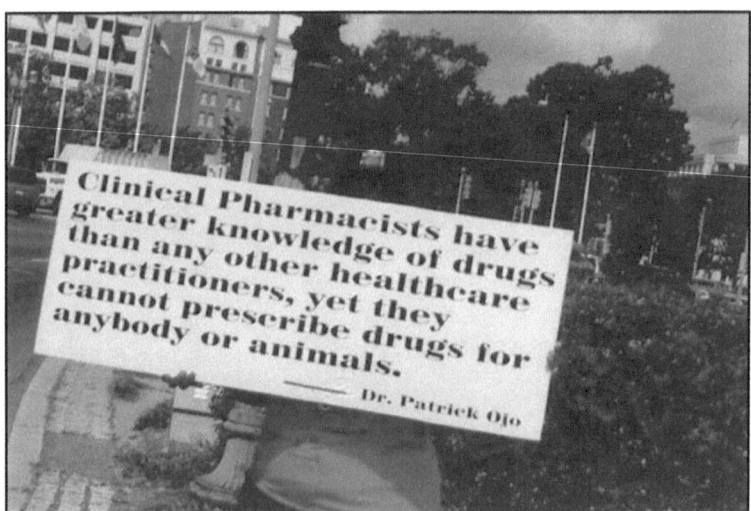

Top: Part of the speech;
bottom: some of the protesters with banners in Washington, D.C.

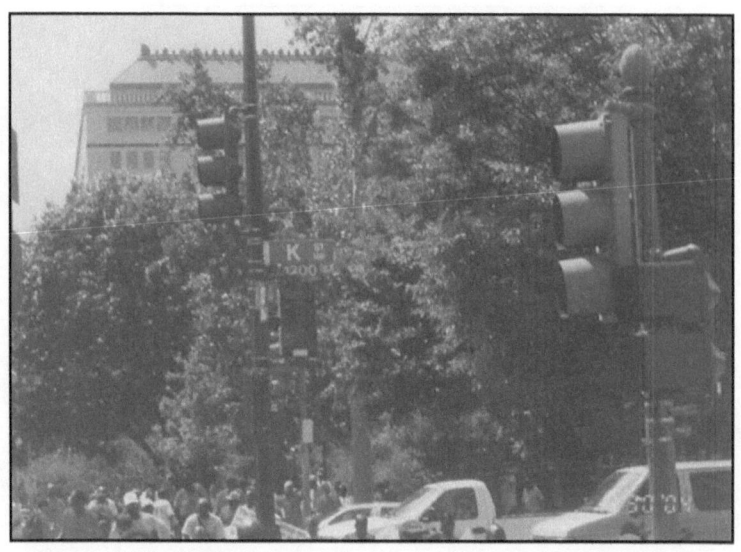

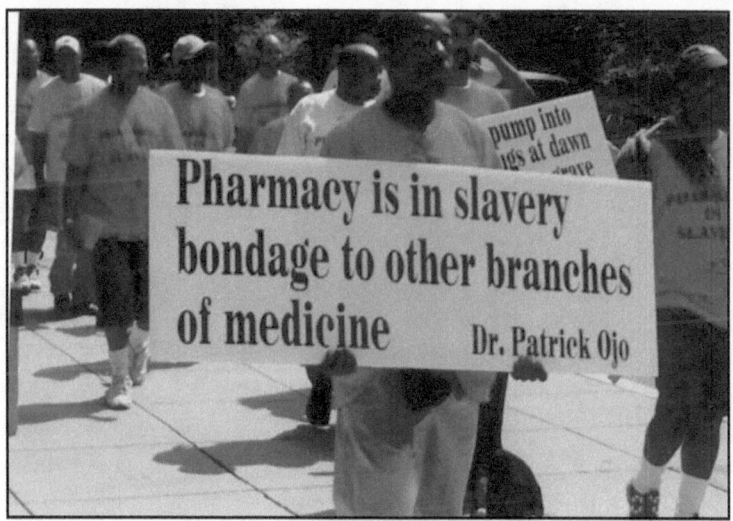

Top: Protesters on K Street,
bottom: one of the protesters with a banner in Washington, D.C.

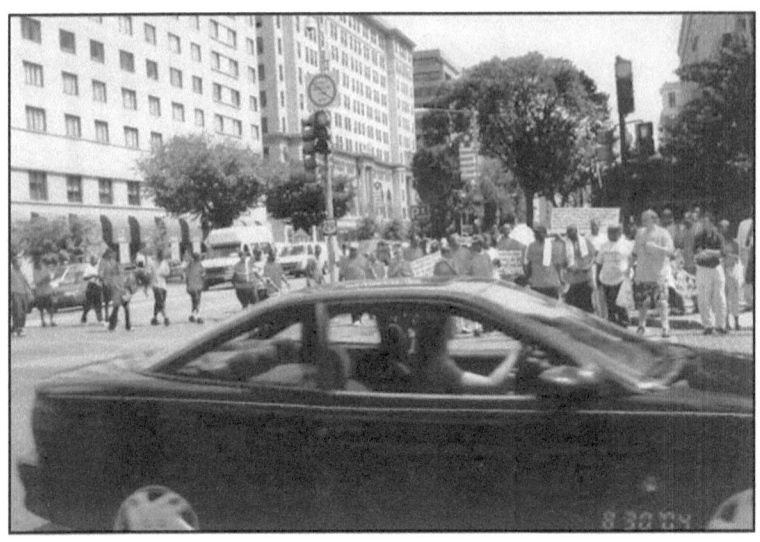

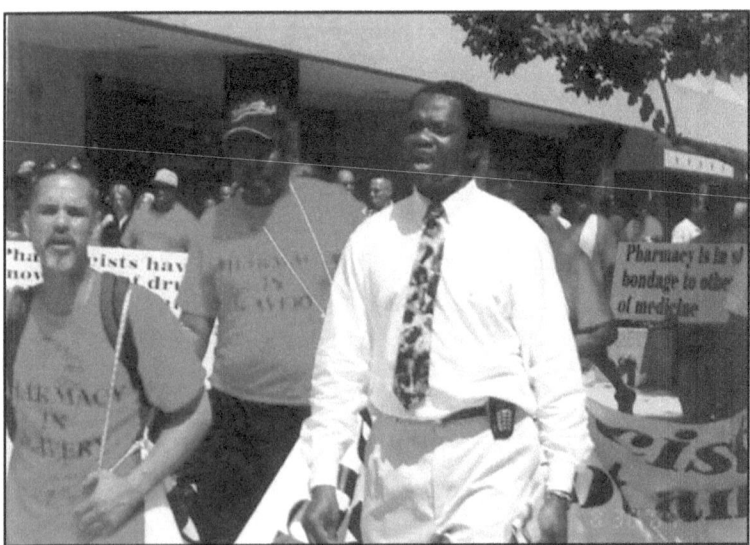

Top: Protesters crossing the Street;
bottom: a march through some of the streets in Washington, D.C.

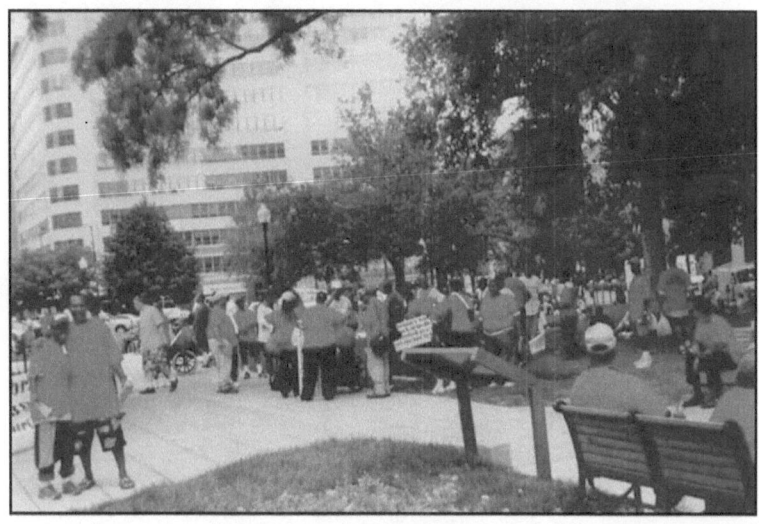

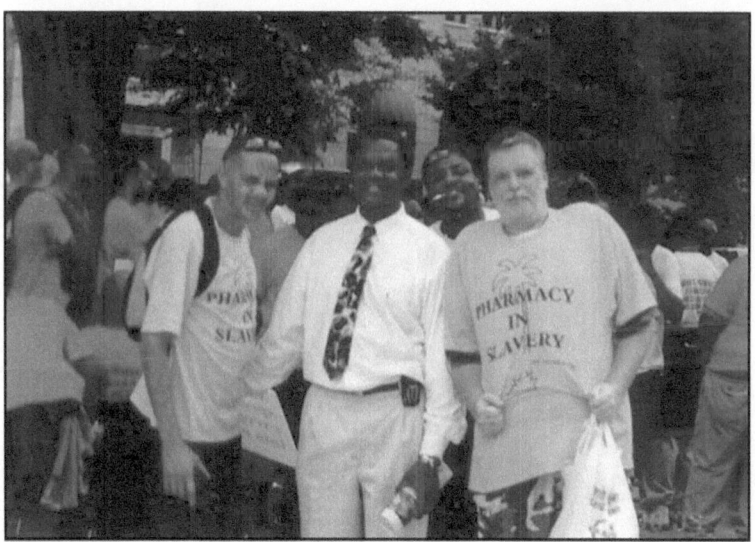

Protesters and Ojo in one of the national parks in Washington, D.C.

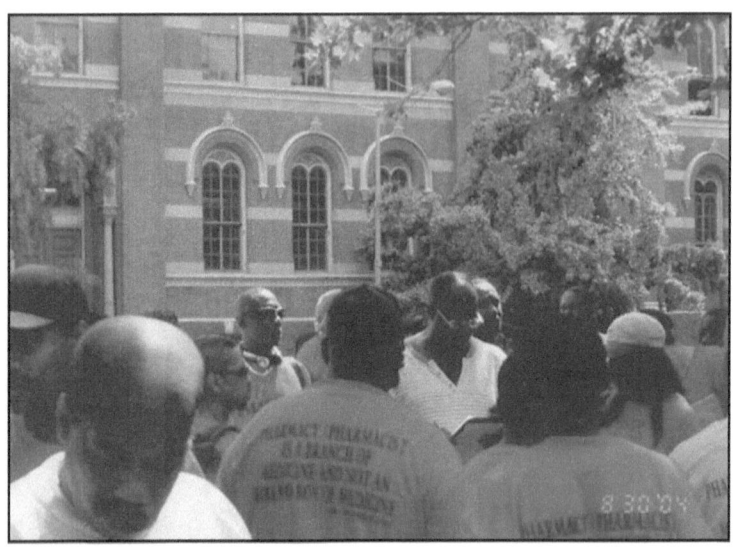

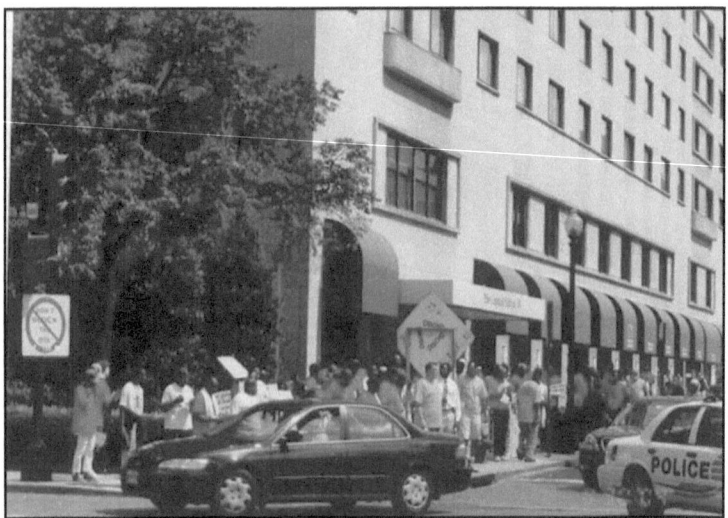

Protesters in one of the parks and on the street
with police control in Washington, D.C.

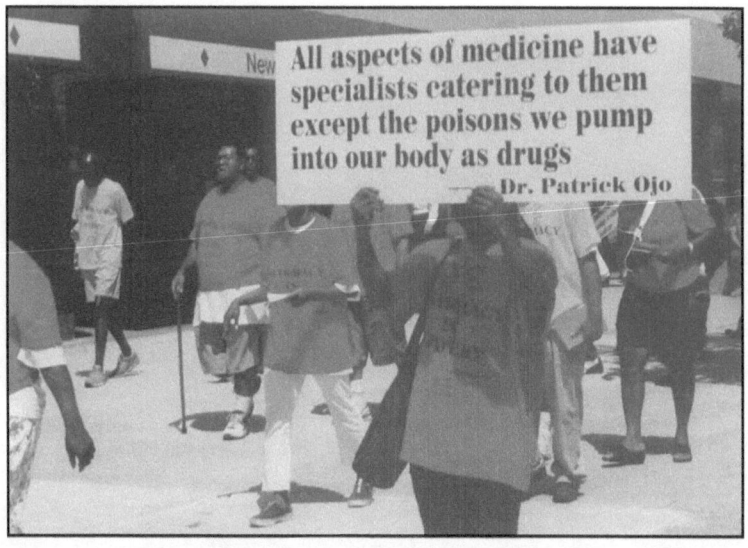

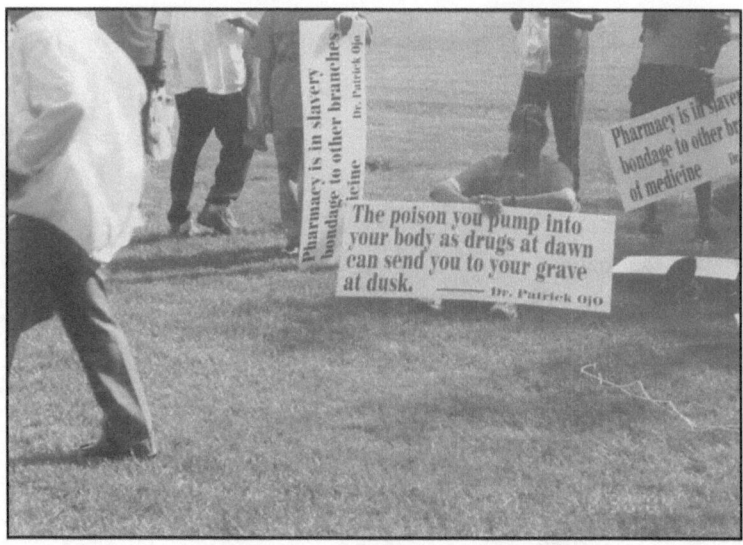

Top: One of the protesters with banners in Washington, D.C.
bottom: Protesters with banners in front of Capitol
Hill building, Washington, D.C.

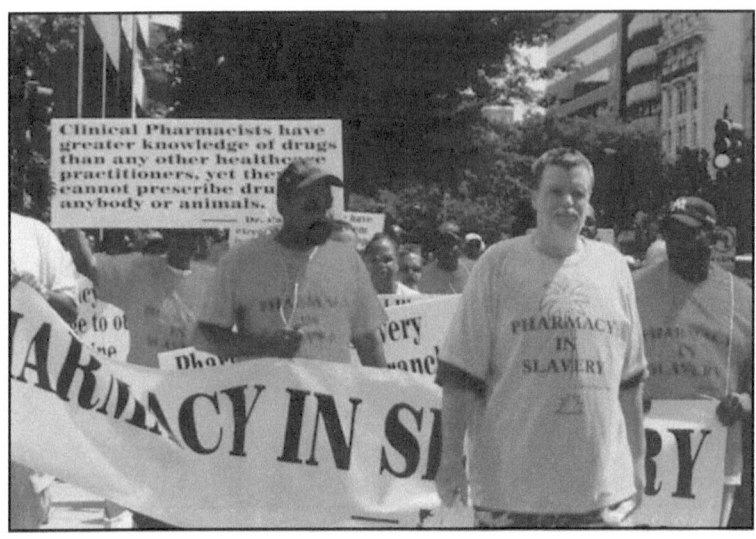

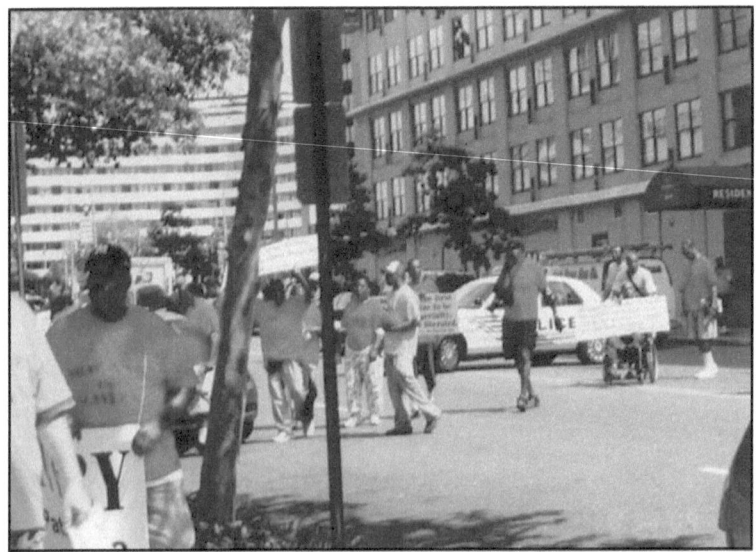

Protesters on the streets with police control in Washington, D.C.

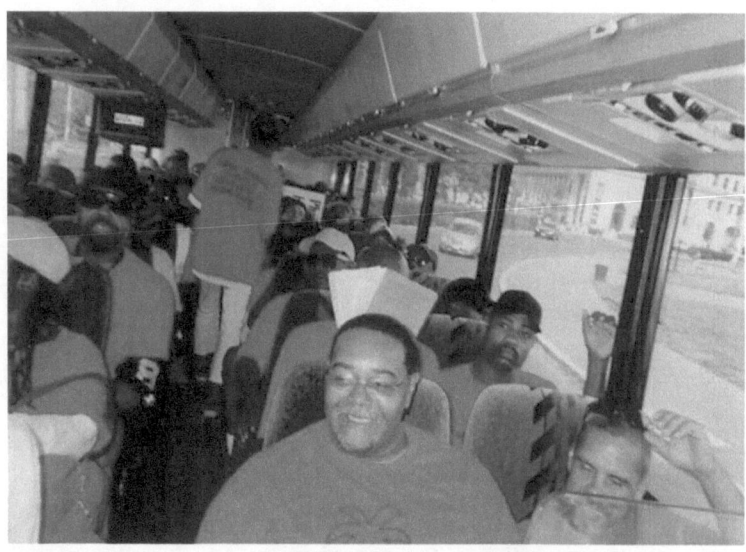

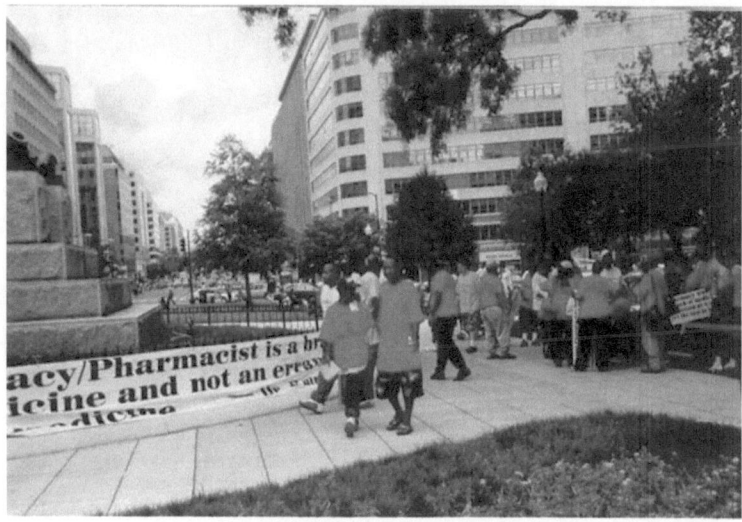

Top: Protesters being conveyed from Capitol Hill to American Medical Association building area in a luxurious bus;
bottom: protesters in one of the parks in Washington, D.C.

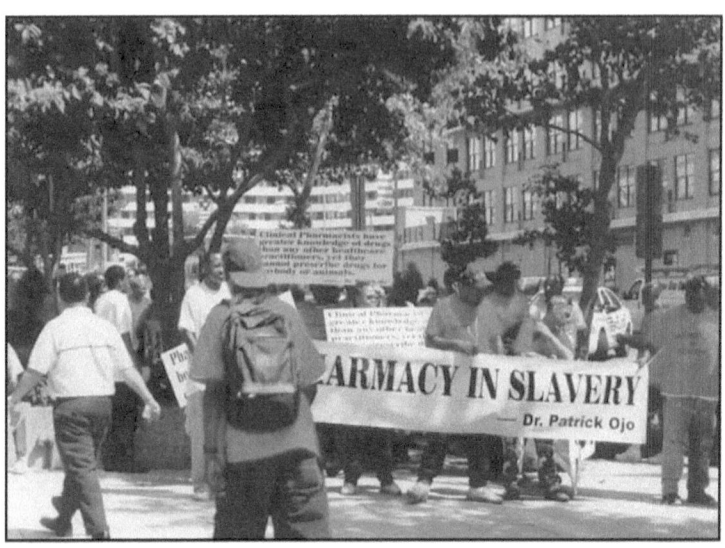

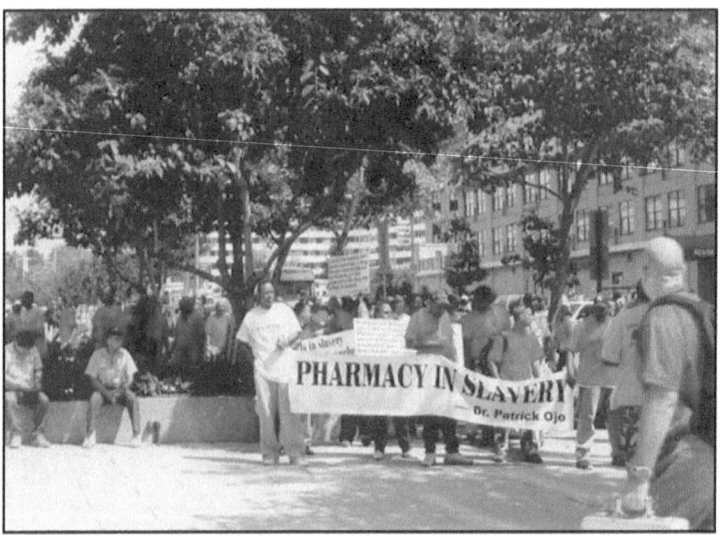

Protesters with banners and police control in one of the streets in Washington, D.C.

At the genesis of the 20th century, pharmacy was dominated by apothecary services, which in part deal with the act of preparing and selling of medicinal drugs. The pharmaceutical industries came into being and took over the role of preparing drugs, while physicians took over the choice of drugs for treatment. The American Pharmaceutical Association (AphA) code of ethics of 1922 to 1969 banned pharmacists from discussing "therapeutic effects or composition of prescriptions with patients." As noted earlier, at the beginning pharmacy was preoccupied with the need and desire to prepare and sell pure and unadulterated drugs to patrons as the first area of specialization in medicine. The acts of prescribing and the need to move close to patients' bedsides for drug monitoring did not receive adequate attention; hence, pharmacy's independence was up for grabs the first time. Pharmacy again failed to move close to patients' bedsides and recognize the fact that the act of prescribing is their right as trained therapeutic physicians or therapeuticians/drug specialists when pharmaceutical industries took over the traditional role of preparing and selling drugs the second time around. The pharmacists were not aggressive enough in demanding their rightful place in medicine; hence, their role was restricted to that of a dispensing function only. The AphA compounded the problem further by prohibiting them from discussing the therapeutic effects of drugs with patients through the enactment of the above code of ethics. These issues as well as others pacified pharmacists for years and prevented the profession from becoming an autonomous branch of medicine till today.

- The role of authority and Flexner's report in subjugating and mollifying pharmacy profession: The government normally functions for the benefit of the people and it is operated by elected officers who are responsive and accountable to the people in a democratic society. Traditional medical doctors have been very powerful, influential, and successful in lobbying elected officials for their own benefits even when such benefits are against the wishes of the people. The above factors, coupled with the enormous power and influence that the traditional medical doctors exerted on the society through elected officials, explains why the plight of pharmacy is comparable to other great struggles for equality in history. The pharmacy officials have exerted enormous strength in dealing with this fragmented issue, and the response has been very poor because of two things which are:
    a. Problem unidentified: They have not yet identified the problem; hence, it appears the organization is beating around the bush rather than tackling the problem in an aggressive manner. One can readily correlate their action to that of a slave who went to

the king to beg for freedom and the king responded by saying I have heard you. When the noise became too much, and the king was determined to mollify the slave, he responded by granting him permission to leave and return to the palace at a certain time during the weekend. The slave was instantly elated; as a result he forgot about every other aspect of his freedom until he discovered that pants without pockets is better than pants with pockets filled with holes. As long as the condition permits the satisfied king will continue to use delay tactics in mollifying the slave. The slave's instant, short-lived joy is exactly how pharmacy organizations and some pharmacists feel when they hear of the fact that they can now prescribe over-the-counter (OTC) and some minor prescription drugs under the supervision of a physician. There were no pharmacy organizations to fight for the profession's liberation the first time around; however, there were pharmacy organizations the second time around, but they failed to identified the problem, push for the profession's liberation, and fight for its autonomy especially during Flexner's move to create specialties in medicine at the beginning of the 20th century.

    b. Enough but insufficient effort: The pharmacy organizations' efforts appear grandiose to the officials, but it is the tip of an iceberg in comparison to the effort and impact of physicians' organizations (e.g., AMA) on elected officials and the society at large. This explains why they feel they are doing their best but the dividend (e.g., highly limited prescribing authority unlike others, even physicians' assistants or CNPs) is relatively small in comparison to the input. For instance, in 1951 while the AphA code of ethics was in place, the Durham-Humphrey Amendment Act of the FDC went further to enhance the code of ethics by restricting pharmacists' role to a dispensing function only.

- Flexner's report: In 1908, the Carnegie Foundation sponsored Abraham Flexner's study of all medical schools in United States and Canada. He published his report in 1910 and made numerous recommendations, as stated earlier. He failed to recognize pharmacy as one of the building blocks of medicine. Moreover, he preached the need for specialties in medicine even when he failed to realize that pharmacy was the first branch of medicine to be conceived out of the necessity for specialties in medicine. Flexner missed a golden opportunity to strengthen and transform pharmacy for good the same way he promoted and transformed other branches of medicine. Prior to Flexner's report and its adoption, the educational basis of medicine and its practice (all branches) was weak, informal, and unscientific in most cases. He came to redeem, redefine, and elevate medicine for good; hence, every aspect of medicine that did not captivate his attention was declared void or immaterial. Flexner's report thus laid the groundwork for the bastardization of pharmacy at a crucial time in history, the second time around for pharmacy as a profession. He humiliated pharmacy, pharmacy organizations, and a few other branches of medicine such as osteopathy. Osteopathy suffered the same fate as pharmacy under Flexner's report. Flexner recognized allopathic medicine as the only sanctioned form of medical practice based on scientific method. Osteopathic medicine according to *Webster's Dictionary* is "a branch of medicine that treats diseases by manipulating joints and bones of the body." Osteopathic medical practice is based on the assumption that diseases occur because of skeletal deformation and its effects on nerves, blood vessels, etc. That is to say that in its pure form, osteopathic medicine abhors the use of chemicals (drugs or prescription) in the treatment of diseases. It has a close resemblance to chiropractic medicine, which is the manipulation of spinal vertebrae in the treatment of diseases or human ailments. Flexner downgraded these branches of medicine because they were not scientifically based.

Unlike pharmacy, osteopathic medicine, after its initial humiliation by Flexner, revamped itself through the practitioners and its organization. Today, osteopathic medicine has branched entirely out of its main domain and incorporates everything about allopathic medicine. It is now difficult to differentiate osteopathic medicine from allopathic medicine. The dictionary meaning of osteopathic medicine has lost its value completely, and in the future there is reason to believe that osteopathic medicine and allopathic medicine will merge in the dictionary to reflect the present-day practice in medical schools and the society. Like every other branch of medicine, osteopathic medicine cannot be exonerated from taking advantage of pharmacy's bondage because it has nothing to do with drugs, which are the centerpiece of the pharmacy profession, yet everything about osteopathic medicine today is diagnosis and drug treatment. Flexner declared alternative medicine such as chiropractic, homeopathic, and acupuncture medicine null and void. They all went into hibernation, revamped themselves, and came back vigorously to attack the medical field, thereby redefining their positions within the medical community. Today, it is easier to go into any of these alternative medicine offices and see the practitioners being addressed as medical doctors even when the curricula of some of these alternative medical schools do not match what the clinical pharmacists go through in school training. Clinical pharmacists are Doctor of Pharmacy degree holders yet people hold them in contempt. This is peculiar not only to clinical pharmacists but also to almost all pharmacists irrespective of the number of doctorate degrees they have; even their closest allies (e.g., colleagues, other staffs, and colleges of pharmacy) want to hold them in contempt. They prefer to address him by his name rather than by his title in his office. This has nothing to do with aggrandizement but simple respect, which is the norm in all medical offices. For example, how many physicians are addressed by their names without their title in their offices throughout the country? Pharmacy is a medical office, and it is by no means different from other medical offices with its peculiar paraphernalia. Anesthesiologists are addressed as medical doctors, yet their specialty is an integral part of pharmacy.

It is astonishing to see how anesthesiology, the study of anesthetics, became a branch of medicine while pharmacy, the parent body, remained after eleven centuries a fetus in the womb of medicine or in bondage with other branches of medicine. Anesthetics are an infinitesimal part of pharmacy, but how did it become an independent branch of medicine? This enigmatizing question can only be answered by putting together the pieces of the puzzle in a simple and complex manner. The simple part of the puzzle is the fact that the surgeons demanded its creation. As reflected in later chapters, surgery was one of the first branches of medicine that took advantage of Flexner's report and recommendations. Flexner's report in 1910 created specialty and/or specialization in medicine. The American College of Surgeons was subsequently founded in 1913, and its board was created in January 1937 as a result of the recommendations. Shortly after the creation of the American Board of Surgery, the surgeons began to agitate for the creation of the American Board of Anesthesiology through the American Medical Association. The struggle paid off with the creation of the American Board of Anesthesiology as an affiliation of the American Board of Surgery in June 1937 and as an autonomous, separate body in 1941. The complex part of the puzzle then arose: why did the surgeons demand the creation of anesthesiology as a branch of medicine when they, like the rest of their colleagues, were vehemently opposed to the uplift of anesthetic's parent, pharmacy, as a branch of medicine? One can reasonably question the rationale by making the following deductions:

— Is the surgeons' medical training different from the rest?
— Is the surgeons' drug knowledge inferior or different from the rest?
— Are the surgeons less competent as therapeuticians in terms of drug treatment than the other branches of medicine?

— Are the surgeons telling the world that they are not smart enough to handle drug treatment?
— Is the world correct to assume that surgeons are not smart enough to offer drug treatment to their patients?

The answer to these questions will reveal a lot about the surgeons' intention and goodwill message to the medical field. As far as smartness is concerned, surgeons are some of the smartest people on the surface of the Earth. They are in the top echelons of medical intelligence, because each time the surgeon performs surgery with the human life in his palm, he plays God. Smartness and intelligence are therefore out of the way. The issue of difference in training can best be answered by using the modus operandi of the U.S. (citadel and home origin of specialization) standard of medical training. In the United States, surgeons go through medical training similar to other branches of medicine until they specialize. Specialization in medical schools varies; however, most students go through all available branches (specialties) in medical school of their choice in a similar manner during clinical rotations, internship, and residence. They exploit their area of interest (specialty) and concentrate on it at the latter part of their training (internship or residence). In some cases, students go through all available branches in the medical school of their choice in a similar manner up till clinical rotations or internship, and then they specialize during residence. In a nutshell, all medical students have similar medical training especially in terms of drug knowledge until they specialize. They go through same pre-clinical didactic class work that laid the foundation for later academic development in medical school. As specialization begins to take control at the latter part of the training, students devote more and more attention, expertise, and knowledge in exploring their area of interest (specialty), thereby neglecting other areas. Licensure and daily practice enhance further a medical practitioner's skills in his area of specialization and the end result is such that with time he drifts into oblivion in terms of other branches of medicine. Specialization thus makes medical practitioners forget everything they learn from other branches of medicine in medical school and concentrate their efforts on their area of specialization, thereby leaving the task of fulfilling these other branches of medicine to the respective specialists. This is a normal human reaction: you perfect your skills in whatever you do every day and forget about whatever you don't do every day, so medical practitioners are no exception.

Consequently, specialty makes surgeons concentrate on human or animal operations in neglect of other branches of medicine. Human or animal operation in itself is a complex phenomenon that demands the utmost attention with the highest degree of human skill/perfection. As noted earlier, each time a surgeon performs surgery, he or she plays God and the slightest mistake or distraction could result in loss of human or animal life. Be that as it may, every operation puts human life in the palm of the surgeon, and knowing full well that the utmost care/precaution is required for the operation, the least thing the surgeon wants to be bothered about is drug mechanism of action, knowledge, and/or intricacy resulting from drug administration. Drug administration during a surgery/operation is a complex issue that demands specialty because of numerous factors and the intricacy involved. Some of these factors are:

— Will the patient be sedated (sleep or unconscious) on time for the surgery to proceed? (Onset of anesthesia action.)
— Will the patient wake up (regain consciousness) during the surgery? (Duration of anesthesia action.)
— Will the patient feel some degree of pain during surgery?
— Will the patient's blood flow, heart rate, blood pressure, respiratory rate, kidney function, and others be normal during and after the operation?
— Will the patient suffer from dizziness, fever, headache, seizure, nausea, vomiting, stomach cramps, cough, hiccups, apnea (breathing problem), twitching (muscle problem), and others after surgery?
— What is the right drug (anesthetic), dose, frequency, distribution rate, plasma protein binding, clearance, metabolic rate, half-life, elimination rate, and other characteristics?
— Will a smaller dosage result in subtherapeutic, or over-dosage (toxicity) result in bradycardia (slow heart rate), hypotension (low blood pressure), cardiovascular collapse, tachycardia (fast heart rate), arrhythmia, or other complications or death?

All these issues and others made the surgeons demand for anesthetics as a branch of medicine. Moreover, surgeons' skills and perfection in human operations made them relegate drug treatment/knowledge/therapy and other branches of medicine to the background, thereby forgetting them. The goodwill message from the surgeon is that we realize the importance of specialization in medicine and Flexner's having created the opportunity for us to excel through specialization; it is therefore incumbent upon us to extend the goodwill gesture to other branches of medicine such as anesthetics. Anesthetics are agents (drugs) used to reduce or abolish feeling/sensation in certain parts of the body (local anesthetic, e.g., lidocaine, cocaine, etc.) or in the whole body (general anesthetic, e.g., versed, propofol, etc.). Anesthetics, like many other drugs, are part of pharmacy and they are taught in various schools of pharmacy. Students' curriculum and studies in schools of pharmacy do not start and end with drugs. There are many other aspects of pharmacy such as pharmacokinetics, pharmaceutical statistics, medicinal chemistry, pathophysiology, microbiology, physical pharmacy, pharmacoeconomics, pharmacy calculations, biochemistry, and others that lay the groundwork for drug knowledge. Drug knowledge constitutes the bulk of disease-state management and pharmacy schools' curriculum.

One can readily assess the degree of importance of anesthetics in pharmacy by looking at various pharmacy books that deal with drugs only. Some of these books are: *The Pharmacological Basis of Therapeutics* by Goodman and Gilman allocates about 2% of the entire book to anesthetics; *Pharmacotherapy: A Pathophysiologic Approach* by Dipiro et al. allocates less than 1%; and *Drug Facts and Comparisons*, a commonly used book by many pharmacies (hospital, institutional, community, etc.) and the otherwise tagged pharmacy dictionary or Bible before the advent of clinical pharmacology on the Internet, devoted about 1% to anesthetics. As of 2003, *Drugs Facts and Comparisons* contains fourteen major headings, and out of this, anesthetics falls under central nervous system (CNS) drugs. CNS drugs comprises of CNS Stimulants; Analgesics; Anti-Emetic/Anti-Vertigo Agents; Anti-Anxiety Agents; Antidepressants; Anti-Psychotic Agents; Cholinesterase Inhibitors; Sedatives and Hypnotics—Non-Barbiturate and Barbiturate, General and Local Anesthetics, Anticonvulsants, Muscle Relaxants; Adjuncts to Anesthesia; Skeletal Muscle Relaxants; Anti-Parkinson's Agents; Adenosine Phosphate; Cholinergic Muscle Relaxants; Anti-Alcohol; Smoking Deterrents; Riluzole; and Physical Adjuncts. In some pharmacy textbooks, anesthetics are treated under the hypnotics and sedatives class of drugs, making it a category of drugs under a class that is in turn under a heading.

The 14 major headings in *Drugs Facts and Comparisons* are Nutrients and Nutritional Agents (e.g., TPN, Vitamins); Hematological, Endocrine, and Metabolic Agents; Cardiovascular, Renal, and Genitourinary Agents; Respiratory Agents; Central Nervous System Agents; Biological and Immunologic Agents; Dermatological, Ophthalmic, and Otic Agents; Antineoplastic (cancer) Agents; and Diagnostic Aids such as the CNS drugs. Other headings equally encompass numerous classes of drugs; for example, cardiovascular drugs contains the following classes of drugs: Inotropic Agents, Antiarrhythmic Agents, Calcium Channel Blocking Agents, Vasodilators, Antiadrenergics/Sympatholytics, Renin Angiotensin System Antagonists, Antihypertensive Combinations, Agents for Pheochromocytoma, Agents for Hypertensive Emergencies, Antihyperlipidemic Agents, Vasopressors Used in Shock, Cardioplegic Solutions, Agents for Patent Ductus Arteriousus, and Sclerousing Agents. Each class of drugs contains numerous categories, combinations of drugs, and individual drugs that are expanding every day with new drugs, recent discoveries, and approval by various government agencies (such as the Federal Drugs Administration (FDA) in the U.S.) throughout the world. It is important to note that each category or subcategory of drugs is worthy of a textbook in pharmacy.

Many will argue that ophthalmic and dermatological agents like anesthetics and others are purely drug treatment, which fall under pharmacy and pharmacists as drug experts or trained therapeuticians. This is correct perception except that unlike anesthesiology, ophthalmology and dermatology involve diagnosis and treatment. In anesthesiology, the surgeons make the diagnosis for surgery/operation, and once that has been done, then anesthesiology comes into play in most cases. This case example typifies how the clinical pharmacist is supposed to operate in relation to other branches of medicine, because drug treatment is to pharmacist as diagnosis is to other branches of medicine. Moreover, medicine in practice involves cross-carpeting; thus, the existence of pediatricians has not stopped family practice, internal medicine, and other physicians from taking care of children. However, when children's ailments become complex they are referred to pediatrician, and that is how it is supposed to be with clinical pharmacists and drug treatment.

Later chapters will reveal that the pharmacy curriculum does not operate in isolation without diagnosis but incorporates it as an integral part, the same way other branches of medicine incorporate drug treatments as an integral part of their studies. How is it that osteopathic physicians, chiropractors, surgeons for anesthesiologists, and others were able to fight for their liberation and there was nobody to identify the problem and fight for pharmacy liberation? Are people right to say that pharmacy stood aside, hands akimbo, waiting for others to fight for him, run his course, and liberate his ingenuity? At any rate, pharmacy has come a long way (11 centuries), and no matter what we do to trivialize the profession, restricting pharmacist's role to a dispensing function only and asking other branches of medicine to prescribe drugs while pharmacists stand aside can only be likened to the following scenarios:

— asking a general practitioner to perform surgery while the surgeon supplies surgical equipment and watches the operation (some will probably say that a GP would do a better job...).
— asking the general practitioner to perform midwifery functions or attend to women's genital/reproductive problems while the gynecologists/obstetricians supply equipment and watch;
— asking the general practitioner to perform eye surgery or treatment while the ophthalmologist/optometrist supplies equipment and watches;

— asking the pharmacist to diagnose complex disease cases while the general practitioner prescribes medication for treatment;
— asking the general practitioner to perform dental surgery or treatment while the dentists supply equipment and watch;
— asking the general practitioner to attend to neurological problems while the neurologist or psychiatrist watches patients for behavioral problems;
— asking the general practitioner to attend to heart problems while the cardiologist watches patients' heart performance (strength);
— asking the general practitioner to attend to debilitating children's health problems/disease while the pediatrician baby-sits and medicates the children;
— and many other, similar situations.

CHAPTER TWO

HISTORY OF THE VARIOUS BRANCHES OF MEDICINE

Medicine began with the dawn of humanity, and so did the various branches of medicine. However, the various branches of medicine were imbedded in one practice; thus, all practitioners were expected to play God and heal human ailments. The practitioners had no standardized forms of practice and education at the beginning, so they acquired their knowledge and technical know-how from old, experienced practitioners through apprenticeships. This form of medical practice prevailed throughout history including the era of Hippocrates of Cos (father of medicine—ca. 460 to 377 BC) until human advancement, technological developments, and growth in knowledge about the human body forced mankind to adopt specialties in medicine for good. Hippocrates stressed the need for medicine to be scientifically based through rationalized study and clinical observation of the human body and its functions. In response to Hippocrates's preaching, scientific study and clinical observations produced an enormous body of knowledge that was just too much for any human being to comprehend and make wise decisions about clinical practice. Specialization became inevitable, and the dawn of a new era in medicine unveiled itself. Initially, specialization was a strange phenomenon; hence, its popularity occurred through a gradual process. The various branches of medicine therefore gained their degree of freedom and autonomy through specialization at different times in human history.

The United States of America has become the pace setter for mankind in numerous human developments, and medicine is no exception. Most specialties in practice today sprang up in the U.S., and nearly all branches of medicine are in existence in the country. Few specialties had their roots in other parts of the world even before the American War of Independence in 1776. The American Medical Association was formed in 1846 and it became a nationalized body of state medical societies in 1901.[17] Certain factors such as practitioners'/pioneers' vision, desire, quest, agitation, determination, and aggressiveness play a key role in the initiation, recognition, and maturity of all specialties in medicine. At the beginning of the millennium, the year 2000, the following specialties were in existence in U.S. according to the official ABMS Directory of Board Certified Medical Specialties and other major sources: allergy and immunology, anesthesiology, dentistry, dermatology, emergency medicine, family practice, internal medicine, genetics, psychiatry and neurology, nuclear medicine, obstetrics and gynecology, ophthalmology, optometry, orthopedic, otolaryngology, pathology, pediatrics, physical medicine and rehabilitation, plastic surgery, radiology, preventive medicine, surgery, urology, and veterinary medicine.

A shift towards specialties in medicine began in the early 20th century, and it was formalized with the institutionalization of various boards in the U.S. The army, as well as the introduction of Medicare in 1965, played a prominent role in the development of specialties in medicine. Specific developments that were meant to enhance strategy, military capabilities, war victories, and minimize casualties and damages from war in the U.S. military spread to other spheres of human endeavor and dominated daily life activities. Some of these developments include Internet services and improvement of medical specialties. The U.S. surgeon general's office reported that the army's general hospital treated World War I casualties with specialists even though these specialists were of little or no value to the war. In the fall and winter of 1944, about 180,000 war casualties returned to the U.S. from World War II and the need to plan for the treatment of these soldiers heralded a breakthrough in the advancement of contemporary medical specialty. There were about 45,000 commissioned physicians and 65 to 70 army general hospitals in the country during World War II. The number of available board-certified specialists was relatively small; hence, the army decided to use various incentives such as higher rank, preferred assignments, and short duration of training (90days) for general practitioners to meet the growing need of psychiatrists, and more pay for commissioned specialists to attract specialists. The short duration of training is said to have done greater harm than good because the so-called "90-day wonder" psychiatrists promoted the early discharge of 750,000 draftees and the release of 1.5 million draft-eligible men who were diagnosed with supposed psychiatric disorders or classified as being mentally/emotionally unfit. In 1943, the surgeon general's office opened six amputation centers; five centers for thoracic and plastic surgery each; twelve neurosurgery centers; two centers for blind, deaf, and vascular surgery each; and various medicine and neuropsychiatry centers. All these centers were staffed with specialists, and they continued to grow until the end of the war.[1,2]

In 1944, the U.S. Congress passed the G.I. bill in anticipation of the end of World War II. The bill made provisions for school fees and personal expenses for any military personnel (soldiers and officers) who chose to further their education/training in civilian professions after an honorable discharge. The incentives provided for specialists within the army had a big impact on the soldiers and officers, many of whom decided to avail themselves of the G.I. bill's opportunity and train in specialized medical care. Specialization in medicine, the future of medical practice, was thus not only encouraged by the shrinkage of the army's specialty hospitals and subsequent release of the army medical specialists to civilian practice life, but also by the G.I. bill that enhanced specialization at the end of the war in August 1945. In addition, the 1965 introduction of Medicare to the nation's health care system led to another wave of increased specialization in the medical field within the country. Medicare provided for liberal funding of graduate programs in medical education and a lot of medical students/practicing physicians availed themselves of the opportunity of upgrading their knowledge and professional skills to become specialists. Besides the nation's desire to promote specialization, all branches of medicine went through series of humiliations, struggles, and exaltations, so pharmacy is no exception to the rule. A brief discussion of the origin and nature of the various specialties listed above would enable us to comprehend the true meaning of each specialty.

Allergy and Immunology

Allergy and immunology is a branch of medicine that deals with the diagnosis and treatment of immune system disorders. There is no much information about the history of this medical specialty; however, its conception and formation appears to be related to the crucial role played by allergy/immunology or antigen-antibody in the diagnosis, treatment, and prevention of anaphylaxis, dermatitis, rhinitis, asthma, hypersensitivity pneumonitis, urticaria, angioedema, autoimmune diseases, adverse drug reactions, gene replacement therapy, bone marrow transplants, hereditary or acquired host resistance defects, and organ transplants. Health care practitioners probably realized this area was crucial in the '60s and began to campaign for the specialty. Their agitation paid off with the establishment of the American Board of Allergy and Immunology (ABAI) as conjoint of the boards of the

American Board of Pediatrics (ABP) and ABAI in 1971. ABAI is one of the 24 board members of the American Board of Medical Specialties and it was sponsored by the American Medical Association (AMA), the Clinical Immunology Society (CIS), the American Academy of Allergy, Asthma, and Immunology (AAAAI), the American Academy of Pediatrics (AAP), and the American College of Allergy, Asthma, and Immunology (ACAAI). Specialists in this field are physicians who have successfully passed the American Board of Internal Medicine or the American Board of Pediatrics certification examination before going through ABAI certification process.[3]

ANESTHESIOLOGY

Anesthesiology is a branch of medicine that deals with relief of pain and stabilization of a patient's condition during and/or soon after surgery, obstetrics, and diagnostic processes. The use of surgery to alleviate human suffering, ailments, and external organ (e.g., skin) damage has been documented since the time of Caius Celsus (25 BC–AD 50). Serafeddin Sebuncuoglu (AD 1385–1468) is, however, credited as the pioneer of all surgical endeavors/fields. Surgery and pain are twin sisters, and the endurance of pain during surgery is a dreadful experience for all patients; hence, no one in his right mind wants to go through surgery a second time because of pain. Pain, therefore, was a major obstacle to surgery, and surgeons realized it. They knew that if any meaningful impact was to be made with successful surgeries something must be done about pain. The discovery of ether anesthesia and its use in the first operation in 1846 by Dr. J. C. Warren in the now-popular Ether Dome or hospital dome at Massachusetts General Hospital helped to resolve this medical dilemma. Other anesthetics were discovered, and surgical pain soon became a manageable condition with little or no sensational feelings. The close relationship that existed between surgery and pain transformed into a professional propinquity between surgery and anesthetics. As noted earlier, shortly after the establishment of the American Board of Surgery on January 9, 1937, the surgeons' agitation led to the formation of a committee consisting of the American Medical Association (surgical section), the American Society of Anesthetists, and the American Society of Regional Anesthesia. The committee was charged with the responsibility of forming an organization whose purpose was to certify physicians in the field of anesthesiology. At the end of the day, the American Board of Anesthesiology (ABA) was created as an affiliation of the American Board of Surgery on June 2, 1937. The American Board of Medical Specialties advisory committee approved the ABA as a separate body in 1941. There are subspecialties within the American

Board of Anesthesiology and two of them are the Society of Critical Care Medicine, which requested recognition of its members/practitioners from the ABA in 1977, and their request was granted on March 21, 1985; and pain management, which was requested by the ABA in 1989 from the ABMS and was approved in 1991. Physicians certified in these areas are free to practice the subspecialties.[3,4,5]

DENTISTRY

Dentistry is a branch of medicine that deals with diagnosis and treatment of tooth, gum, and other oral diseases. Like pharmacy, dentistry can be described as the downtrodden and bastardized branch of medicine because it went through centuries of humiliations, derogatory remarks, denigration, professional floundering, and pandering to define its position in the medical field. Today, despite its indomitable functions, grandiose evolution, remarkable contributions to human welfare/health, enormous progress, indispensable role, and awesome contribution to medicine, dentistry is yet to be recognized as a medical specialty by the American Board of Medical Specialties.[3] McCauley traced dentistry problems to the system of "deep-rooted cultural tradition that relegated surgeons and those engaged in the dental art to a class deemed socially, intellectually, and economically inferior to the physicians."[6] Dental ailments have been part of human health problems right from the dawn of human history, and it was treated much like an integral part of surgery for many years until the early 17th century. The dental part of surgery focuses on tooth extraction, cautery, fumigation, and bloodletting as an art that was elevated by Ambroise Pare, a master barber-surgeon of the French Army and a man commonly referred to as the foster father of dental surgery. Around the mid-16th century, surgeon Pare advanced dentistry through prosthetic replacement, jaw fracture reduction, toothache amelioration, palatal obturation, irregular dentition remedy, and occlusal correction. Fauchard, a French naval surgeon and dental practitioner, is credited as the founder of modern dentistry. He wrote two books that detailed his dental experience and the dental knowledge of his predecessor, thereby dismantling the barrier to dental evolution and advancement. In 1614, a regulatory decree that defined dentistry as a profession by examination was passed for the first time in history in France. Fauchard's book was translated into German in 1733, and most of his successful work was attributed to the invention of the printing press by Gutenberg in 1436. The printing press helped to catalyze society's development and promote dentistry like other professions. Dentistry thus became a separate profession capable of existing on its own feet in the 19th century.

Surgery and medicine went through some ups and downs at various times in history. There were times the profession fell in wrong hands such as street hawkers, quacks, and impostors. This type of situation caused Germany to demand the certification of its Zahnbrecher (tooth-breaker) through *collegium medicum* examination in Berlin in 1685 ("Great Elector edict"); France to ban barbers from practicing surgery in 1743; and Prussia similarly to demand certification for its Zahnarzt (dentist) under the rule of William I in 1725. These attempts were aimed at controlling surgery and dentistry in Europe during the 18th century. Dentistry gradually moved from the streets to the health professional's office or patient's residence, and by 1800 there were 34 registered surgeon dentists in Paris (100 in 1825) and 20 "tooth surgeons" (all foreigners) in Russia. Around the mid 18th century, mass immigration to the United States (the New World) from Europe, especially England and France, witnessed the arrival of some professionals such the barber-surgeons, tooth drawers, tooth operators, and surgeon-dentists. The first dentist to practice in New York was surgeon-dentist Robert Woofendale, who came from London in 1766. Dentistry problems relegated the profession to the background until the 16th century when human advancement and development in surgery as well as medicine caused a resurgence of dentistry from a trade to a medical specialty in Europe in the next two centuries. This phenomenon (birth and resurgence) laid the groundwork for the widespread growth of dentistry in America in the 19th century. The introduction of better pain control, esthetics, functional prostheses, new materials, and techniques invented between the 1700s and the 1900s enabled dentists to perform miracles in both tooth retention and restoration.[7] The profession began to gather momentum with better education and the coming of more dentists to the U.S. In June 1805, the first gesture to recognize dentistry in America took place during the annual convention of the medical and chirurgical faculty of the state of Maryland. The convention participants amended their by-laws by granting licenses to dentists and oculists to practice their respective branches through the Board of Examiners. Horace H. Hayden was the first dentist to receive such a license in 1810. Others such as Chapin Harris, Solyman Brown, and Eleazar Parmly received their licenses and proceeded to form the first short-lived dentist organization, the Society of Surgeon Dentists of the city and state of New York, in December 1834 in U.S. The society was disbanded in 1839 because of "amalgam war"; however, members continued to unite against impostors and quackery through periodic publications in U.S. medical and surgical journals at first; later such publications resulted in the formation of a dental journal, *American Journal of Dental Science*, in 1839. The practicing dentists later rallied around dentistry and transformed it from a system of untutored/untrained practitioners to that of an organized institution of dental education. Some of these practicing dentists are pioneers like Hayden and Harris, who proceeded to create the first dental school, the Baltimore College of Dental Surgery, which was chartered by the governor of Maryland's signature on March 6, 1840. The school was originally founded with four departments: dental physiology and pathology, anatomy and physiology, practical dentistry and special pathology, and therapeutics. Encouraged by the creation of the first dental school, Horace Hayden pushed forward the idea of forming a national body, the National Association of Dental Surgeons, by convening 15 dentists from various parts of the country in New York in August 1840. Hayden served as the first president of the association, the world's first dentist association, which lasted for 16 years.[6]

Dermatology

Dermatology is a branch of medicine that deals with the diagnosis and treatment of skin disorders, sexually transmitted diseases, hair, nails, mouth, and external parts of the genital organs. Cutaneous diseases have affected man right from the dawn of history, but the desire to have specialized physicians cater to man's dermatological needs grew in the 1920s probably because of the devastating effects of syphilis. Aspiring dermatologists are expected to posses experience, sufficient training, adequate knowledge, and technical know-how in handling dermatological immunology. The pioneers of dermatology were members of the American Dermatological Association and the American Medical Association Branch of Dermatology and Syphilology. These pioneers incorporated the American Board of Dermatology and Syphilology in 1932 and changed its name to the American Board of Dermatology in 1955. In order to become a dermatologist, a candidate must be a graduate of an accredited medical school or osteopathic school before proceeding to four years of residency in dermatology in the U.S.[3]

Emergency Medicine

Emergency medicine is a branch of medicine that deals with urgent decisions and action purposely to avoid greater harm, disability, and death. The desire to provide emergency medicine has not been easy on the part of the receiver or provider. In Europe, for example, early English common laws were formulated in England as far back as the 18th century purposely to deal with professional legal responsibility and ethical issues. Most of these laws were published in *Commentaries on the Laws of England* by William Blackstone in 1765. Early American common laws dealing with professional and ethical issues during emergency were patterned after the British system. There was an initial melee over the standard of emergency care undertaken by physicians in America, and this was exemplified by the Richie vs. West case decided in 1860 in Illinois. Abraham Lincoln, then an Illinois lawyer representing the plaintiff, succeeded in prosecuting Dr. West for medical malpractice requiring "ordinary or reasonable care." This problem led to the locality rule, which compared physician's professional conduct to that of his fellows in the defendant's own city, town, or village, and the reinstatement of the law of torts section dealing with emergency. The law states:

> In determining whether conduct is negligent towards another, the fact that the actor is confronted with a sudden emergency not caused by his own tortuous conduct, which requires rapid decision, is a factor in determining the reasonable character of his choice of action.

The latter part of the section made provision for modification of the general rule in a situation where the defendant has "special training" in the encountered emergency situation. However, this provision did not seem to persuade the courts on medical malpractice in the 1930s and 1940s because of the nonexistence of emergency medicine specialty in the medical field. The general public was on the losing end because physicians needed to be encouraged to perform philanthropic gestures in emergency situations without fear of a malpractice suit. Many public officials realized the detrimental effect of this; as a result the Good Samaritan law was passed in 1959 in California, and other states followed. The law gave physicians protection or partial immunity against malpractice suit whenever they responded to emergency situations. A few other states, such as Vermont in 1973, went further to make it mandatory for everybody including physicians to respond to emergencies or pay a penalty with fines or criminal prosecution. In order to enhance training and reduce malpractice suits, the American College of Emergency Physicians was formed in 1968, and in 1969 the federal government with the aid of its tax authorities demanded that all charitable tax-exempt and community general hospitals open a functional 24-hour emergency service to the community regardless of patient's ability to pay. The American Board of Medical Specialties established the American Board of Emergency Medicine in 1979 at the request of the American College of Emergency Physicians, the Society for Academic Emergency Medicine, the American Medical Association, and others.[3,8,9]

FAMILY PRACTICE

Family practice is a modern form of general practice and it deals with prevention, diagnosis, and treatment of various human ailments with a major focus on family care. They receive fragmented training in pediatrics, surgery, internal medicine, psychiatry, geriatrics, obstetrics, and gynecology. Family practice suffered a few humiliations that characterized pharmacy and dentistry for centuries during its transformation from general practice (GP) to a specialty at the turn of the 19th century. David Adams commented about the end of the 19th century general physicians by noting "changes within medicine mirrored a broader social trend, specialization, and professionalization of many other disciplines." Up till the late 1800s medicine was truly family practice because many families dwelled in rural areas, and a physician that treated the father's diabetic condition would deliver the mother's baby, attend to the children's otitis media or fractured arm with no x-ray, and could be requested later in the evening to amputate a servant or slave's hand mangled in a farm's thrasher. He enjoyed fame, prestige, and popularity. In 1912, Charles Dana, a renowned New York physician, noted in a speech before the New York Academy of Medicine that a general practitioner is "a splendid figure and useful in his day; however, he was badly trained; he was often ignorant; he made many mistakes; for one cannot by force of character and geniality make a diagnosis of appendicitis or recognize a streptococcus infection." Dana concluded bluntly that "the ill-educated old family doctor, idealized perhaps less by our memories than in our storybooks, is going and it is a good riddance."

The popularity of general practice started dwindling in the late 1800s because of the following: a shift towards specialization, lack of prestige resulting from exaltation of specialists and hospital relegation of general practice to the background, rural/urban migration of the early 1900s, scientific advancement, and widespread complaints by students about the vast body of knowledge and the inadequacy of four-year medical school training plus a one-year internship in dealing with such an astronomical body of knowledge needed for a GP. The dramatic impact of these issues are well exemplified by the drop in the number of graduates going into general practice from 47% in 1900 to 19% in 1964 in the United States. General practice became the medical field subject of ridicule, while the specialists were showered with praise as wartime and postwar heroes of medicine. Some of these comments were credited to Morris

Fishbein, *JAMA* editor, who made a list of medical specialties officers with no mention of general practitioners in his 1945 monument to wartime medicine *Doctors at War*. In 1941, the American Medical Association's study questioned the rationale behind supporting the GP when an average physician identified himself as a specialist. Some other studies revealed that the GP was moribund in the 1950s and '60s. The public was not left out of these satirical remarks about GPs. Some of these remarks and concerns were expressed in movies of the 1930s, such as *Dark Victory*, which typifies a young socialite with endless inoperable brain tumor, and *Sex Madness*, which typifies a syphilis patient who seeks treatment and believes that she was cured by an incompetent physician, presumably a GP. She went on to marry and ended up with a syphilitic baby and a blind husband. *Sex Madness* showed that the devastating effects of syphilis can only be handled and treated by specialists. A Missouri physician marveled at the extremities of specialization in American cities in 1880 to the point that he claimed "the body is so nicely mapped out and divided that there is only left to the general practitioner the umbilicus."

Judging by the above it is clear that all odds were against general practice as jack-of-all-trades, master of none. The practitioner knew that they had to do something about the plight of GP by looking for ways to revamp it. The initial move to change general practice to family practice as a specialty started in 1940. In 1941, the National Board of Medical Examiners (NBME) formed a special committee to look into certification of general practitioners. This view did not see the light of the day because some members of the committee believed that any acts of consideration of certification for general practitioners would amount to deprivation and suffering of other boards of specialties. In 1946, the AMA sent the same issue to a subcommittee of the postwar medical service committee, which expressed a similar view that the general practitioner's certification does not represent the best views of the profession. Undaunted by the topsy-turvy fate of general practice, the practitioners decided to form the American Academy of General Practice (AAGP) with state and local branches across the country in 1947. A journal named *General Practice* was later created in 1950 to foster solidarity and to address other concerns, especially the creation of specialty board that seemed to divide the ranks and files of general practice. The AAGP emphasized the need for its members to maintain good standards of postgraduate education in form of continuing education. The AMA formed another committee consisting of the American Academy of General Practice, the American Association of Medical Colleges (AAMC), and the Council on Medical Education. In 1959, the committee published its final report that stressed the need for a two-year graduate medical education and the creation of a special proficiency program in place of continuing education. The physicians fought among themselves over what was expected of the new family practice specialty. Some wanted to retain the status quo of the old GP while others wanted a new platform. The AMA formed another two committees in 1963 and 1966 that finally paved the way for the formation and approval of family practice as the 20th board of specialty in February 1969. Family practice now required a three-year residency program and a six-year recertification process for board certification.[3,10]

INTERNAL MEDICINE

Internal medicine is a branch of medicine that deals with diagnosis and nonsurgical treatment of diseases such as skin, eyes, ears, reproductive organs, nervous system, and nose problems. The American Board of Internal Medicine (ABIM) is a private, nonprofit organization that gained its autonomy in 1936. The board certifies physicians who have gone through medical or osteopathic school, completed his /her internship, and passed the board examination. ABIM certification has no special privileges; hence, it is not required to practice internal medicine.[3] An internist is expected to complete clinical rotations in cardiovascular, critical care medicine, endocrinology, diabetes, metabolism, oncology, nephrology, treatment of lungs, sports medicine, and rheumatology.

MEDICAL GENETICS

Medical genetics is a branch of medicine that deals with diagnosis and treatment of diseases on the basis of genetic linkage. The advent of medical genetics transformed medicine from generalized patterns to individualized approaches in dealing with human ailments/diseases. Genetics sprang from the days of Mendel's publication about a green pea's hybridization in 1866, and its rediscovery in the study of heredity in 1900 to the mapping of human genome. It is now projected that all of the 3 billion or more nucleotides and 60,000 to 70,000 genes that constitute the haploid genome will be known by 2005. The desire to understand the molecular basis of the living structure, biologic systems, and the maintenance of such systems is the centerpiece of medical genetics. Medical genetics seems to unite teratologists, dysmorphologists, molecular geneticists, clinical geneticists, drosophila geneticists, pediatrics, internal medicine hematologists, obstetrics, and metaphysicists. Medical genetics is also on a quest to find solutions to various human ailments such as cancer, malformation, sickle cell anemia, hypertension, coronary artery disease, infectious diseases, allergies, cystic fibrosis, Down syndrome, phenylketonuria (PKU), neural tube defect, rheumatoid arthritis, diabetics, Huntington's disease, and others.

In 1945, McCarty, McLeod, and Avery published their work that detailed DNA as the major building block of genetic material. This was followed by Watson and Crick's similar publication in 1953, and Yanofsky decoding of the DNA base pairs in amino acids/proteins in 1960s. The subsequent coding, transcription, and translation of DNA material revealed genes as specific determiners of protein units; consequently, it is now possible to describe mutation and its clinical impact. Extraction and isolation of gene fragments became feasible in the 1970s and '80s with the discovery of restriction enzymes. Drosophila geneticists worried about the future of human genetics; the need to have skillful physicians who knew genetics take over control led to the foundation of the American Society of Human Genetics in 1947 and *American Journal of Human Genetics* in 1949. The popularity of human genome/genetics started with the foundation of the American Society of Human Genetics and spread to the other parts of the world. In the U.S., the number of medical schools offering medical genetics spread from 16 departments in 1975 to almost all medical schools by the year 2000. In the United Kingdom, Manchester University's medical school was the command center for medical genetics, which centered on antenatal testing for Down syndrome and neural tube disorder in the 1970s. Alan Emery founded the genetic clinic in Manchester in 1964 shortly after receiving human genetics training at John Hopkins Medical School in Baltimore. In 1979, the American Board of Medical Genetics (ABMG) was created as a specialty with little or no resistance because of the crucial role of human genetics in finding solutions to human ailments. The American Society of Human Genetics made the formal request for the creation of the board, and it was incorporated in Texas as a nonprofit organization in 1980. The ABMG offers certification in PhD medical genetics, clinical molecular genetics, clinical genetics, clinical biochemical genetics, and clinical cytogenetics.[3,11,12,13]

NEUROLOGY

Neurology is a branch of medicine that deals with diagnosis and treatment of diseases of the brain, spinal cord, peripheral nerves, and autonomic nervous system. Throughout history, man has been fascinated by the mystery of the human brain and its connection with soul and body. Numerous propositions have been made since the days of Hippocrates, but not much was known about the human brain until the mid-19th century. However, Albrecht Von Haller of Switzerland made a little scientific effort to study the cerebrospinal fluid in the mid-18th century. The history of neurology had its roots in Europe and the U.S. around the 1860s, and it can be traced as follows: In France, Jean-Martin Charcot is credited as the founder of neurology; most of his research work on Parkinson's disease, tabes dorsalis, and multiple sclerosis was published in the 1860s, and he was made the world's first professor of neurology in 1882. In Britain, the National Hospital for the Relief and Cure of the Paralyzed and Epileptic was established in 1860 in London, and John Jackson, British father of neurology, began his work in the hospital in 1862. In America, the American Medical Association initially failed to recognize neurology as a specialty; they raised great opposition because such a move was considered anti-general practice. Hammond formally established a training center for diseases of the nervous systems at New York State Hospital in Manhattan in 1870, and by 1875 the American Neurological Association was formally launched. Hammond and Mitchell are regarded as the founders of American neurology.

Journal publications of nervous and mental diseases started in 1874, while similar publications on the brain commenced in 1878. These journals helped to propagate the need for medical board specialty for neurology and American Neurological Association's goodwill messages. Finally, a committee consisting of the American Neurological Association, the American Psychiatric Association, and the AMA section on nervous and mental diseases was formed in the early 1930s. The purpose of the committee was to look into ways and means of creating the American Board of Psychiatry and Neurology. They held several conferences and submitted their findings to ABMS. The ABMS approved the findings, and the American Board of Psychiatry and Neurology was finally created as a nonprofit corporation in 1934. The board presently certifies physicians in neurology, child neurology, pain management, psychiatry, child and adolescent psychiatry, geriatric psychiatry, addiction and forensic psychiatry, and clinical neurophysiology.[3,14,16]

NUCLEAR MEDICINE

Nuclear medicine is a branch of medicine that deals with diagnosis and treatment of diseases with the use of radionuclides such as positron emission tomography (PET), single proton emission computer tomography (SPECT), radioisotopically antibody, and radioimmunoassay. A liaison committee for specialty boards was established around 1970 purposely to explore the modalities for forming the American Board of Nuclear Medicine. The committee made their findings known to the American Board of Medical Specialties and the AMA Council on Medical Education approved the establishment of the ABNM in June 1971.[3] The ABNM is sponsored by the Society of Nuclear Medicine and the American boards of Pathology, Radiology, and Internal Medicine. The ABNM certified 4,454 physicians in the U.S. between 1972 and 1998.

Obstetrics and Gynecology

Obstetrics and gynecology is a branch of medicine that deals with the care of women's reproductive systems and associated disorders. Obstetrics is mostly concerned with women's care during pregnancy, childbirth, and shortly after childbirth. The practice of obstetrics was based on a craft with no scientific basis for years until John Whitridge Williams saw the need to radicalize the profession. Williams reviewed European and American obstetrics and published his work in 1903. Williams's work led to the abolition of obstetrics' craft and its subsequent replacement with science. He believed that the fetus should be treated as a patient.[15] Sponsoring organizations like the AMA's section of gynecology and abdominal surgery, the gynecologists and abdominal surgeons, the American Association of Obstetricians, and the American Gynecological Society initiated the move to establish the American Board of Obstetrics and Gynecology in 1927, and their wish was finally granted with the establishment of the board in 1930. The board presently certifies physicians in obstetrics, gynecology, gynecological oncology, maternal-fetal medicine, and reproductive endocrinology.

Ophthalmology/Otolaryngology

Ophthalmology is a branch of medicine that deals with diagnosis, monitoring, and treatment (medical or surgical) of eye diseases and visual problems. Otolaryngology, on the other hand, is a branch of medicine that deals with the diagnosis and treatment (medical or surgical) of the larynx, ears, head, neck, respiratory system, and upper alimentary canals. Initially a committee was formed by the Triological Society around early 1910. The aim of the committee was to figure out modalities for teaching standardized otolaryngology in medical schools and at the postgraduate level. The committee published its reports in 1913, and shortly after the publication the American Academy of Ophthalmology and Otolaryngology set up two separate committees to examine ungoverned specialty education. The ophthalmological committee was sponsored by the AMA section on ophthalmology, the American Ophthalmological Society, and the American Academy of Ophthalmology. The committee made recommendations for the establishment of a board that will be responsible for organizing and supervising examinations and other criteria for admitting physicians into the practice of ophthomology. The committee's recommendations were accepted in 1915, and the American Board for Ophthalmic examination was created in May 1916. The board became a nonprofit corporation in May 1917, and in 1933 the name changed to the American Board of Ophthalmology. The first regularized ophthalmic examination was conducted in New York in June 1917.

The otolarynlgological committee was sponsored by the AMA section on otolaryngology, the Triological Society, the American Otological Society, the American Academy of Ophthalmology and Otolaryngology, and the American Laryngological Association. The committee recommended the adoption of uniform curriculum and admission requirements to the practice of ophthalmology and otolaryngology. The recommendations were later modified to avoid the double-standard admission requirements. The establishment of the Board of Ophthalmology tremendously influenced the four sponsoring organizations. They decided to select two representatives each in combination with the American Laryngological, Rhinological, and Otological Society to constitute the American Board of Otolaryngology. The American Board of Otolaryngology was eventually established in Chicago in November 1924. The American Board of Ophthalmology was the first specialty board to be instituted, followed by the American Board of Otolaryngology in 1924 and the American Board of Obstetrics and Gynecology in 1930.[3,17]

Optometry

Optometry is a branch of medicine that deals with eye examination in relation to refractive faults and correction of the faults with prescription lenses (spectacles). Optometry is, therefore, concerned with correcting eye defects through the use of lenses (spectacles). The major difference between ophthalmology and optometry lies in the fact that ophthalmology deals with physiology and anatomical features of the eye (eye diseases and visual problems), while optometry deals with physiology, refraction (changes in light rays as it goes through the eye), and lenses. Generally speaking, correcting eye defects with lenses (contacts or spectacles) offers greater choice, fewer risks, fewer side effects, less damage, less expense, greater manipulations and adjustments than correcting eye defects from inside the body. This explains why optometry today is outpacing ophthalmology, and there is evidence to prove that ophthalmology will one day merge with optometry. Optometry started as a commercial trade/business at the turn of the 20th century and gradually evolved into a medical profession that has now incorporated much of the didactic classroom works/curriculum of ophthalmology.

The struggle between ophthalmology and optometry typifies the American Medical Association (AMA)'s dilemma, the great opposition, and what it tried to avoid by creating specialties such as clinical medicine/pharmacology (against pharmacy) and dentistry (against dentistry). The fact is that the medical school curriculum is just too broad in dealing with various aspects of the body and too narrow in dealing with specific aspects of the body to make a meaningful impact on students/graduates. A good number of ophthalmologists attest to this by turning against AMA (especially its views that it was unethical for physicians to teach optometrists in the 1940s and '50s), deriding the profession (ophthalmology), and seeking to propagate optometry at the expense of ophthalmology. Wilber M. Brucker, former governor and attorney general of Michigan, in his 1939 book *The Story of Optometry*, reflected most of these assertions; some of them will be reported here, though not necessarily in sequential order.

> "Eye disease abnormal. Only 7% of all cases presenting themselves to the 'optometrists' office have any disease complications. The other 93% are trying to see better.

> "A comparison of catalogues of medical schools and colleges of optometry discloses that the modern optometrist concentrates far more upon visual defects than any other practitioner on the eye before either is admitted to practice. As a matter of fact, studies such as geometric optics, physiology optics, ocular mycology, and orthoptics are extremely important in the practice of optometry and are listed in the catalog for the optometry students, but are not taught by medical schools. By comparison, we find that the medical students receive an average of 64 hours of classroom and clinical instruction in ophthalmology in the regular four-year course as contrasted with 4,000 hours of classroom and clinical instruction required of an optometry student. That medical training is insufficient to meet present-day needs in regular medical schools seems to be recognized *by* doctors themselves."[24]

The first bulletin of Los Angeles Medical School of Ophthalmology and Optometry after it incorporated on July 2, 1911, defended its usage of the term "medical school," which was meant to justify optometry as a specialty like dentistry. The school taught and graduated professional refractionists (optometrists), a subject that the medical doctor knows nothing about. Part of the bulletin reads

> "The average MD knows nothing at all about this subject. The MD who has taken up and made treatment of diseases of the eye his specialty soon found that a great percent of his cases had defective vision, and he supplied them with glasses finding in due time that what was formerly regarded as a medical case requiring medical treatment was nothing more than a reflex, local or systemic disturbance through nerve exhaustion owing to defective vision, and that there was actually no truly disease condition; and he has appropriated this physical science unto himself while at the same time his medical brother who has not studied optometry wholly ignores its and goes on treating headaches and other distressing conditions in the same old way.
>
> The average four-year graded course in a medical college covers about 40 different subjects while the time of attendance is a little over 4,000 hours, averaging 100 hours to a subject; but only about 75 hours is really devoted to the study of the eye, and no optometry is given at all. In this school our six-month course covers fully 1,500 hours. With the proper teaching, training and drilling during this long period, doesn't it stand to reason that a graduate of this school should be superior to any MD that ever lived who hasn't had such a training?
>
> ... Formerly all non-medical refractionists called themselves "opticians." Since the different states passed law regulating their work and gave them an exemption certificate, a great many have assumed the title "Doctor of Optometry."[26]

Most of this bulletin was the handiwork of Dr. Marshall B. Ketchum, MD, an ophthalmologist, founder, and first president of the school till 1920. The school was founded in 1904. Dr. Ray Lyman and his committee on the costs of medical care published their findings in 1929. Part of the findings reads:

> "The existence of optometry on its present basis is due to the failure of the medical profession to recognize the importance of this field, in its failure to provide needed services. The training received by the medical students does not qualify them to do refraction. The curriculum devotes relatively little time to the eye—all the optometry laws exempt physicians from their

restrictions—while optometry is not considered the practice of medicine, any physician is considered qualified to practice optometry. Optometry is a profession, which the medical men had entered by exemption, never proving to the public or to any one at all their fitness to do the work.[24]

Dr. Jackson Edward, an MD and editorial member of the *American Journal of Ophthalmology*, in his comment observed:

> "The most important thing the medical profession has to do is provide for the adequate teaching of ophthalmology including optometry, in the medical schools, to meet the needs of the practitioner of other branches of medicine and to build up a definite class of practitioners especially trained to recognize and treat the defects and disorders of the eye. It is the failure properly to perform this duty towards the public that is responsible for the optometry question, and the larger issue of a division in the medical profession. Ophthalmology cannot be learned without special school or systematic courses of teaching. Medicine and surgery were so learned by apprenticeship for hundreds of years. But the apprentice system has gone from medicine as it has gone from the mechanical arts. As matters stand now, the graduate, after a scanty introduction to ophthalmology in the medical school, is permitted to pick up ophthalmic knowledge and skill here and there from desultory reading, by study of chance cases, in the unsystematized clinics of post graduate schools, from the courses of self-constituted teachers, and by a partial return to the apprentice system through assistantship in the eye clinic or private office. Preparation for a specialty must begin with fundamental studies. The anatomy, physiology, and pathology of the visual apparatus should be studied, with a detail and thoroughness impossible in the undergraduate study required before formal entrance to the medical profession." [24]

In April 1931, Dr. O'Brien, an ophthalmologist, wrote in the *American Journal of Ophthalmology* about variation of hours, an average of about fifty to sixty hours devoted to ophthalmology in various medical schools, and argued the need to increase such hours for meaningful impact. In August 1933, Dr. Verhoeff, a renowned ophthalmologist, wrote in the *American Journal of Ophthalmology*:

> "In ophthalmology, the need of further requirements is particularly obvious. At present, any licensed physician may treat diseases of the eye and even proclaim himself an eye specialist

however inadequate his training in ophthalmology may have been. Most of us here have seen many cases in which actual loss of sight has resulted from improper treatment by physicians untrained in ophthalmology." [24]

In April 1935, Dr. Post L. T. made a similar observation in the *American Journal of Ophthalmology*.

> "Most ophthalmologists enjoy operative work and, even if they do only a small amount of it, like to discuss this phase of their practice. Histology, pathology, and optics, though much needed, are not much wanted. They are too foreign to the thoughts of most ophthalmologists who have little background of knowledge in these subjects but no great yearning to increase it." [24]

Optometry is a Greek combination of two words: "opto" for eye and "metron" for measure. Optometrist as a word was first used in 1870 German textbooks then adopted in America for connotation of "nonmedical refractionists" in 1903. Optometry deals with laws of physics and mathematics, and it has a lot in common with the use of glass. Opaque glass was invented in Egypt around 3000 BC. The Greek and Romans made use of glass around 600 BC and 423 BC. Spectacles originated in China around 7th century AD; however, the earliest documentation of it dates back to Marco Polo's reports of optometric use of lenses in AD 1260. It has been argued that if you take away spectacles from the world, civilization will degenerate to the Dark Ages. Islamic scholars like Al Hazen, a mathematician, were the first people to study the eye and its refraction around AD 1000. Rogers Bacon (1214–94), an English monk, is reputed to be the first person to use lenses for vision purposes, and he talked about concave lenses in his *Opus Magnus* (1268). In Holland, two Jansens discovered the compound microscope in 1590, and in 1610 Galileo discovered the telescope by using lenses. Anthony Leeuwenhoek (1632–1723), a janitor of Delft Town Hall in Holland, improved the microscope and began the study of microbes. Professional associations of contemporary societies are like the guilds of yesteryear societies. Guilds of spectacle makers existed in Italy, England, France, and Germany at the tail end of the 16th century. Snell, a Dutch astronomer, established a mathematical formula in 1621 illustrating changes in light rays as they go through a lens. He discovered the laws of light refraction. In 1623, Devaldes wrote the first book about optics, and Christian Huyghens (1629–95) in Holland later proved that light acts like undulating waves. Isaac Newton (1642–1727) found the laws of light and thus established physics as a branch of science. Others such as

Joseph Fraunhofer (1787–1862) discovered the spectral lines; David Brewster (1781–1868) discovered the kaleidoscope; John Dalton's (1766–1844) work revealed color blindness and atomic theory; Thomas Young (1773–1829) discovered astigmatism and the optometer; Benjamin Franklin invented the bifocal lens in 1784; George Bidell Airy (1801–92) used cylindrical lenses to correct astigmatism; Hermann Von Helmholtz (1821–94) invented the ophthalmoscope in 1851; William Crookes (1832–1919) invented radiometer and tinted lenses; Garrett made frames of silver, tortoise shell, etc., in 1815 in Philadelphia.[24]

Like dentistry, optometry is not recognized as a medical specialty or branch of medicine by the American Board of Medical Specialties and the American Medical Association (AMA, the brain behind all medical specialties in the United States). Governor Brucker claims that

> "By reason of its specialization solely in matter of vision, optometry is not a part of medicine, although like dentistry it is a related profession, but again like dentistry, a separate one. Its lineage lies in physics, physiology, psychology, mathematics, and optics and not through pathology, pharmacology, or surgery."[24]

It is glaring from this little piece of writing that Governor Brucker was merely responding to indoctrinations by medical doctors, medical schools, the AMA, and the powers that be. Whatever stands the test of time, serves humanity best, justifies its purpose with facts and figures, and not just societal indoctrination or a superstitious belief dominates human life and becomes the modus operandi for life activities. Governor Brucker's contradictory message noted that physiology that deals with structure and functions of the human body especially eye (for optometry) is part of optometry. Physiology reveals normal structures and functions of the body, and by learning normal features of the body one becomes acquainted with and dexterous in abnormal features (disease state or pathology) of the body. The only thing outside optometry in Governor Brucker's assertion in contemporary society is surgery, and there are reasons to believe that in the future when ophthalmology merges with optometry to become one, centralized body/specialty caring for eye diseases/treatment, surgery will become part of optometry. Optometry in the U.S. (North America), Australia (Australia), the United Kingdom (Europe), Nigeria (Africa), Japan (Asia), and Brazil (South America) has incorporated limited pharmacology as part of its curriculum, and optometry physicians in these countries can prescribe a variety of drugs (limited to some extent in some countries) and glasses to their patients. Later in this book, we will discover that optometrists and ophthalmologists are exposed to the same number of pharmacy/pharmacology or drug-treatment courses in the U.S. Dental ailments and vision problems are human pathological conditions that deserve medical treatment by medical specialists like every other part of the body; consequently, dentists and optometrists are medical doctors with specialization in these areas. If eye ailments or poor vision are not medical condition, what is a medical condition? If resolving poor vision is not a medical treatment, what is a medical treatment? A driver with poor vision can kill himself or another person because of his ailment. If the same driver has a simple cough, mild diarrhea, or minor skin cuts that would not endanger his or another person's life and a medical doctor treats him, his ailment would be classified as a medical condition with medical treatment. If we say that dentists and optometrists are not medical doctors because their curriculum is not taught in "traditional medical schools," which is too broad to include detailed aspects of these areas of the body, we might as well forget about specialization and allow medical advancement to degenerate into oblivion (the days when medical doctors were jacks-of all-trades, masters of none). Alternately, we might as well say that surgery is not a branch of medicine because most dentists in contemporary society practice dental surgery with tooth extraction, root canals, etc. Surgeons, like dentists and optometrists, use foreign objects (to the body) to correct human ailments/pathology, and this is based on their knowledge of human physiology.

Judging by the assertions and declarations made by medical doctors (mostly ophthalmologists) above, it is glaring that they are disenchanted and chagrined to know the degree of medical school's inadequacy in dealing with specific curricula, yet arrogate these privileges to themselves with no justification. The public, on the other hand, accepts whatever the medical doctors dictate to them with no qualms or justification because they are alpha and omega. If the ophthalmologists are saying that they do not receive enough training in these areas, what else do we want? When is humanity going to wake up and smell the coffee by realizing that not all that glitters is gold? Just because an MD is an MD does not make him God; if medical schools do not offer enough courses to justify specialization in any area of the body then they don't merit or deserve the credit. If others offer enough courses to justify specialization in any area of the body then they deserve the credit, and honor should be given when and where it is due.

The American Academy of Optometry (AAO), which later became American Optometry Association (AOA), was established in 1898. At the beginning of the 20th century, optometry was purely a commercial business and the business owners only needed trading techniques acquired through apprenticeship. Nobody needed to prove to anyone the ability to practice optometry before entry into the trade. There were no laws regulating optometry until Minnesota passed the first statue in 1901. About 60 schools teaching refraction were in existence in the U.S. around the 1900s, and some of these schools offered two-week courses. Some of these schools are the Spencer Optical Company; the King Optical Company of Cleveland, Ohio; the Foster School of Optics, Boston (1888); Moore's College of Optics, Atlanta, Georgia; Southwestern Optical College, Kansa City, Missouri; and others. After 1901, state laws required a passing grade on a very short, written examination without education requirements. In 1904, Dr. Ketchum opened the Los Angeles School of Ophthalmology and Optometry as a six to eight-week-long course, which later changed to six months of coursework in 1909 and two years of coursework in 1912. A two-year nationwide adoption was introduced in 1922, and later the affiliation of the school with University of Southern California (1929–1933) catalyzed the four-year program because universities' programs at this point in time were mostly four years in duration. Optometry affiliation with a university curriculum proceeded stepwise with three-year program first then four-year program that became fully operational in 1935. The Los Angeles School of Ophthalmology and Optometry, later known as the University of Southern California College of Optometry, was consistently ahead of the national education standard for optometry. Optometrists, often referred to as nonmedical refractionists, were classified as opticians at the beginning. Passage of various state laws regulating optometry granted practitioners an exemption certificate, and this exemption certificate made many assume the title of a doctor or doctor of optometry even with less training. Today oculists and ophthalmologists are considered the same thing, while an optician is classified as a maker of lenses and spectacles according to specification or prescription order of oculist/ophthalmologist/optometrist. Optician is a trade with no license requirement in contemporary society. The optical journal *The Optician* published by Frederick Boger first appeared in 1891 and continued to publish articles about optometry or opticians. Jewelers' magazines used to publish these articles before the advent of *The Optician*.[24,25,26]

Pathology

Pathology is a branch of medicine that deals with causes and nature of disease by sheer observation of blood, urine, diseased tissue, feces, and other samples obtained from a living or dead person (autopsy). Pathology began with the performance of autopsies on patients in Renaissance Italy in the 15th century. Both physicians and patients recognized the importance of pathology with their views and expressions. For example, in 1490, Bernardo Toni, a Florentine physician, in his letter of grief to a bereaved family expressed comfort in the great benefit of examining the patient's organs at autopsy. In 1486, Rinieri's diary revealed the dying wishes of Bartolomea, who requested an autopsy of her body so that her daughters could be treated. Clinical pathologists in Italy, France, the United Kingdom, and Germany between the 15th and 19th century were mostly concerned with the causes of signs and symptoms and deaths of patients. They believed that opening up patients' bodies could reveal more information than sitting by the bedside. The discovery of a microscope in Germany opened a chapter and an era of remarkable improvement in the field of pathology because the microscope became almost an agent of diagnosis. Rudolf Virchow, a German biologist who took advantage of the newly invented microscope to understand the basis of disease, is credited as a scholar who almost single-handedly revolutionized pathology by transforming it. He describes pathology as "the science that studies the causes, mechanisms, and consequences of diseases." He taught pathology and made many of his pupils/followers believe that pathology is the scientific foundation of medicine. Some of his followers such as Welch, Prudden, and Delafield brought pathology to the United of States of America. These followers are the founding fathers of pathology in the U.S.; they organized and formed the American Society of Pathology and the organization's *Journal of Experimental Medicine*. Subspecialties such as surgical pathology later developed and explored the latest technology such as immunohistochemistry, molecular biology, and electron microscopy to advance its development. The desire to establish a certifying board led to the formation of a committee consisting of the American Society of Clinical Pathologists (ASCP) and the AMA section on pathology and physiology in June 1935. The committee published its findings, which were adopted and approved, thereby leading to the creation of American Board of Pathology in May 1936. The board became a nonprofit, incorporated body in Chicago in July 1936.[3,18]

PEDIATRICS

Pediatrics is a branch of medicine that deals with the social, psychological, and physical health of children from genesis (birth) to adolescence. The American Board of Pediatrics became a private nonprofit organization in 1933. The AMA publication of the *American Journal of Diseases of Children* and a private publication of the Archives of Pediatrics helped to nurture the establishment of the American Academy of Pediatrics (AAP) in Detroit in 1930. Two years later, the AAP *Journal of Pediatrics* was created, in July 1932. The AAP provided its members with quality educational material, continuing education, news bulletins, and other vital issues. A committee, consisting of the three sponsoring bodies—namely the AMA section on pediatrics, the American Academy of Pediatrics, and the American Pediatric Society—was formed purposely to look into the modalities for establishing the Board of Pediatrics. The committee published its reports, which were adopted in 1933. Subspecialties became a major issue that plagued the American Board of Pediatrics in the 1940s; consequently, about 13 of them were later established in addition to the American Board of Allergy and Immunology, which it co-sponsored in 1971. The current subspecialties certified by the board are pediatric hematology-oncology, sports medicine, pediatric nephrology, pediatric pulmonology, pediatric critical medicine, pediatric gastroenterology, medical toxicology, neonatal-perinatal medicine, pediatric endocrinology, pediatric infectious diseases, and adolescent medicine.[19]

Physical Medicine and Rehabilitation

Physical medicine and rehabilitation (PMR) is a branch of medicine that deals with diagnosis, management, treatment, and prognosis of cognitive impairment and physical disability of patients. The history of PMR in the U.S. centers on Dr. Frank Krusen's career activities. At the end of the 19th century, the use of physical agents for therapeutic purposes was often correlated with novice and unskillful acts because it was not scientifically based like medicine. It became obvious to the pioneers of PMR that it was necessary for them to document their therapeutic outcome in order to justify the scientific basis of PMR, if it was to survive as a specialty of medicine. Dr. Krusen began his physical therapy research after completing some physical therapy classes. He established the first physical medicine department with his developed curriculum at Temple University's medical school in 1929. Krusen made his initial remarkable success in physical medicine as a Temple University football team physician. He worked diligently to have his injured players return to competition as quickly as possible; hence, he became the darling of football fans. Shortly after his appointment to the AMA Council on Physical Therapy, he joined with Drs. Bierman and Coulter to establish the American Registry of Physical Therapy Technicians in 1934. Krusen later became chairman of the department of physical medicine at the Mayo Clinic, University of Minnesota, a position he used to promote the creation of physical medicine as a specialty.

Dr. Krusen and nine other physiatrists established the Society of Physical Therapy Physicians with the sole aim of creating the specialty later during the 1938 annual convention of the American Congress of Physical Therapy. The society became known as the Professional Association for Certified Physiatrists and later the American Academy of Physical Medicine and Rehabilitation. Krusen published the first comprehensive textbook on physical medicine, entitled *Physical Medicine,* in 1941, and he helped to train army and navy physicians in 1942, with a 90-day program at the Mayo Clinic. Krusen and other pioneers' tireless efforts resulted in the creation of the American Board of Physical Medicine in 1947. The board of directors of PMR is currently drawn from the American Medical Association (AMA), the Association of Academic Physiatrists (AAP), the American Academy of Physical Medicine and Rehabilitation (AAPM&R), and the American Board of Physical Medicine and Rehabilitation.[3,20]

PREVENTIVE MEDICINE

Preventive medicine is a branch of medicine that deals with the maintenance of health and well-being and the prevention of disease, disability, and premature death. Preventive medicine involves issues like immunization and elimination of vectors, e.g., mosquitoes (malaria) or tsetse flies (sleeping sickness). A committee consisting of the Professional Education of the American Public Health Association and the AMA section on preventive and industrial medicine and public health, was formed purposely to look into the certification of the board of preventive medicine. The committee published its report and it was adopted in Delaware in June 1948 by the Advisory Board of Medical Specialties.[3] It was incorporated as a nonprofit organization in the name of the American Board of Preventive Medicine and Public Health; the name was later changed to the American Board of Preventive Medicine in 1952. The American Board of Preventive Medicine can now certify specialists (physicians) in undersea and hyperbaric medicine, aerospace medicine, medical toxicology, occupational medicine and public health, and general preventive medicine.

PSYCHIATRY

Psychiatry is a branch of medicine that deals with diagnosis and treatment of emotional, mood, addictive, and mental disorders. Human history is full of fascinations, various propositions, magic, and mystical rites about the human brain. Ancient medical practitioners used psychology in combination with magic and mysticism to explain and treat what is now regarded as mental illness. Great philosophers such as Buddha, Socrates, and Confucius once made various propositions about the brain and a human's ability to think, act, rationalize truth, and conceptualize sensations and perceptions into thoughts and ideas. Hippocrates believed that psychiatric illness or psychosis was the result of a chemical imbalance in the brain. William James is reputed as the founder of experimental psychology in the U.S.[21] Around 1931, a committee consisting of the American Psychiatric Association, the American Neurological Association, and the AMA section on nervous and mental disease was formed. The committee published its findings and they were adopted by the ABMS in 1934. The American Board of Psychiatry and Neurology was formed as a nonprofit corporation in 1934.[3,21]

RADIOLOGY

Radiology is a branch of medicine that deals with diagnosis and treatment of diseases with radiology. Wilhelm Roentgen, discoverer of the x-ray and father of radiology, was born in Germany in 1845. He has been described as a troublesome youth who later became an erudite scholar. He was expelled from Utrecht Technical School for planning a classroom prank and refusing to disclose his cohorts. He got his Doctor of Philosophy (PhD) degree from Zurich Polytechnic in 1869 and later became a professor at the University of Wurzburg in 1888. Dr. Roentgen started his cathode rays study in 1894 by passing an induction coil that produces high-tension electrical charges through platinum wire contained in a vacuum tube. He observed that cathode rays in the form of colored lights were produced and easily absorbed in the vacuum tube. The rays were capable of darkening photographic plates, so he went further to observe the penetrating effects on solid objects such as cards and books. The experiment revealed that the rays could penetrate most objects except lead. He later performed the experiment on his wife's hand for 15 minutes and published his report in December 1895. Roentgen described his newfound ray as an x-ray, and it became the center of the world's attention.

Dr. Gocht founded the first x-ray department after inventing the first x-ray machine at Berlin Hospital. The use of the x-ray spread from a hands-only device to other parts of the body (organs, skull, arms, legs, feet, etc.) and it soon became a diagnostic tool especially in surgery. Crile was the first person to use x-rays to show a fracture before and after treatment in March 1896. In Boston, Williams used x-rays to differentiate healthy lungs from tuberculosis-infected lungs in April 1896. He found that x-rays could easily penetrate healthy lungs, while the masses of tuberculosis were impervious. Freund used the x-rays to treat a young girl's congenital hairy nevus in November 1896 and thus became the first person to discover the therapeutic effects. X-rays have since been used to treat mouth cancroid's nodules, cancer patients (breast), and gastric carcinoma. Some of the side effects of x-rays such as skin burns, hair loss, scaling, skin discoloration, burning eyes, and retarded growth of fingernails were first notice in Vanderbilt University, Minnesota, and some other places.

Radiology continued to spread and its journal, named *Radiology*, was established in 1924. The journal in combination with various radiological societies began to work for the establishment of a certifying board for Radiology. In 1932, a committee consisting of the AMA section on radiology, the American College of Radiology, the American Roentgen Ray Society, the American Radium Society, and the Radiological Society of North America was formed purposely to review the concept of establishing the board. The committee met in Milwaukee in 1933 and agreed that it was time to create the board. The American Board of Radiology (ABR) was established as a nonprofit, incorporated body in May 1934 in Washington, D.C. The American Board of Radiology has expanded to include the American Society for Therapeutic Radiology and Oncology, the Association of the University Radiologists, and the American Association of Physicists in Medicine. The ABR certifies physicians in diagnostic radiology, radiation oncology, neuroradiology, pediatric radiology, nuclear radiology, radiologic physics, and others.[3,22,23]

SURGERY

Surgery is a branch of medicine that deals with diagnosis and treatment of injuries, deformities, or disease by operation. The surgeon provides adequate care for the traumatized patients as well as the critically ill patients by engaging in preoperative, operative, and postoperative care. There are currently six different certifying boards of surgery in the U.S. They are the American Board of Orthopedic Surgery (1934), the American Board of Colon and Rectal Surgery (1935), the American Board of Surgery (1937), the American Board of Plastic Surgery (1941), the American Board of Thoracic Surgery (1950), and the American Board of Neurological Surgery (1970). Unlike herbs and/or drug treatment, which were part and parcel of medicine from the beginning, surgery is an integral part of medicine that came into being later as a result of human advancement. Although Sushrutha Samitha (800–600 BC) made mention of flaps without details, the earliest documentation relating to the advent of surgery in medicine dates back to the time of Caius Celsius (25 BC–AD 50), a physician who used the skin flap technique for plastic surgery.[5] The first illustrated textbook in surgery was written by Serafeddin

Sabuncuogu (AD 1385–1468), an Islamic physician who is often credited as the pioneer of all branches of surgery. Sabuncuogu described in his book the treatment of gynecomastia with the aid of C-shaped incision in the removal of glandular tissue and the use of eyelid surgery in the treatment of trichiasis, ectropion, symlepharon, and entropion.[4] He is known to have performed surgery on all parts of the human body. A brief description of the various branches of surgery is as follows:

- Orthopedic surgery: Orthopedic surgery involves the correction of deformities caused by diseases/damage to the bones, joints, extremities, and spine. This correction could be in form of surgery, manipulation, traction, and other physical or medical methods. A committee was set up to look into possibilities of establishing the American Board of Orthopedic Surgery in the early 1930s. The committee submitted its reports, and it was adopted in 1934. The American Board of Orthopedic Surgery was chartered as a private nonprofit organization in 1934.[3]

- Colon and rectal surgery: Colon and rectal surgery involves diagnosis and treatment of intestinal tract, colon, anal canal, and rectum with surgery. Members of the American Proctological Society paved the way for the foundation of the American Board of Colon and Rectal Surgery by agitating for its autonomy as a certifying board from the American Board of Medical Specialties (then the Council on Medical Education and Hospitals and the Advisory Board for Medical Specialties) in 1934. The request made by the American Proctologic Society was approved in August 1935, and the American Board of Proctology thus became an incorporated nonprofit organization.[3] The name was subsequently changed from the American Board of Proctology to the American Board of Colon and Rectal Surgery in 1961.

- Surgery: Surgery is a generalized term for surgical treatment of any ailment as defined above. A committee consisting of regional and national surgical society representatives was set up purposely to look into the possibilities of forming the American Board of Surgery. The committee published its report and the findings were adopted by the cooperating societies. The adoption of the findings of the committee led to the foundation of the American Board of Surgery in July 1937 as a nonprofit incorporated organization.

- Plastic surgery: Plastic surgery involves the replacement, modification, and refurbishment of the skin, genital area, face, hand, trunk, breasts, and other parts of the body with surgery. In 1937, various groups with a common interest in plastic surgery formed a committee to work on the establishment of the American Board of Plastic Surgery. The committee met and made their proposal known to the Advisory Board of Medical Specialties. The proposal was approved in May of 1941, and the American Board of Plastic Surgery became a nonprofit incorporated body.[3]

- Thoracic surgery: Thoracic surgery involves the use of surgery to correct any anomalies or pathological conditions of the chest such as cardiovascular disease, heart valves, congenital defects, lung cancer, diseases of the diaphragm, and trachea. The initial move for thoracic surgeons' certification began with the Rochester meeting of 1936. Shortly after the meeting, momentum began to grow and a committee was eventually formed in 1946. The aim of the committee was to evaluate the issue of board certification and publish its reports. The committee published its report, and it was adopted in 1948. The American Board of Thoracic Surgery became a nonprofit incorporated organization in 1950.[3]

- Neurological surgery: Neurological surgery involves the use of surgery to correct anomalies or pathological conditions of autonomic, central, and peripheral nervous systems. The American Association of Neurological Surgeons was previously know as the Harvey Cushing Society. The desire to expand the scope of knowledge, training, and specialized form of practice led members of the Harvey Cushing Society and the Society of Neurological Surgeons to hold their first meeting in March 1939. The meeting grew to embrace others such as the AMA section on surgery, the American College of Surgeons, the AMA section on nervous and mental diseases, and the America Neurological Association, who started agitating for the creation of the American Board of Neurological Surgery. The board was approved by the American Board of Medical Specialties probably around 1970.[3]

UROLOGY

Urology is a branch of medicine that deals with diagnosis and treatment of reproductive and urinary tract diseases. Reproductive and urinary tract diseases include anomalies of the genitourinary tract system and the adrenal gland. The first meeting of the American Board of Urology consisting of members of the American Urological Association and the American Association of Genito-Urinary Surgeons took place in September 1934 in Chicago. The members of these two associations elected officers to conduct the affairs of the organization and agitate for its independence as a certifying board. The elected officials made a formal request for the recognition of the American Board of Urology as a certifying body. The request was granted in May 1935 and the American Board of Urology thus became a nonprofit incorporated body.

Veterinary Medicine

Veterinary medicine is a branch of medicine that deals with diagnosis, treatment, and prevention of animal diseases. Animals have been part and parcel of human history from genesis to the present day. They work the fields (agriculture), provide comfort and companionship to some people, guidance (e.g., guild dogs), protection, entertainment (circus animals), a good source of religious worship and investigation (drug- or bomb-sniffing dog), transportation, warfare (e.g., horses), food, and others. According to the Kahun veterinary papyrus, Egyptians domesticated cats, used cattle for muscle power, and treated livestock diseases about 5,000 years ago. Religious priests in Mesopotamia treated animal diseases because they were seen as good sources of their deity's annoyance, displeasure, and curses. The Greek and Roman empires used animals as a good source of food, transportation, and warfare. Aristotle (384–322 BC), student of Plato and teacher of Alexander the Great, like Hippocrates is at times considered the father of veterinary medicine. Some of the works of Aristotle include *Organon* (Logic), *Ethics*, *Politics*, *Poetics*, *Metaphysics*, *Historia Animalium*, and *Departibus Animalium*, which revealed his works on animal physiology, comparative anatomy, and pathology.[29,30]

Animals may have been a good part of human history, but they are also notorious in degrading the environment and bringing sanitary conditions to a deplorable situation when left uncontrolled. At the turn of the 20th century, urban residents in places such as New York and New Orleans in the U.S. experienced some of these poor sanitary conditions according to the following excerpt:

"Residents of even fashionable districts in New York and New Orleans, pressing handkerchiefs to their noses, would hardly have been surprised to hear that their cities contained such dense populations of horses and mules. Well-to-do ladies crossing streets commonly paid boys stationed with brooms at the corners to precede them and sweep manure out of their way; manure piles at the sides of streets sometimes reached proportions so monumental that sidewalks were impassable. The bodies of horses that fell and had to be killed, or actually died while in harness, often lay unmoved for days, bloating and stinking by the sides of the streets. Urban residents worried that manure and rotting horse carcasses long believed to be a source of disease—causing fumes or miasmas, also harbored the germs of tuberculosis and other diseases, which were thought to be spread by dust and flies.[27]

Charles Dickens, in his comment, considered American pigs as city scavengers of the 19th century. These deplorable situations permeated many developed societies of the world until technological advancement, professional expertise, bureaucratic management, and evolving educational standards helped to improve civilization and curtail animal messes. Animals' needs and their owners' interests spurred veterinarians to rally round the profession, catering to the most economically valuable animals at first, then later all animals. The study of poultry was included in the veterinary medicine curriculum in 1930s. Like medicine and law, veterinary medicine was based purely on an apprenticeship mode of training until the late 18th century in some parts of the world and the 19th century in the U.S. There were no laws governing veterinary medicine in many states, and anybody could be a veterinary medical doctor provided the person could convince animal owners of his ability. Dr. R.J Dinsmore, a graduate of Harvard Veterinary Medical School, said in early 1890s,

> "Nobody was laughed at more than the horse doctor. Horse doctors were supposed to be a coarse, ignorant group who had made a failure of blacksmith or farming and had turned to doctoring. That they actually knew anything about medicine was an absurd notion.... Most were not real veterinarians but farriers.... The same brush of low social status tarred competent and incompetent practitioners alike." [27]

In 1883, Robert Jennings had problems establishing the first veterinary school in Philadelphia because young men or women considered veterinary medicine as a low-social status profession. He was unable to attract young scholars to purse a career in veterinary medicine. Traditional veterinary medical education had it roots in 1762 in Lyons, France, because of Rinderpest disease (cattle plague). The need to control other animal diseases lead to the creation of other veterinary medical schools such as Veterinary School of Edinburd in the UK, Veterinary School of Berlin in Germany, Veterinary School in Mexico in 1853, Ontario Veterinary College in Canada in 1862, Cornell University in the U.S. in 1868, Iowa State Veterinary College in the U.S. in

1879, the University of Pennsylvania School of Veterinary Medicine in the U.S. in 1884, and others. There was little or no formal education (lectures) in most of these schools that were located in or near livery barns or private horse hospitals. Professors'/students' relationship in most of these schools depended on instructions given or learned during provision of medication, dentistry, and surgery to ailing animals and even during feeding at times. The duration of study in 1879 when Iowa State College opened its doors to students was one and a half years consisting of two terms 9 months each. The duration of study later increased to 3 years, then 4 years in 1904. In the U.S., the Bureau of Animal Industry (BAI) raised the veterinary education standard nationally in 1908 when the organization made a 3 years graduation requirement from a reputable veterinary school as the minimum job-entry requirement. There were 25 schools of veterinary medicine in the U.S. between 1880 and 1900; however, the decrease in the economic value of horses, probably because of decreased demand for horses as an effective means of transportation, threatened the profession and resulted in decreased veterinary medical school enrollment from 1,300 in 1917 to 500 in 1925. An agricultural boom after the end of World War II in 1945 brought the profession back to life.[28]

The U.S.'s exports, especially livestock, food, animals, and meat, declined drastically in 1870s and 1880s because of poor standards. European nations such as Germany protested un-inspected American products because they did not meet their high regulatory standards. At home American cattlemen suffered a great loss because of bovine pleuropneumonia and other plague epizootics. Commissioner William G. LeDuc estimated in 1878 that animal losses from disease cost $30 million or more and requested that Congress act promptly to control pleuropneumonia before it spread to other herds (e.g., in the Allegheny Mountains). Animal farm owners began to pressure Congress for a solution to the great threats of animal disease. Finally, in 1881, Congress requested the treasury department to establish a cattle commission and build quarantine stations. Three years later, this commission was transferred to the United States Department of Agriculture (USDA), and the Bureau of Animal Industry (BAI) was created and signed into law on May 29, 1884, by President Chester A. Arthur. Dr. Daniel E. Salmon was appointed as chief of BAI with a budget of $150,000 and 20 employees to start with. The creation of BAI is often correlated with the professionalization of veterinary medicine in the U.S. BAI and the American Veterinary Medical Association are the 2 organizations that shaped the development and growth of veterinary medicine. Even though the U.S. Army depended on horses and mules in some of their war campaigns, they refused to commission veterinarians until 1916. The U.S. Army decision was probably due to the low social status, little public respect, and the reputation of the uneducated or illiterate horse doctor.

Rinderpest's (cattle plague—disastrous between 1774 and 1843) devastating effect in Europe taught many that the easiest, quickest, cheapest, safest, and most effective way to curtail animal epizootics was by the eradication or stamping out of the disease. Gamgee, a popular English veterinarian, and others are reputed to be major forces in propagating this theory to English-speaking countries including the U.S. Gamgee recommended Dr. James Law, another English veterinarian, to Andrew White, president of Cornell University, and he became head of the new veterinary department at Ithaca, New York, in 1868. Dr. James Law was Dr. Salmon's teacher, and together they campaigned against foot and mouth disease in 1870, hog cholera in 1878, and pleuropneumonia in 1879. Dr. Law wrote different books including *Lung Plague* in 1879. The germ theories of the 1870s coupled with the training of veterinarians in Louis Pasteur's, Joseph Lister's, and Robert Koch's laboratories helped to reveal many things about the pathological mechanism of diseases. When Dr. Salmon became chief of BAI at the age of 34, it was glaring that he had been thoroughly schooled in veterinary medicine and was prepared to propagate the legacy of his predecessor, mentor, and teacher, Dr. Law, and Gamgee at the long run.

Professional regulation for veterinary medicine in the U.S. began in a few states in 1890s. Young veterinary medical doctors, together with their mentors, lobbied politicians in various states to pass laws differentiating veterinarians from quacks and prohibiting quackery through licensing and registration of practitioners. At the beginning of the 20th century, some existing state law began to get a grip on veterinary medicine by ensuring that the majority of licensed veterinary medical doctors were graduates of one of the recognized veterinary medical schools. Most veterinary medical doctors at this time felt the imperative need to earn their living as general practitioners of medicine according American Veterinary Medical Association's President Tait Butler in 1901. This was merely due to the fact that the majority of the veterinary medical doctors (80–90%) and veterinary schools were in urban centers, where many people lived, as opposed to rural areas, where many animals lived. Other reasons probably were epizootic disease and decreased economic value of horses as an effective means of transportation. In late 1872, city and town dependence on horses as an effective means of transportation is said to have created a lot of problems such as the collapse of mass transit, Boston's downtown conflagration (poor response by fire crews), grounded street car service in Cleveland, and others because of an epizootic or epidemic of equine catarrh. These problems made officials look at alternative means of public transportation without animals; consequently, there was a simultaneous decrease in the demand for horses.[27] Today some people hide behind their animals to obtain medical services for their ailments from some veterinary medical doctors, or divert medications meant for animal treatment for their own or other people's use with or without the knowledge of the veterinary medical doctors. Later in this book we will see how many pharmacy/pharmacology or drug-treatment courses the veterinary medical doctors are exposed to in comparison to the clinical pharmacists or pharmacists. The number of pharmacy/pharmacology or drug-treatment courses available in veterinary medical schools' curricula shows their preparation for this arduous task for animal or human (in case of necessity or emergency) treatment.

Veterinary medicine like dentistry and optometry is not considered a specialty of medicine by the American Board of Medical Specialties and the American Medical Association (the brain behind all medical specialties). However, traditional medical doctors and the AMA are more receptive to veterinary medical doctors or seem to recognize veterinary medical doctors more than dentists, optometrists, and clinical pharmacists because they know medical schools' curricula couldn't embrace the health problems and treatment of animals. There are presently about 20 boards of certified veterinary specialties in the U.S. and some of these are anesthesiology, cardiology, dentistry, dermatology, radiology, clinical pharmacology, surgery, theriogenology (animal reproduction), and zoology. Veterinary medicine has evolved from a male-dominated profession to a contemporary, female-dominated profession. The *American Veterinary Review* editors in 1897 said, "Veterinary surgery is of all the learned professions the one least adapted for women." The general view was that any woman who engaged in the practice of veterinary medicine ran the risk of losing her feminine feelings. In 1855, the first journal about American veterinary medicine appeared, and eight years later the American Veterinary Medical Association was formed, in 1863.[27,28,29]

OTHERS

Other branches of medicine without recognized boards that are not described in this chapter include hematology, pulmonology, oncology, endocrinology, podiatry, nephrology, gastroenterology, cardiology, rheumatology, and others. Like the 13 subspecialties under pediatrics (e.g., pediatric hematology-oncology, nephrology, pulmonology, gastroenterology, rheumatology, etc.), these branches of medicine are classified as subspecialties not worthy of specialty status as per the ABMS. Thus, an internist or family practice physician could be certified as a pulmonologist as well as an endocrinologist, but an internist cannot be a family practice physician.

REFERENCES

1. Ginzberg, E. The shift to specialism in medicine: The U.S. Army in World War II. *Acad. Med.* 74 (1999): 522-25.

2. Debakey, M. E. Military surgery in World War II: A backward glance and forward look. *New England Journal of Medicine* 236 (1947): 341-50.

3. *Marquis who's who: The official ABMS directory of board-certified medical specialists.* 32nd ed. New Jersey: A division of Reed Elsevier, Inc., 2000.

4. Dogan, T., M. Bayramicli, and A. Numanoglu. Plastic surgical techniques in the fifteenth century by Serafeddin Sabunuoglu. *Plastic and Reconstructive Surgery* 99 (May 1997): 1775-79.

5. Santoni-Rugiu, P., and R. Mazzola. Plastic surgery of the face in the fourth century. *Plastic and Reconstructive Surgery* 102 (September 1998): 1274-80.

6. McCauley, H. B. Professional dentistry's road to autonomy. *Journal of the History of Dentistry* 46(2) (July 1998): 59-64.

7. Ring, M. E. Dentistry: A look backward and a peek into the future. *New York State Dental Journal* 63(1) (January 1997): 40-45.

8. William, J. C. Legal history of emergency medicine from medieval common law to the AIDS epidemic. *American Journal of Emergency Medicine* 15 (1997): 658-670.

9. *Reinstatement of the law of torts* §29. St. Louis, Mo.: American Law Institute, 1934.

10. Adams, D. P. Evolution of the specialty of family practice. *Journal of the Florida Medical Association* 76 (March 1989): 325-29.

11. Van Allen, M. I. Dysmorphology in the next millennium: History of medical genetics. *Pediatrics Annals* 26(9) (September 1997): 540-45.

12. Coventry, P. A., and J. V. Pickstone. From what and why did genetics emerge as a medical specialism in the 1970s in UK? A case history of research, policy, and services in the Manchester region of the NHS. *Social Science and Medicine* 49 (1999): 1227-38.

13. Childs, B. The entry of genetics into medicine. *Journal of Urban Health: Bulletin of the New York Academy of Medicine* 76(4) (December 1999): 497-508.

14. Scott, G. E., and J. F. Toole. History of Neurology: Neurology was there (1860-Neurology was there). *Archives of Neurology* 55 (December 1998): 1584-85.

15. Vasicka, A. John Whitridge Williams' contribution to democracy abroad. (The fetus treated as a patient). *Ceska Gynekologie* 64(2) (April 1999): 118-25.

16. Schiller, F. The cerebral ventricles (History of neurology). *Archives of Neurology* 54 (September 1997): 1158-63.

17. Cantrell, R. W. Joseph H. Ogura and the American Board of Otolaryngology: Development of a specialist: Development of specialty. *Laryngology* 102 (May 1992): 532-37.

18. Rosai, J. Pathology: A historical opportunity. *American Journal of Pathology* 151(1) (July 1997): 3-7.

19. Strain, J. E. The birth and evolution of pediatrics. *Pediatrics* 102(1) (July 1998): 163-67.

20. Opitz, J. L., T. J. Foltz, R. Gelfman, and J. D. Peter. The history of physical medicine and rehabilitation as recorded in the diary of Dr. Frank Krusen. Part 1. Gathering momentum (the years before 1942). *Archives of Physical Medicine and Rehabilitation* 78 (April 1997): 442-45.

21. King, L. J. A brief history of psychiatry: Millennia past and present. *Annals of Clinical Psychiatry* 11(1) (1999): 3-12.

22. O'Leary, P. J., and L. Boyd. Roentgen and his ray: An early impact on modern medicine. *American Journal of Surgery* 65(3) (March 1999): 292-94.

23. Frush, D. P. What of the past—What of the future. *Radiology* 210(1) (January 1999): 3.

24. Bucker, W. M. The story of optometry. *Journal of the American Optometric Association* 13(31) (1939): 37–49.

25. Gregg, J. R. History of the American Academy of Optometry, 1922-1986. New York: The American Academy of Optometry, 1987, 3-16.

26. Gregg, J. R. *Origin and development of the Southern California College of Optometry, 1904–1984.* Fullerton, Calif.: Southern California College of Optometry, 1984, 1-24, 51-55, 71-74, 106-109.

27. Jones, S. D. *Valuing animals, veterinarians, and their patients in modern America.* Baltimore: The Johns Hopkins University Press, 1964, 10-34.

28. Stalheim, O. H. V. *The winning of animal health: 100 years of veterinary medicine.* Des Moine, Iowa: Iowa State University Press, n.d., ix-xvi, 3–21, 35-39.

29. Wick, J. Y., and G. R. Zanni. Patients large and small: Role of the pharmacist in veterinary medicine. *Journal of the American Pharmaceutical Association* 44 (3): 319-23.

30. *New Webster's comprehensive dictionary of the English language.* Deluxe Edition. Lexicon Pub. Inc., 1990.

CHAPTER THREE

HISTORY OF PHARMACY

"Before Abraham there were men, so can pharmacy say to other branches/specialties of medicine."

Long before the 1908 Carnegie Foundation that sponsored Abraham Flexner, and the subsequent 1910 publications that led to specialization, or the advent of the American College of Surgeons in 1913 and its specialty board in 1937, or various committees that led to the foundation of the American Board of Ophthalmology in 1917, Otorlaryngology in 1924, Obstetrics and Gynecology in 1930, and the most recent American Board of Genetics in 1980; pharmacy had been conceived as a specialty and left in the womb of medicine.

As noted earlier, some branches of medicine including pharmacy started with medicine in the form herbal/drug treatment and later became an embodiment of general practice. Others like surgery, anesthesiology, genetics, nuclear medicine, neurology, pathology, psychiatry, radiology, physical medicine, and urology emanated from medicine as a result of human advancement, evolution, and technological developments. At the genesis of humanity, when life was in the most primitive, crude, and simplistic form, there was a direct relationship or correlation between medicine and pharmacy or drugs/herbs. At this stage, medicine was synonymous with pharmacy (drug/herb treatment) because the most important thing was any active ingredients (drugs or herbs) that could resolve human ailments. Sickness was a bad omen because it bred agony, sadness, weakness, pain, and malaise; hence, anything (from plants—in the form of extracts from herbs or purified extracts that were made into drugs—soil, animals, and water resources) that could ameliorate the situation was plausible. As medicine grew to embrace other terms, drugs made from any resources including extracts from plants or herbs became an embodiment of pharmacy.

Pharmacy is a branch of medicine that deals with the treatment of diseases and the science of drugs. Pharmacists are drug experts who specialize in dealing with all the intricacies of drugs and disease-state management. Drug intricacy involves drug/drug interactions, drug/food interactions, pharmacokinetics, pharmacodynamics, therapeutic effects, idiosyncratic reactions, and others. The history of pharmacy is synonymous with the cradle of mankind even though it took thousands of years to define its place in the medical world. Archeologists revealed that man's quest for tools and active ingredients (drugs or medicine) from plants and other resources to resolve his ailments occurred simultaneously during the Stone Age.[1] People were predominantly hunters, fishers, and gatherers of food including medicinal plants during the Paleolithic or Neolithic period—600,000 to 10,000 BC.[5] Shaman, the oldest known priest or witch doctor in human history, originated among Ural-Altaic people (Shanidar settlement) around 30,000 BC.[1,4] The shaman's knowledge of illness, disease, and healing power had a direct correlation with evil, spirits, good and bad supernatural forces, superstitious beliefs, and the use of medicinal plants. After diagnosis, the shaman used active ingredients from medicinal plants in combination with magic and incantations to treat excruciating diseases and chronic illness. The mere fact that these people, such as the elders in every household and shaman especially, were able to identify the healing power of plants' extract or active ingredient in this settlement, which is considered the first recognized, most primitive form of life, goes a long way to show the kind of relationship that existed between pharmacy and medicine from the beginning. This relationship demonstrates the fact that pharmacy and medicine have been part and parcel of human life from the beginning.

The two first great human civilizations, which occurred in Egypt around 4500 BC and in Mesopotamia around 3000 BC, played a great role in bringing medicine or pharmaceutical acts to new heights as seen below[4,5,6]:

- Egypt: Compounding of drugs from active ingredients in plants occurred in various dosage forms in Egypt, and those dosages were expanded with recipes/formulas. People made drugs and perfected their skills in the act. They explored other routes of administration besides the mouth because of patients' needs; thus the making of enema for rectal administration is believed to have originated in Egypt. Egyptians realized the usefulness of documentation in people's lives (for present and future generations); hence, papyrus and clay were used to record important information including the use of drugs. The invention of paper from papyrus plants and the availability of ink and expensive ostrich feather pens helped to facilitate writing, human skill, development, and improve drug production in Egypt (southern Ethiopia) during the reign of Mentuhotep, the 11th dynasty in the first intermediate period (2181-2040 BC).[6] Egyptians administered drugs with some magic terms and incantations even when the influence of gods degenerated at a certain time in the empire.

- Mesopotamia: The Sumerians founded the Mesopotamia kingdom around 3000 BC but were later captured and absorbed by the Babylonians. The Babylonians absorbed the Sumerian culture and established their own system of government, which among other things partitioned medicine into two forms of healings. The two forms of healings were experienced healing guided by Asu and spiritual/magical healing guided by Asipu. Unlike the Egyptians that combined both forms of healing into one practice, the Asu used active ingredients from plants to formulate various dosages such as enemas, ointments, suppositories, and tablets for the purpose of healing patients, while the Asipu believed in the usage of incantations, magical spells, and spirituality in healing patients. There was peace and tranquility among these two sets of healers; hence, the patients could oscillate between them and resolve their ailments.

- Greek Empire: The Greek practice of medicine was similar to Egyptians and Mesopotamians except that the traditional healers, the Demiourgoi, went a little further to diagnose diseases on the basis of natural causes in the early stages. Incantations, magic, and spirituality played a great role in Greek medicine until Hippocrates of Cos (460 BC) came on the scene to advocate the separation of medicine from superstitious beliefs, supernatural forces, divinity, and magic spells. Hippocrates established the basic foundation for today's medicine by emphasizing the need for rationalized medicine and the need to understand, diagnose, and treat diseases on the basis of cause and effect. According to historians and writers, the humoral theory that came out of the Hippocratic, rational means of explaining diseases connected the four basic elements of the environment, namely water, earth, air, and fire, to four basic humors of life, namely phlegm, black bile, yellow bile, and blood.[1,5] In Greece, physicians compounded active ingredients from plants to treat human ailments when lifestyle modification failed. Dioscorides emulated the good work of Theophrastus (370-285 BC) in studying plants and thus came up with the publication of the first standard encyclopedia of drugs called *Materia Medica*.

- Roman Empire: The work of a Greek physician and philosopher, Galen, dominated medicine in Rome until the Middle Ages. He wrote various books on human anatomy and physiology. Galen and his followers were noted for their heresy against Hippocratic principles. They argued that the humoral theory of illness can only be balanced with the opposite, including the treatment of ailments with opposite gestures or drugs. Some of these gestures were the use of onion or pepper to treat colds, a bag of ice to treat fresh fire burns, bleeding of excess blood to treat illness or swelling body parts, and other treatments. Galen's theory blended superstitions and magical spells with drugs to achieve favorable outcomes in treating patients[1,4]. The fall of the Roman Empire around AD 476 heralded the coming of the Middle Ages. The antiquity period started with Egypt and ended with the Roman Empire. The early Middle Ages is often correlated with the Dark Ages. This was the period when the barbarians invaded Europe from the north and west, and humanity was almost strangulated by the loss of contact with learning, science, and the medical advancements of the previous great empires. The fall of the Roman Empire led to the degeneration of central authority, civil disobedience, social and political chaos. Anarchy prevailed until the church and feudal lords rose to the occasion to take control of authority and displace the disintegrated central government. More information about the Roman Empire below.

Conception of Pharmacy as a Specialty

Some people in the medical world prefer to regard this phenomenon as the birth of pharmacy. It is ironic to refer to this age (9th century) as the birth of pharmacy when the profession is still struggling to define its position and stand on its own feet in the medical world by the year 2004, over 11 centuries later. In the words of Charles Darwin and his popular writings about survival of the fittest, pharmacy could be described as a profession on the verge of extinction, at least at the end of its first century (10th century). The situation is further compounded by the sad fact that it took anesthesiology (an integral part of pharmacy) less than six months; urology, colon, and rectal surgery and nuclear medicine less than one year; and the majority of the other branches of medicine less than a decade to define themselves and fight for their liberation as separate entities within the medical field. Other branches of medicine can correctly use the terms conception (the time the ideal of specialty was conceived), birth (the time the specialty was born as a defined, independent board of specialty capable of shaping its own destiny without interference from others), and maturity (the time the newly born/defined specialty was left in the hands of its practitioners to shape its future and nurture it to maturity).

Pharmacy was conceived as a specialty and left in the womb of medicine. Like a fetus whose jerking and kicking movements in the womb of a pregnant woman cause distress, discomfort, and pain, pharmacy, with its concomitant adverse drug reactions (ADR), side effects, toxicities, inadequate drug monitoring, drug utilization review (DUR) problems, drug efficacy problems, therapeutic dosage problems, and other problems, has been known to cause distress, discomfort, and pain in the medical community and the world at large. These problems have resulted in numerous deformations, liability suits, increased morbidity and mortality rates, around the world. The conception of pharmacy has historical connotations that can be traced from the fall of Roman Empire to the rise of Islam.

Roman Empire under the reigns of the five "good emperors"—Nerva (AD 96-98), Trajan (AD 98-117), Hadrian (AD 117-138), Antonius Pius (AD 138-161), and Marcus Aurelius (AD 161-180)—began to decline and face massive invasion threats from the east by the Iranian dynasty (AD 224) and from the west and north by the barbarians of the Germanic tribes. Constantine's rise to power after Diocletian's retirement in AD 305 led to the unification of the empire and the founding of Constantinople as capital of the empire. Constantinople became the center of Christendom and the preservation center for civilization and classical culture until the fall of the empire in 1453 to the Turks. As Roman Empire declined in Western Europe, the rise of Islamic religion began in the Middle East with his leader Mohammed (AD 570-632). Mohammed was a poor orphan who later married an older, wealthy widow, Khadija, from Mecca. He preached the need for morality; social justice for the weak, poor, orphans, and women; and warned against idol worshipping and blasphemy against God. Mohammed nurtured the religion from birth till his death in AD 632. He was succeeded by Abu Bakr (AD 632-634), Umar (AD 634-644), Uthman (AD 644-656), and others who spread Islam to other parts of the world including Byzantine (AD 640), Egypt (AD 642), Spain (AD 716), Sicily, Eastern Europe, and other places, through Arab Islamic armies at first and later jihad. While jihad (an Islamic quest to conquer the world) was going on, there were erudite scholars and physicians who were busy trying to develop Islamic culture and civilization. The Islamic religion taught its followers to respect, learn, translate, and enhance the writings of previous great civilizations such as in Egypt, Mesopotamia, and the Greek and Roman empires. Islamic scholars learned vigorously the medical works of

Hippocrates and Dioscorides of the Greek Empire, and Galen's works in the Roman Empire. They translated their works into Arabic and sought to develop the medical field further except anatomy and surgery, which did not agree with the preaching of Islam. They rejected the notion that the more bitter a pill is or the more foul-tasting a concoction is, the better it is in achieving the desired result/purpose. They made various dosages of drugs in a more fragrant, palatable, and attractive form. As the need to make various dosages (e.g., strength), improve existing dosages, prepare sophisticate medicine and invent new dosage forms grew so does the desire to have specialists within the medical field compound these dosages and advice patients about its uses.[1,5,29]

One of the Islamic physicians, a scholar and perhaps the first known pharmacist to rise to the occasion and conceive the idea of having specialists within the medical field compound drugs and advise patients about its usage, was Rhaze (AD 860-932). Rhaze founded pharmacy in Baghdad, a cosmopolitan city in the 9th century (around AD 890), out of basic necessity. Like Rhaze, other physicians who took the initiative summoned enough courage and rose to the occasion of establishing various specialties of medicine in the 20th twentieth century deserve commendations for leading humanity to the path of greatness. Shortly after the conception of pharmacy, trained medical personnel or specialists (mostly physicians) took over the preparation of sophisticated medicine (compounding). These specialists are the forefathers of today's pharmacists. They became dexterous in the acts of compounding and dispensing of drugs for all forms of ailments with or without prescriptions from physicians. There is evidence to show that pharmacy operated on a professional level in Arab cities in the 9th century, with physicians like Ibn-Imran writing prescriptions to be filled in private pharmacy stores.[2] The hospital helped to nurture the newly conceived profession by emphasizing its separation from medicine. By the 12th century, hospitals in Damascus grew herb gardens that were used by pharmacists to compound drugs. Arab's conquest, academic achievement, and scholarship influence began to degenerate by the 11th century because of the conquest of the Byzantium Empire by the Turks, and much of it became history by 1492 with the Saracens' expulsion from Spain by Ferdinand.

In Western Europe, the period stretching from the fall of Roman Empire in the 5th century (AD 476) to the medieval period is characterized by the barbarians' (from Germanic tribes) conquest, the Vandals' victory, confusion, incessant warfare, civil disobedience, feudal instability, the Crusades, and the pope's absolute power at its zenith. The Roman Catholic Church was the centerpiece of the Crusade and papal power (the pope's authority). Monasteries, an integral part of the Roman Catholic Church, became the center of academic learning, healing, medical knowledge, intellectualism, scholastics, and religious purity (piety). Monasteries came with the church. At the beginning, the act of healing was an essential feature of spirituality, and there was a direct link between disease and sin according to the doctrines/teachings of the church. Besides church, there were also pagan temples, where healing of ailments were said to be similar to those of the Egyptians and Greeks in the Roman Empire. Therapeutic forms of healing with drugs declined during this period because of the monks' adherence to church doctrines. Monks are hermits who sought to imitate Jesus Christ through self-denial by withdrawing from the rest of the society to pursue a perfect way of life. Athanasius and Martin of Tours introduced the concept to the West, while John Cassian (ca. 360-435) and Jerome (ca. 340-420) shaped the values and practices. Benedict of Nursia (ca. 340-420) organized and wrote the rules of monasteries. The monks, their assistants, and trainees were responsible for medical practices. They dispensed medical and surgical care; however, the use of surgery was banded in most parts because it was considered ungodly and incompatible with church doctrine, preaching, and morality.

Pope Alexander III initiated the ban in 1163 and Innocent III in 1215 as well as papal regulation in 1239 intensified it. As the only surviving learning center in the West after the fall of the Roman Empire, the monasteries did encourage pharmaceutical growth as part of its learning culture in spite of the adherence to church doctrines. Cassiodorus, a monk who established the monasteries in Italy, encouraged the study of the learning culture of previous great civilizations. The works of Hippocrates, Dioscorides, and Galen were taught, and the importance of herbs in making and compounding drugs was deciphered and elaborated in the learning center. Monasteries grew their own herb gardens for pharmaceutical use. Two monastery learning centers, at Salerno in Italy (often referred to as the first university in Europe, founded in 10th century) and at Toledo in Spain, played vital roles in the transfer of pharmacy from the Arabic to the Western world. An African erudite scholar and a converted monk by the name of Constantine is said to have been responsible for the major transfer of Arabic work into Latin with the aid of his students in Salerno. Constantine was particularly fluent in Persian, Greek, and Arabic languages. Gerard, a European, on the other hand, performed similar acts in Toledo. The subsequent influence of Salerno on medicine and pharmacy had a great impact on Donnolo's production of antidotary. Donnolo is a Jewish physician who used Arabic data to produce one of the first drug formulary books, *Antidotary*, in the 10th century. Two revised versions of the book, named *Great Antidotary* and *Antidotarium Neolai*, contained about 485 and 115 drugs formulary respectively, and the later version used medical students in the thirteenth century in Paris. These books were also used as a standard reference in recipes for compounding drugs in the "statio." Statio was the original named used to describe a pharmacy shop, and those responsible for operating it were regarded as stationarius or confectionarius (present-day pharmacists). The stationarius or confectionarius made the concoctions (drugs) with honey or sugar in bulk to last for a considerable length of time, possibly for 6 months or a year. Other notable, outstanding works with Arabic influence include *Regimen Sanitatis* and *Grabadin*. *Grabadin* was used as a standard medical reference for compounding in every pharmacy in Europe for many centuries. The emergence of the universities at Fez (Morocco—AD 859), AL-Azhar (Egypt—990, 10th century), Paris (1150), Oxford (London—1167), Salerno (Italy—1180), Cambridge (London—1284), Padua, Timbuktu (Mali—around 1320), Sankore, Prague (1347), and Bologna (11th century) contributed immensely to the enhancement of writings and the expansion of medicine/pharmaceutical work.[1,2,4,5,7,8,29]

The invention of movable-type printing in 1436 by Johannes Gutenberg (1397–1468) revolutionized writings and forever change printing for good. There were enormous requests for Bibles, hymnals, and religious pamphlets, and these requests were balanced by supply-side movable-type printing (e.g., the Gutenberg Bible). Printers improved their works to meet the ever-increasing demand for printing and later focused on medical and pharmaceutical works. Printing thus enabled chemists, botanists, and physicians to illustrate their investigative works of plants for medicinal purposes. Valerius Cordus was one of the erudite medical scientists who took advantage of printing to publish his work *Dispensatorium* in 1546. *Dispensatorium* is recognized as the first pharmacopoeia in general use in compounding drugs in Nuremberg City, Germany, in the mid 16th century.

During the Renaissance, one particular radical voice was noted for his heresy and reactionary views against traditional medicine. This was Paracelsus, the father of toxicology. Paracelsus Phillipus Aureolus (1493–1541) was a Swiss physician, surgeon, alchemist, and philosopher who vehemently opposed the medical doctrines of Galen and Avicenna. Born Theophrastus Bombastus Von Hohenheim, he was an intriguing, complex fellow who preached against university education of physicians. Paracelsus believed that God had placed a healing sign on substances that were expected to cure diseases, such as liverwort for liver disease, and he persistently implored others as well as himself to adhere strictly to the principle of observation of chemical processes of drugs. He claimed that drugs are poisons that have limitations in their usefulness —"all are poisons"; the only thing that differentiates drugs from other poisons is dosages (therapeutic dosage: the range within which a drug is effective in the treatment of human ailment; toxic dose or toxicity: the range above therapeutic dosage after which the drug becomes harmful to the body).

The Renaissance marked the beginning of modern Europe, and Paracelsus as a product of the Renaissance helped to conceive and nurture modern pharmacy. Paracelsus and his followers started the use of distillation in the extraction of active ingredients from plants and minerals. The distillates (extracted drugs) were found to be effective in the treatment of diseases, and medical literature began to enlist these drugs as standard reference for pharmacy. Though critical of pharmacy practitioners, Paracelsus and his followers, with the discovery of distillation and the subsequent effective drugs, became the front-runner of pharmacy and chemistry for three centuries, from the 16th to the 19th century.

Distillation empowered some pharmacists such as Wilhelm Scheele, who discovered oxygen (1773), phosphorus, chlorine, and glycerin; Schelle, who discovered citric acid (1784); Friedrich, who discovered morphine from opium (around 1805); Joseph Pelletier and Joseph Caventous, who discovered quinine from cinchona bark (1820); and Henri Moissan, who discovered fluorine and won the Nobel Prize in Chemistry in 1906. Martin Klaproth eventually started analytical chemistry, and other drug products such as guaiac, cascara, ipecac, and sagrada obtained as active ingredients from plants found themselves in the market and were widely used for treatment of various ailments. Pharmacy's remarkable contribution to the science of drugs, chemistry, and medicine was so great that it became impossible to deny its full place as a profession in Europe during Renaissance. In most parts of Europe, pharmacy (apothecary) was seen as equal to medicine. Pharmacists (apothecaries) and physicians were similar in terms of status quo even in England. At this point in time, pharmacy missed another golden opportunity to liberate itself and define its place in medicine, because medicine was seen as a holistic ideal embracing all terms including surgery (no room for specialization).

The term apothecary according to *Webster's Dictionary* is used to describe "someone who prescribes, prepares, and dispenses medicine and drugs." It is difficult to say exactly where and when apothecary came into existence. However, the need to include pharmacists' activities in the rules and regulations of medicine sparked debate and eventually resulted in the creation of oaths and ordinances in various cities at different times during the medieval period. Some of these cities, with dates pertaining to the creation of these oaths and ordinances, are Montpellier, France, in 1180, where an oath was created for *especiadors* or *apothecayres* (the earliest mention of the term apothecary in history); Marseilles in 1231; Avignon in 1242; and Venice in 1258. Apothecaries were pharmacy practitioners who by the 17th and 18th centuries had emerged as a formidable group of medical practitioners providing medical services to the poor, downtrodden, less privileged, less fortunate, and deserving members of the society who couldn't afford the high medical fee of university-trained physicians. In addition, the number of university-trained physicians was so small that they couldn't meet the demand for medical services. This was the state of affairs when the apothecaries came to the rescue of the society. By the 19th century, apothecaries had elevated their status in most parts of Europe through university education, scientific research in laboratories (research that resulted in the discovery of elements, compounds, drugs, and chemical substances of vital interest to mankind), manufacturing of drugs, compounding of active ingredients from plants, and vested interest in chemistry and analytical chemistry. Apothecaries subsequently became general practitioners basking in fame that catapulted them into the upper middle class through their scientific discoveries and dedicated service to human welfare in England and other parts of Europe. The Apothecaries Act of 1815 in Great Britain established apothecaries as general practitioners of medicine. The physicians at this time felt the need to practice like apothecaries. They prescribed and compounded drugs and dispensed them in their offices (shops), at times with the aid of an apothecary who worked with them either directly as a partner or indirectly as an employee. Apothecaries eventually left behind the job of manufacturing and selling drugs and medicines to the chemists and druggists.[1,2]

The guilds were like contemporary professional associations. The formation of guilds dates back to the 12th century, when pharmacists and physicians formed one guild in Florence around 1199. The formation of a guild in Paris around 1210, "College of Saint Come," helped to organize the barber-surgeon, which was made up of two groups: laymen and clergy. The clergy group separated in 1268 to form the guild of surgeon-barbers, which dominated the profession and later transformed into "Fraternity at the Church of Saints Cosmos and Damian" the patron saints of physicians and apothecaries, in Paris.[2,9] The establishment of Montpellier University in 1289 and the subsequent creation of a school of medicine and pharmacy laid the groundwork for formal education in pharmacy in France. The pharmacists' guilds in Paris followed suit with two failed attempts because of the vicious attack by the school of medicine at the University of Paris. However, the royal decree of 1777 finally created the *college de pharmacie* (school of pharmacy). Some pharmacists' guilds in the 13th century were in Verona, Avignon, and Rome. Others are Colegio in 1441, Valencia in 1445, in Barcelona, and the Society of Apothecaries in 1617 in London. The guild in Rome was created as Universitas Aromatariorum and was later named Corporazione degli speziali di Roma in 1429 by papal decree. The guilds spelled out rules and regulations to maintain professional dignity and integrity, protocol for operating a pharmacy, standards for maintaining price control and monopoly, and the procedures for educating, training, and executing examinations in some cases to the would-be pharmacists (apprentices). The examinations that were conducted in 13th century Marseilles and 15th century Paris showed that the apprentices were required to perform compounding of complex prescriptions, and it was tagged a masterpiece demonstration. The 1777 royal decree equally placed pharmacists' guilds in the hands of the *college de pharmacie* in France. The college became the sole body responsible for regulating pharmacy, pharmacist education, and pharmacists' activities in France. Later the pharmacist's title gradually changed from *apothicaire* to *pharmacien*, and the sale of drugs and medicine was restricted to pharmacy only, thereby putting an end to hospitals and religious bodies' past practices of selling drugs and medicine. In Germany, where the earliest known pharmacy shop was created from a town hall conversion in Lemgo City in 1559, pharmacists' monopoly suffered a great setback in the 18th century because their activities were restricted to pharmacy products only. However, the inspection of pharmacies was removed from physicians' jurisdiction and placed under the auspices of pharmacists. Shortly after the unification in 1871, Germany established pharmacy examining boards at all universities in the country by 1875.

In 1725, King Frederick William I of Prussia enacted a medical edict that can be said to be the genesis of modern pharmacy education. The medical edict delineated two requirements for pharmacy practice in the country. First, the pharmacist needed to serve a three to five years of apprenticeship, seven years as a journeyman, take the *processus pharmaceutico-chymicos* at Collegium Medico-Chirurgicum in Berlin, pass a board examination conducted by the professor of chemistry, the royal apothecary, and two practicing pharmacists, and get approval from the Obercollegium Medicum et Sanitatis before practicing in a large city. Secondly, the pharmacists who wished to practice in small cities or towns needed to serve five years of an apprenticeship, six years of clerkship, and pass a local examination before the Collegiums Medicum. The small city pharmacists were not expected to go through an academically rigorous program, but the situation changed for good in the early 19th century when a three-year apprenticeship was declared as a prerequisite for university pharmacy education.[2] In France, similar gestures required eight years of apprenticeship without pharmacy education, while in the U.S., the College of Philadelphia School of Pharmacy required four years of apprenticeship in 1808.

In the early 19th century, pharmacy education went through some changes because of the preponderance of scientific research in pharmaceutical works and advances in educational materials and literature. Pharmacy courses were predominantly chemistry (inorganic, organic, and applied chemistry) with some mathematics, physics, mineralogy, zoology, botany, pharmacy, and pharmacognosy. Students went to various universities and polytechnics to pursue pharmacy with the aim of preparing for state board examinations in Germany. The universities in Montpellier, Paris, and Strasburg changed their admission requirements to include baccalaureate degrees as entry-level requirements in 1840. The universities of Bordeaux, Lille, and Lyons had mixed courses in the schools of pharmacy and medicine to the point that it was difficult to differentiate between both schools around 1882. In Spain, three-year pharmacy degree programs at the universities of Barcelona, Granada, and Madrid later metamorphosed into five-year programs around 1850.[2] In Great Britain, the Apothecaries Act of 1815 legalized apothecaries as general practitioners of medicine. As noted earlier, apothecaries eventually left the job of manufacturing and dispensing drugs to the chemists and druggists. Initially, the chemists and druggists had no formal education, and pharmacy was left without regulation in Britain. They eventually formed the British Pharmaceutical Society in 1841 and later founded the School of Pharmacy in 1842 in London. The chemists and druggists realized the urgent need for a school of pharmacy because an apprenticeship was not sufficient to meet the demands of pharmacy profession in Britain. The School of Pharmacy later became an integrated member of the University of London, offering Bachelor of Pharmacy or Science in Pharmacy with a one-year clerkship or apprenticeship before board certification. There were instances where pharmacists' inadequacy in training during the 19th century led to the establishment of second-class pharmacists programs. Some of these programs such as the *écoles préparatoires* and *école de plein exercice* were created in France in response to legalization of the program in 1803, and it was abrogated barely more than a century later in 1906. The program involved apprenticeship and a few offered courses in training school; however, the recipients were restricted to their locality in practices.

Pharmacy in the United States of America resembled that of its colonial authority and culture in Britain at the beginning. The apothecaries had advanced in Britain to a high level of pharmacy practice and, as noted previously, they provided effective medical services for less-privileged members of the society and left behind the job of dispensing and manufacturing drugs to the druggists and chemists. This was the state of affairs when pharmacy was imported to some British colonies in the 17th century. The earliest available record showed that some pharmacists like Bartholomew Brown of Massachusetts kept a ledger account book that revealed his medical services and charges as an apothecary in the late 17th century. The same is true of Robert Talbot, whose records showed a "catalogue of medicine sold around 1725 in New Jersey." The practice of medicine was a mixture of medical services rendered by physicians, surgeons, and apothecaries. There were no effective distinctions between these three groups of medical practitioners because all of them could own, prepare remedies, compound drugs, and dispense medicine from their shops to patrons or patients. There were few or no laws regulating pharmacy and medical practice. The ownership and operation of a pharmacy was a combination of luck and wealth. Anybody could open a pharmacy even by mere conversion of his home to a shop, provided he had enough money to do so. Some of the pharmacy owners regarded themselves as apothecaries and druggists with little or no medical knowledge or a pharmaceutical background. The end result was that some of these apothecary shops (fourteen in 1720 in Boston) had saturated all American cities by the end of the 18th century.

The druggists and chemists took over the job left behind by apothecaries and served as wholesalers/retailers of medicine and drugs to physicians, apothecaries, surgeons, and members of the public. A few druggists were known to be involved in the foundation of some colonies like Perth Amboy of New Jersey in 1685 and John Johnstone. These druggists helped to propagate the British form of pharmacy practice in the new colonies of America. Most of the other druggists and chemists who later came to the American colonies from Europe were employees of physicians, surgeons, and apothecaries who had left for the colonies in search of a better life, prosperity, and independence. The economic growth of the colonies as well as a high demand for medical professionals attracted these otherwise second-class medical professionals to the colonies, where they could practice independently like their former employers without any restriction. The druggists and chemists were aided in their desire to dispense drugs by some physicians such as John Morgan, an apothecary who in 1760 started preaching the need to separate pharmacy from medicine. He wrote *Discourse on Medical Education*, which emphasized physicians writing prescriptions for pharmacists to dispense. However, he ended up running an apothecary shop in which he prescribed and dispensed drugs at the same time. The first law created in America in relation to pharmacy was the February 12, 1770 proclamation, which separated pharmacy as a branch/specialty of medicine. In 1769, Louisiana, a colony of France, became the first colony in America to authorize pharmacy practice after examination. As in Britain, the apothecaries in America practiced medicine like other physicians and surgeons. They went on rounds in the hospitals to treat patients and dispense medication. This is evident in the 1804 "Brief account of New York hospital." There was a resident physician who was the superintendent of the hospital, and his assistant was the apothecary, a term used to describe a recent medical school graduate who was appointed to serve one year only. The term apothecary was later replaced by house physician or surgeon in 1828 and house pupil in the late 1840s.[30]

Apprenticeships dominated American society during the colonial era and well into the 19th century. Apprenticeships by then were three to four years of practical experience programs in which the preceptor gave thorough and detailed information in all branches of medicine such as the preparing and dispensing of medications, attending to the sick, performing minor surgical operations, extracting/bleeding teeth, and other medical procedures. The preceptor and his office were limited in scope, size, and space in illustrating chemistry with experiments, clinical observation of disease at the bedside, showing anatomy with dissection, studying physiology with laboratory display, and studying pathology with a cadaver (human specimen). After independence in 1776, it was said that about 400 out of the 3,000 to 4,000 practicing physicians had received their medical degrees and the rest acquired their skills through apprenticeship. One of the apprentices was Dr. John Warren (1753-1815), the founder of the third medical school in the nation (the first medical school after the Revolutionary War), Harvard Medical School, established in 1783. With no medical degree, Warren's medical knowledge came from barely two years of apprenticeship training with an older brother who was a physician in Boston. Medical schools in the United Kingdom (for example, the University of Edinburgh) served as role models for the establishment of the first two medical schools in colonial America: the medical department of the College of Philadelphia in 1765 and the medical department of King's College New York in 1768. John Morgan (1735-1789) and William Shippen Jr. were the brains behind the creation of the first medical school in Philadelphia.[30] Harvard Medical School, created by Warren, was initially a two-year program and later it became a three-year-curriculum program, operating without a hospital for clinical instruction for years until Almshouse, an eight-bed hospital, opened its doors to students in 1810. As expected, an eight-bed hospital was not sufficient for the students' clinical instructions; hence, it was moved to Massachusetts General Hospital in 1821. Massachusetts General Hospital was the first hospital to be organized after 1810, and its organization was considered too radical to be adopted by other hospitals until many years later. Dr. James Jackson and J. C. Warren were the major brains behind the establishment of the hospital, and in 1846 Dr. J. C. Warren, the visiting surgeon, performed the first-ever known operation with ether anesthesia in the popular Ether Dome at the hospital. Warren was the advisor and assistant of Jackson, the resident physician.

The first hospital to be established in the nation was St. Philip's Hospital, Charlestown, South Carolina, established in 1736. Others are Pennsylvania Hospital, founded by Dr. Thomas Bond in 1750; New York Hospital in 1771; Charity Hospital of New Orleans, Louisiana; and Bellevue Hospital in New York. Bellevue Hospital is of particular interest in that it reflected the haphazard operation of most hospitals in the latter part of the nation's first century. The hospital was an old prison that was later converted into an almshouse in 1816. In 1871, there were 7,514 patients, out of which 1,102 patients died (14.7%) and the maternity death rate due to puerperal sepsis was 8.7% in the hospital. In 1876, Dr. W. Gill Wylie's Boylston Prize essay decried the deplorable situation of the hospital by alerting the nation to the conditions. Among them was the fact that the nurses were ignorant and worthless characters in some cases; the patients were at the mercy of three night watchmen, for there were no nurses on duty in the 800-bed hospital; and the sanitary conditions were pathetic, so patients died easily from the slightest operations or injuries—about 40 to 60% of all amputations were fatal because of sepsis and other infections. Some of the results of this outcry were that overcrowding in the hospital was reduced, Lister's method of antiseptic dressings was instituted, and trained nurses were hired. For the first time in American history a school training program for nurses started in the latter part of the 19th century at Bellevue Hospital.[30]

Initially, the druggists and chemists imported most of their wholesale drugs from Britain but later revised the mission by tapping their own ingenuity to improvise the drugs locally. They patterned their locally made medicine after the British model of patent medicine and sold the medicine below the prices of apothecaries in order to attract customers. The systematic approach aimed at relegating apothecaries' role as general practitioners of medicine to merely dispensing functions appears to have started in America in the early 19th century. The physicians' battled fervently to restrict the apothecaries to a dispensing function, while the modalities for training new physicians gradually changed from preceptorships to hospital clinical experience. One of the major focuses of the hospital clinical experience was prescription-writing skills. The hospital thus became the only preceptorial form of apprenticeship and the major focus for teaching new physicians (interns) drugs and how to prescribe them through writing. Apprenticeship and acquisition of drug knowledge in the hospital showed a striking resemblance to preceptorship because the preceptor's preference of drugs, bias, and experience (broad or narrow) was carried forward to the interns. The act of compounding was left as part of the dispensing function of apothecaries. However, a growing concern over accurate compounding of drugs arose in the early 19th century and led to the publication of a state guide for standardization of drugs in Massachusetts in 1808. Twelve years later, in 1820, the National Convention of Physicians approved the United States Pharmacopoeia (USP). The USP became the national guide for drug standards, aiding physicians' writing skills and guiding pharmacists' (apothecaries') desire to compound and dispense drugs accurately. It took years for the federal government to recognize the USP as the official medical textbook.

In 1820, the Medical College of Philadelphia, the first medical school in the country, attempted to incorporate pharmaceutical education as part of the medical school curriculum when the school merged with the University of Pennsylvania. The attempt was foiled by pharmacists who anticipated that such a move would further broaden the medical school curriculum, thereby compounding the already complex case of making general practitioners jacks-of-all-trades, masters of none. They went further to argue that such a mission would be tantamount to the elimination of pharmacy schools; hence, they decided to form the first local societies such as the Philadelphia College of Apothecaries (later Pharmacy) in 1821 and the Massachusetts College of Pharmacy in 1823. These groups of apothecaries in combination with some druggists and chemists rose to the occasion of national call for an increased level of professionalism and thus formed the American Pharmaceutical Association (AphA). The thought of forming a national body had its roots in a conference sponsored by the New York College in 1851 purposely to address the issue of adulterated medicinal goods importation. Participants were only pharmacy societies, and at the end of the conference the major focus was the formation of the national body. William Procter Jr., one of Philadelphia College of Pharmacy's representatives; George Coggeshall of New York; and Samuel Colcord of Boston were charged with the responsibility of organizing a national body consisting of local pharmacy groups. They responded by organizing the first national pharmacy organization called the American Pharmaceutical Association in Philadelphia on October 6, 1852.

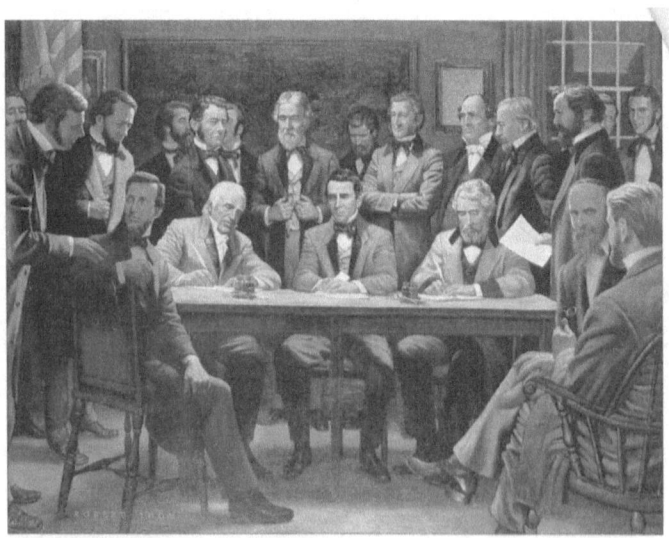

Robert Thom's painting from original portrait photographs of 20 (5 are missing) founding fathers of the American Pharmaceutical Association gathered from eight states around a table in the Philadelphia College of Pharmacy in 1852.

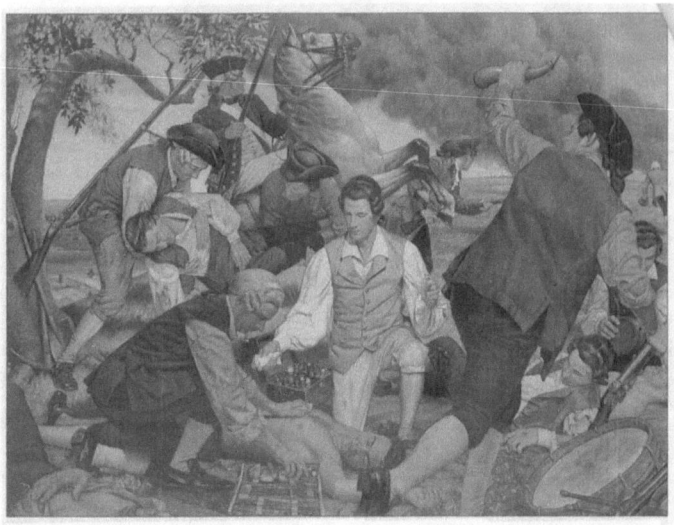

Robert Thom's painting of Andrew Craigie, Boston's pharmacist and America's first apothecary general, attending to the wounded at the Battle of Bunker Hill, June 17, 1775.

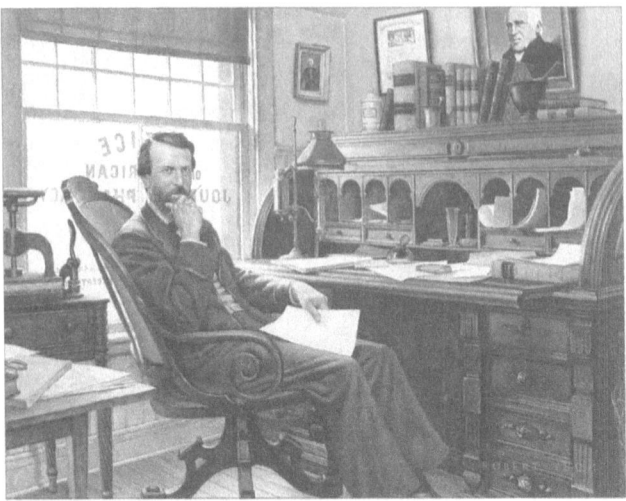

Robert Thom's painting of William Procter Jr. (1817-1874), a man often credited as the father of American pharmacy. William was the first corresponding secretary of AphA and he is shown here in his office as the first editor of the *American Journal of Pharmacy*.

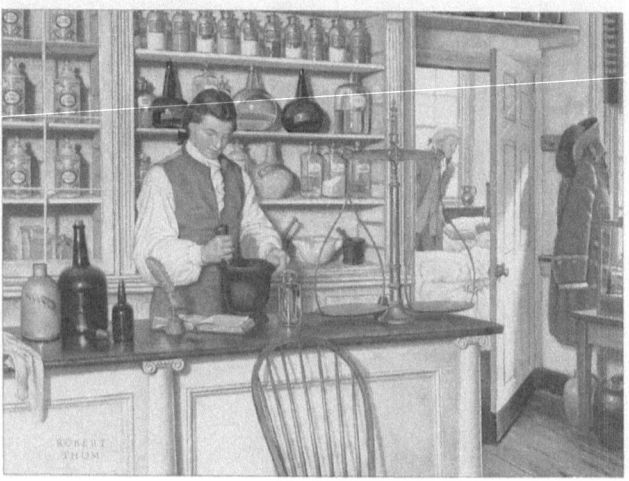

Robert Thom's painting of John Morgan (1735-1789) as apothecary in colonial America's first hospital pharmacy at Pennsylvania Hospital. John later became a medical doctor and was appointed as physician-in-chief of the Continental army in 1776. He preached the need to separate pharmacy from medicine even though specialization wasn't common in his day.

The Industrial Revolution brought rapid development and advanced technology, and forever changed our perception of the world, life activities, and the pace of progress. Pharmacy as an integral part of medicine and human life experienced these changes as well. Industrialization led to the decline of apothecary and the metamorphosis that resulted in the era of count and pour and clinical pharmacy. In pharmacy, industrialization brought large-scale production of drugs by pharmaceutical industries. These drugs, which were previously produced by individual apothecaries (pharmacists), were now better produced on a large scale in a more refined manner, with better quality, and for less cost. Mass production of drugs meant more drugs, and more drugs meant greater market share and subsequent economic gains. The pharmaceutical industry expanded its horizons by discovering new drugs and producing them to meet public demand. The pharmacists filled their shops with these drugs for dispensing purposes as vendors. They engaged themselves in cutthroat competition for customers, and as the drug market became more and more saturated with pharmaceutical goods, pharmacists' knowledge, education, and direct patient's impact became more and more irrelevant as well as restrictive. Many pharmacists rejected the notion that formal education was needed in order to function as a well-rounded pharmacist. Pharmacists' leaders, on the other hand, argued that the major difference between merchants or quack drug sellers and pharmacists was the latter's ability and skill in compounding drugs or official preparation in the shop/in-house. Pharmacists' view about formal education denigrated the profession to the point that around 1860 only 1 out of 20 American pharmacists was formally educated. The situation began to change for the good for numerous reasons. Some of these factors were:

- the advent of new professionals such as the engineers, agriculturists, accountants, and others whose claims of professionalism and competency lie squarely on the acquisition of a university degree and state license in their respective discipline. These new professionals attracted public attention because of the skills they acquired in the university and their ability to produce new inventions and improve and repair existing ones, which differentiated them from the roadside mechanics, farmers, ledger account bookkeepers, and other tradesmen;
- the promulgation of state laws that required passing the state board examination and subsequent registration in the 1870s; and
- discrimination against pharmacists in commissioning military officers as medical practitioners; and others.

Pharmacists became convinced that if they were to forge ahead as professionals, they must not only use their knowledge and skills to differentiate their proficiency and expertise but also back their claims with university degrees and state licenses. Initially university degrees weren't prerequisites for states' licensure. There were educational variations, with students emerging from different backgrounds focusing on passing state boards examinations and becoming pharmacists rather than enhancing their professional image. Numerous local, small, and short-term cram schools emerged, canvassing for students and taking advantage of the situation. The traditional schools of pharmacy such as the University of Michigan's School of Pharmacy refused to just give out degrees, instead emphasizing high standards of education and scholarship for students as far back as 1868. They laid the groundwork for the scientific transformation of pharmacy from vocational courses to full-time courses with laboratory experience. In 1905, New York State preceded others by passing state laws that required diplomas as prerequisites for state licensure. Vocational courses declined and so did the three-year pharmacy program. Pharmacy professional leaders began to articulate their views about pharmacy educational reforms in various local and national associations. In 1928, the American Association of the Colleges of Pharmacy (AACP) adopted a four-year Bachelor of Science/Pharmacy degree (BSc) program as a national requirement for entry-level pharmacists. Four years later, the BSc degree became a criteria/prerequisite for state board examinations and licensure. As technological advancements and the quest for greater drug knowledge accelerated during the mid-20th century, it became obvious that pharmacy professional status deserved more than a four-year program in school. Pharmacists needed to raise their practicing standards, match the status of their colleagues in other branches of medicine, meet public expectations, and gain public confidence. All these factors, coupled with the 1949 pharmaceutical survey and special consideration, led to the proposal of a 6-year doctorate program in pharmacy. A Doctor of Pharmacy degree, otherwise tagged PharmD, had an initially poor response from many pharmacists and others. Pharmacy employers such as the National Association of Chain Drugstores and others argued that there was no market for PharmD because the program would increase labor costs, hike pharmaceutical product (e.g., drug) costs, decrease the number of available pharmacists especially new graduates (they reasoned that students would prefer to add one more year and spend seven years to become graduates in other branches of medicine with higher remuneration than pharmacy), and create a scarcity of pharmacists.

The National Association of Retail Druggists (NARD) was formed in 1898 purposely to cater to the welfare of its members, who were predominantly independent, community pharmacy owners and pharmacists. The aim of the association was to protect its members and drugstores from the encroachment of the ever-expanding large retailers and chain drugstores. Right from the beginning, the leaders of NARD had maintained a low profile in terms of advancing the course of the pharmacy profession scientifically and educationally. Unlike AphA, their vested interest in the commercial success of their members downplayed every other aspect of pharmacy, notably longer years of scholarship in the school of pharmacy. Left alone, the NARD leaders would prefer a shorter duration of pharmacy coursework (e.g., cram schools), which would in turn result in more drugstore owners, more memberships, greater revenue, and a role in national affairs/politics. Little wonder then about the opinion of NARD leaders when the issue of a 6-year doctorate program in pharmacy was proposed. Like the pharmacy employers, NARD leaders argued that a PharmD program was counterproductive. They did not see any advantage in the execution of the program because it would not benefit their members. In spite of the obstacles and horrendous impediments, the University of Southern California started the program in 1950. Pharmacy educators, on the other hand, wondered where they could find the resources, tools, equipment, and laboratories necessary to teach students for the 6 -year program, but gradually they came to terms with reality and comprehended the fact that the pharmacy profession had no alternative but to forge ahead in the direction of change and keep pace with other branches of medicine. Initially, pharmacy educators settled for a 5-year first-degree (BSc) program in order to please both sides: the employers, NARD, and advocates of the PharmD program. The five-year controversial degree program started in Ohio State University two decades earlier before the official commencement in 1960. The program was controversial because neither the employers nor the advocates of the PharmD program were satisfied with the outcome.

Three decades after the commencement of the 5-year program, the AACP was again faced with the reality of time, choice, and the need to advance pharmacy in the interest of posterity. They finally adopted the 6-year PharmD program as entry level for pharmacists, and all colleges of pharmacy are expected to be in full compliance by the year 2005. This is likely to increase to about 8 or 9 years (4 years for the first degree, four years in the school of pharmacy, and probably a one-year or more residence program) in the future so as to even up pharmacy with the other branches of medicine. Besides the economic consequences of prolonged pharmacy coursework, many people have supported the views of NARD by questioning the rationale behind spending 5 or 6 years in school for a job that restricts one's professional performance and practice to mere dispensing functions—the throwing of pills from a large bottle into smaller ones. All the years of college work had little or no impact on the profession. This restrictive role of the pharmacist was further compounded by the controversial stand of the AphA with the adoption of the code of ethics in 1922. The 1922 code of ethics prevented pharmacists from discussing the therapeutic effects of drugs with patients. Pharmacists were asked to send such patients to the physicians for adequate response, and more than four decades later the code of ethics was repealed in 1969. Pharmacists were now asked to use their drug knowledge to impact patients' health care needs.[1]

A decline in the number of dispensing shops owned by physicians, an increase in the number of prescriptions written by physicians, an increase in number of pharmaceutical industries, and production of industrial pharmaceutical products (drugs etc) coupled with a decrease in act of compounding by pharmacists led to the robotic approach of pharmacists to professional practices. Compounding of active ingredients specifically made for each patient as prescription drugs constitutes 75% of the pharmacist's dispensing act in 1930, about 25% in 1950, 4% in 1960, 1% in 1970, and 0.01% in 1990. As compounding degenerated into oblivion, the robotic era of count and pour came into being with a pharmacist pouring pills from a large container into a well-labeled, smaller container, otherwise called a vial. The above situation resulted in astronomical growth of dispensing prescriptions by pharmacists; consequently, pharmacists didn't feel the economic crunch of the compounding disappearance. Economic growth of dispensing prescriptions compensated pharmacists well enough for their job performance that they trivialized their clinical skills and patients' health impact. The appearance of newer, safer, and more effective drugs from the early to mid-20th century helped to boost the sales of prescription drugs dispensed by pharmacists and resulted in gravitation of big companies, retailers, and chain drugstores to the pharmacy business. These big companies and chain drugstores came to the pharmacy business and spread their wings and tentacles across localities, cities, counties, districts, states, and now across international boarders. They grow in size and shape and eventually displace the independent or community pharmacy, otherwise known as the corner drugstore. Competition for patrons/patients stiffens and it becomes increasingly difficult for independent corner drugstores to compete favorably with the chain drugstores. The chain drugstores have large assets to canvass for customers and overcome any shortcomings or depression in any store. The corner drugstore in sharp contrast has limited resources to canvass for customers and overcome any depression; consequently, they are being weeded out of the national economy. This is one of the major reasons why NARD was formed in 1898, to help protect these independent community drugstores against the ever-increasing encroachment of chain drugstores. NARD may have played their role and performed their function in the leaders' view but very little has been done to stem the tidal wave causing the extinction of the community pharmacy. The downward trend continues and no one knows what the end result will be. It might be difficult to eradicate completely the independent community pharmacy but bad omens continue to plague the individual community pharmacy owner.

New drug phenomenon is a relative term in that today's exciting new discovery could become tomorrow's nightmare: old and obsolete drugs. An exciting new drug discovered in 1945 is an old drug in 1990; the same is true of a new drug in 2003 in reference to the future. Throughout human history, the desire to discover new ways and means of resolving human ailments, thereby gaining public recognition, praises, and financial reward, has been a motivating factor for humanity. Consequently, there has always been a new drug (active ingredients) discovered from microorganisms, animals, plants, soil, water, and chemical substances. However, the concepts of new drugs became more evident with the coming of pharmaceutical industries into drug business. The pharmaceutical industries expanded the drug business horizon in terms of both research and discovery of new drugs. Research is the bane of discoveries, and it is championed by scientists. Scientific research by Pasteur and Joubert in 1877 led to the discovery of certain bacteria that can kill anthrax bacilli when cultured.[10] Led Vullemin later used the outcome of this research and other microbiologists' research to define the term "antibiosis," which means the destruction of one organism by another in order to preserve itself (a biologic view of "survival of the fittest" theory). Waksman in 1942 modernized the concept to reflect the term "antibiotic," which means the production of certain substances that are capable of inhibiting growth or the destruction of other microorganisms by one microorganism.

Humoral theory of diseases served humanity for millennia, until the 19th century when the search for agents of diseases led to cellular biology and germ theory of disease. The formation of the American Medical Association (AMA) in 1847 by allopathic medical practitioners helped to propagate and strengthen the germ theory of disease and weaken the scientifically baseless humoral theory of disease. The AMA goal was to stamp out medicine not based on empiricism and science by replacing the humoral theory of disease with germ theory. Louis Pasteur's laboratory research produced other great discoveries such as the rabies vaccine, thus making him one of the front-runners of the germ theory of disease. Like Pasteur, Paul Ehrlich (1854-1915) is another great pillar of germ theory. He is often described as the founding father of chemotherapy, molecular pharmacology, and medicinal chemistry. Ehrlich's major research work started with dyes in the late 19th century in Germany. He successfully stained some human white blood cells—leukocytes (beginning of modern hematology)—and thought that it would one day be possible to selectively stain and probably kill microscopic pathogens without destroying the host ("magic bullet" theory). Ehrlich and his cohort produced several organoarsenic drugs such as typan red, the first synthetic antimalaria drug, in 1904; atoxyl in 1905; salvarsan #606, the first antisyphilitic drug, in 1909, after identifying treponema pallidum as the causative agent (spirochetes) in 1906; suramin in 1917 for African sleeping sickness; pamaquin, an antimalaria drug, in 1926; prontosil, the first antimalaria-antibacteria sulfonamide drug, in 1932; the first broad-spectrum antibiotic-chloramphenicol in 1947 from S. venezuelae; and revealed quinine's structure in 1908.[10,11,25] Ehrlich's success and mission may not have achieved his set goals of a magic bullet, but he did turn out a lot of new drugs for resolving human ailments.

Alexander Fleming's name is almost synonymous with the term antibiotic today because of his awesome discovery of penicillin. In 1928, Fleming stumbled upon the antibacterial properties of penicillium when he discovered the effects of a penicillium mold colony he accidentally placed in a petri dish. Florey and Chain later developed the discovery and made penicillin into therapeutic forms in 1938. The threat of World War II at the tail end of the 1930s made the British embark on large-scale production of the drug penicillin.[1,10] Waksman and his cohort discovered the first aminoglycoside, another class of antibiotic, streptomycin in 1944, and in combination with Lechevalier they discovered neomycin from S. fradiae in 1949. Umezawa isolated kanamycin in 1957 in Japan, and Weistein discovered gentamycin in 1958. In 1945, Giuseppe Brotzu discovered that the cultures of C. acremonium, a cephalosporium fungican, inhibited both gram-positive and negative bacteria. Abraham and his cohort later developed the concept in Oxford in 1948 and isolated three different types of cephalosporin. Duggar discovered chlortetracycline, the first tetracycline, from S. aureofaciens in 1948; Finlay and others isolated oxytetracycline in 1950 from S. rimosus; Conover later found tetracycline and patented it in 1955; and Stephens et al. found doxycycline in 1958. Picromycin was the first macrolide to be isolated in 1950; this was followed by McGuire and others' discovery of the erythromycin in 1952. Magerlein and others discovered clindanycin in 1967. In 1963, nalidixic acid was introduced first as quinolones; this was followed by others like cipro in 1987, floxin and penetrex in 1991, and omniflox and maxaquin in 1992. In 1939, Dubos found tyrothricin in Bacillus brevis culture, and gramicidin was later isolated from it; Meleney and others isolated bacitracin from B. subticis, an organism obtained from the tissue of 7-year-old Margaret Tracy's compound fracture in 1945. Koyama and coworkers discovered colistin from Aerobacillus colistinus in 1950. In 1956, McCormick and others obtained vancomycin from S. orientalis.

Other anti-infectives include the discovery of polymyxin B sulfate in the U.S. and Britain in 1947; amphotericin B in 1956 as antifungal from streptomyces nodosus by Gold and others; nystatin from S. noursi by Hazen and Brown in 1951; griseofulvin from penicillium griseofulvum by Oxford and others in 1939; isoniazid as an antitubercular drug in 1952; and zidovudine as an antiviral by Lin and Prusoff in 1978. The other classes of drugs are antineoplastic agents (e.g., methotrexate in 1949, mechlorethamine in 1946, mercaptopurine in 1952, fluorouracil in 1957, etc.); anesthetics (e.g., halothane in 1956); anxiolytics (e.g., benzodiazepines, buspirone); sedatives/hypnotics (e.g., barbiturates, phenobarbital in 1912, meprobamate); antipsychotics (e.g., phenothiazines, chlorpromazine in 1954, haloperidol); anticonvulsants (e.g., phenytoin in late 1930s, valproic acid); antidepressants (e.g., imipramine in 1959, amitriptyline, fluozetine); bronchodilators (e.g., albuterol, metaproterenol); antihypertensives (e.g., reserpin in 1953, hydrochlorothiazide in 1959, metoprolol in 1978); cardiovascular drugs (e.g., nitrogylcerine, verapamil in 1962); antiarrhythmics (e.g., quinidine, amiodarone); antihyperlipidemics (e.g., gemfibrozil, lovastatin); anticoagulants (e.g., warfarin in 1954, streptokinase); hypoglycemics (e.g., guanidine in 1918, tolbutamide in 1957); thyroid hormones (e.g., thyroxine in 1916, levothyroxine); antithyroid drugs (e.g., propylthiouracil); antihistamines (e.g., diphenhydramine or benadryl by Park-Davis in 1946, clemastine, terfenadine); antiacids (e.g., famotidine, omeprazole); anti-inflammatory (e.g., corticosteroid-hydrocortisone in 1952, ibuprofen, naproxene); contraceptives and hormone therapy (e.g., estrogen, diethylstilbestrol DES in 1946, progesterone in the 1940s, testosterone, oxandrolone); analgesics (e.g., aspirin in 1899, morphine in 1806, meperidine in 1938); neuromuscular blocking agents (e.g., tubocurarine by Squibb in 1946); thrombin (by Upjohn in 1946); and others.

These drugs as an integral part of pharmacy have saved millions of lives around the world since their discovery. As noted, it is important for people to know how and when these drugs came into being so that they will comprehend and appreciate the fact that there was time when humanity existed without these wonder drugs. These drugs have helped to sustain human life, improve the quality of life, and prolong life for all. Most of the antibiotics came to the market in the 1940s and 1950s. Their success in shaping the outcome of diseases as anti-infectives changed people's view and concepts about annexing the environment for the benefit of mankind. Pharmacists wasted no time in stocking their pharmacies with these drugs and making them available whenever requested by the patrons with or without prescriptions (Pharmacists can recommend and sell over-the-counter medications). As many pharmacists avail themselves of these new drugs and depend solely on dispensing them from the shelves, a few other optimistic pharmacists realized the fact that the future of pharmacy does not depend on a pharmacist's restrictive role as a dispenser but on clinical functions and the ability to impact patients' health outcome as a health care provider. This is because computerization and automation are in the making, ready to take over pharmacists' role as dispenser of drugs, and it is cheaper to acquire, maintain, and own computers for a considerable length of time than to shoulder a pharmacist's financial responsibilities. These optimistic pharmacists are the forerunners of clinical pharmacy. They perceived health care reforms because of the need to reduce health care costs, dispense pharmaceutical care, and improve patients' well-being/health outcome as a future goal of pharmacy. This is the driving force behind many pharmacies' innovative efforts including the initiatives of the director of hospital pharmacy in New York City, who decided to train pharmacists for patient care on a one-on-one basis in 1996.

Until the 1960s, the health care delivery system in America since independence was predominantly twofold: the part that belongs to the rich, affluent, and powerful members of the society and the part that belongs to the poor, downtrodden, and less fortunate members of the society. The latter were at the mercy of volunteer groups, churches, and philanthropists. There were no medical services for the poor in the absence of these three groups; consequently, if you were sick and you had no means of paying for medical services, you could not go to the hospital or any other medical facilities, or else you would be sent back home. The Great Depression of 1929 and subsequent ravaging economic impacts deepened the problems further and revealed the inadequacy of these three groups in meeting the social needs, including health care provisions for the poor, needy, and elderly people of the society. The situation persisted with no end in sight until the election of Franklin D. Roosevelt as president of United States of America, which ushered in a new era of social reforms in 1933. Part of these social reforms was the enactment of the Social Security Act in 1935. The Social Security Act guaranteed every member of society some degree of protection against unemployment and provision toward retirement benefits and health insurance. This marked the beginning of government's central role in the regulation and provision of social services. Medicare was not originally part of the Social Security Act, but its roots can be traced to the program.[13,14] Rhode Island's representative Forand first introduced the Medicare bill in the house during Harry Truman's regime in August 1957. The bill was meant to cater to the health needs of millions of aged Americans who were facing an uphill battle in securing health insurance for themselves. The hearing that followed enumerated a myriad of problems and pathetic health conditions of senior citizens. The bill did not pass into law until Arkansas's representative Wilbur Mills sponsored a compromise bill, which combined health insurance for the elderly paid for by payroll tax deductions and state-administered health insurance for the poor. It passed through the house in 1965 during Lyndon Johnson's era. The bill was tagged the Social Security Amendment Act. It was signed into law in July 1965 and became effective in 1966. Wilbur Mill's compromise bill heralds the genesis of Title XVIII of the Social Security Amendment Act (Medicare) and Title XIX of the Social Security Amendment Act (Medicaid). Medicaid, a state means-tested program designed to guarantee health insurance for the poor, was crafted as a last-minute resolution in the form of grants to the states and state governments. Medicare and Medicaid are twin brothers, and the former is financed entirely by the federal government.

There is no doubt that Medicare and Medicaid changed the health care delivery system in America for good and forever resulted in a soaring demand for health care products and services, and increased drug usage by the populace. Increased demand for health care products, services, and drugs led to price gouging that escalated out of hand and went beyond anything ever predicted or envisaged by the originators of the programs. As noted in chapter one, the astronomical high price of health care eats deeply into the fabric of the society to the point where all and sundry, including citizens, employers, businesses, and federal and state governments, became concerned and worried. The nation's concern was not only about rising costs of health care but also the fact that rising costs of health care did not necessarily mean better health care services. At the turn of the millennium, by the year 2000, there was no doubt about the fact that the U.S. without rivalry was the number-one country in the world in terms of technological advancement, production of effective new drugs, medical advances, education, and many other issues; however, a comparative data analysis reveals that the U.S. is not necessarily the best country as far as health care delivery to citizens is concerned. For instance, by the year 1992, the U.S. spent the highest gross domestic product (GDP) on health care but ranked eighteenth in the world in terms of longevity. The world's best health care delivery statistics as reflected by longevity/increased life span showed that:

- Japan spent 6.8% of its GDP on health care and ranked 1st with a 78.6-year life expectancy.

- Sweden spent 8.8% of its GDP on health care and ranked 4th with a 77.7-year life expectancy.

- Canada spent 9.9% of its GDP on health care and ranked 7th th with a 77.2-year life expectancy.

- France spent 9.1% of its GDP on health and ranked 12th with a 76.6-year life expectancy.

- United Kingdom spent 6.6% of its GDP on health care and ranked 14th with a 75.8-year life expectancy.

- Germany spent 9.1% of its GDP on health care and ranked 17th with a 75.6-year life expectancy

- USA spent 13.3% of its GDP on health care and ranked 18th with a 75.6-year life expectancy.

In the U.S., the health care fraction of gross national product or gross domestic product (GDP) rose from 5.2% in 1960 to 13.9% in 1993 and 14.4% in 2001. *Grandfather Economic Health Care Report* showed that America spends 82% more per person on health care than other nations, yet rank 37th in the world in terms of quality of health care as per the June 2000 *Bradenton Herald-Tribune*. Japan spends $1,750 per person and France spends $2,100 per person, while the U.S. spends $3,724 per person on health care. France's health care system ranked the best in the world according to this report. The top ten nations along with France were Italy, San Marino, Andorra, Malta, Singapore, Spain, Oman, Austria, and Japan. The United States along with Finland, Australia, Chile, Denmark, Dominica, Costa Rica, Slovenia, Cuba, and Brunei ranked the 4th-ten best nations in the world. The report added a 1997 statistical abstract of life expectancy in 13 nations: U.S.—76 years; Australia—about 79.5 years; France—about 78.5 years; Germany—76 years; Hong Kong—about 82.3 years; Italy—about 78.2 years; Japan—about 79.2 years; Canada—about 79.3 years; Switzerland—about 77.9 years; England—about 76.3 years; Holland—78 years; Greece—78.2 years; and Mexico—74 years. A 1998 total health care spending statistic as a percentage of GDP in 11 nations showed: U.S.—14.2%; Germany—10.5%; France—9.7%; Canada—9.5%; Australia and the Netherlands—8.5%; Italy—7.8%; Spain—7.7%; Sweden—7.5%; Japan—7.4%; and Britain—7.0%. Medical fraction of consumer price index (CPI) rose by 7.3% when other goods and services rose by only 2.8% annually. Prescription drug expenditure was found to greatly outpace overall health care spending. Total prescription drug spending rose from $12 billion in 1980 to $103.9 billion dollars in 1999. In February 2003, federal centers for Medicare and Medicaid services (CMS) showed an updated record of health care expenditure in the country as $1.42 trillion in 2001, and this represents a total increase of 8.7% over the previous year. Prescription drug expenditure alone in 2001 was 15.7% more than in

2000, and the overall increase in 2001 resulted in the U.S. spending 14.4% of its GDP on health care. The same source showed that Americans spent $1.6 trillion or $5,440 per person on health care in 2002, and this represents an over 9% increase from the previous year. To worsen the situation, countries such as Canada, the United Kingdom, Germany, Japan, and Cuba with lower health care expenditures have universal health coverage for their citizens, while Americans belong to the category of "pay for medical services or drop dead."

In spite of Medicare and Medicaid, the number of Americans without health insurance rose from 27 million in 1977 to 41.5 million in 1993 (45 million by the 2004). 85% of those without health insurance are adults (with families) working as low-income earners (working poor—the majority of whom have income below 200% poverty level). The myriad of problems facing politicians about the American health care system has no end in sight. It shows that health care costs will continue to eat deeply into the fabric of the society. Americans are demanding not only a reduction in health care cost but also a way to make the health care system more effective and responsive to patients' health needs. Some programs such as hospital capital expenditure control, voluntary planning, utilization review, and price and wage freezing were enacted and put into practice but couldn't bring health care costs under control. Other methods include the Health Maintenance Organization (HMO) Act that was signed into law by Richard Nixon in 1973, diagnosis-related groups, and the Medicare Catastrophic Coverage Act of 1983 (MCCA). The MCCA couldn't stand because of drug benefits that taxed the wealthy elderly and passed little or nothing to the poor elderly. The wealthy elderly vigorously attacked treatment inequalities in the program; hence, the MCCA was eventually repealed and later incorporated in the 1990 Omnibus Budget Reconciliation Act (OBRA).

OBRA '90 was the first legislative act that mandated pharmacists to perform drug utilization reviews (DUR) and to counsel patients before dispensing prescribed drugs. OBRA '90 provided a forum for pharmacists, especially the optimistic ones, to expand their clinical role in the health care delivery system and to make a meaningful impact on patients' health care needs. One of the major factors responsible for enacting OBRA '90 was the result of numerous studies that showed how pharmacists' intervention saved human lives, reduced health care costs, prevented drug-related morbidity and mortality, ensured effective use of drugs, and promoted adequate health outcomes. One of these studies, as noted in chapter one, is the mental analysis study conducted by C. D. Hepler and L. M. Strand in their project entitled "Opportunities and Responsibilities in Pharmaceutical Care." Although clinical pharmacy was already in existence before the enactment of OBRA

'90, pharmacists had no legal backing for direct impact on patients' health care needs. OBRA '90 thus provided the first limited legal backing for pharmacists' direct impact on patients' health care needs through counseling. Pharmacists are expected to spend 2 to 4 minutes counseling per prescription at the supposed rate of $1 to $2. Some studies (the 1992 survey, for example) showed an increase in pharmacists' counseling 6 out of 10 patients after enactment of the act in 1990. The state of Georgia is said to have experienced a 16% increase, from 55% to 71%, since the enactment of the acts. There has been a lot of controversy surrounding counseling from both the pharmacists' and patients' point of view. Counseling is a limited form of practice because it doesn't guarantee pharmacists' autonomy. Many pharmacists are frustrated by the fact that most patients come to the pharmacy with the traditional outlook of it performing a dispensing function only. They believe that the traditional medical doctor has done the major work, so all that the pharmacist has to do is give them the drug. In most cases they are not ready to listen to any conversation or waste time on counseling, and this explains why the best time to capture a patient's attention is during recommendation. Recommendation time represents a "window of opportunity" to discuss vital issues about drugs that will sink into a patient's memory and last for the entire duration of therapy. The long-lasting nature of anything discussed during this window of opportunity is enough for many patients to ignore pharmacy drug labels and directions while keeping track of therapeutic requirements as dictated by the physician. In short, some patients resist or show indifferent attitudes to a pharmacist's counseling because they don't want anything to confuse them further or interfere with their first impression of therapy. The importance of the window of opportunity as a first impression about therapy lies in the fact that once a patient has been told what is wrong with them (diagnosis) the next thing they want to know is what to do in order to rectify the problem and improve the condition (therapy). Once any health care practitioner misses the window of opportunity to discuss therapy, it is difficult to build trust in the patient again. It appears that many pharmacists do a better job at counseling and recommending over-the-counter (OTC) drugs to patients than the legend drugs because of this issue.

Counseling may or may not have achieved its intended goal, but it aided pharmacists in the provision of pharmaceutical care to patients. Pharmaceutical care has been defined by Hepler and Strand as the responsible provision of drug therapy for the purpose of achieving definite outcomes that improve patient's quality of life. These outcomes are the curing of disease, elimination or reduction of patients' symptomatology, arresting or slowing of disease processes, preventing a disease, or symptomatology.[15] Pharmaceutical care was adopted as the profession's goal after two conferences were convened by pharmacy leaders in 1984 and 1989. The aim of the conferences was to define "pharmacy in the 21st century."[3,16] Pharmaceutical care became the rallying point for the profession and every pharmacist was expected to incorporate it into their daily functions. Pharmacists were implored to use the SOAP format (Subjective, Objective, Assessment, and Plan) in every encounter with patients. The SOAP format entails going through the following steps:

- SUBJECTIVE: Pharmacists are expected to establish a relationship with patients; collect patients' information based on their observation or complaints; list patients' drug-related problems; and allow patients to express their views, understanding, concerns, expectations, and fears about drug therapy including over-the-counter medications. All necessary information has to be documented.
- OBJECTIVE: Pharmacists perform their tasks such as measuring vital signs and lab values; physical assessments; checking prescription orders for appropriateness and irregularities; checking a patient's profile for DUR, if any; and calling other health care professionals to clarify issues if need be. All necessary information must be documented.
- ASSESSMENT: Pharmacists analyze information gathered from subjective and objective data about patients, diseases, and drug problems (such as drug/drug interaction, drug/disease interaction, drug/food interaction, or concern about drug therapy). The pharmacist will note present and future problematic areas and make adequate documentation.
- PLAN: This involves two steps, which are choosing therapy and intervention, and follow up until the end. In choosing therapy and intervention, the pharmacist will ensure that all disease states are adequately treated with or without drugs, ensure cost effectiveness of the drug choice, set reasonable goals that aim to maximize the objective of therapy, resolve drug therapy problems with or without drug and disease research, avoid drug/drug interactions, avoid therapeutic duplications, counsel patients about drug therapy, give patients supportive education materials, and make referrals to other health care professionals if need be. Follow-up plans involve monitoring treatment (through efficacy or patients' improvement, urine tests, etc.); adequate contact with patients either through planned office visits or by phone; results of therapeutic outcome; and if unsuccessful, repeat the process again, starting from assessment, with some necessary change. The end will be determined by the patient's cure of his medical condition, relocation, refusal to accept

further treatment, or death. Most chronic illness with successful therapeutic outcome requires continuation of therapy till a patient's death (end) and all steps require adequate documentation. The pharmacist must aim to decrease emergency room visits, clinic or physician office visits, and others.

As laudable as it sounds, pharmaceutical care confronted greater problems than its twin sister, counseling. Counseling and pharmaceutical care came into being simultaneously around the early 1990s. Pharmaceutical care confronts the problems of pharmacists' autonomy in greater magnitude than counseling. The Law et al. study of patients, physicians, and pharmacists' opinions about improving medication use shows that pharmacists accepted federal and state laws that mandated medication use counseling as a mainstay of professional practice; but physicians and patients vehemently opposed the idea, arguing that pharmacists' role should be restricted to a dispensing function only. Law and others blamed pharmacists for their inability to convince people of their mandated services through communication. The truth of the matter is that pharmacy autonomy is the major barrier. Pharmacy is the only profession in the world that is held captive by its own fate and is prevented from doing what it does best as specialists in their own field. Many might want to shy away from reality, but the truth of the matter is that pharmaceutical care as defined and presented above will only be meaningful if and when pharmacists start operating as independent health care practitioners in terms of therapeutic choice, adjustment, and elimination of irrelevant treatment. The above SOAP modalities are not different from physicians' protocol in dealing with patients' health care needs except that much of its emphasis is on therapy as dictated by specialist protocol in the medical field. Clinical pharmacists are trained therapeuticians, while most physicians are trained diagnosticians by virtue of the training protocol in schools. This training protocol in schools is explained in later chapters. Except for the law that is a lagging indicator, pharmacists, especially clinical pharmacists, are prepared to take full responsibility for this act as shown by numerous studies. These studies showed that pharmacists who are granted various degrees of freedom to choose drugs, eliminate unwanted ones, and adjust therapy to suit and impact a patient's health outcome through pharmaceutical care have statistical data to prove their worth. Some of these data are available in Veteran Administration Medical Centers (hospitals), correctional facilities (prisons), nursing homes, the pharmacy project ImPACT in Asheville, North Carolina, and others. Pharmacy is probably the only profession in the world that can be held responsible for other people's mistakes. As close as it seems, no siblings (brothers and sisters) or adults are held responsible for each other's mistakes in most societies in the world, yet the pharmacist can be held liable in the court for blunders committed by physicians. Collective responsibility or liability in the American health care system is an indication that one branch of medicine can be held responsible for another's mistakes if it fails to detect the blunder irrespective of the volume of work, the nature of business, and other commitments.

The implementation of pharmaceutical care has other barriers besides autonomy, which is the centerpiece of all problems. Other notable barriers are excessive workload, pharmacy layout, inadequate privacy, lack of financial reward by third parties, difficulties in contacting physicians and physicians' negative attitude, inadequate references and supporting education materials for patients, patient's attitude, peer pressure, fear of litigation, and pharmacy legal regulations. Recognition of pharmacy as a specialty like every other branch of medicine would eliminate or reduce most of these problems to the barest minimum. For instance, pharmacy autonomy would eliminate difficulties contacting physicians and physicians' negative attitude because their relationship would not be different from any other interdisciplinary cooperation in which professionals act independently without need for each other's decisions. Pharmacists as therapeuticians (therapeutic physicians) or drug specialists will focus their attention on disease-state management, the effective combination of drugs with minimal risks or side effects, resolution of drug therapy problems, and selection of cost-effective drugs for simple or complex cases. This phenomenon will eventually carve out a niche for the pharmacists and force other practitioners such as general practitioners, dentists, internists, dermatologists, ophthalmologists, and others to refer patients to them the same way they refer patients to other specialists when patients' health care problems are beyond their expertise level. Pharmacists, on the other hand, will recognize the fact that they are therapists; consequently, general practitioners and other specialists will be recognized for reference purposes for cases outside the pharmacists' jurisdiction (e.g., complex diagnosis, dental, ophthalmic, etc.).

Other issues such as financial rewards will follow suit because third-party payers will be forced to recognize pharmacy as an autonomous medical specialty and reward the practitioners accordingly for their services. Financial reward will help to create a better pharmacy layout with adequate privacy, references, and supportive education materials for patients. Initially, pharmacy autonomy will create two sets of pharmacists but as time goes on, market forces will resolve the problems by eliminating one set of pharmacists at the expense of the other. The two sets of pharmacists that will be created initially are the clinical pharmacists, otherwise know as therapeuticians (therapeutic physicians) or drug specialists, and the archaic pharmacists, those that wish to remain with the old, traditional form of dispensing function only. The archaic pharmacists are definitely going to be eliminated at the expense of the clinical pharmacists; however, pharmacists should be made to play by the rules until the market forces take control. The rule is that, like other health care practitioners/specialists, no pharmacist should be allowed to play both roles as a clinician and dispenser. The pharmacists with a PharmD who want to be dispensers cannot be clinicians. However, the pharmacists with a first degree (BSc) who want to be clinicians must first and foremost go back to school and upgrade their educational status to Doctor of Pharmacy (PharmD) or be content with the role of dispenser for the rest of their lives. It is obvious that as pharmacists become clinicians, market forces are going to readjust in such a way as to make contemporary pharmacy technicians, dispensers. In the long run, after decades if not centuries, pharmacy technicians will be upgraded to first-degree-level (BSc) jobs while pharmacy will even up with the other branches of medicine requiring first degrees (BSc) for entry into pharmacy schools and four years of didactic class work/rotations before residence.

This gesture will decrease the workload for physicians and pharmacists alike, create more time for patients, and give room for better job performance. It is however, not clear if there will be laws regulating health care practitioners' volume of work or if the market forces will be allowed to control the situation irrespective of job performance/effectiveness. The fear of litigation and pharmacy legal requirements that are bound to come with pharmacy autonomy plague some contemporary pharmacists, but they should be rest assured that pharmacy is not alone or an exception because it applies to all branches of medicine. However, those pharmacists who thought that the dispensing-only function shields them from legal action might find themselves in hot water in the future if they want to be clinicians, because the pharmacy profession is fast becoming a case of "if you can't stand the heat, you might have to excuse the kitchen." For example, an Illinois pharmacy organization's pleas help to explain this issue to some extent. Around the mid-1990s, the Illinois Pharmacists Association and the National Association of Boards of Pharmacy (NABP) implored the Illinois Supreme Court to declare as null and void the "no duty to warn" rule because it is dialectically opposed to pharmacists' mandate by prevailing social attitudes and state and federal laws to counsel patients about proper use of drugs. They claimed that pharmacists are professionals by all standards and should be treated as such by the law. The NABP quoted a 1988 survey which revealed that 92% of members of the public or general population "express a desire to have a pharmacist available for personal consultation" and "wanted advice" on storage of drugs, side effects, how to medicate themselves, drug/drug and drug/food interactions. Attorneys William J. Cremer and Thomas R. Pender in their article for *For the Defense*, the monthly journal of the Defense Research Institute (the largest civil litigation defense attorneys association in the U.S.), noted the increasing nature of pharmacists' liability because of judicial expansion of their duty to warn (recall OBRA '90) and the desire to extend their patient care role.[22]

In November 2004, an appellate court in Tennessee state reinstated the *Dubois v Haykal's* case, a lawsuit filed by a patient against her physician and pharmacy. The plaintiff (patient) was treated for bipolar disorder with carbamazepine (Tegretol) by her physician. During the office visit or counseling with the physician she revealed the fact that she was on oral contraceptives to prevent pregnancy and her medical condition was due to divorce and her son's developmental problems because of significant birth defects. She filled the carbamazepine prescription in her regular pharmacy where she gets her oral contraceptives on a routine basis. Two months later she became pregnant despite the oral contraceptive medication. A gynecologist told her during an office visit that carbamazepine is a known teratogenic (causes birth defects) drug after reviewing her regimen. She immediately terminated the pregnancy in order to prevent the birth of another child with birth defects. The abortion clinic employees informed her that carbamazepine compromised the effectiveness of oral contraceptives there by raising the therapeutic issue of combining both drugs in a patient's regimen. She sued the physician and pharmacy for refusing to warn her about the dangers of combining both drugs. The plaintiff produced two expert witnesses, and the defendants implored the court to dismiss the case for lack of merit in their motion. The trial court dismissed the case after reviewing the record and experts' testimonies, claiming that the plaintiff had failed to established her case of inaction by the defendants. The court ruled that the expert's testimonies was unreliable and inadmissible. The plaintiff appealed the judgment to the appellate court in Tennessee. One of the expert witnesses in the trial court was a clinical pharmacist who asserted that in the absence of a gastrointestinal problems that can interfer with patient's absorption of the oral contraceptives, assuming that the patient took the medication, the only thing that can reduced the effectiveness of the oral contraceptives is carbamazepine. The clinical pharmacist cited peer review and studies that justified carbamazepine as a known liver (hepatic) enzymes inducer that can metabolized oral contraceptives and may reduce the effectiveness of the drug. The appellate court reviewed this testimony and the physician's expert similar testimony and ruled that the experts' data and research were trustworthy as a result the trial court erred in it judgment. The judgment was reversed and the case was reinstated.[33] These issues send a good will message to the "dispensing function only" pharmacists that there is no room for them in the profession, nor will there be legal backing by professional organizations for dispensing-only function.

Besides legal backing, these pharmacists need to realize the issues at stake with the pharmacy profession. The profession is feeling the heat of dispensing functions only like a fish out of water or tea without sugar. Employers of labor are already shrugging their shoulders and shaking their heads that pharmacists' salary for dispensing functions only is unrealistic. They can't understand why they have to pay pharmacists so much if they can pay pharmacy technicians to perform the same functions with little or no difference. For instance, the president and vice president of the Florida Pharmacy Association in the November 2004 issue of *Florida Pharmacy Today* highlighted employers' viewpoint and perturbation about pharmacists' salary. President Glenn Boyles (2004–2005) in his article "It's Time to Make Our Case for the Value of Pharmacy Services" said that technology and hardware are already in place to efficiently and cost effectively replace pharmacists' role, and these trends are difficult to reverse, according to him. He implored pharmacists to consider the possibilities of a greater demand for pharmacist-technician ratios, remote medication order processing, central prescription-filling services, Internet prescription services, and automated dispensing machines in hospices, long-term care facilities, and prisons. Vice President Michael Jackson in his article "Working to Preserve Our Profession" echoed employers' sentiments by using the word "unsustainable." He said employers would likely use this term to describe pharmacist salaries and reimbursements. They both claimed that employers are staying late at night or burning night candles to determine how to reduce manpower costs.[31,32] The good news for these "dispensing function" only pharmacists is that pharmacy autonomy will take time to materialize even when everything is all right with the law; consequently, some of them will be dead; many will face retirement, if they are not already retired; and schools of pharmacy would have saturated the job market with clinical pharmacists (PharmD holders) in America by the time pharmacy takes its proper place in the medical field. The number of operating pharmacists with a first degree (BSc) will be infinitesimally low in the society, and market demand for them will be little or nothing. All first-degree holders have good options in upgrading their educational status to doctorate level, so if they failed to utilize the golden opportunity, it is their funeral and nobody else's making.

Regulation of health care policy in America went into full gear at the beginning of the 20th century. Prior to the 20th century there were no laws governing food and drugs; however, numerous adulteration of food and drugs with resultant consequences of civilian casualties culminated in the creation of various laws. In 1902, twelve children died in St. Louis as a result of tetanus-contaminated diphtheria vaccine, and there was spontaneous public outcry that eventually led to the creation of several laws including the 1902 Biologics Control Act for vaccines. The other laws were meant to prevent the selling of adulterated drugs in the country, and the secretary of agriculture was asked to investigate all drugs suspected of adulteration. In order to conduct this investigation in an effective manner, a drug laboratory that later became the Food and Drug Administration (FDA) was carved out of what was the Agriculture Bureau of Chemists in Washington, D.C., under the leadership of Dr. Harvey Wiley. Dr. Wiley used his strategic position to launch a volunteer "Poison Squad," an organization whose aim was to test food with chemical preservative treatments. The findings of the Poison Squad led to the publication of *The Jungle*, an Upton Sinclair novel, in February 1906. Another public outcry led to the "pure food movement" and eventually resulted in the enactment of the Pure Food and Drug Act by the Congress in mid-1906. The growing need for the safety of food and drugs among the public culminated in the separation of the Food and Drug Administration from the department of agriculture in 1927.[17,18]

The 1906 acts required food and drugs to be pure but not necessarily safe, so certain products met the requirements but weren't safe. Some of these products contained ethylene glycol (antifreeze) and thallium. Ethylene glycol is a sweet liquid and solvent that is capable of enhancing drug flavor and dissolving chemicals. However, ethylene glycol is a deadly chemical that is capable of causing severe liver and kidney damage, central nervous system (CNS) depression (neurotoxin), coma, and death. The publication of *100,000,000 Guinea Pigs: Dangers in Everyday Foods, Drug, and Cosmetics* (1933) exposed the inefficiency of the FDA by revealing the calamities of thallium, a rat poison, and diethylene glycol, an antifreeze contained in eyelash (mascara), weight-loss drugs, and sulfanilamide drugs. Women who used the eyelash paint (mascara) with thallium became blind. The Massengill Company of Bristol, Tennessee, publicized sulfanilamide, a new antibiotic drug, in 1937. The drug is almost insoluble in water and alcohol but soluble in diethylene glycol. Massengill chemists discovered this fact and decided to use diethylene glycol as an industrial solvent for dissolving sulfanilamide to make an elixir: a drinkable form of the drug. The drug was immediately launched and sent to the market without any research work or testing with animals or human beings. Within a short period of time the drug became popular as a wonder drug, and the *Journal of American Medical Association* (*JAMA*) was forced to warn against indiscriminate use of the drug by doctors. Later, small children from the South who used the drug developed severe liver and kidney damage resulting in an inability to produce urine (anuria) and premature death. Drug research ordered by FDA and AMA revealed that the causative agent was diethylene glycol, which had never been used or tested in humans before marketing. Animals, such as rats, that took the diethylene glycol developed red urine, became sick, and died. One hundred innocent people died as a result of this drug misadventure, and Massengill, owner of the company, could only be prosecuted for mislabeling the drug as an elixir with no alcoholic content. Massengill later committed suicide because of the episode. At any rate, the unfortunate incident led to the enactment of the Food, Drug, and Cosmetic Act by the Congress in 1938.[18,25] This act is an amendment that was meant to strengthen the 1906 act by requiring food, drug, and cosmetics producers to prove that their product is pure and safe.

ORIGIN OF CLINICAL PHARMACY

Clinical pharmacy started long before pharmaceutical care, but the origin of the latter in the early 1990s accelerated the development and spread of the former. In 1912, there were a series of changes in the government's attitude and interest in public health, and this eventually resulted in the transformation of the U.S. Marine Hospital Service into the U.S. Public Health Service. At this stage, clinical pharmacy began to surface with a four-year baccalaureate pharmacy degree holders rationalizing their position and how to fit into the changing health care system. There was a paradigm shift in pharmacy education from the traditional mode to hospital practice setting, and many pharmacists were impressed with the change. In the 1930s, some pharmacists went into the hospital for post-baccalaureate training programs, otherwise tagged "internship," and this marked the beginning of clinical pharmacy. In 1944, Professor Waite L. Rising of the University of Washington gave credence to clinical pharmacy by introducing college credits for students who performed supervised pharmacy professional work either in the community or in the hospital. In 1950, the University of California pharmacy department became the first school in the world to initiate a Doctor of Pharmacy degree (PharmD) program. By then the program was considered too radical and revolutionary to be adopted by other schools of pharmacy, even though the profession was fast approaching an end to the era of compounding/preparation of drugs and the days of count and pour were numbered. A decade later, in 1960, the College of Pharmacy at the University of Michigan adopted the PharmD program and one of the first sets of pioneer students was David Burkholder. Dr. Burkholder graduated from the program in 1962 and proceeded shortly afterwards to practice at the University of Kentucky Medical Center, Lexington, where he established the first ever known academic Drug Information Center. With this single act, Dr. David thus pioneered the first direct participation of pharmacists with patient health care leading to a greater outcome. The Drug Information Center became known for its quality dissemination of drug information to all medical personnel including physicians, medical students, and nurses. Drug information centers eventually spread to other parts of the country and became a formidable part of the health care delivery system in America by the end of the 20th century and the beginning of the 21st century.[16,19,20]

Drug usage in America was without classification until the enactment of the Durham-Humphrey amendment to the Food, Drug, and Cosmetic Act, which finally separated drugs into two categories (prescription and nonprescription) in 1951. This drug separation aided pharmacists in stocking their shelves, partitioning the store, and knowing which drugs could easily be recommended by them without prescription from other medical professionals. Amid criticism Mr. Eugene White, a practicing pharmacist from Berryville, Virginia, was one of the very few pharmacists that made a move to incorporate elements of clinical pharmacy in 1960. He transformed his pharmacy from the traditional style into the office practice setting, with prescription and nonprescription shelves partitioned separately. He promoted the newly conceived clinical pharmacy in the community by setting up patients' profiles and attending to patients' needs in a private office. Mr. Donald Francke and others in the late 1950s conducted a study that showed the benefits of annexing the expertise of the pharmacy profession in an institutional setting. The study published as a mirror to hospital pharmacy in 1964 was titled "The Audit of Pharmaceutical Service in Hospitals."[3,16]

The early 1960s were characterized by the medical misfortune of the thalidomide episode in Europe. The thalidomide event gripped Europe with its devastating consequences when pregnant women who consumed the drug during pregnancy delivered babies with mutilated limbs. In 1960, Frances Kesley became the FDA medical officer in charge of auditing drug application for human consumption before approval. The first assignment she came in contact with was Merrel Company's application for the thalidomide approval, and she had sixty days to highlight any problem or consider it approved. She went through the company, bound four volumes of paperwork, and notified them of the study's deficiencies. She took a wait-and-see attitude, which eventually paid off. In the interim, she found a letter about thalidomide drug-induced peripheral neuropathy in the *British Medical Journal*. In July 1961 the drug was withdrawn from the German market, and in November 1961 Dr. Lenz Widikundi, a German pediatrician, explained the cause of his country's epidemic of birth defects to his colleagues in Düsseldorf. He highlighted that 50% of the babies' mothers had taken thalidomide during pregnancy. News about the drug's danger spread to America and became widely known through publication in the *Washington Post* and a satirical drama on television about the saga. At the end of the episode, 10,000 innocent babies paid a severe price with various deformities in twenty countries because their mothers had consumed thalidomide during pregnancy. Dr. Kelsey was hailed as an American heroine for keeping the drug out of America's market. The FDA eventually took over postmarking surveillance of drugs from the America Medical Association (AMA). The 1938 Food, Drug, and Cosmetic Act did not require efficacy proof by drug companies prior to approval; consequently, in April 1961, Kefauver-Harris sought to amend the law by sponsoring a bill that required efficacy proof as a modification. Initially, the AMA opposed the bill and Kefauver accused them of neglecting drug analysis because they relied heavily on a company's advertisements. The thalidomide episode heightens the efficacy view and played well into passage of the bill into law in 1962. By the passage of the bill into law, manufacturers were now required to prove that their drugs are effective for the intended use in addition to purity and safety requirements. That same year, 1962, pharmacy leaders in conjunction with the preceptors of the internship program in the hospitals decided to change the name of the program from internship to residence. A year later in 1963, the American Society of Hospital Pharmacists (ASHP) began a site visit of hospital residency programs for the purpose of accreditation.[16,18]

In 1966, the pharmacy department of the University of California, San Francisco Medical Center, took clinical pharmacy a step further by initiating the Ninth Floor Project. The pharmacy department decided to put into practice various aspects of pharmacy like drug information center, patient drug profiles, decentralized pharmacy, and unit dose pharmacy technicians' concept of advanced hospital pharmacy at the Medical center's ninth floor.[3] The result of the ninth-floor experiment was astonishing; hence, many other hospitals' pharmacy leaders took the initiative of developing clinical pharmacy by implementing the advanced hospital pharmacy program. At the beginning, the schools of pharmacy were reluctant to incorporate clinical pharmacy programs in their curriculum, as noted earlier. The school courses were a conglomeration of physical sciences (inorganic chemistry, organic chemistry, physical chemistry, mathematics, and physics), laboratory classes, and pharmaceutical sciences (medicinal chemistry, pharmacology, pharmacognosy, pharmaceutics, and others) because of pharmacy professional demands in the 1950s. Moreover, all professors at the schools of pharmacy were taught these physical and pharmaceutical sciences with an end result of a Doctor of Philosophy (PhD) in various disciplines. These professors had little or no firsthand experience as professional pharmacists operating in the communities or hospitals; as a result they perpetuated the system that schooled them thoroughly by emphasizing to other generations the materials they used. Many young pharmacists were schooled in this system, with all the academic rigors and demands, only to end up with professional practices of count and pour (moving pills from one bottle to another). They burnt out easily and were frustrated by the profession that limits their talents, educational output, and knowledge. They began to question the essence of going to a school of pharmacy in an era of count and pour. The professors at the schools of pharmacy just didn't understand the difference between what they were teaching in classrooms and the reality of life for the practicing pharmacists.[19] The young/new pharmacists were looking for escape for the profession and some found it in clinical pharmacy.

In 1969, the AphA repealed its code of ethics that barred pharmacists from discussing drug therapy with patients. Around 1975, the situation began to change for good when the American Council on Pharmaceutical Education (ACPE) and the federal government forced schools of pharmacy to institute clinical pharmacy in their educational programs. The federal government used clinical education as criteria for reimbursing schools of pharmacy and the availability of pharmacy in hospitals as criteria for Medicare reimbursement. Clinical pharmacy excelled; pharmacists began to expand their role in the hospitals by taking up new tasks. They went on rounds and provided information on drugs and drug/food interactions, pharmacokinetics services and evaluations, consults, parental nutrition evaluation and services, pharmacodynamics, and pharmacological in-services to physicians mostly, nurses, and other health care providers. In 1992, the American Association of Colleges of Pharmacy in combination with the American Council on Pharmaceutical Education moved to implement its 1989 letter of intent, which implored all schools of pharmacy to adopt the 6-year Doctor of Pharmacy degree (PharmD) program as entry level for practicing pharmacy.[16] All schools of pharmacy are expected to be in full compliance with the new regulation by the year 2005. With the advent of clinical pharmacy the traditional medical doctors now rely more and more on pharmacists for clarity and resolution of drug problems especially in institutional settings. In addition, Courts, jurors, judges, lawyers, patients and others relied heavily on evidence produced by clinical pharmacists as drug experts/therapeutic physicians in court proceedings to make sound or good judgment.

More discussion on the impact of clinical pharmacy on the health care system will be seen in later chapters.

CLINICAL PHARMACY IN PRACTICE

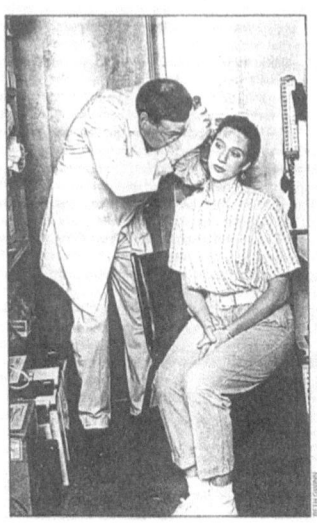

In a privately owned, independent community pharmacy, Manchester, Tenn., Pharmacist Ray Marcrom provides clinical pharmacy services. He examines a patient, Kim Roberts, above for ear infection.

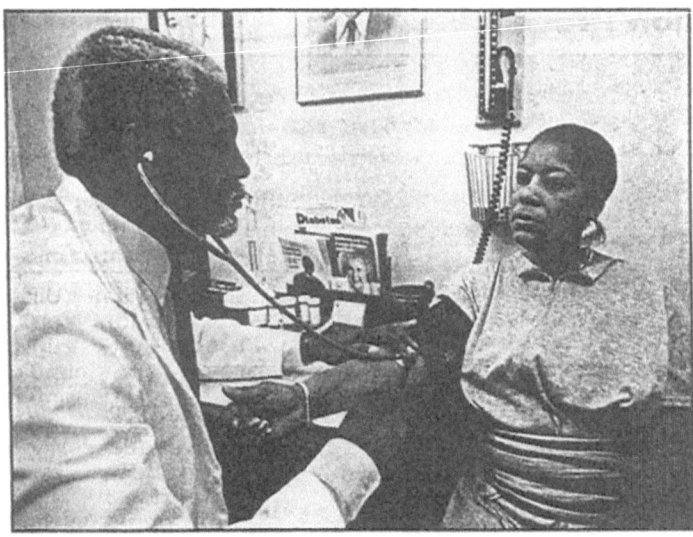

Pharmacist Ozelle Hubert provides clinical pharmacy services to his patient as seen above in Pharmacists Officentre, Chicago, Ill.

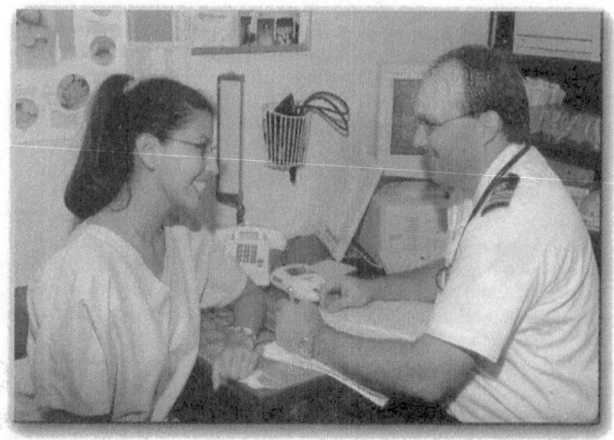

Dr. Watts, with a stethoscope around the neck, talks to a patient in his cardiovascular risk-reduction clinic. The clinic provides disease-state management including anticoagulation management service.

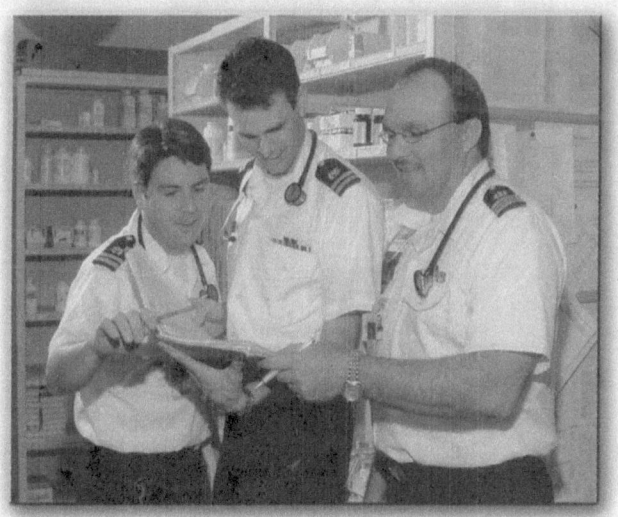

Dr. Travis Watts, right, confers with Dr. Robert Hayes, center, and Dr. Brian Wren, left in the clinic.

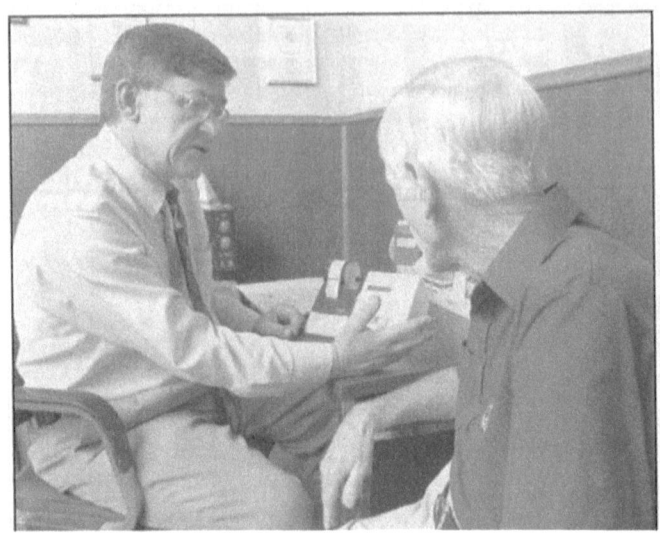

Pharmacist Lowell Anderson provides clinical pharmacy services to one of the Project ImPACT patients in a privately owned, community pharmacy, Bel-Aire Pharmacy, White Bear Lake, Minn.

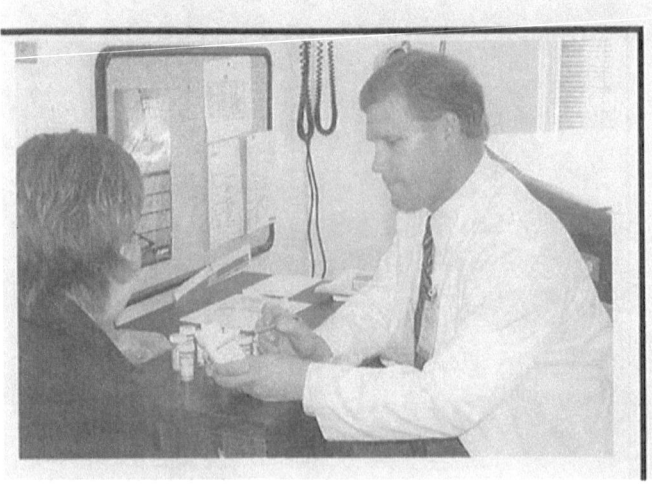

A clinical pharmacist provides clinical pharmacy services to a patient at Kern Medical Center, Bakersfield, Calif.

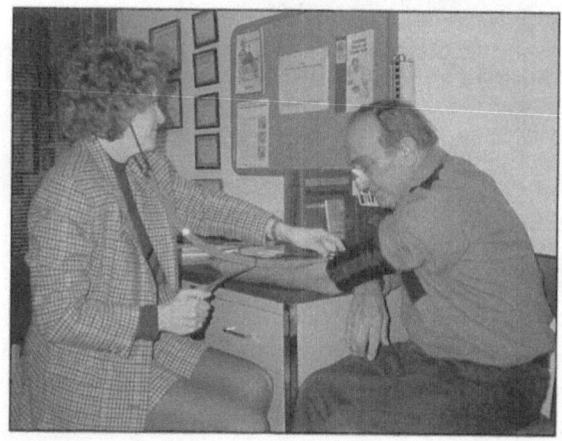

Pharmacist Julie Eggerman provides clinical pharmacy services to a patient in a semi-private pharmacy counseling area, Taylorville, Ill.

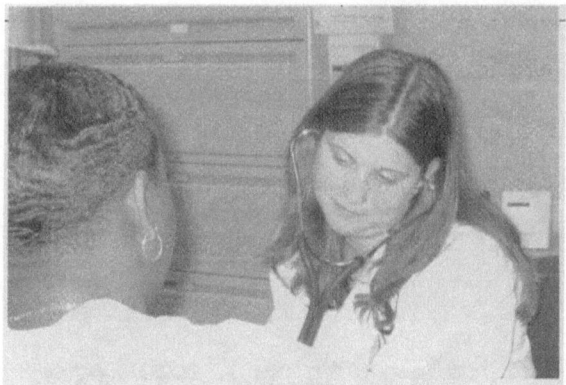

Dr. Stacey McNeal of University of Cincinnati/Kroger Pharmacy provides clinical pharmacy sevices to her patient in Kroger Patient Care Center.

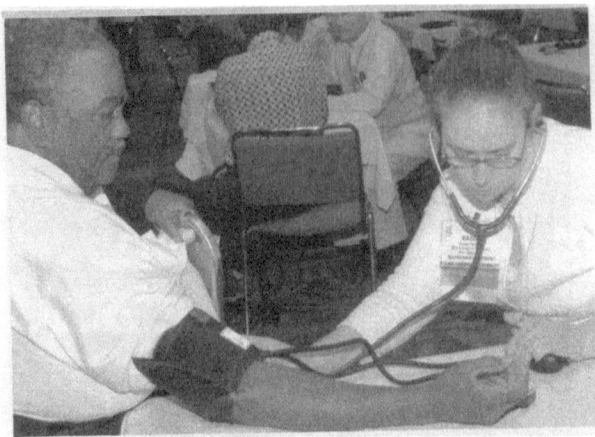

A Pharmacist renders clinical pharmacy services to a patient during health care expo tagged family caregiving in the 21st century, Washington, D.C.

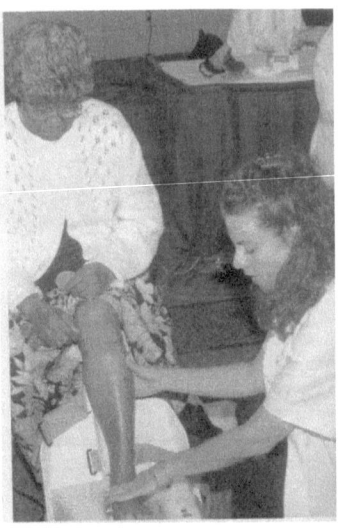
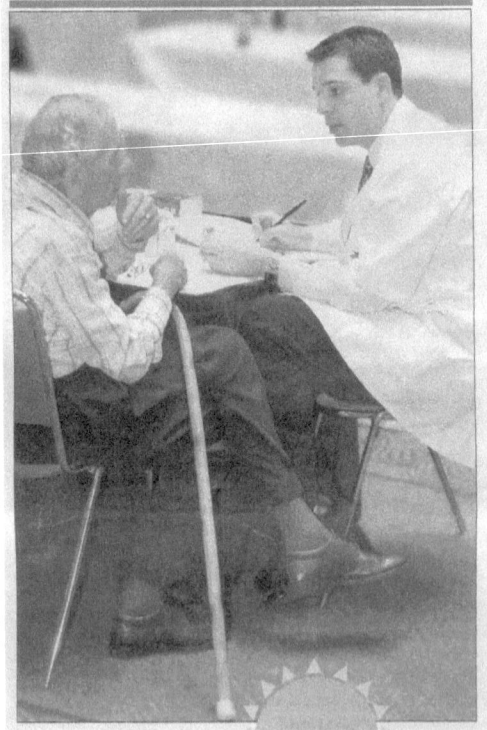

A Pharmacist renders clinical pharmacy services to a patient by checking the bone mineral density during health care expo tagged family caregiving in the 21st century, Washington, D.C.

Pharmacy In Bondage 131

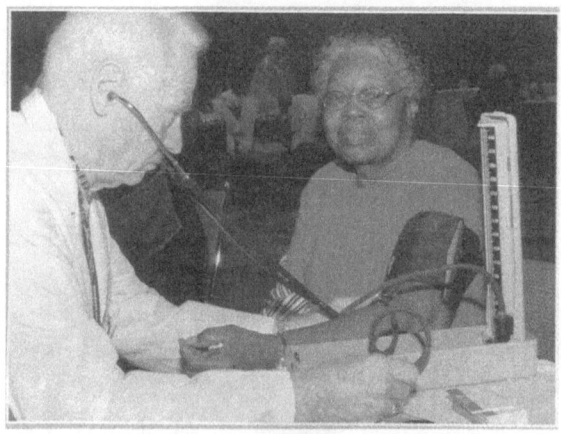

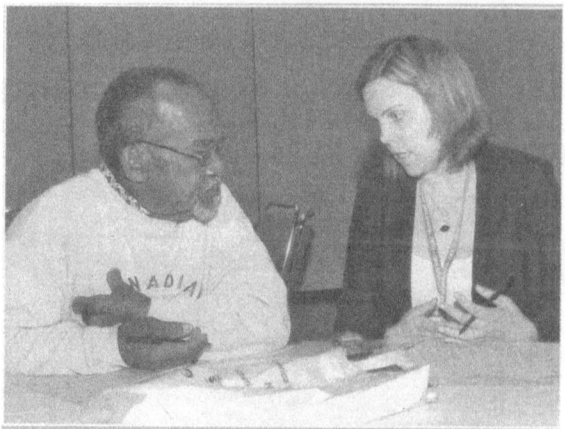

Clinical Pharmacy in progress in Medicare Today, a program that is designed to assist patients, employers, and health care providers in understanding Medication Therapy Management (MTM) and the complexities of Medicare Prescription Drug, Improvement and Modernization Act (MMA) - A new Federal Government program.

Pictures 4,5,6

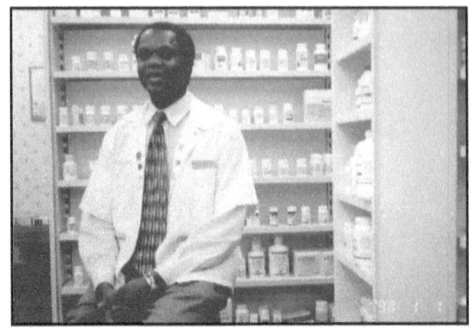

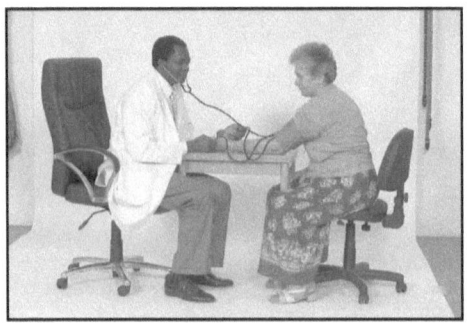

Dr. Patrick Ojo in a typical community pharmacy (*last 4 photographs*) in the U.S., where, in spite of a layout barrier and legal limitations, he provides some patients with clinical services.

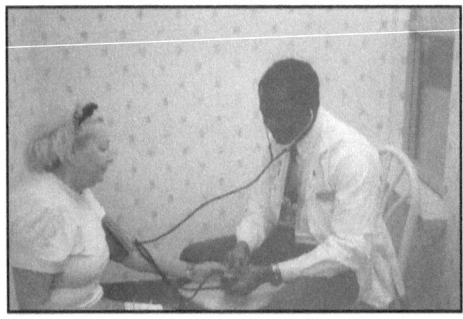

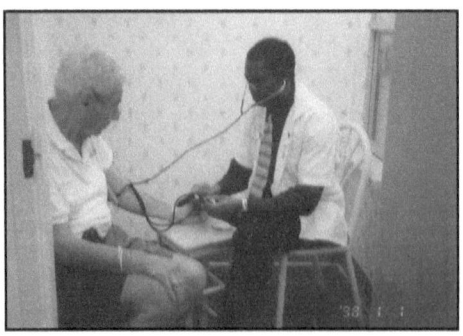

REFERENCES

1. Higby, G. J. *Evolution of pharmacy in Remington: The science and practice of pharmacy.* 19th ed. 1995, 1, 7-28.

2. Cowen, D. L, and W. H. Helfand. *Pharmacy: An illustrated history.* New York: Harry N. Abrams Inc.

3. Higby, G. J. American pharmacy in the twentieth century. *American Journal of Health-System Pharmacy* 54 (1997): 1805-15.

4. *New Webster's comprehensive dictionary of the English language.* Deluxe Edition. Lexicon Pub. Inc., 1990.

5. Craig, A. M, et al. *The heritage of world civilizations.* 2nd ed. 1990; Vol. A 3-16, 173-178, 342.

6. Williams, C. *The destruction of black civilization: Great issues of a race from 4500 BC to AD 2000.* Rev. ed. 1988, 96-106.

7. Rodney, W. *How Europe underdeveloped Africa.* Rev. ed. 1981, 238-41.

8. Abiola, E. O. *A textbook of West African history (AD 1000 to present day).* Rev. and enl. ed. 1984, 9-10.

9. Marti-Ibanez, F., and E. Henry. *Sigerist on the history of medicine.* New York: MD Publications, Inc.

10. Martin, A. R. *Antibiotics: Wilson and Gisvold's textbook of organic medicinal and pharmaceutical chemistry.* Edited by J. N. Delgado and W. A. Remers. 9th ed. 1991, 227-310.

11. Fullerton, D. S. *Antimalarials: Wilson and Gisvold's textbook of organic medicinal and pharmaceutical chemistry.* Edited by J. N. Delgado and W. A. Remers WA. 9th ed. 1991, 205-15.

12. Martin, A. R. *Anti-infective agents: Wilson and Gisvold's textbook of organic medicinal and pharmaceutical chemistry.* Edited by J. N. Delgado and W. A. Remers. 9th ed. 1991, 151-88.

13. Pedersen, C. A. Healthcare reform. In *Introduction to health care delivery: A primer for pharmacists.* Edited by Robert L. McCarthy. An Aspen Publication, Gaithersburg, Maryland. 1998, 331-53.

14. Wolfgang, A. P. Medicare and Medicaid. In McCarthy, *Introduction to health care delivery.* Edited by Robert L. McCarthy. An Aspen Publication, Gaithersburg, Maryland. 1998, 229-61.

15. Hepler, C. D., and L. M. Strand. Opportunities and responsibilities in pharmaceutical care. *American Journal of Pharmaceutical Education* 53 (1989): 7s-15s.

16. Broeseker, A., and K. K. Janke. The evolution and revolution of pharmaceutical care. In McCarthy, *Introduction to health care delivery.* 1998, 393-416.

17. Tebbe, J. L. Healthcare delivery in America: History and policy perspectives. In McCarthy, *Introduction to health care delivery.* 1998, 3-28.

18. Fried, S. *Bitter Pills.* A Bantam Book, 1998.

19. Miller, R. R. History of clinical pharmacy and clinical pharmacology. *Journal of Clinical Pharmacology* 21 (1981): 195-97.

20. Sapienza, A. M., and A. Broeseker. Health care professionals and interdisciplinary care. In McCarthy, *Introduction to health care delivery. : A primer for pharmacists.* Edited by Robert L. McCarthy. An Aspen Publication, Gaithersburg, Maryland. 1998, 31-61.

21. Maldow, H. E. Preparing for expanded and changing roles (president's message). *New York State Council of Health-System Pharmacists* (1996): 3.

22. Pharmacists' liability exposure on the rise. *New York State Council of Health-System Pharmacists* (1995): 8-9.

23. Scott, D. M., and M. J. Wessels. Impact of OBRA '90 on pharmacists' patient counseling practices. *Journal of the American Pharmaceutical Association* NS 37 (1997): 401-406.

24. Lai, Leann. Pharmacoeconomics, student reading assignment. Fort Lauderdale, Fla.: Nova Southeastern University. Fall 1999.

25. Worthen, D. B. The pharmaceutical industry, 1902-1952. *Journal of the American Pharmaceutical Association* 41(5) (2001): 656-59.

26. Eckel, F. M. Editor's note: Health care spending rises 8.7%. *Pharmacy Times* (February 2003): 4.

27. Shaw, K. L. "Improving medication use: Patients, physicians, and pharmacists offer opinions." *Pharmacy Today* (June 2003): 6, 30.

28. Worthen, D. B. William Procter Jr. (Heroes of pharmacy). *American Journal of Pharmaceutical Education* 42 (2): 363-64.

29. McCauley, H. B. Professional dentistry's road to autonomy. *Journal of the History of Dentistry* 46(2) (July 1998): 59-64.

30. Bordley, J., III, and M. A. Harvey. *Two centuries of American medicine (1776 to 1976).* W. B. Saunders Company, 3-16, 53-61.

31. Boyles, Glenn. The president's view point: It's time to make our case for value of pharmacy services. *Florida Pharmacy Today* (November 2004): 5-6.

32. Jackson, Michael. Executive insight: Working to preserve our profession. *Florida Pharmacy Today* (November 2004): 7-9.

33. Brushwood, David. Failure to warn of drug interaction at issue. *Pharmacy Today* (January 2005): 11, 21 and 23.

CHAPTER FOUR

DOCTOR OF PHARMACY (PHARMD) DEGREE

"Pharmacy has become a professional hot place where if you can't stand the heat, you might excused the profession or kitchen."

This is true of those who, for one reason or the other, join the profession with the aim of making quick money with minimal performing functions as a dispenser; and, to make matters worse, they are not prepared to follow the profession in the direction of change. Many of these dinosaur pharmacists (those not ready for change) joined the profession between the 1950s and 1990s when pharmacists were stripped of compounding functions by pharmaceutical industries and prescribing functions were out of their reach. The end results were such that they became functional dispensers with little or no avenue for practicing their acquired skills/expertise on patients and the health care system. The profession began to change for good with counseling and pharmaceutical care. Pharmaceutical care became the rallying point of the profession, and the Doctor of Pharmacy degree (PharmD) emerged as a professional tool/weapon to drive home a professional message and eventually led the profession to its final destination. The degree equally nurtured and enhanced pharmaceutical care.

PAST

Initially many wondered why pharmacy as a profession needed a doctorate program (PharmD) in order to dispense drugs. Today some critics still share this view especially in light of the numerous specialties in the medical field. Many critics of pharmacy as a specialty in the medical field are unaware of the fact that pharmacy was the first branch of medicine to be conceived, as previously enumerated. In spite of being the first branch of medicine to be conceived, there are numerous other reasons why pharmacy deserves a doctorate program, and many of these facts will be discussed here. First and foremost, the father of toxicology, Paracelsus, born Philippus Aureolus Theophrastus Bombastus Von Hohenhein (1493-1541), said it right when he ascertained that all substances are poisons. As noted earlier, he claimed that the only thing that differentiates poison from a remedy is the right dose. He proposed the need to differentiate between the therapeutic and toxic properties of chemicals on the basis of dose, by examining responses to chemicals on the basis of experiment and by determining chemical specificity in therapy or toxicity.[1] All branches of medicine including dermatology (skin), dentistry (teeth), optometry (Eye), and many other non-life-threatening phenomena have specialists catering for them except the poison that we pump into our bodies on a daily basis. The poisons we pump into our bodies at dawn in the name of pills or injections can send us to our graves at dusk because all are poisons and poisons exterminate lives. If Paracelsus was a product of the nineteenth or twentieth century, it is easy to envision that pharmacy would have been liberated by now. The idea of medical specialties was a strange phenomenon in his day. However, it is easy to visualize his ideas because we are all living witnesses of various medical mishaps/misadventures; and it is obvious that we seek specialists every day to perform many things including car repair, but when it comes downto the poisons we consume in the name of drugs, we simply do not care.

According to Paracelsus, these chemicals are poisons (all are poison). We can consume them at dawn for various ailments with the intention of getting better at dusk. Ironically, instead of feeling better at dusk the poison can send us to our grave. All chemicals including drugs are poisons, and once inside the body they have no master. They do not respond to people's directions, thinking, or propositions as people wish. That is to say, a drug once popped into the human body through the mouth, anus, vein (injection), or other means does not say that the cardiologist, internist, general practitioner, president, homeless fellow, or others want me (drug) to do this task; as a result, I have no business elsewhere; I must go directly to accomplish the task at the site of action. Chemicals or drugs have definite patterns like every other thing on earth. If a drug is taken through the mouth, it must proceed through various parts of the body (pharmacokinetics) before accomplishing its task at the site of action (pharmacodynamics).

PHARMACOKINETICS involves absorption, distribution, metabolism, and excretion (ADME). Each of these steps is a complex phenomenon that involves other processes. For instance, in:

- Absorption: A specialist would want to know if the drug is a salt or a compound, ionized or non-ionized, an acid or a base, a solid (e.g., tablet) or a liquid (e.g., suspension). These qualities affect drug dissolution and absorption rate in the stomach and without these two steps, you might as well forget about taking any drug through the mouth. Body functions such as gastric motility, emptying time, splanchnic blood flow, and rate of absorption decrease with age and need to be taken into consideration during therapy.[14] Moreover, drug/drug interactions or drug/food interactions interfere with dissolution and absorption processes; thus, diary products will chelates ciprofloxacin as well as other quinolones and prevent effective absorption in the stomach or bile acid sequestran such as questran can reduce the absorption of lipid-soluble drugs like lipitor, synthroid, propranolol, warfarin, etc.
- Distribution: Once a drug has been absorbed through the stomach, it goes into the bloodstream. Many will be taken by the liver and metabolized before going into blood circulation (first-pass effect), while others will go directly through blood circulation to the site of action (e.g., injectable drugs). Certain factors such as protein-binding ability, lipid solubility, hydrophylicity (water solubility), etc., do affect drug distribution through blood circulation. Thus, a specialist will wants to know the bioavailability of a drug or the amount of a free drug that will be available for pharmacological action (e.g., if a free drug is 0.1 that means 1 out of every 10 aspects of the drug is available for therapy and the rest are bounded in protein—warfarin has 0.03, phenytoin has 0.10, digoxin has 0.70, etc.). Certain drugs (e.g., versed-general anesthetics) penetrate blood brain barriers easily and are more easily distributed in the brain than others (e.g., levodopamine—anti-Parkinson's drug). Drug/drug interactions also affect distributions; for instance, salicylates, glyburide, and others can displace warfarin from protein-binding sites and cause undue increase in plasma concentration of the drug or toxicity. Body fat increases while total body water, lean body muscle mass, apha-1 acid glycoprotein, and serum albumin (protein) decreases as human age increases.[14] Gentamycin dosing in small-framed individuals is different from obese patients because of weight, fat/water content of the patient, which needs to be taken into consideration. A sick patient might have low albumin (plasma protein), which will make a drug such as phenytoin ineffective and create problems for epilepsy/seizure patients. Other factors such as idiosyncratic reaction of the body and bioequivalence of drugs also affect drug distribution in the body.

- Metabolism: The absorbed drug is carried by the blood to the liver for metabolism. Many drugs are converted into an active form (metabolite), while others remain unchanged. Metabolism occurs in the liver by way of oxidation, hydrolysis, conjugation, reduction, and methylation. Conjugation in the liver takes place with glycine, sulfate, glucuronidation, and acetylation. Metabolism is affected by many factors such as condition of the liver; drugs (e.g., ketoconazole, etc.) that inhibit liver enzymes and cause other drugs to increase in plasma concentration; drugs (e.g., carbamazepine, etc.) that enhance or induce liver enzymes and result in decreased concentration of other drugs; ethnicity; and cultural variation, which affects certain drugs.

How do ethnicity and culture affect drugs' metabolism? Polymorphic metabolism is a term used to describe ethnic variation in biological response to medications. Biologists revealed that individual DNA differs from a random stranger (i.e., someone from a different ethnic group) by 0.2% and less than 0.2% for family members or someone from the same ethnic group. Culture is often defined as a way of life that encompasses religion, language, rituals, eating habit, values, attitudes, family structure, and social interaction, which affects physical and biological responses to drugs. For instance, most Caucasians are slow acetylators but have high levels of rennin. Most Africans have low rennin levels and a glucose-6-phosphate dehydrogenase (G6PD) deficiency but they are fast acetylators. Most Asians are fast acetylators with glucose-6-phosphate dehydrogenase (G6PD) and alcohol dehydrogenase isozyme deficiency.[2] Slow acetylators or most Caucasians are predisposed to high plasma levels and the toxic effects of some drugs such as isoniazid, procainamide, sulfonamides, dapsone, caffeine, and hydralazine. Low rennin levels make beta-blockers and angiotensinogen-converting enzyme (ACE) inhibitor drugs less effective in blacks than whites. G6PD deficiency predisposes most Asians and Africans to hemolytic anemia because of the oxidation of hemoglobin to methemoglobin. Alcohol dehydrogenase deficiency causes Asians to have alcohol toxicity such as flushing, tachycardia, and palpitation even at regular doses for other ethnic groups. Caucasians and Asians are at greater risk for osteoporosis. Others are cytochrome P-450 deficiency that occurs in 5% of Caucasians, 2 to 10% in other groups, and is nonexistent in Africans and Japanese. The P-450 2D6 isoenzyme that is responsible for metabolizing codeine, beta-blockers, tricylic antidepressants (TCA), tamoxifen, etc., are absent in 10% of Caucasians and hyperactive in up to 30% of East Africans. Asians have about a 52% higher haldol plasma level than Caucasians at the same dose; the same is true of TCAs and other neuroleptic drugs because Asians are slower in metabolizing these drugs. Infants metabolize caffeine in an ultra-slow manner resulting in toxicity; men metabolize propranolol faster than women; as a result they need higher doses, and women's menstrual cycle affects drug metabolism; hence, a drug like lithium needs almost two times the regular dose (a toxic level at another time) to achieve a therapeutic level during the premenstrual period. Antibiotics reduce oral contraceptives' effectiveness, which in turn affects the metabolism of antidepressants.[2,12]

In addition, human physiology has been known to decline with age. Reserved functional ability of different organs in the body, for example, decreases after the age of 30 years at an average rate of 0.85%, blood flow to the liver decreases by 0.3-1.5% annually after age 25 years; and as a result it is estimated that at the age of 65 years the reduction rate climbs to about 40-45%. The elderly patients in America presently account for 25% of total drug expenditure (estimated to be 40% by 2030) and they are highly susceptible to adverse drug reaction (ADR) when their physiological conditions and individualized dosing are not taken into consideration in prescribing drugs/drug regimens. This perhaps explains why, in this population, inadequate dosing according to their pharmacokinetic changes accounts for a 70 to 80% ADR, a 17% hospitalization rate, and $20 billion in hospital costs annually.[14]

- Elimination: Metabolized drugs are more soluble and ready for elimination from the body than nonmetabolites. There are various routes of elimination, but the two most important ones are renal and fecal elimination via hepatic clearance. The renal elimination is more frequent than fecal and it relies on good kidneys for maximum effect. Creatinine clearance, an effective way of measuring renal functions, decreases at the rate of 0.5 - 1ml /min/70kg annually after reaching a level of 120ml/minute at age 25 years. Creatinine clearance (Clcr) that is less than 30ml/minute can inactivate certain drugs such as hydrochlorothiazide—HCTZ. The creatinine clearance of females is 0.85 or 85% of their male counterparts. Certain drugs such as probenecid can interfere with the renal elimination of other drugs such as penicillin, thereby causing an increased plasma level and half-life in the latter; oral contraceptives decrease clearance and volume of distribution, thereby increasing the half-life (t1/2) of other drugs such as prednisolone; and Non-steroid anti-inflammatory drugs (NSAID e.g., Motrin) can decrease renal functions by inhibiting prostaglandin, thereby reducing effectiveness of other drugs (e.g., anti-hypertensive drugs such as furosemide-lasix). Asians have lower clearance rates of benzodiazepines (e.g., Valium) and benadryl than others; consequently, they need smaller doses of the drugs. Hepatic functions, alcoholism, renal function, creatinine clearance, smoking, drug abuse, ethnicity/polymorphism as in metabolism, patient weight (e.g., slender people clear certain drugs slower than others), age, gender, hydration status, and other factors affect elimination and, consequently, the toxicity of drugs.[2,12,13]

Individualizing doses instead of a one-dose-fits-all model helps to maximize outcome and improve patient's health. This is the single reason why pediatric drug therapy ranks the best while others such as psychiatric and geriatric drug therapy rank the worst in terms of reducing/increasing ADR and ADR-related deaths.

Pharmacodynamics like pharmacokinetics is affected by numerous factors. Some of these factors are receptors and age-related issues. Generally traditional medical practitioners think of drugs in a pharmacodynamic manner and their view of pharmacodynamics is restricted to effectiveness. Drug effectiveness is directly related to receptors, and the functions of receptors depend on several factors including age. Receptors are found in various cells, organs, tissues, and other places in the body, and they are responsible for immediate action of the drugs at the site of action. Receptors have binding affinities/sensitivities, quantity limitations that determine their ability to bind to drugs and translate the biochemical reaction of drugs into cellular responses. These three factors may increase or decrease with age and thus result in increased or decreased dosages of drugs, frequency of administration of drugs, and quantity of drugs in order to reach a therapeutic level.[14] If a medical doctor recommends a drug and it fails to work, the rule of thumb in most cases is to add more drugs in combination or increase the dosage until the patient complains of side effects. The only thing that matters to the general practitioners in all cases that result in changes is effectiveness; however, the drug specialist will consider the rationale behind the failure and drug mechanism of action. Thus, a drug specialist will look at a diabetes type II patient and ask or find out if he/she is producing enough insulin or not. If the patient is producing enough insulin, why is he or she diabetic? And that narrows his thoughts/ views to receptors and resistance problems. The next issue is how to combat the resistance with diet modifications, exercise, and the use of drugs such as glucophage, avandia, and others if necessary. If the patient does not produce enough insulin, then the use of drugs such as sulfonylurea (e.g., glucotrol, diabeta, etc.), insulin (e.g., humulin, novolin) for severe cases, and others, if necessary, will be required. The same is true of patients who develop tachphlaxis (decreased effect of drugs because of continuous/repeated usage). These patients, such as asthmatic patients using beta-agonists such as albuterol, benefit from using steroid-like vanceril, pulmicort, flovent, aerobid, and others that reduce receptors' resistance and enhance receptors' sensitivity among other functions. The same is true of Angina or cardiovascular disease patients who developed a nitrate tolerance because of receptors' resistance, which can be overcome with adequate dosing, adjusting dosage intervals, and implementing free nitrates period. Drug specialists in all these cases would comprehend the problems and the best way to resolve it, while other specialists would throw pills like candy bars at patients, leaving problem resolutions at the mercy of a game of chance. Unlike pharmacokinetics, pharmacodynamics research, study, and publications are very much limited and things would only improve when trained therapeutic physicians or therapeuticians/drug specialists take charge of their destiny and guide the profession they love dearly.

Contemporary problems demand contemporary solutions, and in our jet (speed) age society where technology is the bane of the society, longevity/extended life spans have become common life processes. Longevity/extended life spans bring with them chronic illness in addition to the well-known acute illnesses. Most elderly citizens find themselves dealing with chronic illness in the proportion of two or more simultaneously occurring sicknesses. Some find themselves besieged with new and inexplicable illnesses that deserve a great deal of attention. We on a daily basis are discovering that many elders confront multifarious chronic illnesses in an unprecedented manner in the history of mankind. Many patients on a routine basis confront three or more chronic conditions, four or more chronic medications, 12 or more pills per day, four or more changes of drug regimen per year, three or more physicians per year, cognitive or physical impairment, a low level of education, poor compliance, and other conditions. Chronic illness demands chronic therapy, much of which entails the use of drugs, be it antineoplastic (anti-cancer), antihypertensive, antilipidemic, anti-hyperglycemic, etc. Chronic therapy involves the use of two or more drugs and more than one pharmacy (polypharmacy) at times by the patients. As a matter of fact, it is not uncommon to see a patient taking twenty or more pills in a day to cure or alleviate their illness these days. The most astonishing aspect of this multi-drug and polypharmacy therapy is that many of these drugs interact with each other (drug/drug interactions), food (drug/food interactions), disease (drug/disease interaction), and produce various side effects in the body. Some patients have had their drug treatment regimen skyrocketed because of the treatment of side effects. Instead of removing the causative agent or reducing dosage and/or the frequency of the culprit agents and many other options, many prescribers find themselves confronting a dilemma they are unprepared for because of inadequate medical school training in terms of drug treatment. Many prescribers are apt to increase drug regimen as a way of dealing with side effects. For instance, in a symposium organized by the New York City Society of Hospital Pharmacists at LaGuardia Marriott Hotel on April 18, 1996, entitled "Ethics Issues in Contemporary Health System Reform: Issues Facing the Institutional Pharmacists," Dr. Kenneth Freedman (MD), the keynote speaker, spoke of a chronically ill patient who was on many drugs including phenothiazine. This patient's condition was deteriorating fast, with his white blood cells and other hematological conditions going down the hill at an alarming rate in the face of the best medical doctors. Dr. Freeman said doctors upon doctors were at a lost road, and some were in a state of dilemma; they didn't know what to do because they did not know what was going on with the patient. He went further to say that all it took was for one Doctor of Pharmacy (PharmD) degree holder or a clinical pharmacist to appear on the scene. The clinical pharmacist looked at the patient's medical profile and requested that the phenothiazine be taken out of the regimen at once. The phenothiazine was taken out and within days the patient's health condition improved dramatically. The patient's white blood cell and other hematological conditions were on their way back to a normal level. The issue here appears simple, but many prescribers in various settings may opt for the addition of neupogen and procrit that would have cost the patient an average of $3,000 to $4,000 per month as an additional therapy and medical expense for the two drugs alone. Dr. Freeman is the president/chief executive officer (CEO) of Managed Care Solutions, Leesburg, Virginia, and attending physician at Alexandria Hospital, Alexandria, Virginia.

Dr. Janet Engle, a clinical pharmacist, associate dean for academic affairs, and clinical professor of pharmacy practice at the College of Pharmacy, University of Illinois, Chicago (UIC), had a similar but different experience from Dr. Freeman. She wrote about her experience in "Mounting Evidence of the Need for Change" as part of the article "150 Years of Pharmacy: Our Patients, Our Passion," published in the October issue of the *Journal of the American Pharmacists Association*. At the age of seven months her daughter became sick and the pediatrician recommended Dimetapp. Based on her knowledge of drugs as a clinician she demanded to know the type of Dimetapp (drops or elixir), and the pediatrician responded by saying it doesn't matter. She reminded him that there were different ingredients in the two products, and he didn't know that. Dr. Engle then wondered how the pediatrician could recommend pediatric dosing if he didn't know the active ingredients in the products. With most over-the-counter (OTC) medications requesting parents and guardians to contact their physicians for dosing children under age two, she could estimate the predicament of parents. Dr. Engle's mother is an asthma patient with high blood pressure, and she was given samples of a nonspecific beta-blocker at the doctor's office to treat the high blood pressure.

Dr. Engle's mother's asthma was exacerbated because of the nonspecific beta-blocker, and the physician that treated her had no clue about what was going on. Mum was given an inhaler (another sample) she didn't know how to use. After a while she called her daughter, Dr. Engle, about 600 miles away for assistance. Dr. Engle began to probe her mum's treatment through questions and answers and she was able to identify the nonspecific beta-blocker as the causative agent. Mum was switched to another antihypertensive medication by the doctor and her condition improved dramatically without the prescribed inhaler. Dr. Engle asserted how pharmacists' knowledge, if well tailored, can help turn things around and improve the health care system for the patients and make enormous savings for many sectors. She noted that doctors are in the habit of giving out samples to patients without thinking about other complications that can accompany such gestures (money-saving gestures become money-spending gestures as in Diana's case). She stated that patients, not physicians or pharmacists, control the health care system.[43]

Some pharmacists have taken the initiative to ask some elders to bring all of their medications from the medicine cabinet to the pharmacy for review. The brown bag of the elderly is of great interest to the pharmacy profession because of the many revelations contained in the bag. It is astonishing to see how many expired drugs, inadequately stored drugs, noncompliance leftover drugs, and self-medicating over-the-counter drugs are available for them for immediate use in the event of any ailment, even if such ailment is slight and capable of readjusting itself within hours. In 1995, it was estimated that half of the 1.8 billions drugs prescribed in the U.S. are not taken adequately. The present-day prescribers are too busy to confront this problem. Drug problems in America have taken on a different dimension and it has gotten to the point where people, prescribers, and patients alike are now beginning to get nervous about prescribing and using medications. Statistics about drug problems are staggering and scary. It is unreasonable to blame the consumers who, as a result of mass media coverage, discovered that drug-related problems are now between the fourth and sixth leading cause of death in the country. How is it that medication(s) that one takes to alleviate an ailment ends up killing the person? It is therefore not unusual to find patients wondering and questioning themselves if left alone will the ailment have caused the deceased death sooner or the treatment aggravated the ailment and compounded the problem thereby precipitating premature death. But the treatment was supposed to solve and not compound problems for patients. The prescribers, on the other hand, worry about litigations and probably some of the carry over inadequate pharmacological training in medical school. All these conditions created instability and put medicine at the mercy of politics. In order to understand drug problems in America and the reason why therapeuticians/drug specialists need a Doctor of Pharmacy degree to deal with the problem here and in other parts of the world, a little light on the issue will be shed here.

American Pharmacists Association (AphA) celebrated 150 years of existence in 2002, and one of the events commemorating the sesquicentennial celebration was a symposium titled "Critically Examining Pharmaceutical Care." During the symposium, Dr. Hepler quoted a recent research study that showed 5 out of every 1,000 hospital admissions are due to preventable drug-therapy problems. This statistical data puts hospital admission due to drug-therapy problems ahead of hospital admissions due to heart disease and diabetes mellitus and next to cancer patient admission. Dr. Strand, on the other hand, reiterated the fact that safe and effective drug therapy is every patient's right.[44]

In 1995, Dr. Bootman and J. F. Johnson of the University of Arizona conducted a study on drug-related morbidity and mortality and projected that the ambulatory care patients spent well over $76 billion on drug-related illnesses every year. This study was only focused on ambulatory care alone without hospital inpatients or nursing home/correction facilities residents and others. The $76 billion was the result of expenditures on patients' visits to physicians' offices, emergency rooms, drug usage that cost $73 billion the same year, and hospital days. Dr. Bootman noted the failure of Omnibus Budget Reconciliation Act of 1990 because of poor management by pharmacy owners, supervisors, and pharmacy benefits-management administrators. He blamed them because he felt their aim was to decrease drug costs and increase profitability instead of looking at the overall health care costs. Dr. Bootman and Johnson came to the conclusion that pharmacists' services in ambulatory care, if fully utilized, could save up to 120,000 human lives by preventing mortality, and reduce medical expenses by 60%, which would have resulted in $45 billion instead of the $76 billion in this case.[3] The $76 billion serves as a wakeup call for various states including California, whose senate insurance committee on May 8, 1996, unanimously passed the SB 1596 bill that authorizes pharmacists to be paid for non-dispensing functions by managed care plans.

In 1977, a *JAMA* report showed that adverse drug events cost the nation 4 billion dollars, and 2 billion dollars of this was preventable. The study describes percentage errors as overdose—41.8%, underdose—16.5%, allergy—12.9%, dosage form—11.6%, wrong drug—5%, duplicate therapy—5%, wrong route—3.3%, wrong patient—0.4%, and miscellaneous—3.3%. The National Forum for Health Care Quality Measurement and Reporting described adverse events of health care errors as the number-one fear of patients, with a 2% hospitalization rate and a more than $5,000 cost increase for every admission. A Harvard study, on the other hand, showed that most errors occured in intensive care units (ICUs), surgical floors, and medical floors with culprit medications such analgesics, antibiotics, cardiovascular, psychotropic, and sedative drugs. The Harvard study went further to claim that preventable errors were mostly associated with ordering—56%, administration—34%, transcription—6%, and dispensing—4%. When the ADR was compared at the rate of 0.1% with other life eventualities in the airline industry, it correlates with 84 unsafe landings per day in America.

In 1994, Lazarous et al. conducted meta-analysis prospective studies of incidence of adverse drug reactions in hospitalized patients. The study focused on the WHO (World Health Organization) definition of ADR, which is "any noxious, unintended, and undesired effect of a drug which occurs at doses used in humans for prophylaxis, diagnosis, or therapy." The study did not include errors in drug administration, possible ADR, subtherapeutic doses, retrospective studies, drug abuse, therapeutic failures, noncompliance, and overdose. The study analysis was based on ADR occurring while the patient was in the hospital (ADRIN) and ADR resulting in hospitalization (ADRAD). The inclusion criteria used in the study eliminated 114 studies, thereby narrowing the 153 to 39 studies. The results revealed that in 1994, an average of 702,000 patients (95% CI, 635,000-770,000) experienced ADRIN, while 1,547,000 patients (95% CI, 1,033,000-2,060,000) experienced ADRAD, making a total of 2,216,000 patients (95 percent CI 1,721,000-2,711,000) that experienced serious ADR. This value represents 6.7% of hospitalized patients. The study went further to estimate that 63,000 patients (95% CI 41,000-85,000) experienced fatal ADRIN, and 43,000 patients (95% CI 15,000-71,000) experienced fatal ADRAD, making a total of 106,000 deaths (95% CI 76,000-137,000) in 1994. Fatal ADR is ADR that resulted in death.[4] There were 2,286,000 deaths in the country in 1994; hence, ADR is said to be responsible for 4.6% (95% CI 3.3%-6%) of the total deaths. Judging by the confidence interval range, the study discovered that a conservative figure of 76,000 deaths placed ADR as the sixth leading cause of deaths and a liberal figure of 137,000 deaths placed ADR as the fourth leading cause of death, and these statistics have been relatively stable for three decades. In 1994, deaths due to heart disease were first with a figure of 743,460, followed by cancer with 529,904, stroke with 150,108, pulmonary disease with 101,077, accidents with 90,523, pneumonia with 75,719, and diabetes with 53,894 deaths.

The study noted that the emphasis on decreased hospital stay may have contributed to an increased number of drugs per day because of the need to expedite recovery. They quoted research, which asserted a direct hospital cost per year due to ADR as $1.56 to $4 billion. This study, published in *JAMA* on April 15, 1998, may have revealed various issues about ADR but it must be noted that the study was mostly restricted to serious and fatal ADRs. The study did not include mild, moderate, and severely moderate ADRs, which are capable of becoming serious at a later date; community ADRs; and nursing homes ADRs (homes of many elderly citizens who are much more susceptible to ADR than the general public). Dr. Bates in his editorial comment about this study noted that hospitals have high incentives not to report ADR because of public reaction and regulators' scrutiny. Another study by Generali et al. highlighted the facts that spontaneous reporting system (SRS) is belittled in the country, with less than 1% reported cases of serious and/or fatal ADRs to FDA; and pharmacists who are supposed to be the ADR reporting programs' caretakers in nursing homes and hospitals are underutilized. Dr. Bates said most hospitals depend on spontaneous reporting, which accounts for only 1 in 20 ADRs, thereby trivializing the episodes. He went further to delineate the fact that patient's known allergic reactions and sensitivity are in most cases not recorded, and many drugs revealed their risks by using them in sicker patients after approval in required trial setting. Above all, he asserted that there was not enough research in this area in comparison to other major causes of death (e.g., heart disease, cancer, stroke, etc.).[4,5,32] Dr. Bates hit the nail on the head with this last comment, because the various branches of medicine cannot shy away from the fact that they knew the consequences of ADRs for many years. They knew if they had encouraged research in the area, they would have been the culprit and the end results would not be kind in regard to their status quo. If there had been such research in the past, pharmacy by now would have been liberated. It appears these are all part of an effort to sabotage pharmacy and keep it perpetually checked in bondage.

Grizzle and Ernst conducted another study between July 1999 and March 2000 purposely to revisit and update the 1994 study of the annual cost of drug-related problems (DRPs). The above 1994 study estimated $76.6 billion cost for drug-related morbidity and mortality; Grizzle and Ernst used this estimate assuming the problems, morbidity, and mortality, remained the same (an almost impossible phenomenon because there is almost no standstill in life; you are either progressing or retrogressing). They conducted the update on the basis of changes in cost increase and the additional cost of attending to ADR in the emergency room, hospital admissions, physicians' visits, long-term care admissions, and acquisition of more drugs. Other changes are initial treatment cost, treatment failures (TFs) cost based on the assumption that 10% of prescriptions are not filled within a year, new medical problems (NMPs) cost, and total cost. Grizzle and Ernst duplicated Bootman and Johnson's decision-analytical model and data set by using the average cost of emergency room visits, hospital admission, physician visits, long-term care (LTC) admissions, and prescription drugs based on the most recent available data before March 2000.[17] The results showed that, using 2000 dollars adjustment, the average cost of hospitalization was $12,646 obtained from 1998 total inpatient admission hospital revenue of $407,650,369,271divided by total number of admissions 33,776,000; LTC was $9,489 per stay obtained from 1999 LTC length of stay by dividing 5,224,710 patient days with 62,610 total admissions, and a monthly average of $3,135 per LTC resident; additional prescriptions cost was $42 obtained from 1999 total sales of $111,101,894,000 divided by 2,712,456,000, the total number of dispensed prescriptions; physician visits was $109 obtained from a total cost of $13,826,275,829 divided by 126,846,567, the number of visits according to the Center for Disease Control; emergency room visits was $308 obtained from a 1996 total revenue of $5,760,780,460 divided by 18,703,833, the number of visits; and the total number of deaths was 218,113. The overall cost due to drug-related morbidity and mortality was estimated to be $177,407,869,681; that was 131.7% higher than the 1995 Bootman and Johnson's estimated $76.6 billion.[17] The data showed that the majority of the soaring health care costs resulting from ADR were due to physician visits, which were 1.9 times greater than the 1995 estimates; LTC admission, which was 2.3 times greater than the 1995 estimates; and the hospital admission, which was 2.6 times greater than the 1995 estimates. The study is however limited by the fact that it is a projected estimate based on the most recent data, and the $177.4 billion estimates are due to ambulatory care settings. This projection might appear large and unrealistic to many, but we might be surprised to see the merging nature of the estimate if the actual study that takes everything into consideration were done and published.

An earlier study of 91,574 patients who were admitted to LDS, Salt Lake City, revealed that 2,227 developed an adverse drug event (ADE). A comparison of the ADE group with a control group showed that the former had a mortality rate of 3.5% and an average of 7.69 days length of stay while the later had 1.05% and 4.46 days. The ADE group spent an average of $10,010 for the total cost of hospitalization compared to $5,355 for the control group. This study was published in *JAMA*, January 22, 1997.

In 1996, the Senate special committee on aging chaired by Senator William Cohen (R-Maine) decided to study adverse drug reaction in the elderly in a bid to raise public consciousness about the devastating effects of adverse drug reaction and the subsequent human suffering and cost. The committee summoned a hearing composed of organization, government, managed care, and pharmacy representatives. Ms. Linda Golodner, president of the National Consumer League, cited poor communication and lack of coordination among health care providers, cost containment by managed care, and patients' incorrect use of medication as well as multiple-drug usage. AphA president Knowlton blamed pharmacists' inability to provide pharmaceutical care on a lack of financial incentives by health insurance plans. He noted that pharmacists are forced to dispense more and more drugs more quickly in order to make a living, thereby leaving no room for counseling. Knowlton suggested Medicare payment for pharmaceutical care and retention of drug safety programs in federally funded nursing homes and state Medicaid programs. Cohen, on the other hand, noted pharmacists' ability in controlling ADR and improving patient's health outcome through counseling by citing an 82 year old multiple-drug patient in Iowa who immediately experienced improved health outcome by seeking a pharmacist's consultation.[6] He concluded by noting that Medicare and consumers will save billions of dollars in addition to saving lives or improving the health status of senior citizens if only there could be positive improvement in physicians' prescribing habits, managed care formulary, patients' compliance, and counseling by pharmacists. In November 2000, Senator Tim Johnson (D-South Dakota) in his comments during pharmacists' role recognition on the Senate floor noted how pharmacists' interventions in various anticoagulation, asthma, diabetes, and pain control studies are saving health care costs and improving patient outcomes. He observed that pharmacists' involvement increases effectiveness with fewer ADRs. In January 2002, Joann Emerson (R-Missouri) and Mike Ross (D-Arkansas) sponsored HR 3626, the Medicare Drug and Service Coverage Act of 2002 (MEDS Act). This bipartisan Medicare drug benefit bill guarantees pharmacists reimbursement for medication therapy management and services. The bill was expected to assist senior citizens, especially those with multiple disease states and medications, manage their health in the most effective, safe, and cost benefit manner through education and monitoring of medication use. AphA endorsed the bill because it would save not only lives but also money for the senior citizens (beneficiaries), the government, and pharmaceutical industries.[41] As of May 2002, the Social Security Act only recognized dieticians, social workers, nurses, midwives, physicians, nurse practitioners, and physician assistants as providers. Pharmacists are nowhere to be found on the list even though they have greater training in drug treatment as therapeuticians than any other group cited as providers on the list.

In September 2003, the House and Senate Medicare conferees concord that the Medicare Prescription Drug and Modernization Act of 2003 (HR 1 and S 1) should include medication/drug therapy management services (MTMs). The conferees noted that MTMs provided by pharmacists would ensure appropriate use of medications, improve therapeutic outcomes, and reduce adverse drug interactions for patients having multiple chronic conditions, using multiple prescription drugs, and at risk of incurring high drug expenses. The Medicare bill was approved in the House of Representative by a margin of 220 to 215 and in the Senate by a margin of 54 to 44 in

November 2003. This was the first major landmark legislation since the inception of Medicare in 1965. The law is expected to go into effect by the year 2006, and it provides coverage for outpatient prescription drugs for Medicare beneficiaries. Beneficiaries who wish to participate in the program will pay (1) average monthly premium of $35, (2) deductible of $250, (3) co-payment of 25% up to $2,250, and (4) out-of-pocket coverage between $2,250 and $3,600 and after $3,600 out-of-pocket expenses, the catastrophic coverage sets in with patients paying either $2 generics/$5 brands or a 5% co-payment. Pharmacists were recognized for the first time in the history of Medicare as providers with the passage of this bill into law and they are expected to provide the MTMs as outlined by the conferees.[51]

A 1995 National Ambulatory Medical Care Survey (NAMCS) of medication-related morbidity visits to physician-based offices showed that 2.01 million visits (95% CI, 1.69 to 2.34 million) were made to physician-based offices because of ADR. This shows a total of 7.7 visits per 1,000 persons or 0.29% of all visits or that 2.57% of all injury-related visits are due to medication problems. These statistics were provided by the National Centers for Health Statistics (NCHS). A breakdown of the statistics revealed that whites accounted for 85.69% of the cases; women accounted for 56.30%; patients 65 years and older accounted for 30%, with 22.94 visits per 1,000 persons for patients between 65 and 74 years; blacks accounted for 12.89% (in comparison to the black population and their ability to seek medical help, the rate was different from that of whites); visits by other races were lower, primary care physicians (internists, family or general practitioners) attended to 55.98% of the cases; and specialists such as pediatricians and dermatologists attended to 15.96% of the cases. Further analysis showed that nurses attended to 29.69% while physician assistants attended to 16.60% of the medication-related visits at the physician's office. The medications that were responsible for most visits were antibiotics, cardiovascular drugs, hormones, and synthetic substitutes. The signs and symptoms mostly associated with these effects were skin rash, nausea, shortness of breath, leg symptoms, menstrual irregularities, and others. Dr. Aparasu, who conducted the study, noted that physicians frequently attend to patients with drug-related problems, but research in the area is scanty. He reported that an estimate of 0.86-2.9% of emergency room visits, 0.2-21.7% hospital admissions, and 2.6-50.6% of adverse drug effects in outpatients are drug-related problems. The study did not, however, include ambulatory care patients in outpatient and emergency departments. The patients in this study had a subsequent scheduled follow-up visit, and less than 1% resulted in hospitalization because of inadequate documentation and the fact that the study excluded outpatients and emergency department visits.[7]

A 1992 study conducted by Fink, a professor of pharmacy at the Kentucky College of Pharmacy, about counseling patients on prescription therapy and over-the-counter medications revealed that a total of $76.5 billion was spent on drug-related morbidity and mortality. Ironically, $75 billion was spent on prescription drugs alone in 1992. A breakdown of the drug-related morbidity and mortality rate revealed that $7.459 billion was spent for physician visits for a total of 1.15 billion events; $5.32 billion was spent for emergency room visits for a total of 17.05 million events; $47.445 billion for hospital admissions for a total of 8.7 million events; $14.398 billion was spent in long-term care visits for total of 3.149 million events; and $1.93 billion as additional cost for prescriptions for a total of 76.35 millions events. The number of recorded deaths due to drugs was 198,815 in 1992, and various issues such as compliance, changes in dosages of medication, inappropriate directions by health care professionals, and others were cited as reasons for the problems. The study called on pharmacists to uphold the Omnibus Budget Reconciliation Act of 1990 (OBRA '90) by using various body language (forward leaning, eye contact, nodding, humility, and others) to encourage counseling. Dr. Srnka Quentin predicted that in the future, pharmacies will have laboratories, reception areas, waiting areas, counseling centers and pharmacists will be providing product supervision, disease-state management (be it in primary, self-care, or preventive services), and drug research programs.[8]

Berg et al. studied noncompliance and discovered that businesses lost over $50 billion, hospital admissions cost of $25 billion (Gans et al. study noted about 10 to 30%), nursing home admissions cost of $5 billion, and pharmacies lost revenues totaling $8 billion annually because of noncompliance. Other studies have shown that CAP, noncompliance, non-adherence, and non-persistence cost the nation about $100 billion dollars. Realizing pharmacy's crucial role in researching and improving patients' compliance, Hoechst Marion Roussel decided to launch patient health first program by encouraging pharmacists to document improvements with reimbursement.[9] Noncompliance has been linked to low income, inadequate drug knowledge, forgetfulness, ADR, regimen complexity, and patient-provider relationship.

In 1990, the World Health Organization's report showed that ADR cost the U.S. 1.6 million in hospitalization and 160,000 deaths. Aspirin alone caused 2,000 deaths. NSAID-induced GI complications caused 26,000 deaths and 20,000 hospitalizations every year in rheumatoid arthritis patients, more than those that died from illegal drug use. An average family has 29 different drugs in its bathroom cabinets, and drug companies spend $13 million/day for television advertisements. Smalley et al. conducted a study and discovered that the hospitalization rate for serious ulcer disease among the elderly varies from 4.2 for non-NSAID to 16.7 for NSAID users per

1,000 people per year. This condition was said to be worst for new users and it deteriorated further as the NSAID doses increase. Poison control centers in the late 1990s reported over 130,000 cases per year involving children less than five years old being overdosed with gastro-intestinal (GI), cold, pain, and cough medications. Some statistics claim that 40% of nursing home residents receive inappropriate medications, 25% of elderly drugs are dangerous or unnecessary, and death-related ADR is more than 50% among the elderly. In 1993, suicide was the ninth leading cause of death and depression has been linked to a majority of the cases. Some studies have shown that only 33.3% of patients taking antidepressants receive a therapeutic dosage.[16,17,32]

Bacteria resistance has grown since the discovery of penicillin and other antibiotics in the 1940s. In 1950s staphylococcus resistance led to the discovery of penicillinase-resistant penicillin such as methicillin (or condom drugs). Bacteria became resistant to these condom drugs including methicillin-resistant staphylococcus aureus (MRSA) in the 1980s, and this climbed to a level of 40% in some localities. Researchers have found that streptococcus pneumonia resistance to penicillin and other antibiotics (like meropenem, erythromycin, and bactrim—3 different classes of antibiotics) has grown from 1 in 11 in 1995 to 1 in 7 in 1998 in the U.S. This translates into an increase of 9 to 14 percent, and penicillin-resistant isolates are said to have grown from 21 to 25%. In 1998, 24% of the 4,013 (963) reported cases of streptococcus pneumonia were said to be penicillin resistant, and this was 4% higher in whites (26%) than in blacks (22%). Vancomycin came on the market to combat these resistances, yet resistance developed especially the multidrug resistant or vancomycin-resistant enterococci in the 1990s. The trend continued unabatedly and the danger now is that we might one day run out of effective antibiotics to combat diseases such as communicable tuberculosis and other infections. Antibiotic resistance has been blamed on a number of factors such as misuse and overuse, patients' unnecessary demands and failure to complete regimen, prescribers' inappropriate choice of drugs, subtherapeutic dosing, inadequate dosing, inadequate dosing frequency, inappropriate combination of drugs, inappropriate monitoring of patients' dependence on drugs (antibiotics), side effects, unexplained danger in other drug usage, inability to withstand patients' and pharmaceutical companies' pressure through education, patients' problems in knowing how and when to medicate themselves, inadequate monitoring of patients' regimen, and writing of unnecessary prescriptions. The Centers for Disease Control and Prevention claimed that Americans used 2 million pounds of antibiotics in 1954 and 50 million pounds in 1999, and the article claimed that resistance problems were due to about 50 million unnecessary prescriptions written out of 150 million outpatient antibiotics prescriptions in a year. There is a call for all health care practitioners and patients to do everything within their reach to combat this problem, but the pharmacist will do better if they are allowed to put their drug expertise into use. According to the March 20, 2001, broadcast of *Good Morning America*, doctors issued a warning against the use of antibiotics for sinusitis and other minor aches where the antibiotics have been proven to be ineffective and unwise, thereby giving room for resistance. In midst of the bad news, one report showed that the campaign against antibiotic misuse appears to be yielding some dividends because of a decrease in antimicrobial prescriptions written by office-based physicians for children younger than fifteen years, from 46 million in 1989 to 30 million in 1999.[11,40,42]

A Doctor of Pharmacy degree (PharmD) would enhance pharmacy's status in the medical field and help to catalyze its liberation. If pharmacy had been liberated before now, many of the incidents above would have been reduced to the barest minimum, because it is impossible to eliminate them. Many people such as Franklin Horner, who lost his life to a drug misadventure, would have been alive today. Franklin Horner is a resident of Kansas City, Missouri, who was prescribed diazepam 10mg, 1 tablet every 8 hours, and ethchlorvynol 750mg, 1 capsule every 8 hours. The pharmacist, Anthony Spalitto, noticed a discrepancy in the ethchlorvynol dosing instructions when the two prescriptions were presented. The normal dose of ethchlorvynol is 500 to 1000mg at bedtime, and a sedative dose is 100 to 200mg up to three times daily when used alone. The two drugs have a cumulative effect of sedation when used together. Spalitto summoned the courage to call the doctor's office for verification and an unidentified fellow told him that everything about the two prescriptions was correct because the doctor meant to sedate the patient for a whole day. Spalitto filled the prescriptions, and six days later Horner died. Blood analysis revealed that his blood plasma level of ethchlorvynol was closed to toxicity, which is an indication of the fact that he experienced toxicity at the point of death. Horner's family sued the pharmacist and the case was dismissed on the grounds that the prescription was filled correctly according to Kampe's rule in Missouri; the appellate court, however, set aside Kampe's rule claiming that it denigrated the pharmacist's expertise, especially with the recognition of OBRA '90, and the battle goes on.[15] Kentucky had a similar incident when a five-foot-five, 257-pound diabetic patient was prescribed fen-phen for weight loss. The patient filled the prescription several times in more than four months before her death. The last script was filled nine days before her death, and her weight had dropped to 112 pounds. The patient's estate sued the pharmacist and physician for damages because there were some restrictions against such prescriptions based on body mass index and health risk factors in 1997. These problems raised ethical issues facing a pharmacist who, on one hand, is told that his function is to dispense drugs only and, on the other hand, is told no he has a collective responsibility in the event of a drug misadventure. Pharmacists cannot worship God and Mammon at the same time; it is either one or the other. Is it reasonable to expect a pharmacist to set aside hundreds of prescriptions in a busy store of 400 to 800 scripts per day to go and weigh a patient in order to verify the authenticity of one prescription? Moreover, patients or their agents can drop and pick up their prescriptions in the pharmacy without the knowledge of the pharmacist at times so the issue of estimating or weighing the patient does not arise when the prescription is ready to be filled.

In another scenario in Florida, a nurse, Elizabeth, called in Tussi-Organidin, four ounces, one teaspoonful every six hours for a one-and-a-half-year-old child, Jose. The pharmacist took the order, and at the point of dispensing medication to the patient's mother, counseling revealed that the medication was intended for a child's running nose. The clinical pharmacist informed the mother that there is nothing for running nose in the order, so she called the doctor's office for clarification. The nurse then called the clinical pharmacist to change the order to tanafed, same quantity and directions. The clinical pharmacist noticed something unusual with the dosage because the maximum dose per day of tanafed is 8ml. He called the nurse to find out if she meant the dosage of 20ml per day. The nurse realized the consequences of her order; hence, she decided to change the order to one teaspoonful daily. The question being asked here is will Dr. Jose (coincidentally the same first name as the patient) have accepted full responsibility for this order if anything had gone wrong with the child? Any rational human being will question where is the doctor in all these transactions, and, as anyone would rightly predict, the answer was "he is busy." This issue sounds odd, and to many Doubting Thomases it is an isolated case. Believe it or not, this is the usual scenario in most physicians' offices especially those with certified nurse practitioners (CNP) and physician assistants (PA). Written and phoned-in prescriptions to pharmacies fly out of the offices without the doctor knowing the diagnosis or what was prescribed to the patients. This explains why some of these surrogate physicians, especially some CNPs, operate independent offices without the supervising physicians. In a few cases the supervising physicians might not even know the location of the offices. Many will ask if these people are supposed to be under the supervision of a physician and the best way to answer these people is that the term "under the supervision of a physician" is a theoretical phrase without meaning or reality. Shefcheck et al.'s study proves the fact that "nurse practitioners and physician assistants now have the authority to prescribe independently and deliver many of the same services as physicians at lower cost."[23] These are some of the issues the pharmacists have to deal with on a daily basis. It is pointless to mention the various obstacles pharmacists encounter in contacting doctors about prescription irregularities especially those in hospitals. After going through various ordeals, it is not unusual to hear that the doctor is busy with a patient or is unavailable till 2 or 4 p.m. There are instances where some doctors have told some pharmacists, "My duty is to prescribe and your duty is to dispense; whatever I give the patient is between the patient and me, and you don't question me about it, however polite you may be." It will not be out of place to say that some pharmacists think of a nightmare ordeal whenever they are faced with the option of calling the doctor for clarification, verification, or other purpose. It is easy to pass the doctors' mistakes to the pharmacists because of collective responsibility, which is unheard of in other aspects of life in the world. Ironically, the pharmacists have no one to shift his mistake and blame. He cannot ask the patients to bear the responsibility for his wrong label (e.g., the patient ought to remember what the doctor told him irrespective of the wrong label), nor can he pass such a mistake to the prescriber for a correctly written prescription.

Drug problems have been underestimated for many years until recently. Today, many people still do not consider drugs a poison, probably because they have no direct personal experience of bad drug response, and any drug can fit into this category. If the above issues failed to drive home the intended message, perhaps these people can learn from Stephen Fried's lesson. Stephen Fried's bitter lesson led to the publication of a book titled *Bitter Pills*. He is an investigative journalist whose wife, Diane, was given a free sample of a new antibiotic considered "a wonder drug" by her gynecologist in 1992 for an unnoticeable, minor urinary tract infection. The health problem was a simple/minor problem because Diane didn't even notice it, but the five-year ordeal that followed the administration of the supposed "wonder drug" was not only a nightmare but a catastrophe that was a million times greater than the initial health problem.

Six hours after she had taken the "wonder drug" Floxin (Ofloxacin) that was expected to treat an unnoticeable infection and make the patient feel better, Mr. Fried found himself rushing his wife to the emergency room (ER). She was delirious, disoriented, shaking, convulsing (experiencing seizures), and hallucinating, with tingling feelings in her left arm and difficulty talking. In the ER, a team of emergency medicine specialists and neurology residents conducted several exams to excavate the mystery. The poison control center later responded to an earlier call made by them by informing them that the patient's problem was the result of a documented reaction to the antibiotic Floxin. The ER did a CT scan, which came out negative, and they were sent home with the notion that her condition would improve and she would recover from the devastating effect of the drug as soon as the drug left her body. They were now given a cheaper, milder antibiotic. They went home; some symptoms waned, while new ones emerged with fixed pupils, aggressiveness, insomnia, visual distortions, and aphasia (patient can't make a complete sentence). The drug had gone out of her system yet the problem continued. She underwent further tests including an electroencephalogram (EEG), magnetic resonance imaging (MRI), CT scan, spinal tap, and blood work to diagnose her problem. The results came out again negative, and the doctors concluded that the Floxin had precipitated some genetic abnormality or predisposition to mood disorder, which had led to the neurological disorder. They claimed that her body had not been able to adjust naturally to the drug side effects; consequently, she would be given heavy-duty drugs to combat the problem.

Initially she was given Klonopin to combat insomnia, and lithium for mood swings or manic depression. Klonopin became too sedative for her, making her drowsy (zombie sleep), so it was switched to Ativan. Lithium wasn't quite effective; hence, it was changed to Depakote and later tegretor. Diane gradually metamorphosed into a chronic patient with chronic illnesses such as manic depression and a neuro-ophthalmologic condition, all because of one pill, Floxin. She was given medications to treat the manic depression but the visual distortions remain unabated with no solution in sight. They contacted Dr. Galetta, the best known neuro-ophthalmologist in Pennsylvania, for an examination. Dr. Galetta did the eye examination and came up with the explanation that Diane's visual problem was the result of subacute myelo-optic neuropathy due to halogenated hydroxquinolones. He provided them with literature and further explanation of how this condition can cause permanent nerve damage and visual problems that can precipitate paralysis and blindness. After Galetta's diagnosis, Diane came to the conclusion with a bitter resolution/reality to move on with her life by dealing with the health problems she could handle with treatment and adjusting to those that were untreatable. She angrily said she is now a seriously mentally ill patient, and her husband understandably began to grapple with the fact that he is now married to a chronically ill patient with manic depression and a neuro-ophthalmologic condition for the rest of their life together. On the issue of lawsuit, Diane rebuffed the idea claiming that it is for people that have nothing to lose, and she still has her life. She was conscious of the fact that an earlier consultation with an attorney revealed that the discovery process alone would cost them $50,000. Mr. Stephen, however, decided to move on with the desire to publish a book about the episode, with Diane's blessing.

Mr. Stephen Fried's extensive work highlighted a lot of hidden facts: facts about the health care profession that have been swept under the rug in America, and the world to some extent, for quite a long time. Diane's health ordeal brought Stephen in contact with various health care practitioners, many of whom he had bitter remarks. He exalted the glorious work of clinical pharmacologists (the few present-day physicians who specialize in drug therapy) and implored patients to consult them when they find the need to do so. One of the clinical pharmacologists, Dr. David Flockhart, that attended to Diane's health problems fought relentlessly to explain her condition on the basis of mechanism of action of the drug. He blamed his colleagues for treating all patients in a similar manner with one-dose-fits-all models irrespective of ethnic groups, weight, metabolic and gender differences, etc. Dr. David reiterated the fact that clinical pharmacologists are interested in drug efficacy and safety irrespective of pharmaceutical companies' views and sales representatives' pressure. All drugs have a benefits and risks ratio; these are issues that ought to be taken into consideration in the prescribing act of every drug, but quite too often they are neglected by doctors. Stephen also extended kudos to Ann and Kristen, the young CVS pharmacists who understood drug problems, were involved in patient health care, and were willing to question any doctor about therapy because physicians don't get it. He said these pharmacists knew everything about omniflox, for example, while the doctors who often downplay ADR were clueless.[16] Abbot Laboratories in its congratulatory message to pharmacists for being the most trusted professionals according to a 1992 Gallup poll acknowledged the fact that pharmacists are medication experts.

Dr. Kessler, a medical doctor, lawyer, and former FDA chairman, claims that more than half of the drug-related ADRs are preventable, and as many as 99% of serious adverse drug and device events are not reported because it is difficult for the doctors to say I hurt you, I didn't mean to do so, or you are just one out of many who develop ADR after taking the drug. He blamed the problem on inadequate medical school training in drug therapy and clinical pharmacology. Many medical schools teach only a few hours of clinical pharmacology in the early years of students' training. This is why errors in prescription drugs account for the second cause of malpractice suits and claims. Drug companies at times misrepresent facts and downplay ADR as insignificant in order to get FDA approval, and the FDA can't verify this information until they are in the market because of inadequate funding. For example in 1982, Eli Lilly pleaded guilty for criminally withholding facts about oraflex, and Hoechst did the same about merital in 1986. Ironically, physicians depend on these facts for their knowledge instead of journals. Dr. Flockhart had accused the FDA and pharmaceutical companies of meddling with drugs when they don't know the mechanism of action of the drug. The pharmaceutical companies spend $10 billion every year to persuade the 550,000 physicians to prescribe their drugs as part of their market strategy and $9 billion on research. Some of the pharmaceutical industry sales representatives who used various tactics including hosting MDs in the best hotels/restaurants, free samples, flyers' awards, gift certificates, tickets for luxurious occasions, and sexual manipulations with female sales representatives to drive home their message have expressed dismay and distrust of the medical field. They reportedly claimed that they wouldn't see 90% of the physicians they used for their sales promotions. They said physicians are in the habit of asking a patient, "What is your problem?" and the moment the patient says anything, even coughs, the next thing is "Take this antibiotic." This indiscriminate use of antibiotics and other drugs is creating problems for the medical world and it is further compounded with direct-to-consumer (DTC) advertisement in television and the news media. A 1995 survey showed that 99 out of 100 (99%) physicians will succumb to or consider a patient's request to prescribe a drug when asked to do so. DTC advertisement has been blamed for patient's demand for drugs from prescribers who either succumbed to patient's request or run the risk of losing the patient to another prescriber who will do so.[16]

Stephen went beyond Diane's case to bring to light other people's medical predicaments such as Stacy Phillips, a lawyer who was equally floxed by Floxin. She ended up with a seizure, which forced her to quit her job. Joan Hiddemen's husband died from kidney failure because he was given omniflox for bronchitis (non-FDA-approved indication). Velva Conrad ended up on life support and with kidney and multi-organ failure because she was given omniflox for a simple urinary tract infection (UTI). Lita Cohen, a Pennsylvania state representative, was prescribed Floxin then noroxin after she had a bad reaction to the former, and the doctor didn't know that Floxin and noroxin are in the same class of drug. David was on an antiseizure drug when he phoned the MD about flu and chest cold symptoms and the doctor phoned in Floxin, Imodium D, and cough syrup to a pharmacy with no office visit. Less than an hour after medicating himself he was in the emergency room—the doctor thought it was the cough syrup that was causing the problem because he did not know that Floxin and seizure (or antiseizure drugs) are major contraindications. Alice McGee of the *Oprah Winfrey Show*, Sue, and many others. Diane's health sequeal and many others could have been avoided by mere simple office protocol of asking patients their health history, which would have revealed that Diane once had a concussion and loss of consciousness because of two auto accidents in her youth. As a result she was not a candidate for Floxin or floroquinolones. Moreover, floroquinolones are not the first line of therapy for any infection outside the hospital. They are considered second and third against indiscriminate protocol adopted by many prescribers who now see it as first-line therapy.

Dr. Raymond Woosley and Dave Flockhart had planned to propagate and implement Woosley's Center for Education and Research in Therapeutics

(CERT) program as a way of establishing information and education centers for patients, physicians, and pharmacists. The aim was to rescue the society from inadequate drug knowledge by doing drug research with the FDA and disseminating unbiased information about efficacy, safety, benefit/risk ratios, and the price of drugs to all and sundry. It was expected to be funded by the government with operations in major universities that have a clinical pharmacology department. The plan was first suggested in the 1970s; then in the 1990s, the NIH and FDA regarded it as a laudable idea but there is no money to execute it. The drug industries considered the idea a nightmare because the center was expected to operate independently without their influence. Dr. Woosley may have borrowed the laudable idea from the Netherlands, the world's safest drug country. Netherlands has an effective drug safety program, which is propagated by the universities and supported by the government, and an active adverse drug reaction monitoring system. The program helped to minimize drug casualties. Dr. Ray's desire to include price in the program is born out of the fact that many studies have shown that most prescribers are ignorant of drug prices; consequently, cost-effective therapy is foreign to them.[16]

Though Woosley's plan did not materialize because of funding; however, the schools of pharmacy in various universities across the nation moved in swiftly to fill the vacuum by creating drug information centers as part of its clinical pharmacy program. Like schools of pharmacy, many hospitals' pharmacies left no stone unturned in creating drug information centers within the department or making pharmacy available for drug information to any health care practitioner including physicians and nurses. Drug information centers have helped to provide drug research, disseminate unbiased information about drug efficacy, safety, price, and benefit/risk ratio, as well as educate patients, physicians, and pharmacists. Although its impact is not fully realized because of public unawareness, it is easy to see that much of its silence is linked to pharmacy's bondage to other branches of medicine. Pharmacy liberation will go a long way to enhance its status in the society. Students under the supervision of their professors/lecturers conduct drug research and the government is not directly involved in funding of the program. Besides being the cheapest means of funding such programs, drug information centers in schools of pharmacy have provided a forum for students to explore their talents, tap lecturers/professors' ingenuity, and gain firsthand information about pharmaceutical companies and the real world of drugs. Needless to say that drug information centers have saved the government another bureaucratic and expensive program that is of vital interest to the public.

In spite of the glorious words about pharmacy, this is not an attempt to portray pharmacists as angels or saints while downplaying their weaknesses.

Pharmacists are human, and very human indeed in terms of human flaws. In late 1995, Diane Sawyer of *ABC Primetime* enumerated several issues involving pharmacists' mistakes, their refusal to counsel on dangerous drug combinations such as coumadin and aspirin, fast counseling over the counter with mother gaining nothing, pharmacy unreceptive environments (patients down and pharmacists up), and others. In 1996, Woosley's study revealed that many pharmacists filled every prescription without counseling, and the study was published in *U.S. News and World Report, JAMA,* and other places. Investigators were sent out with three paired contraindicated prescriptions such as seldane and erythromycin, which are not supposed to be taken together. 16 out of 50 pharmacies in Washington, D.C., dispensed seldane 60mg 1BIDX5D and erythromycin 250mg 1TIDX7D with no verbal warning or written precaution for patients about the contraindication, and when questioned about therapy---5 out of 14 said no, you can't take both medications together, while the rest pharmacists said yes, you can. The results demonstrated that seriously contraindicated prescriptions with labels were filled without verbal warning one third of the time; three out of sixty-one pharmacists deemed it necessary to warn about two antihypertensive medications (vasotec and dyazide) with interactions; and more than three quarters (4 out of 17) pharmacists filled birth control pills and antibiotic perscriptions (rimactane-rifampin) without any caution. Pharmacists in lower-income neighborhoods and independent community pharmacies were more likely to be guilty than others. Less than half of the surveyed pharmacies gave out written warnings with dispensed prescriptions, and there were city-to-city variations in terms of warnings about dangerous drug interactions.[16,20,22] Other complaints such as wrong labels or drugs, inaccurate counting, and unnecessary delay have been levied against various pharmacies.

Pharmacists have responded to the above publications by citing computer's inability to differentiate between serious and insignificant interactions---for instance there are about 30,000 drug interactions of which 3,000 - 4,000 are moderate and 1,200 - 1,300 are major (this is beyond the comprehension of one man according to Professor Phillip Hansten of the University of Washington, a known drug interaction authority who came to the aid of the pharmacy by accusing computer systems manufacturers of highlighting all interactions irrespective of their significance or insignificance for legal reasons), managed care pressures (pressure such as adherence to formulary, prior and grudging), patients' apathy in seeking pharmacists' consultation, employers' appetite for increase profit through volume of prescriptions (pharmacists are pressurized to dispense more prescriptions with fewer helps in less time. It is now customary for supervisors/employers to ask pharmacists what happens whenever pharmacies fall short of a new record e.g., 400 instead of 600 scripts per day), patients' interruptions, telephone conversation and frequently ringing phone, phone in-prescriptions and other problems as a major factor. In view of the above reasons, most pharmacists do not consider drug interactions, drug choice, and therapeutic counseling even though the law mandates it through OBRA '90 as their primary responsibilities/functions. They assume that if the prescriber has performed his primary functions (drug choice, interactions, and therapeutic counseling) judiciously then they don't have to worry about it as a secondary function, because filling and dispensing of medications is their primary function in the era of count and pour.[18]

Though it is widely acknowledged that people get drowned in the sea and people still drink water, people get killed in plane crashes and car accidents and people still fly and use cars—humanity's perseverance depends on a benefits/risks ratio in most cases. This explains why we have specialists taking care of every aspect of our lives to minimize risks and increase benefits. For instance, a meteorologist is a specialist in weather forecasting because he has gone through rigorous university training to groom him for the job. In view of this drastic training to perfect his skills in weather reporting, his forecast is not expected to be 100% perfect because he is not God. It is reasonable and realistic to expect 80 to 90% perfect predictions or correct weather forecasts in light of a benefits/risks ratio compared to non-specialists who will be 30 to 40% right (low benefits) and 60 to 70% wrong (greater risks). Consequently, while judging pharmacists' competency in terms of the above human flaws and ability to write prescriptions at the early stage of its liberation whenever it happens, it is important to note that we cannot use the performance of present-day first-degree holders or even Doctor of Pharmacy degree holders to judge the performance of future Doctor of Pharmacy degree holders—the ones who are expected to drag the bull by the horns to the altar and will eventually take pharmacy to its final destination. Contemporary pharmacists' success in the nation's health care delivery system, with the aid of pharmaceutical care, is a fragment of tomorrow's pharmacists' achievements. This is because today's pharmacists find themselves constantly pulled out of the traditional role of the dispensing-only function (be it in the form of government-mandated OBRA '90 counseling or a professional's self-invented pharmaceutical care) to a more deserving position in patients' health care. This is because of an existing vacuum or perpetual state of want that is clamoring for drug experts—experts that have been lying fallow for years. It is important to note that today's pharmacists were not groomed in schools of pharmacy for prescription-writing skills, therapeutic counseling, and drug interactions (non-PharmD holders) and other deserving roles that they are now being called upon to fulfill. Yet study after study has shown that when they perform these roles, they do better than physicians and other health care practitioners put together. We therefore need no soothsayers to predict that the sky would be the limit at the time these functions/roles are taught in schools of pharmacy; pharmacists are free to act independently like other specialists in their respective fields, and clinical pharmacists (Doctor of Pharmacy degree holders) take over control of the profession's fate and destiny. Dr. Hansten spoke about drug interactions and computer industries; it is nice to note that manufacturers of computers are themselves confused about this phenomenon because they do not know who to listen to. They have to cover all loopholes by exposing all drug interactions for legal reasons. They are caught between pharmacists and physicians because they don't know who is in charge or who to tell what is minor, moderate, and major drug interactions or what should be included or excluded from drug interactions in the database. If they know who is in charge as drug specialists then they can comfortably rely on them for data input and be ready to quote them as the final and resolute authority in court whenever they are called upon to do so.

As shown, all enumerated facts about drugs and drug-related problems did not occur simultaneously prior to the commencement of the Doctor of Pharmacy degree. However, it is necessary to highlight them to justify the need for drug specialists and the reasons why these specialists need higher doctorate degrees to prepare them for the arduous task ahead, like every other specialty in the medical field. Judging by the magnitude of drug problems in this country and the world at large, it is obvious that these specialists are needed today and in future societies. Some studies buttress the fact that drug problems in this country have remained fairly constant from the 1960s till the present day. This explains why all hands must be on deck to strengthen the pharmacy rather than impoverish it as is currently practiced in the medical field—robbing Peter to pay Paul. The origin of clinical pharmacy and the Doctor of Pharmacy degree (PharmD) were detailed in the previous chapter. At the beginning, clinical pharmacy and PharmD degrees had no market base; it was difficult to sell them to the patients, third-party payers, and the government because of lack of professional autonomy. These programs, however, were destined for success, if only pharmacy autonomy could be guaranteed and the profession had no alternative. Other issues such as counseling and pharmaceutical care may have served the profession well at one point or the other, but they were merely beating around the bush without hitting the nail on the head. After initial humiliation by market forces, a Doctor of Pharmacy degree and its clinical impact began to creep and ascend to prominence as the years rolled by. Dr. Strand, one of the co-authors of pharmaceutical care, experienced firsthand pharmacy humiliations and lack of professional autonomy when she was forced to face reality as a PharmD student in the 1970s. She questioned herself about the finality of a pharmacist's responsibility (where does it start and end). Dr. Strand's question and views were encroached and imbedded in a questionable answer from Peter Morley, a British medical anthropologist. Peter told Dr. Strand in 1983 that "pharmacy had no niche—the profession could get to the patient only through the drug or the disease or another practitioner."[34]

Peter's opinion correlates well, and every pharmacist can relate to it because this has been the fate of the profession for years after the apothecaries' humiliation and denigration. This impression probably accounts for the daily humiliations that pharmacists encounter in the discharge of their duties in chain pharmacies that are now the protagonist of community pharmacy. Pharmacists' niche is not defined anywhere, even in chain pharmacy where pharmacists are caught between worshipping God and Mammon. Pharmacists are told that their position is below that of the store manager no matter the status of the latter in terms of education and income. If this is true, what is the pharmacist's position in relation to the store manager/management? They cannot define it; consequently, all other defined positions below the store manager, even newly appointed or promoted cashier managers from bag boy positions, start to count their blessings by assessing their positions from the top to know where the pharmacist/pharmacy comes under them. Numerous conflicts have arisen because of this issue, and many pharmacists refused to accept the status dictated to them by top management. They find it difficult to respond to complaints and other issues to someone (store manager, assistant store manager, etc.) whom they feel knows nothing about the running of a pharmacy instead of their immediate supervisor, the pharmacy supervisor, who knows the ins and outs of pharmacy. Few chain drugstores (about one or two) have responded to pharmacists' plight by rerouting complaints to district managers for investigation and resolution, while others remain the same. The majority of the chain drugstores sound indifferent to pharmacy's image and reputation. At one time in Florida, chain drugstores moved to deprofessionalize the profession through enforcing a dress code, and as far as a dress code is concerned, words of elders are words of wisdom that never fade away. Thus, the common sayings that "actions speak louder than words" and "the first impression matters a lot" go a long way to define dressing code. Personal appearance speaks loud and clear about anybody even before the person has any opportunity to defend himself or address anybody/situation through communication. Dress code is the easiest way to demean or uphold the dignity of a profession. All schools of pharmacy in the world need to bear in mind that pharmacy is a branch of medicine and not an errand boy of medicine; as a result, like other branches of medicine, they need to get tough on rudimentary principles of dress code for pharmacy students. Pharmacy students are the future of the pharmacy profession and, like other branches of medicine, they need to imbibe the tenets of a good dress code in school so as to project a good image of the profession to patients, the community, and the world at large.

In our contemporary society, many jobs (e.g., hotel waiters, post office clerks, social workers, and others) that had not previously cared about workers' appearance are moving towards professionalization of the job through a strict dress code at a time when these chain drugstores deem it necessary to move away from such dress code. The chain drugstores claim that pharmacists are no longer required to appear in smart dress with a tie. No matter what we say or do, the first impression matters a lot to patients and patrons of pharmacy because it says so many things about the person and the profession he represents. If for any reason we have cause to doubt this idea, let us ponder over the following scenarios: What is the general opinion of a nation whose president appears in a presidential conference in jeans and a polo shirt? Or a traditional medical doctor who constantly appears in his office with earrings, jeans, and a T-shirt? Even if he is the best medical doctor in the world, would you allow him to continue rendering health services to you? Listen to what people have to say about him in the community. Your outward appearance goes a long way to show the degree of your seriousness and how much you care about yourself, your job, and people's feelings. You are what you make of yourself. If you make a mess out of yourself, no matter your status, be you a doctor, lawyer, engineer, president, homeless person, or other, people will treat you as such. Likewise, if you make gold out of yourself, even if you are the lowest in the society, people will treat you like gold. Thus, if you dress casually to a job as if you're going to a tennis court or working in your backyard garden, you can't expect people to rate you or the entire job otherwise than that which you portray to them. Generally, a dress code, like every other rule and regulation, helps to enhance adherence and people feel compelled to abide by rules and regulations. In every society, there are deviants however tough the rules and regulations may be, but the majority of the people have a civic responsibility and will do everything within their reach to obey the laws. With a strict dress code there are some people within every profession that find it difficult to comply with the rules and regulations, but the situation is better. Personal motivation in the absence of laws is a good idea, but many people forget about it when they don't see it as a personal issue. The tendency to backslide and relapse increases when rules and regulations are rescinded. Pharmacy is better with a tough dress code including use of ties than without a good dress code. At least do not alter the status if you cannot improve it; leave it as it is and allow the situation to take care of itself. You send a wrong message when you rescind good rules and regulations, and that is the situation with pharmacy, because the profession and professionals are role models to millions of people around the world. Outward appearance is one of the good/outstanding qualities of a role model; the affected chain drugstores above are beginning to learn their lessons when they discover that patients/patrons of the pharmacy cannot differentiate between pharmacists and other pharmacy personnel in the pharmacy. It is shameful to discover that yesteryear pharmacists are better groomed in the dress code than contemporary pharmacists in affected areas when the profession is supposed to be moving forward.

PRESENT

The present phase is the transitional phase, an era characterized by professional indignity, shame, feelings of inadequacy, and ego brutalization when addressed as a medical doctor. Yet no one can deny the awesome contribution of clinical pharmacists in improving patients' lives, saving huge amounts of money for the health care system, and saving many human lives. It is therefore reasonable to ask, what do other medical doctors do that is different from clinical pharmacists?

Pharmacists need self-confidence and ego brush up in order to move beyond the redundant era of count and pour, an era that trivialized them, impoverished the profession, sangfroid their knowledge to the point that they doubted even the things they knew, and wasted their intelligence and years of school training.

If Doctors of Pharmacy (PharmD) Degree Holders Are Not Medical Doctors, What Are They?

There are three forms of doctorate degree in the world today and they are honorary doctors, medical doctors, and academic doctors (PhD). Honorary doctorate degrees are conferred on deserving candidates by universities, colleges, or institutions of higher learning. Medical doctorate degrees are conferred on graduates of various branches of medicine, with different titles such as ophthalmology, dentistry (DMD), surgery, internal medicine, optometry (OD), pediatrics, osteopathy (DO), psychiatry, radiology, and others. Academic doctorate degrees are the highest academic honor/degree conferred on graduates in various disciplines such as biology, chemistry, history, mathematics, and others. Academic doctorates, otherwise tagged Doctor of Philosophy (PhD), are research degrees awarded to deserving candidates by institutions of higher learning. The Doctor of Pharmacy degree in all its ramifications is not an honorary degree, neither is it an academic doctorate degree (PhD). Pharmacy is a branch of medicine like every other branch, and a doctorate degree in the field is no different from other medical doctorate degrees. Veterinary doctors, dentists, and optometrists go through four years of professional didactic coursework without residence requirement and they are considered medical doctors. Clinical pharmacists go through four years of professional didactic course work with or without residence, and so what is the difference? As noted earlier, a chiropractor's academic rigor is not as tough as the dentist's, clinical pharmacist's, optometrist's, or veterinarian's, yet they consider themselves medical doctors and people treat them as such. An osteopathic physician was once considered as nonprofessional and unworthy of medical doctors' characteristics, but today the reverse is the case.

The major problem that characterizes pharmacists' professional shame, indignity, inadequacy, and ego brutalization when addressed as medical doctors is the bondage and enslaved nature of his job performance. Pharmacy is the only profession in the world where people can acquire a doctorate degree and still be treated like a baby rather than the master of his destiny. As noted earlier, a teacher goes through four years of college and becomes the great shaper of a student's life by planning his class work as well as lesson notes. Attorneys go through 6 to 7 years of college work (4 years for BSc and 2 to 3 years in law school) and become the planner of his clients' cases. An electrical engineer goes through 4 years of college work and becomes the planner of electrical projects. An architect goes through 4 to5 years of college work and become the designer of building projects, and many other examples. Ironically, pharmacists go through 6 to 7 years (2 years for associate and 4 years in school of pharmacy—6 years for direct students and 7 years for BSc and PharmD) of college work to become a doctor, and he is told at the end that he cannot write in a patient's chart in the hospital, he cannot prescribe any legal drug, he cannot change a patient's therapy without notifying the prescriber, and prior to 1969 he (including Dr. David Burkholder, 1962 PharmD holder and founder of drug information center) cannot speak to patients about drug therapy. The pharmacists are constantly reminded of the need to declare their doctorate degree null and void and be content with increasing their skills as a typist. Little wonder why a Florida congressman in Washington, D.C., asked if pharmacists have college degrees (Florida Society of Health System Pharmacists newsletter, May 2002). Typing skills enable him to spill out as many prescriptions as possible and dispense them within a twinkle of an eye. Unfortunately, typing skills are coursework for the typists and not for the pharmacists; there is nowhere in pharmacy curriculum where the course is encouraged as a prerequisite. It therefore sounds unreasonable to expect pharmacists to be perfect typists, but that is the reality of life for most pharmacists (recall Jerry Seinfeld's satirical remarks) and this is what it takes to be in bondage with others, an ordeal that characterized pharmacists' foot dragging phenomenon, greater delay and more time to liberate pharmacy than other fields like dentistry, osteopathic medicine, and family practice.

"FREEDOM IS A RIGHT AND NOT A PRIVILEGE"

The enslaved must recognize his condition and be conscious of his rights in order to demand for them. If he waits for the enslaver to voluntarily relinquish his privileges and set him free, he might as well forget about his freedom and ponder about his death in bondage. (also in chapter 1).

Many pharmacists have accepted their restrictive job functions as a way of life while some see it as repugnant act. Those who have accepted their restrictive role as a way of life do not only consider the idea of regarding a pharmacist as a medical doctor a strange phenomenon but also an abomination. Respect for a Doctor of Pharmacy (PharmD) degree to these fellows sounds like a prophet that never commands respect in his hometown. Many people, especially those in Spanish and underprivileged neighborhoods, and some within the medical community have recognized Doctor of Pharmacy degree holders as medical doctors. A few dentists, osteopathic physicians, family practice physicians, and those who suffered the same initial humiliations and recognition problems as pharmacy have sympathized with pharmacy and wasted no time in recognizing Doctor of Pharmacy degree holders as medical doctors. Dr. Eric Alvarez's euphemism about his personal experience in dealing with his Doctor of Pharmacy degree, other health care practitioners, and a professional outlook serve as living example to illuminate the issue of revamping pharmacists' image and reputation. Dr. Eric Alvarez is a PharmD holder and former president of the Florida Pharmacy Association (FPA). During his tenure in office, he wrote an article entitled "The Ten Commandments of Pharmacy" in *Florida Pharmacy Today* (a publication of the FPA) in which he narrated his phone-in-prescription ordeal with Dr. Smith himself (not a staff member). At the end of the telephone conversation, Smith asked Eric for his name and Eric responded by saying, "Eric Alvarez." Smith told him, "Thank you, Eric." At this point he decided to ask Smith for his name again and he replied, "Dr. Smith." Eric insisted further, "What is your first name?" and he told Eric, "S. Smith." Eric became a little exasperated and told Smith, "Look, Dr. S. Smith, my real name is Dr. E. Alvarez." He implored him to forget about his first name since they were not operating at the same frequency by using first names simultaneously. Dr. Alvarez said this was a daily occurrence and he reminded his colleagues of the "respect, trust, and credibility" that goes with the title of doctor, which he believed was taught in medical school.[19]

In actual sense there is nowhere the title "medical doctor" is taught as a course in medical schools; it is like every other process in human life, and we can use growth from adolescence to adulthood as a typical example. In every society a child is treated like a child; however, at adolescence the situation begins to change depending on how fast the child matures. The moment people begin to treat the adolescent like an adult and address him as Mister (Mr.) instead of Master in a title-conscious society, the adolescent becomes conscious of his new role as an adult and the need to behave appropriately because society places greater responsibility, trust, credibility, and duty on him now. This process is considered a rite of passage and it is treated as an initiation process with a ceremony in very few societies today. The title "medical doctor" is treated in a similar manner in medical schools; the only difference is that the medical doctor becomes conscious of the new title and their treatment of it, which determines people's response and society's respect. Thus, a young medical doctor that graduates from a medical school but seldom uses the title with his name will notice little or no difference in people's response and society's respect. The fragmented respect that will be passed on to him in his office is the result of societal indoctrination by his colleagues who adhered strictly to usage of the title with their names. In our contemporary society, where titles means a lot to many people in offices especially medical doctors' offices, and pharmacy is not an exception to the rule of medical office. Pharmacy is a medical office by all standards with even more medical paraphernalia (e.g., drugs, medical supplies, testing apparatus, etc.) than some other medical offices. Disregarding the Doctor of Pharmacy degree and the subsequent title that goes with it does not only puts the profession at odds and in an awkward position to others but also alienates it and trivializes its impact on the health care system.

Hence, it is compulsory for the PHARMACIST-PATIENT relationship to change from the PRODUCT-ORIENTED SERVICES to PATIENT-ORIENTED SERVICES on both sides (pharmacist and patient). The pharmacy/pharmacists must initiate the move to change the orientation from PHARMACIST-CUSTOMER relationship to a PHARMACIST-PATIENT RELATIONSHIP. This will enhance the relationship, make greater demands on the pharmacist, increase pharmacist's responsibilities, create greater awareness in society, improve patient's health care, quality of life, and therapeutic outcome. It is absolutely ridiculous that this is a contemporary issue for pharmacists to deal with, because this is the key element in trivializing pharmacists and the pharmacy profession. The patient-health care practitioner relationship does not start and end with one health care practitioner or branch of medicine. As a matter of fact, most healing processes or patient ordeals end with the pharmacists, so why must the patient-provider (health care practitioner) relationship stop just because the patient goes from the traditional medical doctor's office to the pharmacy and the pharmacy or pharmacist is no place or nobody in the healing process? With the exception of very few patients who receive medicinal samples (supplied by drug manufacturers) from the traditional medical doctors' offices, no patients are cured or healed in medical doctors' offices; they (patients) must complete the healing processes with a visit to the pharmacy. Pharmacy and pharmacists must change this orientation through massive education of its staff and the public.

If any pharmacist feels that they are not worthy of the title and society's subsequent image of a medical doctor, they can do themselves, the degree, and the profession a big favor by donating the degree to a nearby library. The degree merits more respect in the library where it can serve better purposes at least to future generations as evidence of what was obtainable in our days. Dr. Alvarez reiterated his mother's views by saying, "If you don't respect yourself, no one else will either" (a popular saying by worthy parents). He ended his note by calling on his colleagues to use Mr. or Dr. in referring patients to other pharmacists because of the need to treat ourselves the way we want others to do.

Another pharmacist with a PharmD degree and whose sole aim of going to a postgraduate Doctor of Pharmacy degree program was to become a clinical pharmacist had a similar but different experience. The use of the title "doctor" was not even an issue before he went into the program, but at the tail end of the course, sometime before the beginning of 2000, an in-depth analysis of the medical field and its relation with pharmacy revealed a lot of facts. Some of which are:

- The origin of pharmacy and other specialties in the medical field.
- The treatment of pharmacy/pharmacist as errand boy of medicine.
- The second-class status of the pharmacy profession in the medical field.
- The impact of pharmacy on the health care system and drug knowledge of pharmacists as drug specialists/therapeuticians (therapeutic physicians).
- The award of a PharmD, which is by no means different from other medical doctorate degrees, yet many recipients feel unworthy of it, inadequate, and genetically inferior to other medical practitioners.
- How pharmacists are treated like women and every other oppressed group in human history.

The pharmacist came to the conclusion that respect is a two-way affair that begins with oneself because respect respect those who respected themselves. For instance, doctors learned how to respect themselves in spite of their professional failures and of their topsy-turvy condition. If a doctor called a pharmacist for drug information (dosage, strength, ingredients, composition, administration, etc.) and in the next 5 minutes or so called the pharmacy back or called another pharmacy to give the same information as a phone-in prescription order or sent a patient home with the information on a prescription, this does not belittle him as a doctor in the public eye or make him relinquish his title. Rather, he addressed himself there and then as a medical doctor and people treated him as such. A 1993 University of Mississippi national survey of pharmacists revealed pharmacists' growing role as physician educators, with 88% of the respondents claiming that physicians depend on them for information about drugs already in the market; 87% said the same thing about a new drug; 85% about drug prices; and 83% claimed that they were asked to select appropriate prescription drugs for a given therapy by the physician.[35] Alternatively, if a patient goes to the doctor's office with therapeutic suggestions or a drug excerpt because he needs a prescription for the drug and the doctor has never heard anything about the therapy or drug in his whole life. The doctor looks at the therapy, examines the patient's complaints, and writes a prescription as dictated by the patient. These are regularly occurring daily issues because doctors are human beings with all human flaws. They are not infallible and these issues do not make them feel inferior, inadequate, or unworthy of their medical doctor's degree unlike many pharmacists. The pharmacist noted these facts and resolved to constantly use the title "doctor" until anybody proved the opposite to him. The resolution has meant various obstacles, but none of these obstacles in the form of hurdles are as disdainful as the ones put forth by his fellow colleagues (pharmacists) and others within the profession. If the law says you are a human being and you say or feel that you do not deserve to be treated as such because you are not as rich as Bill Gates, as pretty as Marilyn Monroe, as smart as Isaac Newton or Albert Einstein, as strong as Mike Tyson, or as powerful as an American president, that is your funeral. Hold no one culpable for your misfortune, because you are the architect. It is important that you keep your beliefs and personal philosophy to yourself rather than use it to destroy others.

The present transitional phase of the pharmacy profession might be characterized with humiliations as seen in the initial stage of every profession, but it has helped to nurture many well-rounded first-degree-holder pharmacists and Doctor of Pharmacy degree holders/clinical pharmacists. Clinical pharmacy had its roots in the early 1930s with the intern students or pharmacists who went into the hospital for additional training/institutional practice of pharmacy. The term clinical pharmacy was hardly used until the mid-1960s, and it has since grown out of pharmacists' desire to search for a new direction for the profession. The new direction has created new and different sets of health care practitioners; practitioners that understand drugs' mechanism of action, drug benefits/risks ratios, adequate dosing, reduction of skyrocketing health care costs, adverse drug reactions, and minimizing morbidity and mortality resulting from ADR. In 1952, two years after the commencement of the radical Doctor of Pharmacy degree program by the University of California in 1950, Dr. Harry Gold, a physician, requested the establishment of a specialty that could handle pharmacology and clinical medicine within the health care field. This set of specialists was classified as clinical pharmacologists.[21] Pharmaceutical industries and some medical schools rationalized Dr. Gold's proposals and came to the conclusion that it was the right thing to do because it is a right step in the right direction. However, the American Medical Association (AMA) and other physicians groups just didn't see the need for it; consequently, the program was almost strangled to death. Clinical pharmacology started on a sluggish note and became a foot-dragging phenomenon for adroit physicians like Drs. Flockhart, Woosley, and others who equally saw the need for a specialty for pharmacology and clinical medicine within the medical field.

Clinical pharmacy has outpaced clinical pharmacology in terms of evolution, growth, impact, and the tendency to spread to various universities and other places around the world through schools of pharmacy. Special grace and thanks to the pioneering efforts of Don Francke, David Burkholder, Paul Parker, Charles Walton, Waite Rising, Eugene White, the University of California School of Pharmacy at San Francisco, the University of Michigan School of Pharmacy, University of Kentucky School of Pharmacy, Kodak Kimble, Philip Hansten, Dipiro, Hepler, Strand, Bonds, Bootman, Johnson, Ralp Small, Daniel Buffington, Osterhaus, Christopher Green, Tara Green, Gouveia, Donald Downing, James Cloyd, and many others. The impact of pharmacists on the health care system will be examined in detail in chapter 8; however, some studies about the needs for pharmacists will be highlighted here.

Shefcheck and Thomas studied the role of pharmacists in initiating and modifying drug therapy. The aim of the study was to examine the status of state laws that allow and do not allow pharmacist initiation and/or modification of drug therapy and the activities of those who facilitate or act as an impediment. The study was conducted with fifty-two revised surveys sent to director of pharmacy associations in all states including Puerto Rico and Washington, D.C., through the mail. Results revealed 84.6% (i.e., 44 States) response rate and there were numerous variations in the statistics/information provided by the states. Sixteen states allowed pharmacists to initiate and/or modify drug therapy. Twelve out of thirteen of those states have such gestures in hospital, while 11 out of 13 of those states permit the gesture in long-term care settings and 11 out of 14 of the 16 states permit pharmacists to do so in community settings. California required clinical residence with no additional education in order for hospital pharmacists to prescribe drugs independently, while Florida required maintenance of state license for pharmacists to prescribe drugs from state formulary such as decongestants (e.g., ephedrine), lindane products, fluoride products, antihistamines (e.g., loratadine, brompheniramine, fexofenadine, carbinoxamine, azelastine), mild pain killers, some topical products (e.g., nystatin cream, ointment, lotion, or powder; erythromycin; hydrocortisone not more than 2.5%), acetic acid (2% in aluminum acetate), antacid (e.g., cimetidine, famotidine, ranitidine), acyclovir, penciclovir, antipyrine, benzocaine, glycerin, and some cough products according to Florida Department of Health in the year 2000. (This is less than fifty drugs minus OTC drugs, and it is absolutely nothing compared to other non-drug specialists' prescribing authority, such as the PA's more than 650 drugs.) Of the forty-four states, 36.4% percent permit pharmacists to perform the above role in a different capacity; another 36.4% currently do not have such laws but plan to do so in the nearest future; while the rest (27.3%) do not have the laws, nor do they plan to allow it in the future. Majority of the 27.3% states (28) cited physicians associations (76.2%), pharmacists' indifferent attitudes (28.6%), pharmaceutical companies (23.8%), pharmacists' prevailing practices and laws (14.3%), pharmacists' inability to grasp what is at stake (19%), insurance or third-party payers (9.5%), and few others as barriers. Majority of the states (19) that allowed pharmacists to prescribe drugs independently or dependently cited physicians' support (57.9%), savings for the health care system (52.6%), pharmacists' initiatives (31.6%), patients' attitude and support (26.3%), legislators' education (5.3%), and others (21.1%) as source of encouragement.[23]

Provision of health care services to citizens of rural areas of the U.S. faces an uphill battle because of inadequate clinics, hospitals, and other health facilities; insufficient health care providers; transportation obstacles; distance problems; traveling inconveniences; and time-consuming effort. In 1994, Knapp et al. conducted a study to determine the numbers of physicians, physician assistants, nurse practitioners, certified nurse practitioners, midwives, and pharmacists in rural areas. The above named health care practitioners, except the pharmacists, are considered as the "four major groups of primary care providers." They use the five-digit zip code mapping statistics or population/ primary care providers ratio of 3,500 to 1 or greater to define the term primary care health professional shortage areas (HPSAs). Results revealed a conservative estimate of 22,127,000 people dwelling in 67% of the primary care HPSAs area and they were rural inhabitants. Most of the states with the greatest number of rural residents have the lowest number of managed care facilities. A statistical analysis in 1994 of population and providers in rural zip code areas per 100,000 rural inhabitants showed a national average of 13.8% rural dwellers; 53.6 physicians (mainly family practice, internal medicine, pediatrics, obstetrics surgery, and obstetrics/gynecology) per 100,000; 66.4 pharmacists per 100,000; 10 physician assistants per 100,000; 7.6 nurse practitioners per 100,000; and 1 certified nurse-midwife per 100,000. There were no pharmacists or other primary health care providers in 6,581 zip codes, with a total population of 4,750,626 over 877,502 square miles.[24]

Another study conducted by Gangeness revealed downward trends of pharmacists' availability in rural area in spite of the fact that their demand is on the rise in these areas. This study was conducted as an integral part of Lake Superior Rural Cancer Care Project in Minnesota, and the result showed that one pharmacist catered to 1,499 rural inhabitants, which included 279 senior citizens aged 65 years and above and 1,022 urban inhabitants including 124 senior citizens aged 65 and above.[25] This research might show a decline in the availability of pharmacists in rural areas, but the fact remains that pharmacists are still the most readily available and accessible health care providers everywhere including rural areas, as per general belief and many studies including the above Knapp et al. study (66.4 pharmacists per 100,000 rural inhabitants). Pharmacy as a medical office operates in different environments, from hospitals, clinics or physicians' offices and other health facilities; consequently, they are able to compensate for shortages of medical facilities. Some studies and the inspector general's report revealed that patients' counseling and drug monitoring can best be practiced at a community pharmacy.[24,31]

One major problem facing contemporary pharmacists and their availability in rural and urban centers is payment for their services outside the dispensing function. Remuneration for dispensing function has dwindled in recent years, and pharmacists find it difficult to sell their services to the public when people are used to the idea of obtaining the services for free. Government and third-party payers are reluctant to grant pharmacists remuneration for cognitive services as health care practitioners. However, some states governments like Mississippi have taken the initiative to pay pharmacists the same rate as physicians ($20 to $25 per hour) for providing disease-state management to patients with diabetes, hyperlipidemia, asthma, and anticoagulation. Pharmacists are expected to meet certain requirements as "other licensed practitioners" in order to provide these services. They must complete a state-approved disease-specific program or be a registered pharmacist who possesses a Doctor of Pharmacy degree (PharmD). The Mississippi Medicaid program requires a physician's referral for disease-state management in order for pharmacists to be compensated for the services. In North Carolina, similar episodes occurred with the passage of HR 1095. The bill recognized clinical pharmacists as clinical practitioners by granting them collaborative practice with physicians, and Governor James B. Hunt Jr. (D) signed it into law in July 1999. The law went into effect on July 1, 2000, and clinical pharmacists can now order laboratory/medical tests, implement and modify drug therapy in the state. Pharmacists must apply for the license with a cost of $100 and $50 renewal fee before engaging in the practice.[26,27,37]

Pharmacists' achievement in these states and the facts that pharmacy and pharmacists have been able to fill the vacuum created by physicians' absence and shortages of health facilities in rural areas and other places deserves commendations. These gestures have been fueled and exerted by the advent of the Doctor of Pharmacy degree (PharmD), a quixotic act that came at the right time, moment, and place in history. PharmD afforded pharmacists the opportunity to upgrade their skills, knowledge, and training as well as embark upon optional residence programs, thereby equating themselves with other branches of medicine. Considering the above facts about pharmacists' demands, accessibility/availability, and valuable knowledge that need to be annexed for the benefit of humanity, one would have expected an accelerated momentum in liberating the profession as an independent branch of medicine. Rather, the idea of robbing Peter to pay Paul seems to work well with all branches of medicine at the expense of pharmacy and it continues to flourish like the bubonic plague. This is a chronic condition and a cankerworm that has eaten deeply into the fabric of medicine and the society at large. As noted earlier, the delegation of prescribing authority from physicians to others with little or no drug knowledge continues unabatedly while numerous studies point to the fact that pharmacists are more dexterous than others in their prescription-writing skills, prudent disease-state management, effective therapeutic choice, drastic reduction of health care costs, etc. It's ironic to note that as smart as the physicians are, they pretend not to see these studies by turning their faces to the other side and raising great opposition to pharmacy's independence and liberty while at the same time encouraging their subordinates with little or no drug knowledge to take over the role of trained therapeuticians—the pharmacists. These subordinates operate independently, as noted in the Shefcheck et al. study: "Nurse practitioners and physician assistants now have the authority to prescribe independently and deliver many of the same services as physicians at a lower cost."[23] The word "physician assistants" has therefore lost its dictionary meaning, as assistants of physicians in most of physicians' offices and other places where these subordinates, including nurse practitioners, operate. Many states have various formularies for the nurse practitioners and physician assistants, and these include many drugs that the pharmacists cannot even dream of prescribing. In some states this formulary is almost the same as the physicians' formulary. For example, the Florida Physicians

Assistants' formulary allows them to prescribe from about 650 drugs by the year 2000 as per Florida statutes (chapter 458.347[4][F] and 459.022[4][F]) and Florida administrative codes chapter 893. The formulary includes the following: alprostadil, azelastine HCL, cefdnir, cerivastatin sodium, clopidogel, grepafloxacin, irbesartan, montelukast sodium, nefazodone HCL, raloxifene, saquinavir, tamsulosin HCl, trovafloxacin mesylate, valsartan, zolmitriptan, acarbose, acyclovir, albuterol, amlodipine, atenolol, bisoprolol, budesonide, captopril, carbidopa, cimetidine, clobestasol propionate, clonidine HCL, danazol, dapsone, desoximetasone, dicloenac potassium, digoxin, doxazosin mesylate, ergotamine tartrate, fenoprofen calcium, finesteride, furosemide, glyburide, hydralazine, indinavir, insulin, isoniazid, isosorbide dinitrate, ketoconazole, lamivudine, levodopa, metformin, mupirocin, nadolol, naproxen, niacin, norgestimate, ofloxacin, omeprazole, oxaprozin, pancreatin, phenytoin, probucol, propranolol HCl, salmeterol, stavudine, theophyline, tramadol HCl, troglitazone, valsartan, zolmitriptan , amprenavir, atropine/scopolamine/hyosyamine/phenobarbital, candesartan cilexetil, cantharidin, capsaicin, celecoxib, cilostazol, citalopram, dihydroergotamine mesylate, efavirenz, fenofibrate, levalbuterol, nicotine, orlistat, polyethylene glycol, rizatriptan benzoate, rofecoxib, rosiglitazone maleate, sildenafil citrate, synthetic conjugated estrogen, tazarotene, telmisartan, tiagabine, etc. The formulary does not include controlled substances, antipsychotics, antineoplastics, radiographic contrast materials, parenteral preparations except insulin and epinephrine, radiopharmaceuticals, and general anesthetics.

These formularies, which vary from state to state, show that pharmacists' (the trained therapeutic physicians or therapeuticians/drug specialists) formulary in the same state, Florida, as shown above is a tip of the iceberg compared to physician assistants' formulary. How much drug knowledge do physician assistants really encounter in their four years post high school—first-degree college work in any area (e.g. history, english, sociology etc) and one year post-baccalaureate-degree didactic class work in a PA program—that prepares them for this Herculean task? The response to this question will be revealed in a later chapter; however, one can conveniently draw an analogy here with proverbial words that say "When a mighty wind blew away stones from the ground, what do you expect of falling leaves from the trees?" If FDA chairman Kesler, a medical doctor and a lawyer, openly declared to the whole world that physicians do not receive enough drug knowledge in school to prepare them for the task of prescribing in spite of their years of school training, what can one expect from a curriculum of one year of didactic class work for physician assistants (plus a one-year rotation, making a total of 2 years post-baccalaureate medical training) to do about drug knowledge? The nurse practitioners have either similar or greater independent prescribing authority depending on the state or local authorities. Some states allow them to prescribe schedule II (C2) drugs. Dr. Rena Coll, director of pharmacy services, University Hospital, Fort Lauderdale, in a May 2001 delivered a lecture titled "Beyond Blame: Medication Safety," said an average nurse has one pharmacology course of 34 hours and physicians have 6 months of pharmacology courses. This explains why some people question the ability of nurse practitioners to function as independent practitioners. Dr. Cathy Worrall, a registered nurse who later became a clinical pharmacist and professor of pharmacology in nurse practitioners school, is one of such voices. Dr. Worrall works as a critical care clinical pharmacist at the Mayo Medical Center, Rochester, Minnesota. She was one of the 12 member multidisciplinary committee that was asked to review the family nurse practitioners' prescriptive role and the pharmacology background that laid the basic foundation for such authority in 1996. 18 out of 42 states that granted nurse practitioners prescribing authority gave them automatic power to do so while others required other forms of approval. The committee discovered that a four-year Bachelor of Science (BSc) graduate in nursing needs two years of work experience and a master's degree in order to become a nurse practitioner. This is for traditional nurse practitioner program; however, there are other cram or crash programs that require four or five years post high school to become nurse practitioners without any work experience.

The traditional program (2 years—MSc) required one pharmacology class in a semester or quarter making a total of two didactic class works. Dr. Worrall claimed that she had only one hour each to discuss anticoagulation, hyperlipidemia, hypertension, and diabetes—the four major topics in her one-quarter-long Pharmacology 1 class.[29] The nurse practitioners downplay their negativity in terms of pharmacology curriculum by emphasizing their strengths in diagnosis and physical assessment, areas in which the pharmacists have little training. They have every right to defend themselves and point out pharmacists' weakness. However, in the interest of humanity, advancement, the soaring cost of treatment/health care, morbidity and mortality due to ADR, cost benefits, cost utilization, cost-effective combinations of drugs, consequential effects of subtherapeutic (low dose)/toxic (overdose) doses, etc., there are growing needs for specialists to take control of drug therapy management. Moreover, blaming pharmacists for inadequate diagnosis or physical-assessment training is like blaming all physicians for inadequate therapeutic training or drug knowledge, blaming a surgeon for not properly managing a diabetic patient when his specialty is surgery, blaming a pediatrician for not properly managing plastic surgery or a dermatological condition when his specialty is pediatrics, and many other similar situations. Nobody in his rightful senses in our contemporary society can judiciously crave for olden days' medicine without specialties, the days when medical schools generally specialized in producing medical doctors that were jacks-of-all-trades and masters of none. Division of labor and the comparative law advantage stresses the need for every individual, group, society, and nation to do whatever it does best.

With physicians, drug therapy management in the country is being questioned, little wondered why the problem is further compounded and complicated with greater health care costs, loss of many human lives, and others as delegation or decentralization of prescribing authority from physicians to non-therapeuticians or drug specialists like physician assistants, nurse practitioners, and others like psychologists goes on unabately. The April 2002 issue of *Pharmacy Today* reported that New Mexico granted psychologists with doctoral degrees the authority to prescribe medications to patients with effect from July 1, 2002. Although psychiatric professional representatives opposed the idea on the grounds of inadequate drug knowledge, the law was implemented. If we feel that physician assistants, nurse practitioners, psychologists, and others have gained enough experience to practice on their own independently because they have spent some years under the practice of physicians then we might as well get rid of all the medical schools, schools of pharmacy, nursing schools, and other schools and revert back to the old system of apprenticeship programs. It is necessary for those prophets and harbingers of doom who specialized in speculating that the liberation of pharmacy will eventually herald the demise of medicine in the world to borrow a leaf from the facts that the existence of pediatricians has not stopped general practitioners and others from attending to children's health problems; dentists have not stopped general practitioners, internists, and others from attending to patients' mouth/tooth problems; psychiatrists have not stopped the general practitioners and others from attending to patients' brain problems; ophthalmologists have not stopped general practitioners and others from attending to patients' eye problems; dermatologists have not stopped general practitioners and others from attending to patients' skin problems; etc.

THE SPREAD OF CLINICAL PHARMACY AND DOCTOR OF PHARMACY DEGREES AROUND THE WORLD.

The spread of clinical pharmacy and Doctor of Pharmacy degrees to other parts of the world is due to three major factors:

- The desire to deal with increasing drug problems through greater drug knowledge.

- The professional desire to practice clinical pharmacy as an independent branch/specialty of medicine.
- The place of origin of the program, which is the U.S., and the U.S. as a role model for the rest of the world.

These three factors are interrelated in most parts of the world. Drug problems, notably adverse drug reactions, inappropriate medications, subtherapeutic dosage, toxicity, misuse of drugs, etc., are world problems and not just the U.S. problems. Numerous studies show worldwide problems with drugs. Some of these studies have been highlighted in previous chapters and a few others will be enumerated here.

AFRICA: The three factors enumerated above are very much alive in Africa because most countries in Africa are in tune with the recent developments in the world. Data about clinical studies involving pharmacists are rare because of a lack of incentives. However, as of January 2001, plans were in advanced stages for the implementation of a Doctor of Pharmacy degree (PharmD) program at the University of Ife and the University of Benin, both in Nigeria, the largest or most populous black nation in Africa. Like the United States of America, the implementation of Doctor of Pharmacy degree programs will no doubt demand additional year(s) of training for attending students/aspiring contemporary pharmacists. Any additional year(s) of training to the present 5 years would level the years of school training for pharmacists with other branches of medicine, which is 6 years in Nigeria. There are graduate programs such as Master and Doctor of Philosophy degrees in pharmacy in many schools of pharmacy in Africa.

ASIA (Thailand): Dr. Sakolchai Sumon, a PhD holder, highlighted issues relating to pharmaceutical care and the Doctor of Pharmacy degree program in Thailand during the sesquicentennial symposium of the American Pharmaceutical Association (AphA). He told the audience that Thailand Ministry of Health collaborated with four regional universities in the country to develop patient-oriented pharmaceutical care services in hospitals in 1990. The project began to grow, and at the time of the symposium in 2002, 50% of large hospitals and 30% of small hospitals monitored adverse drug reactions (ADRs), counseled patients about the use of drugs, and evaluated drug usage in hospitals. Like the hospitals, education reforms led to the introduction of clinical pharmacy and pharmaceutical care in pharmacy schools' curriculum, and finally the first 6-year Doctor of Pharmacy degree program was established in 1997. More than 6,500 out of 8,000 pharmacists in Thailand between 1993 and 2000 have availed themselves of the continuing-education training workshops purposely to upgrade their clinical skills and knowledge. The

Thailand National Pharmacy Council was created in 1994 and has set forth pharmaceutical care as the goal of professional achievement.[44]

JAPAN: Physicians dispense medications/drugs in Japan, and pharmacists are paid as health care providers for services such as taking a patient's drug history ($2.10 per order), counseling a patient about medication ($0.5 or $2 per order), detecting drug interactions ($2.50), detecting therapeutic duplication ($2.50), providing home pharmaceutical services ($55 per month/patient), providing hospital or clinical pharmacy services ($60 per month/patient), and providing hospital pharmacokinetic services ($65 to $335 per month/drug). Payment for pharmacy clinical services in the hospital started in 1988 as part of patient care reimbursement (PCR) policy, while same service for pharmacokinetic consultations began earlier, in 1980. Genesis of these services is the result of the worldwide growth of clinical pharmacy and pharmaceutical care that started in the U.S. Japanese authorities believed that pharmacists can help to reduce health care costs by improving drug therapy and decreasing the hospitalization rate; however, the issue of pharmacy autonomy remains an illusion.[44]

CHINA: Pharmacists in China are commonly referred to as Yodian, and they are independent practitioners especially in the community. Pharmacists might be independent in China but the professional practice is not different from the rest of the world. Pharmacists can prescribe and dispense any drugs in community pharmacies, but the issues of adequate documentation, patient privacy, treatment profundity, monitoring of efficacy, adverse drug reactions, and other disease-state management issues are far from reality. Chinese pharmacy is very much tailored after Western culture; hence, the lack of disease-state management in spite of its autonomy is the result of the trickle-down effect of Western civilization in relation to pharmacy. It is obvious that this is not the direction of change for future pharmacy; however, the autonomy deserves a lot of commendation and emulation by the rest of the world. China's medical education, as shown in chapter 6, is slow in catching up with the rest of the world because of its adherence to its own traditional Chinese medicine.

The liberation movement that came into power in 1949 as a result of the formation of the People's Republic of China, under the leadership of Chairman Mao Tse-tung, attempted to improve people's health by organizing the health care system through socialism. Chairman Mao's government reforms imposed a Cultural Revolution that ended all educational, scientific, and cultural programs in 1966. Peasants joined forces with trained workers, and impoverished facilities and barefoot doctors instead of professionally trained physicians became the main source of primary health care delivery. Hospitals were built and drug production increased especially through hospital pharmacy. China produces about 95% of its drugs today through pharmaceutical companies and hospitals. Many large hospitals produce sterile solutions, and all hospitals' pharmacies have a medical supply committee that performs government-mandated research as well as guarantees safe and effective use of drugs within the hospital. The research work is primarily aimed at merging Western and traditional medicine. Clinical pharmacy came into China through Donald E. Francke (a U.S. hospital pharmacy leader) in 1962 and ended shortly because of the Cultural Revolution. At any rate, the program resurfaced again and dominated the 1981 annual conference of the Society of Pharmaceutics of the Chinese Pharmaceutical Association. Clinical pharmacy in Nanjing hospitals aimed to resolve drug interactions, drug incompatibilities; decrease drug side effects, abuse, and misuse of drugs; and improve drug use. In education, the Ministry of Health mandated all pharmacy schools/faculties to include clinical pharmacy training in their curriculum and employed specialized clinical pharmacists as academic staff in 1977. Students in the last year of their pharmacy school can now specialize in clinical pharmacy as a branch of the pharmacy program. Pharmacy programs are mostly 4 years courses and 5 years in some cases because of the 1981 changes in some programs. Graduate programs (i.e., masters and PhDs) in pharmacy were a nonexistent phenomenon in China prior to 1979 because of the difficulties in recruiting faculty members. The return of advanced, trained Chinese pharmacists from foreign countries began to change the situation for good.[50] Doctor of Pharmacy programs might be a strange phenomenon now in China but the desire to catch up with the rest of the world will eventually change the situation for good.

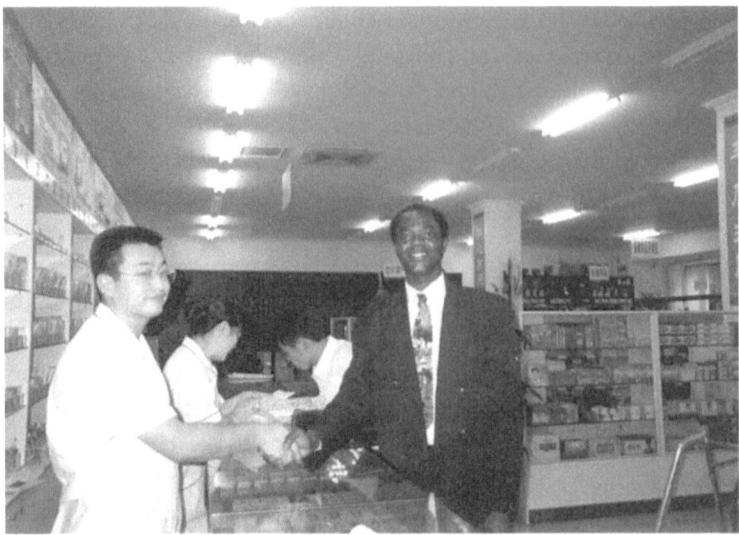

Dr. Patrick Ojo with a Yodian (pharmacist) in a community pharmacy, Beijing, China.

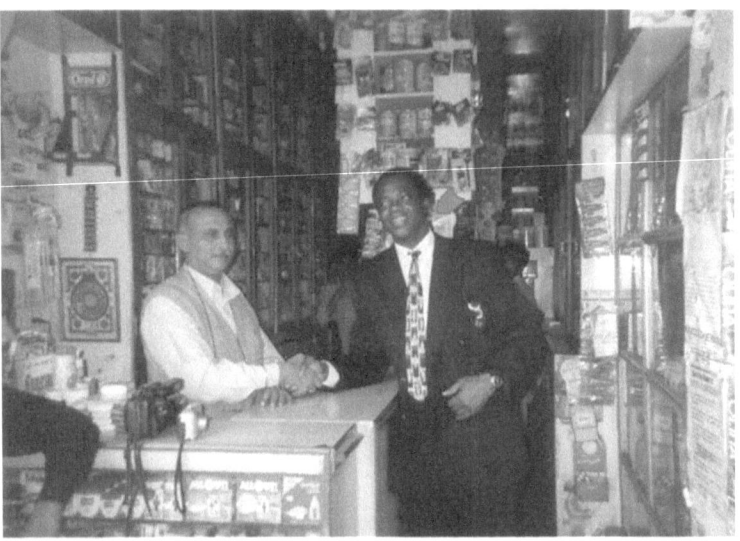

Dr. Patrick Ojo with a surrogate pharmacist in a community pharmacy, New Delhi, India. In India, a surrogate pharmacist is a professional with a diploma or associate degree in pharmacy and he is authorized to open and operate a pharmacy in the country. Pharmacy in India has a lot in common with Chinese pharmacy and most third world countries.

AUSTRALIA: Like Africa, Australia is in tune with the recent developments in the world. Australia is ranked as one of the developed countries of the world. Clinical pharmacy is alive in Australia through various graduate programs in pharmacy at various schools of pharmacy. For instance, there are Master of Pharmacy (clinical) or M Pharm (Clin) degree programs and graduate certificates in clinical pharmacy (Grad Cert Clin Pharm) but clinical studies involving pharmacists are rare. However, one study reported in the July/August 2004 issue of the *Journal of the American Pharmacists Association* showed how implementation and evaluation of Australian Pharmacists' Diabetes Care Services resulted in patients' better diabetes control and health care outcomes. This was the first of it kind in the country, as noted in the study. The 9 months, parallel group, multi-site, control/intervention study was conducted by C. L. Armour, S. L. Taylor, F. Hourihan, C. Smith, and I. Krass. With the exception of Smith (B Pharm) and Hourihan (MPh), the others are professors and senior lecturers with Doctor of Philosophy (PhD) degrees in pharmacy, all on the faculty of pharmacy, University of Sydney, New South Wales, Australia. The design measures were repeated in three different regions in New South Wales as intervention regions and then matched with control regions.

Participating pharmacists were trained and meant to follow clinical protocol over 9 months with roughly monthly intervention site visits by patients. Patient's blood glucose readings were discussed with each patient including goals and the interventions were documented. Only intervention region patients' blood glucose levels were measured throughout the study and the following clinical outcome measures: risk of nonadherence, glycosylated hemoglobin ($A1_c$) values, well-being, and quality of life were recorded at the beginning and end of the study. 106 intervention and 82 control patients completed the study. Patient blood glucose levels were significantly lower in all intervention regions and the pharmacists documented 1,459 interventions during the study. Results showed that patients in both intervention and control regions had similar values at the beginning of the study (baseline); however, different results were recorded at the end of the study. The patients with glysosylated hemoglobin ($A1_c$) values greater than 7 (i.e., > 7%) went up by 7% from 54% baseline to 61% after 9 months (the study period) in control regions (patients received treatment from traditional medical doctors) but the results was classified as similar. Patients in the intervention regions (pharmacists' patients in collaboration with physicians), on the other hand, had a significant reduction of 19 from 72% baseline value to 53% after 9 months (the study period). $A1_c$ values are a hallmark parameter in the measurement of diabetic condition (progress or retrogression). Intervention regions patients equally did better significantly with other parameters like risk of nonadherence, well-being, and quality of life.[51] There is no Doctor of Pharmacy degree program neither are there plans for its implementation in Australia as at October 2002. There is Doctor of Philosophy (PhD) degree program in pharmacy in Australia. Like China, the desire to catch up with the rest of the world is going to push Australia to implement the Doctor of Pharmacy degree program.

EUROPE: In Norway, a multidispliciplinary study examined the 732 deaths out of 13,992 patients admitted over 2 years at Central Hospital of Akershus (Department of Internal Medicine), Nordbyhagen, Norway, and found that 133 deaths (9.5 deaths per 1,000 hospitalized patients) were due to adverse drug events (ADEs). They examined clinical records, autopsy results in 78% cases, and drug analyses from premortem and postmortem results. 75 out of 133 deaths were the results of fatal ADEs, of which gastrointestinal diseases/problems were the highest proportion with 42.2%. It was roughly estimated that about 202 patients were on 12 or more medications at the time of death and the most culprit medications were antithrombotic agents, sympathomimetic medications, and cardiovascular drugs. The authors blamed preventable ADEs and other problems on lack of monitoring drug concentrations, misinterpretation of symptoms and inadequate dosages adjustment in accordance with pharmacokinetics properties (e.g., absorption, distribution, metabolism, and excretion), and age.[47]

PORTUGAL: Hypertension and concomitant cardiovascular disease takes it toll around the world because of uncontrolled hypertension (high blood pressure) and about 58 to 68% of the patients in Portugal have uncontrolled hypertension. Garcão and Carbrita studied the clinical impact of community pharmacists on hypertensive patients in rural (semi-literate) Portugal with the aid of pharmaceutical care in 2000. The study is composed of 100 patients with essential hypertension on less than six months antihypertensive drug regimen. Patients were randomly assigned to a control group of 50 with traditional care, and an intervention group of 50 with research pharmacists. The research pharmacists provided their patients with nonpharmacological control of blood pressure, 6 months regular visits to monitor their BP, treatment adherence monitoring, prevention, detection, and resolution of any drug-related problems (DRPs). 41 patients completed the study in each group and at the end of 6 months, results showed that the number of uncontrolled BP decreased by 77.4% (systolic BP from 152 ± 23 mmHg to 129 ± 15 mmgHg) in the intervention group (P < 0.0001) compared with 10.3% (systolic BP from 148 ± 16 mmHg to 143 ± 20 mmHg) in the control group (P = 0.48) with traditional physician care. 40% of potential DRPs were prevented and 83% detected actual DRPs (24 out of 29) were resolved. Some of the DRPs included therapeutic duplications

(2 diuretics and the same drug), patients with extremely low BP taking 3 antihypertensive medications without justification, high doses of thiazides, short-acting nifedipine, and others. Some potential DRPs were prevented because of pharmacists' recommendations to the physicians; however, the physicians generally refused to change the antihypertensive drug regimen based on pharmacist's recommendations.[48] The two authors of this study are Doctor of Pharmacy degree holders trained in the U.S.

THE NETHERLANDS: Dr. Tromp, a PhD and PharmD (Doctor of Pharmacy degree holder) reflected on the development of pharmaceutical care in Europe during the sesquicentennial symposium of the American Pharmaceutical Association. He noted that in an effort to reduce errors and improve medication management in the Netherlands, pharmaceutical care is gradually becoming a duty for all pharmacists. Patient moves through a sequence of four stations where staff scrutinize patient medications for the correct drug, proper usage instructions, and pharmaceutical care. Dr. Tromp cited other issues such as the availability of pharmacies in 15 European Union countries, a factor that varies from country to country and influences greatly pharmaceutical care practices. Greece has more pharmacies, with rough estimates of 1,143 people per pharmacy, compared to Denmark with estimates of 18,000 people per pharmacy.[44]

Norway, Portugal, and the Netherlands are in tune with the rest of the world and the U.S. in terms of recent developments in pharmaceutical care; however, there is no data to support the availability of Doctor of Pharmacy degree programs in these countries. The United Kingdom has various clinical pharmacy degree programs in schools of pharmacy in Britain and the rest of the country, but the Doctor of Pharmacy degree program is a non-issue as of 2001. The desire to catch up with the rest of the world will result in the implementation of Doctor of Pharmacy degree program in Britain and other parts of Europe.

NORTH AMERICA: Besides the United States, similar problems in Canada were addressed in a different manner. Canadian authorities were motivated by the development of drug problems and pharmacists' intervention in the U.S. Consequently, they decided to mandate pharmacists and compensate them for their intervention on any drug-related problems through various provincial government agencies responsible for health care policies. In Quebec, for example, the province compensates pharmacists through Régie de l' Assurance-maladie du Quebec (RAMQ), a government agency that manages a drug plan for the indigent and elderly. Poirier and Gariépy studied pharmacists' compensation for resolving drug-related problems through pharmaceutical opinions and refusals to dispense in Quebec, Canada. The first program started in June 1992 and ended in May 1993. Results revealed that pharmaceutical opinions were filed because of 8 or more medications—33%; side effects—29%; interactions and noncompliance—11% each; lack of efficacy—8%; additional medication required and benzodiazepine use—3% each; refusal to dispense claims were filed because of wrong dosage—27%; overuse—20%; duplicate therapy and previous drug-related problems—13% each; irrational therapy—11%; irrational quantity or duration of therapy—8%; drug interaction—7%; and falsified prescription orders—1%. Between June 1992 and May 1993, RAMQ paid 5,656 pharmaceutical opinion claims (80% due to patients age 65 and older, and 33% of Quebec pharmacies filed for at least one) and 9,184 refusal to dispense claims (62% due to patients 65 and older and 55% of Quebec pharmacies filed at least one). The claims increased by 9% to 6,189 for pharmaceutical opinions and 90% to 17,444 for refusal to dispense in the second year, 1993 to 1994. The study noted that pharmacists spent an average of 6 to 7.8 minutes in HMO (Health Maintenance Organization) to resolve DRPs, while third- or fourth-year students together with their preceptors spent an average of 17.1 minutes to intervene and document any DRP prevention or resolution; the community pharmacists spent between 9.35 minutes for new order with overdosage to 9.64 minutes for a new order with drug interaction and 4.68 minutes to process an order with no DRP. The pharmacists' intervention value was estimated to be $122.98 per prescription order with DRP, a $3.50 savings for every prescription screened by the pharmacist. The reimbursement rate for pharmaceutical opinion is Canada $15.45, which is twice that of refusal to dispense.[45]

Kassam et al. studied pharmacists' interventions as part of pharmaceutical care research and education project in Alberta province, Canada, over a 4 years period. Five community pharmacies with 9 pharmacists participated in the study, and the results revealed that pharmacists in the treatment group identified 559 DRPs for 145 patients who received approximately 6,309 prescriptions (i.e., 8.2 DRPs per 100 prescriptions). In telephone surveys, pharmacists documented 8.7 intakes of prescription medications per day, while patients reported 4.7 prescriptions per day. The pharmacists identified 131 patients in need of pneumococcal or influenza vaccinations (needs drug and respiratory disorder DRP) and this represented 24% of all DRPs, 109 DRPs relating to cardiovascular system, some musculoskeletal DRPs, and 15 problems for new drug requirements or dosage adjustments. They wrote 551 initial SOAP (Subjective, Objective, Assessment, and Plan) notes and 346 follow-up SOAP notes, with 613 recommendations out of 551 DRPs. Out of the 502 pharmacists' recommendations, patients accepted 76%, refused 12% and modified 5% while the physicians accepted 72%, refused 8% and modified 9% of the 247 pharmacists' recommendations. Pharmacists were much more likely to follow up 75% of the time compared to physicians' record of 10%. 40% of 559 DRPs were resolved, 18% improved partially or remained the same, and 1% grew worse or failed recommendations during follow up. and 40% of all DRPs lacked follow up because of no DRP status, and 39% of the problems were actual DRPs while 60% were potential DRP. The study, PREP, finally identified more DRPs (3.9 per patient) than previous studies that showed 0.8 and 2.0 DRPs per patient.[46]

As of 2003, some pharmacy schools in Canada have upgraded their pharmacy curriculum and school programs to reflect the standards of Doctor of Pharmacy degree programs.

SOUTH AMERICA: Like Africa and Australia, South America is in tune with recent developments in the world for the same reasons. Clinical pharmacy is not very common in Brazil, the largest country in South America, but some of the schools of pharmacy offer clinical analysis with an additional 6 months to the regular 4 years pharmacy degree program. Data about clinical studies involving pharmacists are rare because of lack of incentive. Clinical pharmacy is almost a nonexistent phenomenon in South America, and there are equally no Doctor of Pharmacy degree program, neither are there plans for its implementation as of October 2002. Like Africa and Australia, there are graduate programs in the form of Master and Doctor of Philosophy degrees in pharmacy in South America. The desire to catch up with the rest of the world will lead to the implementation of Doctor of Pharmacy degree programs in South America.

FUTURE

After all said and done, after all talk and various metamorphoses of the pharmacy profession, the dust finally settled and the buck stopped here with prescribing authority and the ultimate liberation of the profession as an autonomous body worthy of all privileges ascribed to other specialties/specialists within the medical field. Pharmacists will be accorded their long overdue recognition as trained therapeuticians or therapeutic physicians.

The fate and destiny of any profession lies in the hands of its practitioners, and pharmacy is no exception—no special interest groups or groups of specialists, however powerful and influential they may be, should be allowed to dictate the fate of others.

The last phrase is not an attempt to undermine collaborative efforts of a health care team in the interest of patients, but rather to call a spade a spade by allowing pharmacy to stand on its feet (like other branches) before it can effectively cooperate with others. The same market forces that killed the Doctor of Pharmacy (PharmD) degree on arrival are also going to raise it to an expected height and equate it with other branches of medicine. Dr. Hepler in a symposium titled "Developing a Market for Pharmaceutical Care," delivered during the Florida Pharmacy Association's 108th annual meeting and convention, enumerated several factors. He quoted Dr. Martin Luther King Jr. by saying that anybody can ride you when you are bent over, but nobody can ride you when you are standing tall. Some of the views expressed by Dr. Hepler include suggestion of ADR as the leading cause of death in the country; the fact that many people encounter ADRs, which escalates health care cost to the tune of billions of dollars; the fact that most ADRs can be avoided by merely changing medication use systems; failures of the present regimen (remedies), which stresses boomerang prescriptions with expensive limitations/formularies; third-party shift towards disease management; and the fact that many studies buttress the view that a change in medication use systems by incorporating pharmacists in drug therapy results in dramatic patient improvement/outcome at same or lower cost.[30]

On arrival, Doctor of Pharmacy degrees meet the cold hand of market forces, and for years the degree made no difference in pharmacists' reputation and remuneration. All pharmacists were treated alike in terms of employment requirements (BSc or PharmD), pay or remuneration, bonuses, vacations, and other benefits provided the pharmacist had a license. Pharmacists with a first degree (BSc) had no financial incentives or enhanced status in terms of a better reputation to look forward to as goals for pursing the Doctor of Pharmacy degree; consequently, many felt there was no need for it. However, a few optimistic ones who saw light at the end of the tunnel realized that the future of pharmacy depends not on the traditional role of dispensing-only function but on patient-oriented clinical services. This set of pharmacists gave up many things including a pharmacy job in some cases to acquire the Doctor of Pharmacy of degree—GLORY BE TO THEM. They weren't after any reward in terms of remuneration and enhanced status other than the satisfaction of their conscience and rendering patient-oriented pharmacy services. At the turn of the millennium, in the year 2000, things began to change for the better because clinical pharmacists' positions that came into being in the 1930s began to gain the attention of the employers.

In the beginning, very few clinical pharmacists' positions were filled by licensed, first-degree holder pharmacists who demonstrated a good clinical background/orientation to their employer. The employers showed no inclination for potential clinical pharmacy or a Doctor of Pharmacy degree because it didn't make any difference to them whether the contesting candidate for the vacant position was a first-degree (BSc) or Doctor of Pharmacy degree holder. With time the beneficial effects of clinical pharmacists with Doctor of Pharmacy degrees in hospitals, managed care centers, home health, and other places became glaring in the form of health care cost reduction, decreased emergency room visits, resolution of drug problems, prevention of ADRs, decreased morbidity and mortality resulting from ADR, and others. These benefits made employers open up more positions for clinical pharmacists and the huge difference between the first-degree (BSc) and Doctor of Pharmacy degree holders made them clamor for the latter at the expense of the former. At the turn of the millennium, all employers that showed no previous inclination for Doctor of Pharmacy degree made a U-turn and started stipulating the requirement/prerequisite of a clinical pharmacy position as the possession of Doctor of Pharmacy degree (no waiver). This time around there was no room for the first-degree holders to show up for an interview for an advertised clinical pharmacist position unless such pharmacist wanted to subject himself to ridicule or rejection. Thus, clinical pharmacists became a direct correlation with Doctor of Pharmacy degree holders. The only few, sporadic exceptions that might still be tenable with first-degree holders and clinical pharmacy positions were employments based on greater, insurmountable power, influence, family ties, or impeccable credentials with years of experience (even then unless the operating bottom power is insurmountable, a fresh-out-of-school PharmD holder can readily knock off the years of experience with relative ease because the young graduate is considered a product of modern-day pharmacy while the old pharmacist is considered a product of old traditional/redundant pharmacy with nothing much to offer).

Shortages of pharmacists make it impossible for employers of labor to discriminate against pharmacists with a first degree in filling a general pharmacist's position in contemporary society. At any rate, some employers deem it necessary to request or ask potential employees during an interview if they posses a Doctor of Pharmacy degree or not in filling certain general pharmacist positions (positions that do not require anything more than the first degree). Judging by the present pharmacy philosophy, it is glaring that the profession is moving forward in the right direction, and for those young pharmacists (fresh out of school) just entering the profession with the hope of retiring in it but who currently possess first degree have a lot of opportunities to upgrade their educational standard to Doctor of Pharmacy. They will be doing themselves a great favor if they decide now to avail themselves of the opportunities of the nontraditional PharmD program before it is too late. All schools of pharmacy in the nation have adopted the ACPE policy, which aims to stamp out the first-degree (BSc) program in place of PharmD in the near future. Most of these schools are offering the nontraditional PharmD program to assist first-degree holders in obtaining the Doctor of Pharmacy degree. Presently there is a market for the nontraditional PharmD program, but as the waves of PharmD graduates from various schools of pharmacy begin to flood the market, most of the current first-degree holders are retired or have died, and others have used the program to upgrade themselves, the demand for nontraditional PharmD program will degenerate into oblivion and the schools will be forced to close the programs. One does not need a soothsayer to prophesize that in the future all pharmacy employers will require PharmD for any pharmacist position.

Pharmacy liberation as an autonomous body worthy of all privileges ascribed to other specialties/specialists within the medical field will no doubt herald a different phase in the profession and medicine in general. All pharmacists presently serving as clinical pharmacists or clinical pharmacy coordinators generally have an edge over others in terms of remuneration and better status. They serve as role models for present and future generations of pharmacists as far as job satisfaction, knowledge, clinical impact on patients' health care/outcome, commensurate payment, and other benefits are concerned. Clinical pharmacists with a Doctor of Pharmacy degree are medical doctors with the specialist title of Therapeutic physician or therapeutician (drug specialist). They may or may not be recognized for their crucial role in our contemporary society, but as time goes on, their impact on the nation's health care system will be obvious and people will accord them due respect (pharmacy has no other destination). The laws of supply and demand works perfectly well in every sphere of life in determining prices and market forces. The shortage of pharmacists in the U.S. at the turn of the millennium resulted in a decrease supply of pharmacists while demand was on the rise. The resultant equilibrium precipitated greater competition among employers for the existing pharmacists. Employers engaged themselves in cutthroat competitions unveiling numerous incentives such as competitive/ higher salaries, sign-on bonuses of up to $15,000 in some cases, excellent benefits (which include vacation pay, health insurance, disability, etc.), shift differentials, overtime pay, continued education assistance/tuition reimbursement, relocation allowance, paid time off, and excellent 401(k) plans. Some employers seek the assistance of recruiters with fabulous reward to help in the employment of pharmacists.

The Department of Health and Human Services described the pharmacist shortage as a dramatic increase in unfilled part-time and full-time positions from 5,000 in 1998 to about 13,000 in 2000.[39] The situation is expected to grow worse before it gets better because of the change in program from BSc to PharmD. The PharmD program takes longer, with emphasis on clinical training, and it is three times more expensive annually than the first-degree

(BSc) program, yet there is no difference in the paycheck of both graduates.[25] Enrollment in schools of pharmacy has plummeted because of the above reasons, and competition for pharmacists with residency and fellowship training has stiffened among pharmaceutical industries, HMO/managed care, and schools of pharmacy, thereby creating greater shortages. Moreover, the adoption of PharmD as a minimum entry requirement in the country is bound to create a vacuum with foreign graduates in the future until the rest of the world catches up with the PharmD program. When PharmD becomes the bane of the American pharmacy practice, foreign pharmacy graduates will no longer be able to come to the country, take the board exams, and join the bandwagon of pharmacists serving the need. These foreign pharmacy graduates will then be required to go back to schools of pharmacy and complete two or more years depending on the situation before joining the bandwagon. Some of the foreign graduates might take the issue with a grain of salt while others will not, but expected shortages in this area will hit the market in the future. These shortages have created scarcity and increased pharmacists' remuneration/rewards but failed to deliver pharmacy or catalyze any movement towards the professional liberation from bondage.

Market forces are beginning to respond to the demands of PharmD; pharmacy liberation will enhance this response and level up the professional status with other branches of medicine. Better remunerations, rewards, and enhanced status will attract young people to the profession because their thoughts and the views of career advisers will change to reflect the new outlook of the pharmacy profession. Young people will no longer have to meditate over spending 6 to 7 years in pharmacy school and end up with second-class fiddle positions when they can spend the same number of years to become dentists, optometrists, and veterinary medical doctors or add two to three years to become other specialists in the medical field and earn more respect with better remuneration. They will comprehend the fact that pharmacy is no longer what it used to be—taking orders, dispensing medication, and playing second fiddle to other branches of medicine—but rather an autonomous medical field with practitioners worthy of similar status as other co-equals. One day the profession might become the backbone of medicine, ranking high on top of the list of medical specialties and attracting more scholars into the field. Market forces in terms of demands, which have always been on the rise, will even out with an increased supply of pharmacists.

Attracting more scholars to the profession with the 6 to 7 year training program will lead to increased demand for pharmacy programs, and schools of pharmacy are quite sensitive to market forces. They are going to respond to high demand for pharmacy programs by raising the entry-level requirements from the present 2 years community college/associate degree to a four-year baccalaureate degree (BSc). The 2 years community college/associate degree entry level was one of the attempts made by schools of pharmacy to prevent pharmacy strangulation by encouraging young scholars to come to the profession with less duration of training before entering the professional coursework/phase in schools of pharmacy. A four-year first-degree (BSc) entry requirement would equate pharmacy's entry requirements with other branches of medicine. Pharmacy courses would be tailored to patients' needs and how best to improve patient outcome. Many of the present-day norms and prescription order directives such as BID (twice daily), TID (three times daily), QID (four times daily), PRN (as needed), HS (at bedtime, which varies because some people sleep and wake up at various time of the night or day), and others might become a thing of the past because they are not specific. Twice daily can be interpreted by different patients in different ways. A patient is right to think that twice daily means he must take the medication two times daily irrespective of the time difference. Thus, a patient might be predisposed to feel that he can take one pill now and the other about 2 to 4 hours later. Taking the medication in this manner is an incentive that makes him forget about the task of taking the medication 12 hours later or allow the task to linger on with the probability of forgetfulness. This patient may not be aware of the problem he has created for himself by overdosing with the medication and precipitating toxicity that can result in ADR, morbidity, and mortality depending on the circumstance. The same is true with other vague directions like TID, QID, PRN, and others. Besides toxicities, a patient's drug plasma concentration needs to be maintained at a certain level for effective therapy; any compromise resulting from inadequate dosing can precipitate subtherapy and ineffective treatment at other times. Patients in this category can be helped with a more specific direction such as between 7 and 8 in the morning and in the evening or 7 a.m. and 7 p.m., and what to do in case of a missed dose. Other problematic areas such as graveyard dosing (disrupting sleep to take medication at midnight or 2 a.m.), which poses a great barrier to compliance, can be avoided with drug selections and better dosing regimens such as 10 or 11 p.m. and 6 a.m. instead of 8 or 9 p.m. and 2 or 3 a.m., etc.

Presently pharmacists are known to be better than other health care practitioners at handling patient compliance; it is therefore reasonable to expect better compliance with pharmacy liberation. Liberated pharmacies will encourage greater research in the form of student projects, literature reviews, course assignments, practice research, assistance of computerized technology, creation of new inventions (e.g., machines), and other research into problematic areas. Pharmacists have assisted the computer industry in creating software models that incorporate identification of patients at high risk of developing drug-related problems. This invention was the result of a two-year study by Daniel Malone and others at the Health Sciences Center, University of Colorado, Denver. They studied patients' records at the Veterans Affairs Medical Center (VAMC) and came up with six criteria for identification purpose:

- "Drug regimens of five or more drugs, twelve or more daily medication doses, change of regimens four or more times in 12 months, the existence of more than three concurrent disease states, history of noncompliance, and drug therapy that requires monitoring."

The study was presented at the 1997 AphA convention. Another invention named the "talking pill bottle" was designed to assist visually impaired patients in taking their medications. The talking pill bottle is constructed with the aid of a device called Script Talk that reads a prescription label, otherwise tagged a "smart label," to blind or vision-impaired patients. Script Talk is able to store computer information from the pharmacy and produce it verbally in English and Spanish (16 other languages are in future plans). However, a pharmacy needs a specialized printer to print labels from the Script Talk system. This system is of great benefit to illiterate patients, memory-impaired patients such as dyslexics, and aging patients with deteriorating cognition. Other inventions include a medication-dispensing machine that keeps a pharmacy abreast of a patient's compliance (an alarm triggers when the patient refuses or forgets to take his medication at the correct time).[36,38]

Compliance problems cost the nation billions of dollars annually and, as seen from the above, it is an issue for pharmacies to deal with as professional challenges. Certain factors such as forgetfulness, lack of drug knowledge, low income, ADR, regimen complexity, work disruption, side effects, disease knowledge (what happens when you refused or failed to comply with treatment against compliance or believe in drug efficacy e.g., Patti Labelle's controlled diabetic condition against amputee's unmanaged condition), poor vision, poor cognitive factors, cost of medications, length of treatment, clinic inconvenience, waiting time, number of medications and multiple-drug regimen (addition of a drug to a regimen or use of more than 5 drugs decreases compliance), social isolation, confusion, severity of disease, chronic disease, patient values, dosage adjustment for all including dialysis patients (instead of one-dose-fits-all as it is currently practiced by health care practitioners; clinical pharmacists are known to do a better job than others in this regard), dosage frequency (the more the frequency of administration of a drug the greater the decrease in compliance) and patient-provider relationship, which has been known to be responsible for most noncompliance, are all key factors in the compliance issue. Some solutions include: the aim of medications (patients monitoring their condition for feelings of wellness, low blood pressure readings, low blood sugar, low cholesterol, etc., which can prevent heart attack, stroke, amputations, etc.); well-designed dosage schedules; simple regimens; the use of simple devices (such as Medi-Planner, boxes for morning-noon-evening-bedtime, Medidot reminder labels, a prescription time cap with an alarm clock, or a Pipeer box/reminder with a digital timer); assigned technicians to call patients and remind them of their refills; monitoring with pill counts; self-reporting; drug detection in serum and excretions; patients discharged from the hospital with dosage adjustment--explanations and answers to questions; and a good patient-provider relationship. The use of patients' complete questionnaire about life history will enable healthcare practitioners get enough information about patients before medicating them in order to avoid incidents like Diane's catastrophe. This gesture is presently in place in some offices; however, most are ineffective in relation to drug and prescribing habits. They are just like the allergy issues, of which pharmacists have been known to do a better job than other health care practitioners because this is their specialty and area of jurisdiction.

Drug choice and effective combination of drugs: this is one area of pharmacy and drug therapy that deserves attention of specialists. It has no limitations yet inappropriate guidance and reckless choices can trigger a cascade of events, send health care costs through the roof, and precipitate ADR, morbidity, and mortality. The liberation of pharmacy would make this issue a top priority in schools of pharmacy, classrooms, internship programs, rotations, residencies, and other pharmacy forums. It is not unusual to see hypertensive or diabetic patients on 5 to 8 medications for high blood pressure or sugar alone, and in many cases these patients come down with ADR or another form of illness that is the direct result of their present treatment (regimen). Various health care practitioners are mesmerized by this situation; consequently, in an attempt to downplay patients' complaints or satisfy patients temporarily, they add another drug instead of scrutinizing the existing one to see what is wrong or the precipitating factor (drug). Thus, a hypertensive patient that comes down with dizziness because of the hypotensive effects of his medications is likely to get antivert or pro-amantine (midodrine) as additional therapy, a depressed patient on antidepressant medications with temporary anxiety mood will end up with Xanax or other anxiolytic agents, psychiatric patients might end up with cogentin or other anti-Parkinson's disease medications, diabetic patients with glucagons, etc. Chronically ill patients with these types of conditions take up to 30 pills a day in some cases, and many elderly patients whose livers and renal functions have degenerated found themselves compounding their problems. One might be surprised to see that dosage adjustment or removal of one or few medications from the existing regimen instead of adding more drugs might go a long way toward resolving the patients' complaints and enhancing compliance. Effective drug management can reduce a regimen from 30 to less than 10 pills a day.

Other issues about drug choice and effective combinations are Cost-effectiveness, cost minimization, cost utilization, and cost-benefit analysis. These issues are presently treated as minor or non-issues. Cost-effectiveness and benefits makes a lot of difference to patients especially when it is a matter of choice between accepting therapy/wellness and putting food on the table for their children/family to eat. Cost-effectiveness measures health benefits/outcomes in relation to resources used to obtain them. It takes a comparative approach to drugs of choice for any given therapy by comparing effectiveness and prices of drugs from the same class or therapeutic group. A therapeutician or drug specialist is able to use his drug knowledge to draw inferences and make logistic conclusions that are commensurate with patients' wallet/economics and effective therapy for the given condition. For instance, if drug A is 10% more effective but 100% more expensive than drug B, a careful analysis of the overall long/short-term effects (e.g., hospitalization cost) and the patient's financial status especially if he is paying out of pocket for his medications would enable the provider to make a sound judgment about probably choosing drug B. Cost benefits are used to identify, measure, and compare benefits and costs of treatment or alternatives and express them in a ratio (B/C). If the ratio is greater than one, the benefits outweigh the cost and the treatment is worthwhile. If, on the other hand, the ratio is less than one the reverse is true, and if it is equal to one then there is no advantage either way. The cost is not necessarily measured in dollars alone; it could be in the form of ADR and other issues. Studies have shown that low prices are not necessarily cost-effective because the whole scenario (e.g., ADR, recovery time, hospitalization rate, if any, etc.) has to be taken into consideration.

Clinical rotations, internship, residency, and fellowship in a liberated pharmacy will help to drive home the above message by intensifying student didactic classwork as in other fields such as engineering, agriculture, law, accounting, and others in which classroom work helps to groom students and lay a solid bedrock of foundation for them to deal with complex issues later and excel. Medical students display this expertise especially in diagnosis during rotations and residencies. As noted previously, rounds with medical doctors, residents, and students of other branches of medicine will no doubt convince anyone that they are diagnosis specialists. You would be amazed by the degree of patience, analysis, and the display of talents and scholasticism that they put into complex cases. They go systematically, peeling layer by layer in a bid to unravel the mystery of diagnosis, and the end results in most cases justifying the means. As noted previously, drug treatment or therapy during these rounds is a complete opposite of diagnosis. A similar procedure by clinical pharmacy instructors or therapeutic physicians (therapeuticians), students, and residents during rounds will no doubt reduce health care costs, improve compliance, enhance drug choice and combination of drugs, decrease morbidity and mortality resulting from ADR, etc. In every complex drug cases, they will simplify the issue by excavating all known side effects of drugs, where they are expected to occur (e.g., skin, brain, eyes, etc.), signs and symptoms of the side effects, and how to combat them through elimination, dosage adjustment, and change of therapy. The effects of stomach physiology, liver functions, number of receptors, biochemical transformation, binding sites, lipophylic and hydrophilic distributions, blood circulation, pharmacokinetic properties, receptors affinities/sensitivity, and others will be routing measurers. Unlike medical schools, these attributes that are associated with drugs are taught in various schools of pharmacy. Pharmacy students just need clinical rotations and residency to reiterate and inculcate the knowledge in them. Pharmacy residency is bound to increase in duration, size, and magnitude the moment pharmacy is liberated. No patients in hospitals or other institutional settings will escape pharmacy rounds by then because most if not all patients take medications, and many have a complex regimen.

Documentation is a cankerworm that has long plagued the pharmacy profession because of its bondage, and many detractors such as third-party payers and others have used the excuse as an opportunity to avoid paying remunerations for services to the professionals. Is documentation actually a problem for pharmacists as many are made to believe, or it is just an artificial condition created by the laws that compel them to forget about writing or using their knowledge and be content with dispensing functions only? If high school graduates can conveniently write letters, essays, and projects; if associate degree holders can conveniently write better than the high school graduates; if school teachers with four years of college work can conveniently write lesson notes for students; if engineers with four to five years of college work can conveniently write projects; if lawyers with 7 years of college work can write volumes of pages in defense or support of their clients; if social workers with 4 years of college work can write about their clients/patrons; if accountants with four years of college work can conveniently write everything about auditing a firm and other situations then what is the big deal about pharmacists' documentations with 5 to 7 years of college work? The pharmacist went through high school and an associate degree program, so he is not a novice in writing letters, essays, and projects talk less of mere patient drug therapy or documentation. Pharmacy liberation will eradicate this obstacle and set pharmacists free to write anything about their patients' drug therapy.

Pharmacy is a diverse profession with many areas of interest and numerous branches such as nuclear pharmacy, disease management, education, research, and others. Various branches of pharmacy will increase in size and scope with pharmacy liberation, and many pharmacists will discover that they have no option but to specialize like other branches of medicine before residencies. Like dentistry, ophthalmology, and others, pharmacy will eventually grow to embrace specialty groups such as infectious Diseases, gastrointestinal, hematological, endocrine and metabolic, cardiovascular, respiratory, renal and genitourinary, dermatological, antineoplastic, psycho-therapeutic drugs, drug information, acute and chronic care therapy, etc. It is going to be impossible for any pharmacists to be well rounded in all these areas and be up to the task. Pharmacy needs to stand on its feet first and foremost, and then portray its good image, improve the professional standard, and accelerate its growth before collaborating with other branches of medicine. Pharmacy might need to modify its degree title or abbreviation in order to remain in line with others. The profession cannot isolate itself from others with 2 to 3-letter degree abbreviations such as BSc, BA, JD, PhD, OD, MD, DO, DDS, MD, MBA, VMD, MSc, MOT, OTD, DMD, etc. Pharmacy with its current 6-letter abbreviation, PharmD, is alone with very few others, if any, and it doesn't argue well for the profession, the spread of its Doctor of Pharmacy degree, and its acceptability in other parts of the world. It might become necessary to shorten the 6-letters to 3 by taking away "har" and leaving the other parts, as PMD (*P*MD) or PmD or pMD. Whatever is chosen between these three options shows that three letters is the maximum of most degree titles. The three letters will not only enhance the status of the degree but identify pharmacy as a specialty of the medical profession like Doctor of Veterinary medicine (VMD) and Doctor of Dental Medicine (DMD). MD already is a degree title used to identify medical doctors all over the world; the addition of "p" as a prefix in front of the MD would help to accelerate pharmacy's liberation, and serve as an easy means of identifying clinical pharmacists as therapeuticians or therapeutic physicians (drug specialists) and a group of medical specialists. Ceteris paribus (all things being equal), a liberated pharmacy in the long run will need the assistance of pharmacy technicians. Pharmacy technicians have no specific requirements other than high school diploma in contemporary society, but this is likely to change in the future to a four-year first-degree (BSc) requirement as a prerequisite for the position with liberated pharmacy fully in operation. (That is, when pharmacy has been fully integrated with other branches of medicine as a specialty and pharmacists have been able to convince the world of their crucial role in treatment as therapeuticians, because treatment is to pharmacy as to what diagnosis is to other branches of medicine or surgery is to a surgeon.) The first-degree holder pharmacists can borrow a leaf from this idea about what is likely to occur in the future, although it might not happen in their lifetime. They are better off taking advantage of the nontraditional PharmD program now than allowing the system to make them subordinates of their colleagues (i.e., they will become what the technicians are to them, to their colleagues—again it might not happen in our lifetime).

To end up with future hope, we might very well be looking at a profession that will one day become the backbone of medicine. The days when contemporary prescriptions will become a diagnosis note for the clinical pharmacist or therapeutic physicians to prescribe drugs.

REFERENCES

1. Klaasen, C. D. 500th Birthday of Paracelcus, Father of Toxicology. International Union of Toxicology (IUTOX) newsletter. 1992/93.

2. Wick, J. Y. Culture, ethnicity, and medications. *Journal of the American Pharmaceutical Association* NS 36 (1996): 556-62.

3. Bootman, L. J. The $76 billion wake-up call: By practicing pharmaceutical care, pharmacists can help patients avoid costly drug-related illnesses. *Journal of the American Pharmaceutical Association* NS 36 (1996): 27-28.

4. Lazarou J., B. H. Pomeranz, and P. N. Corey. Incidence of adverse drug reactions in hospitalized patients: A meta-analysis of prospective studies. *Journal of the American Medical Association* 279 (1998): 1200-1205

5. Bates, D. W. Drugs and adverse drug reactions. How worried should we be? *Journal of the American Medical Association* 279 (1998): 1216-17.

6. Stover, K. A. Senate studies adverse drug reactions in the elderly: Knowlton cities pharmaceutical care as key to improving drug use. *Pharmacy Today* 2(5) (1996): 1, 17.

7. Aparasu, R. R. Visit to office-based physicians in the United States for medication-related morbidity. *Journal of the American Pharmaceutical Association* 39 (199): 332-37.

8. Fink, J. L., III. Counseling patients on Rx therapy and OTC drugs: Legal issues. The Pharmacy Letter 1(student ed.) (1997): 1-6.

9. Vogel, M. R. Compliance program rewards pharmacies' individual successes. *Pharmacy Today* 3 (8) (1997): 8.

10. Garnett, W. R. GI effects of OTC analgesics: Implications for product selection. *Journal of the American Pharmaceutical Association* NS 36 (1996): 565-71.

11. Castiglia, M., A. Raymond, and Smego Jr. The global problem of antimicrobial resistance. *Journal of the American Pharmaceutical Association* NS 37 (1997): 383-87.

12. Berg, M. J. Status of research on gender difference. *Journal of the American Pharmaceutical Association* NS 37 (1997): 43-56.

13. Riggs, M. M. Population pharmacokinetics/pharmacodynamics and individualized drug therapy. *Journal of the American Pharmaceutical Association* NS 36 (1996): 59-61.

14. Steiner, J. F. Pharmacotherapy problems in the elderly. *Journal of the American Pharmaceutical Association* NS 36 (1996): 431-37, 467.

15. McGuire, D. Pharmacy and the law: The pharmacist's duty to the patient. *Florida Pharmacy Today* 65(2) (2001): 10, 19.

16. Fried, S. *Bitter pills*. A Bantam book 1998.

17. Ernst, F. R., and A. J. Grizzle. Drug-related morbidity and mortality: Updating the cost of illness model. *Journal of the American Pharmaceutical Association* 41 (2001): 192-99.

18. Lowers, J. Pharmacists respond to report of missed drug interactions: Workplace distractions, pressure from managed care, and patient apathy are causes, but not excuses. *Pharmacy Today* 2 (10) (1996): 1, 10, 22.

19. Alvarez, E. The president's viewpoint: The Ten Commandments of pharmacy. *Florida Pharmacy Today* (1999): 5, 10.

20. Maltz, G. A. JAMA letter fall out prompts pharmacists to voice their concerns. *Pharmacy Today* 2 (5) (1996): 1, 18.

21. Miller, R. R. History of clinical pharmacy and clinical pharmacology. *Journal of Clinical Pharmacology* (1981): 195-97.

22. Kirk, K. W. What can the public expect of pharmacists? A study in *U.S. News and World Report* sounds an alarm for pharmacists and patients: Will the profession respond? *Journal of the American Pharmaceutical Association* NS 36 (1996): 577, 622.

23. Shefcheck, S. L., and J. Thomas III. The outlook for pharmacist initiation and modification of drug therapy: The concept of pharmaceutical care is becoming a reality, but progress is slow and laws vary widely from state to state. *Journal of the American Pharmaceutical Association* NS 36 (1996): 597-604.

24. Knapp, K. K., et al. Availability of primary care providers and pharmacists in the United States. *Journal of the American Pharmaceutical Association* 2 (1999): 127-34.

25. Gangeness, D. E. Pharmaceutical care for rural patients: Ominous trends: Workforce trends, financial concerns, current curricular, and population demographics are combining to limit rural patients' access to care. *Journal of the American Pharmaceutical Association* NS 37 (1997): 62-65, 84.

26. English, T. Miss Medicaid will pay for pharmacy services: Pharmacists to be recognized as providers. *Pharmacy Today* 17.

27. Nichols B. The president's viewpoint: The power of agreement. *Florida Pharmacy Today* (1998): 5, 24.

28. Brooks, R. G. Florida Department of Health: Update, update, update. Newsletter (1999): 1-5.

29. Worrall, C. Nurse practitioners: Are they trained enough to manage drug therapy? *Journal of the American Pharmaceutical Association* NS 36 (1996): 233.

30. Hepler, C. Developing a market for pharmaceutical care. *Florida Pharmacy Today* 62(7) (1998): 28.

31. Barnette, D. J., C. M. Murphy, and B. L. Carter. Clinical skill development for community pharmacists. *Journal of the American Pharmaceutical Association* NS 36 (1996): 573-80.

32. Generali, J. A., M. A. Danish, and S. E. Rosenbaum. Knowledge of and attitudes about adverse drug reaction reporting among Rhode Island pharmacists. *Annals of Pharmacotherapy* 29 (1995): 365-69.

33. Hartman, T., and Watanabe. Pharmacotherapy of depression: Focused considerations for primary care. *Journal of the American Pharmaceutical Association* NS 36 (1996): 521-32.

34. Posey, M. L. Pharmaceutical care: Will pharmacy incorporate its philosophy of practice? *Journal of the American Pharmaceutical Association* NS 37 (1997): 145-48.

35. Penna, P. M. Managed care and the community pharmacist. *American Pharmacy* NS (1995): 54-60.

36. Maltz, G. A. Computer records can identify patients at risks for drug-related problems. *Pharmacy Today* 3(3) (1997): 11.

37. English, T. Pharmacists recognized in North Carolina Medical Practice Act. *Pharmacy Today* 5(8) (1999): 8.

38. Price, S. Talking pill bottles target visually impaired patients. *Pharmacy Today* 7(6) (2001): 11.

39. U.S. facing shortage of pharmacists. *Pharmacy Digest* 7(1) (2001): 4.

40. Whitney, C. G., et al. Increasing prevalence of multi-drug resistance streptococcus pneumonia in the United States. *New England Journal of Medicine* 343 (2000): 1917-24.

41. Price, S. Pharmacists' services included in Medicare drug benefit bill. *Pharmacy Today* 8 (February 2002): 2, 12.

42. Erickson, M. Message about appropriate used of antibiotics finally hold. *Pharmacy Today* (August 2002): 6.

43. Engle, J. P. 150 years of pharmacy: Our patients, our passion. *Journal of the American Pharmaceutical Association* 42 (5 Supplement 1) (2002): 57-59.

44. Critically examining pharmaceutical care. *Journal of the American Pharmaceutical Association* 42 (5 Supplement 1) (2002): 518-19.

45. Poirier, S. and Gariepy. Compensation in Canada for resolving drug-related problems. *Journal of the American Pharmaceutical Association* NS 36(2) (1996): 117-22.

46. Kassam, R., et al. Pharmaceutical care research and education project: pharmacists' interventions. *Journal of the American Pharmaceutical Association* 41 (2001): 401-10.

47. Erickson, A. K. Study examines drug-related deaths in hospital. *Pharmacy Today* 7(12) (December 2001): 4.

48. Garcão, J. A., and J. Cabrita. Evaluation of pharmaceutical care program for hypertensive patients in rural Portugal. *Journal of the American Pharmaceutical Association* 42 (2002): 858-64.

49. Akaho, E., E. P. Armstrong, and M. Fujii. Pharmaceutical care innovations in Japan. *Journal of the American Pharmaceutical Association* NS 36(2) (1996): 123-27.

50. Guo-jie, L. Hospital pharmacy practice in the People's Republic of China. *American Journal of Hospital Pharmacy* 39 (1982): 1487-90.

51. Armour, C. L., et al. Implementation and evaluation of Australian Pharmacists' Diabetes Care Services. *Journal of the American Pharmaceutical Association* 44 (2004): 455-66.

CHAPTER FIVE

CURRICULUM OF VARIOUS BRANCHES OF MEDICINE IN COMPARISM TO PHARMACY

Members of the public institutions work for the sole purpose of serving public interest, and none of these entities are bound in secrecy like a secret cult. Schools from elementary to the highest doctorate program (PhD) are living examples of such entities; consequently, none fit into the category or definition of a secret cult/society. Schools of pharmacy, dentistry, optometry, medicine, nursing, and others are no exception to this rule; hence, the affairs/curriculum of all schools are public property and should be open to the public. Thus, a parent reserves the right to know everything especially the curriculum of any school, including medical and law schools, before sending their children to the school. This gesture enables them to assist their children in designing/planning a career for them. One good source of information about schools in the U.S. is the *U.S. News and World Report* survey of America's best colleges.

The magazine uses certain criteria, which are three basic steps defined by the colleges' missions and regions, 16 academic excellence indicators, and a ranking of colleges against their peers in each category using score weights. The final overall score is basically judged in terms of seven categories: academic reputation—25%, graduation and retention rates—20%, faculty resources—20%, students' selectivity—15%, financial resources—10%, alumni giving—5%, and graduation rate performance—5%. The school categories are grouped and modified by the Carnegie Foundation for the Advancement of Teaching. This is the foundation that classified schools according to their mission, and there are 228 national universities in the U.S. (147 public and 81 private) that fall within these categories. These universities offer a wide range of undergraduate, master's, and doctorate degree programs.

The schools that have enrollments below 250 or specifically designed specialty schools were excluded from the ranking. The major subheadings under which the schools' grading finally appeared on paper are: overall scores (for top-ranking schools), academic reputation score, graduation and retention rank, average freshman rate, graduation rate, faculty resources rank, percentage of classes under 20 students, percentage of classes of 50 or more students, student/faculty ratio, percentage of faculty who are full-time, selectivity rank, SAT/ACT in the 25th-75th percentile, freshmen in top 10% of high school (HS) class, acceptance rate, financial resources rank, alumni giving rank, and alumni giving rate. *U.S. News* ranks the top schools, then groups others into the second, third, and fourth tier.[1,3]

No single study or rating in the world can be said to be perfect. It will take more than a man to predict schools that will produce the next American president. These ratings do not necessarily predict one's success in school and life. After all, there are people like Bill Gates who either dropped out of school or did not go to school at all and later became an icon, world genius (genius behind computer industry in the case of Gates), erudite fellow, and successful people in life. Moreover, these ratings looked at the broad spectrum of school. Thus, a school might be the national best in one area (top ranking) and a total failure in others; consequently, the end result would be tier four or lower. The authors of how *U.S. News* ranks colleges warned against using this rating to judge winners instead of school choice guidance. Be that as it may, this rating should be taken with a grain of salt. It is the best alternative in the midst of none in the U.S. Many schools have expressed their dissatisfaction with the rating but many families are contented and satisfied with the rating.

U.S. News and World Report has another version of the survey—America's best graduate schools—which focuses on business, medicine, law, engineering, and education schools. Similar criteria are used in rating schools but the major subheadings under which final grading appear on paper for medical schools are: overall score, reputation score by academics, reputation score by residency directors, student selectivity rank, the year 2000 average undergraduate GPA-MCAT score/acceptances rate, NIH research grants, faculty/student ratio, out-of-state tuition and fees, total medical school enrollment, and percentage of 1998-2000 graduates entering primary care. The year 2001 report shows top-ranking medical schools in overall scores, research, and primary care as given below.[5]

#	Schools	Overall Score	Research	Primary Care
1.	Harvard University (MA)	100	1st	11th
2.	John Hopkins University (MD)	94	2nd	18th
3.	Duke University (NC)	90	3rd	21st
4.	University of Pennsylvania (PA)	89	4th	33rd
5.	University of Washington	100	5th	1st
6.	Oregon Health Sciences University	87	35th	2nd
7.	University of New Mexico	82	None top rank	3rd
8.	University of California, S.F.	77	7th	4th

The ratings used in this chapter will be limited to the popular general schools for undergraduate, master's, and PhD programs. Great efforts will be made to use medical schools' curriculum from the top-ranking schools (three choices), average-ranking schools from the second and third tiers (four choices), and low-ranking schools from the fourth tier (4 to 5 choices). The schools' curriculum will include various branches of medical schools and schools of nursing and physician assistants. However, other schools that do not fall within this range will be considered based on available data. It is important to note that many schools were cooperative in the desire to obtain their curriculum, while a few others were either secretive about the issue or limited in their response/approach. Some data were obtained from the Internet. The schools of choice are:

TOP-RANKING SCHOOLS

#	Schools	Overall Score	Academic Resp. Score
1.	Harvard University (MA)	93	4.9
2.	John Hopkins University (MD)	86	4.7
3.	University of Pennsylvanian (PA)	86	4.4

MIDDLE OR AVERAGE-RANKING SCHOOLS

#	Schools	Tiers	Academic Resp. Score
1.	University of Iowa (IA)	2nd	3.7
2.	University of Miami (FL)	2nd	3.0
3.	Arizona College of Osteopathic Medicine	3rd	3.3
4.	University of Maryland (Baltimore)	3rd	2.7

LOW-RANKING SCHOOLS

#	Schools	Tiers	Academic Resp. Score
1.	University of Wisconsin, Milwaukee	4th	2.8
2.	University of Louisville School of Medicine, Kentucky	4th	2.6
3.	University of Alabama School of Medicine, Huntsville	4th	2.4
4.	Wright State University School of Medicine, Ohio	4th	2.3
5.	Nova Southeastern University School of Osteopathic Medicine	4th	1.7

HARVARD UNIVERSITY

Courses offered to students in the four-year professional phase leading to the award of a Doctor of Medicine (MD) degree before residency (information was obtained from the Internet):

YEAR 1 (2000-2001)

1. Human Body; 2. Chemistry and Biology of the Cell; 3. Integrated Human Physiology; 4. Pharmacology; 5. Genetics, Development, and Reproductive Biology; 6. Immunology, Microbiology, and Infectious Disease; 7. Critical Reading of the Medical Literature; 8. Patient/Doctor.

HEALTH SCIENCES AND TECHNOLOGY (HST)

9. Human Functional Anatomy; 10. Pathology; 11. Molecular Biology and Genetics in Modern Medicine; 12. Cellular and Molecular Immunology; 13. Endocrinology; 14. Cardiovascular Pathophysiology; 15. Respiratory Pathophysiology; 16. Renal Pathophysiology; 17. Molecular Medicine; 18. Intensive in Human Intermediary Metabolism; 19. Introduction to Patient Care; 20. Emerging Medical Technologies; 21. Introduction to Business and Management in Medicine; 22. IT and Future Health Care; 23. Statistical Planning and Investigation.

(D: 1, 2, 3, 5, 6, 9, 10, 11, 12, 13, 14, 15, 16, 17, 18, 19, 20; P: 4)

[D = Diagnosis-related courses; P = Pharmacy or drug treatment-related courses]

Number of pharmacy or drug treatment-related courses: 1 out of 23 (all the HST courses might not be compulsory).

Number of diagnosis-related courses: 17 out of 23.

YEAR 2 (2000-2001)

1. Human Nervous System and Behavior Pathology; Human System—Module I--2. Dermatologic Pathophysiology; 3. Cardiovascular/Respiratory Pathophysiology; 4. Hematological Pathophysiology; Human System—Module II--5. Gastrointestinal Pathphysiology; 6. Musculoskeletal Pathphysiology; 7. Renal Pathophysiology; 8. Endocrine Pathophysiology; 9. Reproductive Pathophysiology; 10. Pyscholpathology 700M. J.; 11. Preventive Medicine/Nutrition; 12. Patient/Doctor II.

HEALTH SCIENCES AND TECHNOLOGY (HST)

13. Mechanisms of Microbiology and Pathology; 14. Human Reproductive Biology; 15. Gastroenterology; 16. Introduction to Neuroscience; 17. Hematology; 18. Principles of Pharmacology; 19. Introduction to Clinical Medicine; 20. Real Medicine; 21. Emerging Medical Technologies; 22. Psychopathology; 23. Introduction to Business and Management in Medicine; 24. IT and Future Health Care.

(D: 1, 2, 3, 4, 5, 6, 7, 8, 9, 10, 13, 14, 15, 16, 17, 19, 21, 22; P: 18)

Number of pharmacy or drug treatment-related courses: 1 out of 24 (all the HST courses might not be compulsory).

Number of diagnosis-related courses: 18 out of 24.

YEAR 3 AND 4 (2000-2001)
CORE CLERKSHIPS

1. Medicine I; 2. Medicine II; 3. Neurology; 4. OB/GYN; 5. Patient/Doctor III; 6. Pediatrics; 7. Primary Care Clerkship; 8. Psychiatry Clerkship (under development); 9. Radiology; 10. Surgery Clerkship; 11. Clerkship Lectures; 12. Women's and Children's Health.

ELECTIVE CLERKSHIPS

1. Emergency Medicine; 2. Infectious Diseases.

OTHERS

1. Course Evaluations; 2. Clinical Application of Anatomy; 3. Emergency Medical Care; 4. HMS Transition Course; 5. Injury and Violence Prevention; 6. OED Curriculum Themes; 7. Psychiatry Interest Group; 8. Year III/IV Ind. Study—ECG tutorial.

Number of pharmacy or drug treatment-related courses: None, but they constitute an integral part of the clerkship.

Number of diagnosis-related courses: Constitute a major part of the clerkships.

RESIDENCY AFTER GRADUATION (3 YEARS)

YEAR 1: INTERNSHIP (PGY-1 I.E., POSTGRADUATE YEAR 1)
1. Gen Med—Inpatient General Medicine; 2. Amb Med—Ambulatory Medicine; 3. EU—Emergency Unit; 4. Gen Med; 5. Gen Med; 6. MICU—Medical Intensive Care Unit; 7. WR VAH—West Roxbury Veterans Administration Hospital; 8. Cardiol—Cardiology Step-Down Unit; 9. DFCI or ONC—Dana Farber Cancer Institute or Oncology; 10. Gen Med; 11. CCU—Coronary Care Unit; 12. Gen Med.

YEAR 2: JUNIOR RESIDENCY (PGY-2)
1. MICU; 2. Gen Med; 3. Amb Med; 4. Cardio; 5. Gen Med; 6. Elective—Clinical Elective; 7. Amb Med; 8. Elective; 9. DFCI or ONC; 10. WR VAH; 11. Amb Med; 12. EU.

YEAR 3: SENIOR RESIDENCY (PGY-3)
1. Gen Med; 2. Amb Med; 3. SICU—Surgical Intensive Care Unit; 4. Gen Med; 5. RES—Research Elective; 6. RES; 7. RES; 8. Amb Med; 9. MICU; 10. Elective; 11. EU; 12. Amb Med.

JOHNS HOPKINS SCHOOL OF MEDICINE

Courses offered to students in the four-year professional phase leading to the award of Doctor of Medicine (MD) before residency (information was obtained from the Internet—no brochure; like Harvard University, John Hopkins's school officers constantly refer investigator to the Internet but Internet information was insufficient for the study as a result the school was excluded from data analysis):

YEAR 1
One topic per quarter.

1. Molecules and Cells; 2. Anatomy and Developmental Biology; 3. Neuroscience; 4. Organ Systems; 5. Journal Club Sessions.

(D: 1, 2, 3, 4; P: 0)

Number of pharmacy or drug treatment-related courses: None out of 5.
Number of diagnosis-related courses: 4 out of 5.

YEAR 2

1. Organ System in Human Pathophysiology, History Taking, and Physical Examination. Small-group learning sessions, Laboratory work, and clinical rotation.

YEAR 3 AND 4

Students' individualized two-year plan with faculty member in the following clerkship areas:

1. Ambulatory; 2. Medicine; 3. Emergency Medicine; 4. General Surgery; 5. Pediatrics; 6. Psychiatry and Neurology and Ophthalmology; 7. Obstetrics and Gynecology; 8. Internal Medicine.

UNIVERSITY OF PENNSYLVANIA SCHOOL OF MEDICINE

Courses offered to students in the four-year professional phase leading to the award of Doctor of Medicine (MD) before residency[6] (information obtained from the Internet and brochure):

YEAR 1 (18 WKS)

1. Orientation: Development and Molecular Biology; 2. Genetics; 3. Embryology: Cellular Physiology, Metabolism, and Pharmacological Processes; 4. Biochemistry; 5. Pharmacology; 6. Physiology: Human Body—Structure and Function; 7. Histology; 8. Gross Anatomy: Host Defenses and Pharmacological Responses; 9. Immunology; 10. Pathology; 11. Microbiology; 12. Pharmacology.

(D: 1, 2, 3, 4, 6, 7, 8, 9, 10, 11; P: 5, 12; D and P: 3, 8)

[D and P = approximately equal combination of diagnosis and pharmacy or drug treatment-related courses]

Number of pharmacy or drug treatment-related courses: 2-4 out of 12.
Number of diagnosis-related courses: 8-10 out of 12.

YEAR 2 (40 WKS)
MODULE 2 (JANUARY YEAR 1 TO DECEMBER YEAR 2)

Transition Block (2 weeks); 1. Immunology; 2. Neoplasia; 3. Cardiology (5 wks); 4. Pulmonary (4 wks); 5. Renal (4 wks); 6. Dermatology (1 wk); 7. Connective Tissue (1 wk); 8. Musculoskeletal (1 wk); 9. Hematology and Oncology (2 wks); 10. Gastrointestinal and Nutrition (4 wks); 11. Brain and Behavior (11 wks); 12. Endocrine and Reproduction (5 wks).

(D: 1, 2, 3, 4, 5, 6, 7, 8, 9, 10, 11, 12; P: 0)

MODULE 3

Technology and Practice of Medicine, Concurrent with Modules 1 and 2 (58 weeks)

Introduction to Clinical Medicine: 1. Doctor/Patient; 2. History Taking; 3. Physical Exams; 4. Differential Diagnosis; 5. Doctoring; 6. Professionalism and Humanism: Epidemiology; 7. Epidemiology; 8. Managed Care; 9. Ethics; 10. Emergency Medicine.

(D: 2, 3, 4, 5, 7, 10; P: 0)

Number of pharmacy or drug treatment-related courses: zero (0) out of 22 (module 2 and 3).

Number of diagnosis-related courses: 18 out of 22.

YEAR 3 (48 WKS-12 WKS FOR EACH BLOCK)
MODULE 4 (CORE CLERKSHIP: JANUARY YEAR 2 TO DECEMBER YEAR 3)

BLOCK 1: 1. Internal Medicine (9 wks: 6 wks inpatient and 3 wks ambulatory); 2. Family Medicine (3 wks). BLOCK 2-3: Obstetrics/gynecology (6 wks: 3 wks each for OB and GYN): 4. Pediatrics (6 wks: 3 wks each for inpatient and ambulatory). BLOCK 3-5: Surgery/Anesthesia (9 wks for inpatient and ambulatory): 6. Emergency Medicine (3 wks). BLOCK 4-7: Psychiatry/Substance Abuse (6 wks inpatient and ambulatory): 8. Neurology (3 wks); 9. Clinical Specialists (3 wks: 1 wk each for ophthalmology, otorhinolaryngology, and orthopedic surgery).

Number of pharmacy or drug treatment-related courses: None, but they constitute an integral part of the clerkship.

Number of diagnosis-related courses: Constitute a major part of the clerkship.

YEAR 4 (68 WKS-12 WKS EACH)
MODULE 5 (ELECTIVES, SELECTIVES/SCHOLARLY PURSUIT: JANUARY YEAR 3 TO MAY YEAR 4)

Same as year 3 in terms of medicine/family medicine; pediatrics/obstetrics and gynecology; psychiatry/neurology/otorhinolaryngology/ophthalmology/orthopaedics; surgery/anesthesia/emergency medicine; then radiation oncology and informatics as additions. Alternatively, a breakdown of Module 5 in terms of weeks are: 1. Intersession (1 wk for ACLS and Bioethics); 2. Scholarly Pursuit (12 wks); 3. Sub-internship in General Medicine or Pediatrics (4 wks); 4. Board of Review Course (4 wks); 5. Six Additional Advanced Electives (24 wks); 6. Frontiers in Medicine (4 wks); 7. Open/Unscheduled Time (19 weeks).

Number of pharmacy or drug treatment-related courses: None, but they constitute an integral part of the clerkship.

Number of diagnosis-related courses: Constitute a major part of the clerkship.

Residency after graduation: Not available.

UNIVERSITY OF IOWA COLLEGE OF MEDICINE

Courses offered to students in the four-year professional phase (2000-2002) leading to the award of Doctor of Medicine (MD) before residency are[7]:

YEAR 1
SEMESTER 1

1. Biochemistry for Medical Students; 2. Medical Gross Anatomy; 3. Medical Cell Biology; 4. Medical Genetics; 5. Foundation of Clinical Practice I.

SEMESTER 2
6. Medical Neuroscience; 7. Principles of Medical Immunology; 8. Human Organ Systems; 9. Foundation of Clinical Practice II.

(D: 1, 2, 3, 4, 5, 6, 7, 8, 9; P: 0)

Number of pharmacy or drug treatment-related courses: zero (0) out of 9.

Number of diagnosis-related courses: 9 out of 9.

YEAR 2
SEMESTER 3
1. Medical Pharmacology; 2. Principle of Infectious Diseases; 3. General and Systemic Pathology; 4. Foundations of Clinical Practice III.

SEMESTER 4
5. Foundations of Clinical Practice IV; 6. Health Law; 7. Clinical Pharmacology and Therapeutics.

(D: 2, 3, 4, 5; P: 1, 7)

Number of pharmacy or drug treatment-related courses: 2 out of 7.

Number of diagnosis-related courses: 4 out of 7.

YEAR 3 (49 WEEKS—FIRST CLINICAL YEAR)
Six generalist core clerkships (36 wks): 1. Family Medicine Preceptorship; 2. Internal Medicine (ambulatory and inpatient); 3. Pediatrics; 4. Obstetrics and Gynecology; 5. Surgery; 6. Community-based Primary Care.

Subspecialty clerkships: 12 wks of courses chosen from anesthesia, dermatology neurology, ophthalmology, orthopedics, otolaryngology, psychiatry, radiology, Laboratory medicine, and electrocardiography. Orientation: 1 wk.

Number of pharmacy or drug treatment-related courses: zero (0), but constitute an integral part of the clerkship.

Number of diagnosis-related courses: Constitute a major part of the clerkship.

YEAR 4 (32 WKS—SECOND CLINICAL YEAR)
Generalist core clerkships and subspecialty clerkship (not completed in year 3—first clinical year in year 4): Advanced clerkships—sub-internship; Electives—3 electives.

Number of pharmacy or drug treatment-related courses: zero (0), but constitute an integral part of the clerkship.

Number of diagnosis-related courses: Constitute a major part of the clerkship.

RESIDENCY AFTER GRADUATION IN SELECTED SPECIALTIES:

Family Medicine (offers 72 individual rotations)—three years residency.

Core rotation: Adult medicine, natural child health, surgery, and behavior medicine.

Elective rotation: internal medicine, pediatrics, obstetrics and gynecology, psychiatry, medication and surgical subspecialties, geriatrics, rural family practice, and community medicine. First year in mercy hospital, second and third years at the University of Iowa Hospital and Clinics.
Obstetrics and Gynecology—four-year residency: training in obstetrics, gynecologic surgery, office gynecology, ultrasound, reproductive endocrinology, gynecologic oncology, family planning, and endoscopic procedures.

Pediatrics—three-year residency program.

Otolaryngology (head and neck surgery)—four-year residency program.

UNIVERSITY OF MIAMI SCHOOL OF MEDICINE
Courses offered to students in the four-year professional phase (2000-2001) leading to the award of Doctor of Medicine (MD) before residency[10] (information obtained from the Internet and Catalog):

YEAR 1
CORE MODULE (19 WKS)

1. Genetics and Early Development; 2. Human Structure; 3. Metabolism and Cellular Physiology; 4. Host Defenses and Pharmacological Responses; 5. Microbiology and Infectious Diseases.

(D: 1, 2, 3, 5; P: 4)

YEAR 1 AND 2
(SECOND HALF OF YEAR 1 AND FIRST HALF OF YEAR 2: 49 WKS)
INTEGRATED ORGAN SYSTEMS MODULES

1. Brain and Behavior: Neuroscience and Behavior Sciences; 2. Cardiovascular System; 3. Respiratory System; 4. Renal Systems; 5. Endocrine and Reproductive Systems; 6. Gastroenterology and Nutrition; 7. Hematology and Oncology; 8. Musculoskeletal System and Skin; last 12 weeks used as a problem-based learning segment.

(D: 1, 2, 3, 4, 5, 6, 7, 8; P: 0)

Number of pharmacy or drug treatment-related courses in year 1 and 2: 1 out of 13.

Number of diagnosis-related courses in year 1 and 2: 12 out of 13.

YEAR 3
CORE CLERKSHIPS (50 WKS).

1. Internal Medicine (8 wks); 2. Surgery (8 wks); 3. Pediatrics (6 wks); 4. Generalist: Primary Care (6 wks); 5. OB/GYN (6 wks); 6. Family Medicine/Geriatrics (6 wks); 7. Psychiatry (6 wks); 8. Neurology (4 wks).

Number of pharmacy or drug treatment-related courses: None, but they constitute an integral part of the clerkship.

Number of diagnosis-related courses: Constitute a major part of the clerkship.

YEAR 4

1. Ward Service (sub-internship—4 wks); 2. Surgery Sub-internship (4 wks); 3. Geriatric Medicine-Geriatric Psychiatry (4 wks); 4. Anesthesia (2 wks); 5. Consult Electives (6 wks); 6. Selectives (14 wks); 7. ACLS Certification and Molecular Basis of Medicine (4 wks).

Number of pharmacy or drug treatment-related courses: None, but constitute an integral part of the clerkship.

Number of diagnosis-related courses: Constitute a major part of the clerkship.

Residency after graduation: Available in the following areas:

1. Anesthesiology; 2. Dermatology; 3. Epidemiology; 4. Family Medicine; 5. Internal Medicine; 6. Neurological Surgery; 7. Neurology; 8. Obstetrics and Gynecology; 9. Ophthalmology; 10. Orthopedics and Rehabilitation; 11. Otolaryngology; 12. Pathology; 13. Pediatrics; 14. Psychiatry; 15. Radiation oncology; 16. Radiology; 17. Surgery; 18. Urology.

ARIZONA COLLEGE OF OSTEOPATHIC MEDICINE

Courses offered to students in the four-year professional phase (2002) leading to the award of Doctor of Osteopathic Medicine (DO) before residency (information obtained from the Internet):

YEAR 1 (885 HOURS)
FIRST QUARTER (10 WKS-300 HRS)

1. Interdisciplinary Health Care (5 hrs); 2. Gross Anatomy I (90 hrs); 3. Histology/Embryology I (40 hrs); 4. Biochemistry I (80 hrs); 5. Osteopathic Medicine I (30 hrs); 6. Clinic Correlates/ICM I (30 hrs); 7. OCM/Community Medicine I (30 hrs); 8. Introduction to Human Behavior I (10 hrs).

(D: 2, 3, 4, 5, 6, 7, 8; P: 0)

SECOND QUARTER (10 WKS—310 HRS)

1. Gross Anatomy II (90 hrs); 2. Histology/Embryology II (20 hrs); 3. Biochemistry II (50 hrs); 4. Physiology I (60 hrs); 5. Osteopathic Medicine

II (30 hrs); 6. Clinical Correlates/ICM II (30 hrs); 7. OCM/Community Medicine (15 hrs); 8. Introduction to Human Behavior II (15 hrs); 9. Clinical Correlates/ICM II (30 hrs).

(D: 1, 2, 3, 4, 5, 6, 7, 8; P: 0)

THIRD QUARTER (11 WKS-275 HRS)
1. Physiology II (60 hrs); 2. Neuroscience (80 hrs); 3. Immunology (30 hrs); 4. Osteopathic Medicine III (30 hrs); 5. Topics in Medicine I (20 hrs); 6. Clinical Correlates/ICM III (30 hrs); 7. OCM/Community Medicine (15 hrs); 8. Introduction to Human Behavior III (10 hrs).

(D: 1, 2, 3, 4, 5, 6, 7, 8; P: 0)

Number of pharmacy or drug treatment-related courses: zero (0) out of 24 or 885 hrs (may be an integral part of some of the courses).

Number of diagnosis-related courses: 23 out of 24 or 880 out of 885 hrs.

YEAR 2 (735 HOURS)
FIRST QUARTER (10 WKS-265 HRS)
1. Pathology I (60 hrs); 2. Microbiology (60 hrs); 3. Pharmacology I (40 hrs); 4. Osteopathic Medicine IV (30 hrs); 5. Introduction to Clinical Medicine IV (10 hrs); 6. Clinical Correlates/Case Presentation IV (30 hrs); 7. OCM/Community Medicine (15 hrs); 8. Topics in Medicine II (20 hrs); 8a. Mandatory Elective.

(D: 1, 2, 4, 5, 6, 7, 8; P: 3)

SECOND QUARTER (10 WKS-245 HRS)
1. Pathology II (60 hrs); 2. Microbiology (60 hrs); 3. Pharmacology II (40 hrs); 4. Osteopathic MedicineV (30); 5. Introduction to Clinical Medicine V (10 hrs); 6. Clinical Correlates/Case Presentation V (30 hrs); 7. OCM/Community Medicine (15 hrs); 7a. Mandatory Electives.

(D: 1, 2, 4, 5, 6, 7; P: 3)

THIRD QUARTER (10 WKS-255 HRS)

1. Osteopathic Medicine II (30 hrs); 2. Pharmacology III (50 hrs); 3. Pathology III (50 hrs); 4. Osteopathic Medicine VI (30 hrs); 5. Introduction to Clinical Medicine III (20 hrs); 6. Clinical Correlates/Case Presentations VI (30 hr); 7. OCM/Community Medicine (115 hrs); 8. Topics in Medicine III (20 hrs); 9. Psychopathology IV (10 hrs); 10. Osteopathic Clinical Medicine I (30 hrs); 10a. Mandatory Electives.

(D: 1, 3, 4, 5, 6, 7, 8, 9, 10; P: 2)

Number of pharmacy or drug treatment-related courses: 3 out of 25 or 130 out of 735 hrs (may be an integral part of some of the courses).

Number of diagnosis-related courses: 22 out of 25 or 605 out of 735 hrs.

YEAR 3 (1880 HRS-12 MONTHS)
ROTATIONS

1. Cardiology (4 wks-160 hrs); 2. Family Medicine (12 wks-480 hrs); 3. Surgery (4 wks-160 hrs); 4. Gen. Internal Medicine (4 wks-320 hrs); 5. Pediatrics (4 wks-160 hrs); 6. Obstetrics/Gynecology (4 wks-160 hrs); 7. Psychiatry (4 wks-160 hrs); 8. Maternal/Child Health (4 wks-160 hrs); 9. Osteopathic Clinical Medicine II (integrated—128 hrs); 10. Electives (4 wks-160 hrs).

Number of pharmacy or drug treatment-related courses: Constitute an integral part of the rotations.

Number of diagnosis-related courses: Constitute a major part of the rotations.

YEAR 4 (1880 HRS-12 MONTHS)
ROTATIONS

1. Rural Family Medicine I (4 wks-400 hrs); 2. Surgery II (4 wks-160 hrs); 3. General Internal Medicine II (4 wks-480 hrs); 4. Emergency Medicine (4 wks-160 hrs); 5. Neurology (2 wks-80 hrs); 6. Critical Care (4 wks-160 hrs); 7. Subspecialty Internal Medicine (4 wks-160 hrs); 8. Expanded Primary Care (6 wks-240 hrs); 9. Osteopathic Clinical Medicine IV (integrated-120 hrs); 10. Electives (12 wks-480 hrs).

Number of pharmacy or drug treatment-related courses: Constitute an integral part of the rotations.

Number of diagnosis-related courses: Constitute a major part of the rotations.

UNIVERSITY OF MARYLAND SCHOOL OF MEDICINE

Courses offered to students in the four-year professional phase (2002-2004) leading to the award of Doctor of Medicine (MD) before residency[8] (information obtained from catalog):

YEAR 1 (37 WKS)

1. Medical Informatics (1 wk—Area of Study (AOS): Computing, E-mail, Electronic Resource Databases, Information Management, Internet, Hospital System, UMB Network); 2. Structure and Development (9.5 wks—AOS: Human Gross Anatomy, Embryology, and Histology); 3. Human Behavior (1 wk); 4. Cellular and Molecular Biology (9 wks—AOS: Protein Structure and Function, Cellular Metabolic Pathways, Cell Signal Transduction, Cell Microanatomy, Human Genetics, Molecular Biology); 5. Cell Function Section of Functional Systems (2 wks—AOS: Cell Membrane, Physiology, and Dynamics); 6. Neurosciences (6 wks—AOS: Development, Structure, and Function of Nervous Tissues, Anatomical Organization of CNS, Sensory and Motor Systems, Higher Functions, and Concepts in Clinical Neurology); 7. Intimate Human Behavior (3 days); 8. Functional Systems (10 wks—AOS: Cell, Cardiovascular, Endocrine, Gastrointestinal, Renal, Respiratory, and Integrative Function); 9. Introduction to Clinical Practice (half day per week—AOS: Ethics, Nutrition, Intimate Human Behavior, Interviewing, and Physical Diagnosis Issues).

(D: 2, 3, 4, 5, 6, 7, 8, 9; P: 0)

Number of pharmacy or drug treatment-related courses: zero (0) out of 9.

Number of diagnosis-related courses: 8 out of 9.

YEAR 2 (34 WKS)

1. Host Defenses and Infectious Diseases (10 wks—AOS: Immunology, Bacteriology, Virology, Parasitology, Mycology); 2. Pathophysiology and Therapeutics (24 wks—AOS: Bone, Cardiovascular, Dermatologic, Endocrine, Gastrointestinal, Hematologic, Nervous, Renal and Reproductive Systems); 3. Physical Diagnosis (half day per week—AOS: Fundamental Aspects of History Taking and Physical Examination).

(D: 1, 2, 3; P: 0)

Number of pharmacy or drug treatment-related courses: None, but may constitute an integral part of some areas of study.

Number of diagnosis-related courses: 3 out of 3 or a majority of the areas of study.

YEAR 3 (48 WKS)
CORE CLERKSHIPS

1.Internal Medicine (12 wks); 2. Surgery/Surgical Subspecialty (12 wks); 3. Family Medicine Clerkship (4 wks); 4. OB/GYN (6 wks); 5. Pediatrics (6 wks); 6. Psychiatry/Neurology (8 wks).

Number of pharmacy or drug treatment-related courses: None, but constitute an integral part of the clerkship.

Number of diagnosis-related courses: Constitutes major part of the clerkship.

YEAR 4 (32 WKS)
CORE CLERKSHIPS

1. Ambulatory Care (8 wks); 2. Sub-internal (8 wks); 3. Surgical Subspecialties (4 wks); 4. Electives (12 wks).

Number of pharmacy or drug treatment-related courses: None, but constitute an integral part of the clerkship.

Number of diagnosis-related courses: Constitutes major part of the clerkship.

Residency after graduation is available in the following departments:

1. Anesthesiology; 2. Dermatology; 3. Diagnostic Radiology; 4. Epidemiology and Preventive Medicine; 5. Family Medicine; 6. Medicine; 7. Neurology; 8. Neurosurgery; 9. Obstetrics, Gynecology, and Reproductive Sciences; 10. Ophthalmology; 11. Orthopedic Surgery; 12. Pathology; 13. Pediatrics; 14. Psychiatry; 15. Radiation Oncology; 16. Surgery.

UNIVERSITY OF WISCONSIN MEDICAL SCHOOL

Courses offered to students in the four-year professional phase (2001) leading to the award of Doctor of Medicine (MD) before residency (information obtained from the Internet):

YEAR 1
FALL SEMESTER
1. Gross Human Anatomy; 2. Biomolecular Chemistry; 3. Histology; 4. Patient, Doctor, and Society I.

SPRING SEMESTER
5. Principles of Human Physiology; 6. Pathology; 7. Neuroscience; 8. Medical Genetics; 9. Patient, Doctor, and Society II.
(D: 1, 2, 3, 4, 5, 6, 7, 8, 9; P: 0)

Number of pharmacy or drug treatment-related courses: zero (0) out of 9.

Number of diagnosis-related courses: 9 out of 9.

YEAR 2
FALL SEMESTER
1. Hematology; 2. Infection and Immunity I; 3. Pharmacology I; 4. Cardiovascular System; 5. Renal System; 6. Respiratory System; 7. Patient, Doctor, and Society III.

SPRING SEMESTER
8. Neoplastic Diseases; 9. Infection and Immunity II; 10. Pharmacology II; 11. Endocrine System; 12. Gastrointestinal/Hepatic; 13. Psychiatry; 14.

Autopsy Pathology; 15. Clinical Nutrition; 16. Patient, Doctor, and Society IV.

(D: 1, 2, 4, 5, 6, 7, 8, 9, 11, 12, 13, 14, 16; P: 3, 10)

Number of pharmacy or drug treatment-related courses: 2 out of 16.

Number of diagnosis-related courses: 13 out of 16.

YEAR 3
CORE CLERKSHIPS

1. Medicine; 2. Surgery; 3. Primary Care; 4. Pediatrics; 5. Obstetrics and Gynecology; 6. Psychiatry; 7. Neurology; 8. Anesthesia; 9. Ophthalmology.

Number of pharmacy or drug treatment-related courses: None, but constitute an integral part of the clerkship.

Number of diagnosis-related courses: Constitute a major part of the clerkship.

YEAR 4
CORE CLERKSHIPS

1. Internal Medicine (sub-internship—4 wks); 2. Surgical Area (sub-internship—4 wks elective); 3. Preceptorship (8 wks); 4. Clinical Electives in specialty area and other institutions or countries.

Number of pharmacy or drug treatment-related courses: None but constitute an integral part of the clerkship.

Number of diagnosis-related courses: Constitute a major part of the clerkship.

Residency after graduation: No available data.

UNIVERSITY OF LOUISVILLE MEDICAL SCHOOL

Courses offered to students in the four-year professional phase (2001) leading to the award of Doctor of Medicine (MD) before residency (information obtained from the Internet):

YEAR 1
1. Gross Anatomy; 2. Biochemistry; 3. Clinical Practice Sciences 1a; 4. Clinical Practice Science 1b; 5. Microanatomy; 6. Neurosciences; 7. Human Embryology; 8. Physiology.

(D: 1, 2, 3, 4, 5, 6, 7, 8; P: 0)

Number of pharmacy or drug treatment-related courses: zero (0) out of 8.

Number of diagnosis-related courses: 8 out of 8.

YEAR 2
1. Clinical Practice Sciences 2a; 2. Clinical Practice Sciences 2b; 3. Microbiology and Immunology; 4. Pharmacology; 5. Pathology; 6. CNS; 7. Genetics.

(D: 1, 2, 3, 5, 6, 7; P: 4)

Number of pharmacy or drug treatment-related courses: 1 out of 7.

Number of diagnosis-related courses: 6 out of 7.

YEAR 3
1. Primary Care Clerkship (24 wks); 2. Basic Clerkship (8 wks); 3. Obstetrics and Gynecology Clerkship (8 wks); 4. Psychiatry Clerkship (6 wks).

Number of pharmacy or drug treatment-related courses: None, but constitute an integral part of the clerkship.

Number of diagnosis-related courses: Constitute a major part of the clerkship.

YEAR 4
1. AHEC Rural/Urban rotations in specified disciplines/specialties (selectives); 2. Ambulatory Primary Care rotations in one of three disciplines (selectives); 3. Ambulatory rotations in specified disciplines (selectives); 4. Inpatient General Medicine; 5. Inpatient General Surgery; 6. Neurology Clerkship; 7. Electives (10 wks).

Number of pharmacy or drug treatment-related courses: None, but constitute an integral part of the clerkship/rotations.

Number of diagnosis-related courses: Constitute a major part of the clerkship/rotations.

Residency after graduation: No available data.

UNIVERSITY OF ALABAMA SCHOOL OF MEDICINE

Courses offered to students in the four-year professional phase (2001) leading to the award of Doctor of Medicine (MD) before residency (information obtained from the Internet):

YEAR 1 (40 WKS: 24 HOUR/WEEK—955 HRS)

1. Gross Anatomy (200 hrs); 2. Biochemistry (131 hrs); 3. Behavioral Sciences (56 hrs); 4. Cell and Tissue Biology (152 hrs); 5. Physiology (109 hrs); 6. Neurosciences (108 hrs); 7. Nutrition (49 hrs); 8. Pharmacology I (52 hrs); 9. Introduction to Clinical Medicine I (98 hrs).

(D: 1, 2, 3, 4, 5, 6, 9; P: 8)

Number of pharmacy or drug treatment-related courses: 1 out of 9 or 52 out of 955 hrs.

Number of diagnosis-related courses: 7 out of 9 or 723 out of 955 hrs.

YEAR 2 (35 WKS, 20 HOUR/WEEK—691 HRS)

1. General Pathology (102 hrs); 2. Microbiology (94 hrs); 3. Pharmacology II (66 hrs); 4. Correlative Pathology (386 hrs); 5. Introduction to Clinical Medicine II (43 hrs).

(D: 1, 2, 4, 5; P: 1)

Number of pharmacy or drug treatment-related courses: 1 out of 5 or 66 out of 691 hrs.

Number of diagnosis-related courses: 4 out of 5 or 625 out of 691 hrs.

Introduction to Clinical Medicine I and II is composed of: physical diagnosis, medical ethics, interviewing skills, professionalism, and history of medicine biostatics/epidemiology.

Correlative Pathology is composed of: human systems—nervous, cardiovascular, pulmonary, musculoskeletal, skin, gastrointestinal, hematology, oncology, reproductive, and endocrine.

YEAR 3 (48 WKS)
REQUIRED CLERKSHIPS

1. Internal Medicine (8 wks); 2. Surgery (8 wks); 3. Pediatrics (8 wks); 4. Psychiatry (5 wks); 5. Neurology (3 wks); 6. Obstetrics-Gynecology (8 wks); 7. Family Medicine (4 wks); 8. Rural and Primary Care (4 wks).

Number of pharmacy or drug treatment-related courses: None, but constitute an integral part of the clerkship.

Number of diagnosis-related courses: Constitute a major part of the clerkship.

YEAR 4 (32 WKS MINIMUM)
REQUIRED CLERKSHIPS

Acting Internship (4 wks): 1. Internal Medicine; 2. Selected Inpatient; 3. Selected Ambulatory; 4. Surgical Specialties and Electives (16 wks from tri-campus or other approved locations including international sites).

Number of pharmacy or drug treatment-related courses: None, but constitute an integral part of the clerkship.

Number of diagnosis-related courses: Constitute a major part of the clerkship.

Residency after graduation: No available data.

WRIGHT STATE UNIVERSITY SCHOOL OF MEDICINE

Courses offered to students in the four-year professional phase (2001) leading to the award of Doctor of Medicine (MD) before residency[9] (information obtained from the Internet and catalog):

YEAR 1

1. Human Structure; 2. Molecular, Cellular, and Tissue Biology I and II; 3. Introduction to Clinical Medicine (ICM) I (multi-quarter course with one final grade); 4. Human Development; 5. Social and Ethical Issues in Medicine I and II; 6. Principles of Disease; 7. Evidence-based Medicine; 7a. Electives.

(D: 1, 2, 3, 6, 7; P: 0)

Number of pharmacy or drug treatment-related courses: zero (0) out of 7.

Number of diagnosis-related courses: 5 out of 7.

YEAR 2

1. ICM II (multi-quarter course with one final grade—same as year 1); 2. Infectious Disease; 3. Neuroscience; 4. Blood; 4a. Elective; 5. Cardiology; 6. Respiratory; 7. Gastrointestinal; 8. Renal; 8a. Electives; 9. Endocrine and Reproductive; 10. Musculoskeletal and Integument.

(D: 1, 2, 3, 4, 5, 6, 7, 8, 9, 10; P: 0)

Number of pharmacy or drug treatment-related courses: zero (0) out of 10.

Number of diagnosis-related courses: 10 out of 10.

YEAR 3 (48 WKS)
CLERKSHIPS (1 WK = 2 CRS)

1. Family Medicine (6 wks); 2. Internal Medicine (12 wks); 3. Women's Health (8 wks); 4. Pediatrics (8 wks); 5. Psychiatry (6 wks); 6. Surgery.

Number of pharmacy or drug treatment-related courses: None, but constitute an integral part of the clerkship.

Number of diagnosis-related courses: Constitute a major part of the clerkship.

YEAR 4 (32 WKS)
CLERKSHIPS (1 WK = 2 CRS)

1. Emergency Medicine (4 wks); 2. Neurology (4 wks); 3. Orthopedic Surgery or Surgical Subspecialties (4 wks); 4. Electives (20 wks—chosen from at least 3 different department—5 electives); 5. Primary Care Junior Internship; 6. Senior Seminars.

Number of pharmacy or drug treatment-related courses: None, but constitute an integral part of the clerkship.

Number of diagnosis-related courses: Constitute a major part of the clerkship.

Residency after graduation: 13 programs and 6 other affiliations to chose from.

NOVA SOUTHEASTERN UNIVERSITY COLLEGE OF OSTEOPATHIC MEDICINE

Courses offered to students in the four-year professional phase (2001-2002) leading to the award of doctor of Osteopathic Medicine (DO) before residency[11] (information obtained from catalog):

YEAR 1
1ST SEMESTER CORE COURSES (26 HRS)

1. Medical Histology (4 hrs); 2. Gross Anatomy (8 hrs); 3. Medical Biochemistry (6 hrs); 4. Basic Life Support (0.5 hrs); 5. Osteopathic Principles and Practices (OP&P 1-2 hrs); 6. Medical Informatics (0.5 hrs); 7. Clinical Practicum I (3 hrs); 8. Interdisciplinary Generalist Curriculum Preceptorship I (IGC) (1 hr); 9. Clinical Correlation (0.5 hrs); 10. Principles of Radiology I (0.5 hrs); 10a. Electives.

(D: 1, 2, 3, 5, 6, 7, 9, 10; P: 0)

2ND SEMESTER CORE COURSE (24.5 HRS)

1. NeuroAnatomy (3 hrs); 2. Medical Ethics (0.5 hrs); 3. Medical Epidemiology (1 hr); 4. OP&P II (2 hrs); 5. Violence and Abuse (0.5 hrs); 6. IGC Preceptorship II (1 hr); 7. Ethnocultural Medicine (0.5 hrs); 8. Clinical Practicum II (1 hr); 9. Clinical Correlation II (0.5 hr); 10. Medical Microbiology (7 hrs); 11. Medical Physiology (7 hrs); 12. Principles of Radiology II (0.5 hr); 12a. Electives.

(D: 1, 3, 4, 8, 9, 10, 11, 12; P: 0)

Number of pharmacy or drug treatment-related courses: zero (0) out of 22 or 50.5 hrs.

Number of diagnosis-related courses: 16 out of 22 or 47 out of 50.5 hrs.

YEAR 2
1ST SEMESTER CORE COURSES (37 HRS)

1. Psychiatry (2 hrs); 2. OP&P III (2 hrs); 3. Clinical Correlation III (3 hrs); 4. Clinical Practicum III (1 hr); 5. Hematopoietic and Lymphoreticular System (3 hrs); 6. Substance Abuse and Addiction (0.5 hrs); 7. Cardiovascular System (5 hrs); 8. Respiratory (4 hrs); 9. Endocrine System (2 hrs); 10. IGC Preceptorship III (3 hrs); 11. Integumentary System (2 hrs); 12. Alternative Medicine (0.5 hrs), 13. Renal/Urinary System (3 hrs); 14. Clinical Procedures I (1 hr); 15. Principles of Pharmacology (2 hrs); 16. Principles of Pathology (3 hrs); 16a. Electives.

(D: 1, 2, 3, 4, 5, 7, 8, 9, 11, 13, 14, 16; P: 6, 15)

2ND SEMESTER CORE COURSES (28 HRS)

1. Advanced Cardiac Life Support (1 hr); 2. Pediatric Advanced Cardiac Life Support (1 hr); 3. Geriatrics (0.5 hrs); 4. Medical Jurisprudence (1 hr); 5. OP&P IV (2 hrs), 6. Rural Medicine (0.5 hrs); 7. HIV Seminar (0.5 hr); 8. Clinical Correlation IV (2 hrs); 9. Clinical Procedures II (1 hr); 10. Reproductive System (3 hrs); 11. Nervous System (4 hrs); 12. Musculoskeletal System (3 hrs); 13. Gastrointestinal System (4 hrs); 14. Clinical Practicum IV (1 hr); 15. IGC Preceptorship IV (2 hrs); 16. Human Sexuality (0.5 hrs); 17. Pre-clerkship Seminar (0.5 hrs); 18. Anesthesiology (0.5 hrs); 18a. Electives.

(D: 5, 6, 8, 9, 10, 11, 12, 13, 14; P: 18)

Number of pharmacy or drug treatment-related courses: 3 out of 34 or 3 out of 65 hrs.

Number of diagnosis-related courses: 21 out of 34 or 51.5 out of 65 hrs.

YEAR 3 (11 MONTHS—88 HRS)
CORE CLINICAL ROTATIONS (8 HRS PER MONTH OF ROTATION)
1. Psychiatry; 2. Geriatrics; 3. Family Medicine—Clinics; 4. Internal Medicine (3 months); 5. Obstetrics/Gynecology; 6. Pediatrics—Ambulatory; 7. Pediatrics—Hospital; 8. General Surgery (2 months).

Number of pharmacy or drug treatment-related courses: None, but constitute an integral part of the clerkship.

Number of diagnosis-related courses: Constitute a major part of the clerkship.

YEAR 4
CORE CLINICAL ROTATIONS (8 HRS PER MONTH OF ROTATION)
1. Emergency Medicine; 2. Family Medicine—Preceptorship; 3. Rural Medicine—Ambulatory (3 months); 4. Senior Seminar; 5. Electives.

Number of pharmacy or drug treatment-related courses: None, but constitute an integral part of the clerkship.

Number of diagnosis-related courses: Constitute a major part of the clerkship.

Residency after graduation: data not available.

UNIVERSITY OF PUERTO RICO SCHOOL OF MEDICINE

Courses offered to students in the four-year professional phase (2001) leading to the award of Doctor of Medicine (MD) before residency (information obtained from the Internet):

YEAR 1 (916 HRS)

1. Medical Gross Anatomy (168 hrs); 2. Medical Histology (98 hrs); 3. Medical Embryology (22 hrs); 4. Medical Neuroscience (110 hrs); 5. Introduction to Biochemistry (113 hrs); 6. Human Physiology (160 hrs); 7. Human Development I (60 hrs); 8. Public Health and Preventive Medicine I (20 hrs); 9. Integration Seminar I (54 hrs); 10. Behavioral Sciences (5 hrs); 11. Introduction to Clinical Diagnosis (60 hrs); 11a. Electives.

(D: 1, 2, 3, 4, 5, 6, 10, 11; P: 0)

Number of pharmacy or drug treatment-related courses: zero (0) out of 11 or 916 hrs.

Number of diagnosis-related courses: 8 out of 11 or 678 out of 916 hrs.

YEAR 2 (882 HRS)

1. Pathobiology Introduction to Laboratory Medicine (166 hrs); 2. Infectious Diseases (144); 3. Medical Pharmacology (114); 4. Fundamentals of Clinical Diagnosis (105 hrs); 5. Human Development II (52 hrs); 6. Public Health and Preventive Medicine II (40 hrs); 7. Basic Clinical Clerkship (31 hrs); 8. Mechanisms of Disease (136 hrs); 9. Psychopathology (40 hrs); 10. Integration Seminar II (54 hrs).

(D: 1, 2, 4, 7, 8, 9; P: 3)

Number of pharmacy or drug treatment-related courses: 1 out of 10 or 114 out of 882 hrs.

Number of diagnosis-related courses: 6 out of 10 or 633 out of 882 hrs.

YEAR 3 (48 WKS)
CLERKSHIP ROTATIONS

1. Radiology (2 wks); 2. Psychiatry (4 wks); 3. Medicine (12 wks); 4. Family Medicine (4 wks); 5. Pediatrics (10 wks); 6. Surgery (10 wks); 7. Obstetrics/Gynecology (6 wks); 8. Electives.

Number of pharmacy or drug treatment-related courses: None, but constitute an integral part of the clerkship.

Number of diagnosis-related courses: Constitute a major part of the clerkship.

YEAR 4 (32 WKS)
CLERKSHIP ROTATIONS
1. Dermatology (1 wk); 2. Physical Medicine and Rehabilitation (1 wk); 3. Public Health (3 wks); 4. Legal, Ethical, and Administrative Aspects in Medicine (1 wk); 5. Selective Clerkship (4 wks); 6. Required Clerkship (4 wks—one choice from Internal Medicine, Pediatrics, OB/GYN, or Family Medicine); 7. Elective (18 wks).

Number of pharmacy or drug treatment-related courses: None, but constitute an integral part of the clerkship.

Number of diagnosis-related courses: Constitute a major part of the clerkship.

Residency after graduation: Data not available.

UNIVERSITY OF FLORIDA COLLEGE OF MEDICINE

Courses offered to students in the four-year professional phase (2002) leading to the award of Doctor of Medicine (MD) before residency (information obtained from the Internet):

YEAR 1
1. Clinical Anatomy; 2. Diagnostic Imaging (Radiology); 3 and 4. Essentials of Patient Care I and II; 5. Basic Clinical Skills; 6. Keeping Families Healthy; 7. Medical Cell and Tissue Biology; 8. Medical Neuroscience; 9. Preceptorship; 10. Biochemistry and Molecular Biology; 11. Genetics; 12. Human Behavior; 13. Physiology.
 (D: 1, 2, 3, 4, 5, 7, 8, 10, 11, 12, 13; P: 0)

Number of pharmacy or drug treatment-related courses: zero (0) out of 13.

Number of diagnosis-related courses: 11 out of 13.

YEAR 2

1. Ethics; 2. Evidence-based Medicine; 3. General and Systemic Pathology; 4. Geriatric Cases; 5. Hematology—Coagulation Cascade; 6. Immunology Lectures; 7. Introduction to Clinical Medicine/Clinical Diagnosis/EPC IV; 8. Introduction to Clinical Neurology; 9. Introduction to Clinical Radiology; 10. Medical Microbiology and Infectious Diseases; 11. Oncology; 12. Physical Diagnosis Study Guides.

(D: 2, 3, 6, 7, 8, 9, 10, 11, 12; P: 0)

Number of pharmacy or drug treatment-related courses: zero (0) out of 12.

Number of diagnosis-related courses: 9 out of 12.

YEAR 3
CLERKSHIP

1. Family Medicine/Geriatrics; 2. Neurology; 3. OB-GYN; 4. Pediatrics; 5. Psychiatry; 6. Surgery.

Number of pharmacy or drug treatment-related courses: None, but constitute an integral part of the clerkship.

Number of diagnosis-related courses: Constitute a major part of the clerkship.

YEAR 4
CLERKSHIP

1. Anesthesiology and Critical Care; 2. Emergency Medicine; 3. Introduction to Medical Informatics (CMC 56) Elective; 4. Medical Therapeutics; 5. Special Projects in Medical Informatics (CMC 57) Elective.

Number of pharmacy or drug treatment-related courses: None, but constitute an integral part of the clerkship.

Number of diagnosis-related courses: Constitute a major part of the clerkship.

Residency after graduation: Data not available.

STATE UNIVERSITY OF NEW YORK HEALTH SCIENCE CENTER AT BROOKLYN

Courses offered to students in the four-year professional phase (1995-1996—the only odd date in the data analysis) leading to the award of Doctor of Medicine (MD) before residency[12] (information obtained from the catalog):

YEAR 1
1. Gross Anatomy; 2. Biochemistry; 3. Embryology; 4. Histology/Cell Biology; 5. Introduction to Clinical Medicine; 6. Preventive Medicine: Epidemiology; 7. Human Behavior; 8. Physiology; 9. Neuroscience; 10. Genetics; 11. Preventive Medicine-Biostats.

(D: 1, 2, 3, 4, 5, 7, 8, 9, 10; P: 0)

Number of pharmacy or drug treatment-related courses: zero (0) out of 11.

Number of diagnosis-related courses: 9 out of 11.

YEAR 2
1. Microbiology; 2. Pathology; 3. Nutrition; 4. Preparation for Clinical Medicine; 5. Pathophysiology; 6. Pharmacology; 7. Psychopathology; 8. Preventive Medicine.

(D: 1, 2, 4, 5, 7; P: 6)

Number of pharmacy or drug treatment-related courses: 1 out of 8.

Number of diagnosis-related courses: 5 out of 8.

YEAR 3
CLERKSHIPS
1. Medicine (12 wks); 2. Obstetrics/Gynecology (6 wks); 3. Neurology (4 wks); 4. Surgery (12 wks); 5. Psychiatry (6 wks); 6. Pediatrics (8 wks).

Number of pharmacy or drug treatment-related courses: None, but constitute an integral part of the clerkship.

Number of diagnosis-related courses: Constitute a major part of the clerkship.

YEAR 4
Clerkships

1. Subinternships (4 wks); 2. Ambulatory Care (6 wks); 3. Clinical Electives (20 wks).

Number of pharmacy or drug treatment-related courses: None, but constitute an integral part of the clerkship.

Number of diagnosis-related courses: Constitute a major part of the clerkship.

Residency after graduation: Data not available.

OTHER BRANCHES OF MEDICINE AND ALLIED SCHOOLS

Other branches of medicine and allied health that are associated with prescription-writing authority are dentistry, optometry, veterinary medicine, physician assistant, and certified nurse practitioner. Fewer schools were sampled here because of the need to avoid monotonous readings, which would eventually turn the book into a schools catalog.

DENTISTRY

HARVARD SCHOOL OF DENTAL MEDICINE

Courses offered to students in the four-year professional phase (1998-1999) leading to the award of DMD without residency requirements[14] (information were obtained from the catalog):

YEAR 1

1. Human Body; 2. Chemistry and Biology of Cell; 3. Integrated Human Physiology; 4. Principles of Pharmacology; 5. Genetics, Embryology, and Reproduction; 6. Immunology, Microbiology, and Infectious Disease; 7. Patient-Doctor I; 8. Dental Head and Neck; 9. Scientific Inquires; 10. Oral Structure and Function; 11. Development; 12. Oral Microbiology and Immunology; 12a. Elective: Research International and Exchange Programs.

(DD: 1, 2, 3, 5, 6, 7, 8, 9, 10, 11, 12; P: 4)

(DD = diagnosis and dental-related courses)

Number of pharmacy or drug treatment-related courses: 1 out of 12.

Number of diagnosis or dental-related courses: 11 out of 12.

YEAR 2

1. Human Nervous S and B; 2. Psychopathology—ICP; 3. Pathology; 4. Human Systems: Patient-Doctor II: 5. Introduction to Clinical Medicine/

Dentistry; 6. Diagnosis and Prevention; 7. Orofacial Pain; 8. Oral Pathology and Pathophysiology.

(DD: 1, 2, 3, 4, 5, 6, 7, 8; P: 0)

Number of pharmacy or drug treatment-related courses: zero (0) out of 8.

Number of diagnosis or dental-related courses: 8 out of 8.

YEAR 3

1. Treatment of Active Disease; 2. Restorative Treatment; 3. Treatment of the Child and Adolescent; 4. Advanced Surgical Treatment; 5. Advanced Topics in Dentistry.

(DD: 1, 2, 3, 4, 5; P: 0)

Number of pharmacy or drug treatment-related courses: zero (0) out of 5 (may constitute an integral part of some of the core courses).

Number of diagnosis or dental-related courses: 5 out of 5 (constitute a major part of the courses).

YEAR 4

1. Required Externships in General Dentistry and Oral and Maxillofacial Surgery; 2. Elective Rotations; 3. Research; 4. Research Presentation and Graduation.

(DD: 1, 2, 3; P: 0)

Number of pharmacy or drug treatment-related courses: zero (0) out of 3 (constitute an integral part of the externship and other courses).

Number of diagnosis or dental-related courses: 3 out of 3 (constitute a major part of the externships/rotations/research).

Residency after graduation: Optional as postdoctoral programs.

UNIVERSITY OF PENNSYVANIA SCHOOL OF DENTAL MEDICINE

Courses offered to students in the four-year professional phase (2001-2002) leading to the award of DMD without residency requirements[15] (information were obtained from the catalog):

YEAR 1

1. Biochemistry; 2. Histology/Embryology; 3. Health Promotion I; 4. Introduction to Medicine; 5. Dental Materials; 6. Gross Anatomy; 7. Radiological Anatomy; 8. Microbiology; 9. Restorative Dentistry Lecture I; 10. Restorative Dentistry I Laboratory; 11. Radiology; 12. Anatomy Dissection; 13. Preclinical Periodontics; 14. Health Promotion II: Anatomy Dissection Honors Elective.

(DD: 1, 2, 3, 4, 5, 6, 7, 8, 9, 10, 11, 12, 13, 14; P: 0)

Number of pharmacy or drug treatment-related courses: zero (0) out of 14.

Number of diagnosis or dental-related courses: 14 out of 14.

YEAR 2

1. Basic Clinical Dentistry; 2. Introduction to Patient Evaluation; 3. Dental Care Systems; 4. Pharmacology; 5. Orthodontics Lectures; 6. Anesthesia, Pain, and Emergency; 7. Restorative Dentistry II Lecture; 8. Restorative Dentistry II Laboratory; 9. Adjunctive Orthodontics; 10. Endodontics; 11. Behavioral Management; 12. Pathology Lecture; 13. Principles of Medicine; 14. Periodontics; 15. Diagnostic Radiology; 16. Complete Denture Lecture; 17. Complete Dentures Laboratory. 18. Removable Parts.

(DD: 1, 2, 3, 5, 6, 7, 8, 9, 10, 12, 13, 14, 15, 16, 17, 18; P: 4)

Number of pharmacy or drug treatment-related courses: 1 out of 18.

Number of diagnosis or dental-related courses: 16 out of 18.

YEAR 3

1. Pediatric Dentistry Lecture; 2. Endodontics Lecture; 3. Periodontics Lecture; 4. Health Promotion Seminar; 5. Implant Dentistry Lecture; 6. Preventative and Interceptive Clinic; 7. Restorative Dentistry Lecture; 8. Restorative Dentistry Clinic; 9. Pediatric Dentistry Clinic; 10. Orthodontics II Lecture; 11. Endodontics Clinic; 12. Oral Medicine Lecture; 13. Oral Surgery Lecture; 14. Radiology Clinic; 15. Periodontics Clinic; 16. Practice Management; 17. Clinic Seminar; 18. Honors Hospital Dental Program; 19. Geriatric Dentistry Lecture.

(DD: 1, 2, 3, 4, 5, 6, 7, 8, 9, 10, 11, 12, 13, 14, 15, 18, 19; P: 0)

Number of pharmacy or drug treatment-related courses: zero (0) out of 19.

Number of diagnosis or dental-related courses: 17 out of 19.

YEAR 4

1. Health Promotion Clinic; 2. Grand Rounds Lecture; 3. Adjunctive Orthodontics Clinic; 4. Community Dentistry Clinic; 5. Restorative Dentistry Clinic; 6. Pediatric Dentistry Clinic; 7. Endodontics Clinic; 8. Admissions and Emergency Clinic; 9. Oral Surgery Clinic; 10. Radiology Clinic; 11. Periodontics Clinic; 12. Hospital Assignment; 13. Clinic Seminar.

(DD: 1, 2, 3, 4, 5, 6, 7, 8, 9, 10, 11, 12; P: 0)

Number of pharmacy or drug treatment-related courses: zero (0) out of 13 (constitute an integral part of the clinic).

Number of diagnosis or dental-related courses: 12 out of 13 (constitute a major part of the clinic).

Residency after graduation: No available data.

BALTIMORE COLLEGE OF DENTAL SURGERY DENTAL SCHOOL, UNIVERSITY OF MARYLAND

Courses offered to students in the four-year professional phase (2000-2002) leading to the award of DDS without residency requirements[13] (information was obtained from the catalog):

YEAR 1 (48 CREDITS)

1. Anatomy (13 crs); 2. Biochemistry (5 crs); 3. Conjoint Sciences I (2 crs); 4. Radiology (1 cr); 5. Microbiology (5 crs); 6. Physiology (6 crs); 7. Oral Health Care Delivery (3 crs); 8. Periodontics (2 crs); 9. Dental Anatomy/Occlusion/Operative (9 crs); 10. Dental Biomaterials (2 crs).

1st semester—6 courses and 25 credits.

2nd semester—8 courses and 23 credits.

(DD: 1, 2, 3, 4, 5, 6, 7, 8, 9, 10; P: 0)

Number of pharmacy or drug treatment-related courses: zero (0) out of 14 or 48 crs.

Number of diagnosis or dental-related courses: 14 out of 14 or 48 crs.

YEAR 2 (51 CREDITS)

1. Conjoint Sciences IIA (6 crs); 2. Conjoint Science IIB (5 crs); 3. Biomedicine (12 crs); 4. Pharmacology (5 crs); 5. Oral and Maxillofacial Surgery (1 cr); 6. Endodontics (2 crs); 7. Oral Health Care (3 crs); 8. Orthodontics (1 cr); 9. Pediatric Dentistry (1 cr); 10. Periodontics (2 crs); 11. Dental Biomaterials II (1 cr); 12. Fixed Prosthodontics (6 crs); 13. Complete Dentures (3 crs); 14. Removable Prosthodontics (3 crs).

(DD: 1, 2, 3, 5, 6, 7, 8, 9, 10, 11, 12, 13, 14; P: 4)

1st semester—7 courses and 24 credits.

2nd semester—11 courses and 27 credits.

Number of pharmacy or drug treatment-related courses: 1 out of 18 or 5 out of 51 crs.

Number of diagnosis or dental-related courses: 17 out of 18 or 46 out of 51 crs.

YEAR 3 (67 CRS)
1. Conjoint Sciences III (4 crs); 2. Oral Medicine and Diagnostic Sciences (7 crs); 3. Oral and Maxillofacial Surgery (4 crs); 4. Endodontics (4 crs); 5. Oral Health Care Delivery (6 crs); 6. Orthodontics (2 crs); 7. Pediatric Dentistry (8 crs); 8. Periodontics (11 crs); 9. Operative Dentistry (7 crs); 10. Fixed Prosthodontics (6 crs); 11. Removable Prosthodontics (8 crs).

(DD: 1, 2, 3, 4, 5, 6, 7, 8, 9, 10, 11; P: 0)

1st semester—11 courses and 34 credits.

2nd semester—11 courses and 33 credits.

Number of pharmacy or drug treatment-related courses: zero (0) out of 22 or 67 crs.

Number of diagnosis or dental-related courses: 22 out of 22 or 67 crs.

YEAR 4 (64 CRS)
1. Advanced Dental Pharmacotherapeutics (1 cr); 2. Conjoint Sciences IV (3 crs); 3. Clinic (60 crs); 4. Clerkship I (elective—20 crs); 5. Clerkship II (elective—10 crs)

(DD: 2, 3; P: 1)

1st semester—3 courses and 32 credits.

2nd semester—2 courses and 32 credits.

Number of pharmacy or drug treatment-related courses: 1 out of 5 or 64 crs (constitute an integral part of the clinic or clerkship).

Number of diagnosis or dental-related courses: 4 out of 5 or 63 out of 64 crs (constitute a major part of the clinic or clerkship).

Residency after graduation: Optional as postdoctoral, advanced education programs.

NOVA SOUTHEASTERN UNIVERSITY COLLEGE OF DENTAL MEDICINE

Courses offered to students in the four-year professional phase (2001-2002) leading to the award of DDM without residency requirements[11] (information was obtained from the catalog):

YEAR 1
FALL SEMESTER (25 CRS)
1. Anatomy Lecture/Lab (5 crs); 2. Biochemistry (4 crs); 3. Histology (3 crs); 4. Introduction to the Dental Profession I (1 cr); 5. Introduction to Computers (2 crs); 6. Periodontology I Lecture (1 cr); 7. Restorative Dentistry I Lecture (2 crs); 8. Restorative Dentistry I Lab (2 crs); 9. Dental Materials (4 crs).

(DD: 1, 2, 3, 4, 6, 7, 8, 9; P: 0)

WINTER SEMESTER (25 CRS)
1. Microbiology (5 crs); 2. Physiology (4 crs); 3. NeuroAnatomy Lecture (2 crs); 4. NeuroAnatomy Lab (1 crs); 5. Dental Nutrition (1 cr); 6. Oral Histology and Embryology (3 crs); 7. Periodontology II (3 crs); 8. Periodontology II Clinic (1 cr); 9. Restorative Dentistry II Lecture (operative—2 crs); 10. Restorative Dentistry II Lab (operative—2 crs); 11. Restorative Dentistry III Lecture/Lab OCCL (1 cr).

(DD: 1, 2, 3, 4, 5, 6, 7, 8, 9, 10, 11; P: 0)

Number of pharmacy or drug treatment-related courses: zero (0) out of 20.

Number of diagnosis or dental-related courses: 19 out of 20.

YEAR 2
FALL SEMESTER (21 CREDITS)

1. Pharmacology (4 crs); 2. General Pathology (3 crs); 3. Periodontology III (1 cr); 4. Anesthesia I (1 cr); 5. Endodontics Lecture (1 cr); 6. Endodontics Lab (1 cr); 7. Restorative Dentistry Lecture (2 crs); 8. Restorative Dentistry Lab IV (2 crs); 9. Restorative Dentistry Lecture V (2 crs); 10. Restorative Dentistry Lab V (2 crs); 11. Radiology (2 crs).

(DD: 2, 3, 5, 6, 7, 8, 9, 10, 11; P: 1,4)

WINTER SEMESTER (25 CRS)

1. Radiology II (1 cr); 2. Pharmacology (3 crs); 3. Oral Medicine I (1 cr); 4. Oral Surgery I (2 crs); 5. Periodontology IV (1 cr); 6. Anesthesia II (1 cr); 7. Pediatric Dentistry Lecture (2 crs); 8. Pediatric Dentistry Lab (1 cr); 9. Orthodontics Lecture/Lab (3 crs); 10. Restorative Dentistry Lecture VII (2 crs); 11. Restorative Dentistry Lab VII (1 cr); 12. Restorative Dentistry Lecture VIII (3 crs); 13. Endodontics Clinical Lecture (1 cr); 14. Restorative Dentistry Lecture VI (1 cr); 15. Restorative Dentistry Lab VI (1 cr); 16. Clinic V (1 cr).

(DD: 1, 3, 4, 5, 7, 8, 9, 10, 11, 12, 13, 14, 15, 16; P: 2, 6)

SUMMER SEMESTER (5 CRS)

1. Clinic VI (5 crs)

(DD: 1; P: 0)

Number of pharmacy or drug treatment-related courses: 4 out of 28 or 9 out of 51 crs.

Number of diagnosis or dental-related courses: 24 out of 28 or 42 out of 51 crs.

YEAR 3
FALL SEMESTER (13 CRS).

1. Oral and Maxillary Pathology (2 crs); 2. Oral Medicine II (2 crs); 3. Periodontology V (1 cr); 4. Oral Surgery II (1 cr); 5. Ethics and Jurisprudences (1 cr); 6. Advanced Clinic Lecture: Treatment Planning I (1 cr); 7. Clinic VII (5 crs).

(DD: 1, 2, 3, 4, 6, 7; P: 0)

WINTER SEMESTER (19 CRS)

1. Restorative Dentistry Lecture X (1 cr); 2. Behavioral Science (2 crs); 3. Introduction to the Dental Profession II (1 cr); 4. Periodontology VI (1 cr); 5. Internal Medicine (3 crs); 6. Implant Restorative Dentistry Lecture (2 crs); 7. Cosmetic Dentistry Lecture/Lab (3 crs); 8. Geriatric Dentistry Lecture (1 cr); 9. Clinic VIII (5 crs).

(DD: 1, 3, 4, 5, 6, 7, 8, 9; P: 0)

SUMMER SEMESTER (5 CRS)

1. Clinic IX (5 crs).

(DD: 1; P: 0)

Number of pharmacy or drug treatment-related courses: zero (0) out of 17 (constitute an integral part of the clinic).

Number of diagnosis or dental-related courses: 15 out of 17 (constitute a major part of the clinic).

YEAR 4
FALL SEMESTER (9 CRS)

1. Oral Manifestations of Systemic Disease (1 cr); 2. Advanced Clinic Lecture: Treatment Planning (2 crs); 3. Introduction to the Dental Profession III (1 cr); 4. Clinic X (5 crs).

(DD: 1, 2, 3, 4; P: 0)

WINTER SEMESTER

1. Introduction to the Dental Profession IV (1 cr); 2. Regional Board Prep Course (1 cr); 3. Clinic XI (5 crs).

(DD: 1, 2, 3; P: 0)

Number of pharmacy or drug treatment-related courses: zero (0) out of 7 (constitute an integral part of the clinic).

Number of diagnosis or dental-related courses: 7 out of 7 (constitutes major part of the clinic).

Residency after graduation: Optional as postdoctoral programs; internship or residency experience is preferred but not required in some postdoctoral specialty programs such as periodontics and prosthodontics.

OPTOMETRY

SOUTHERN CALIFORNIA COLLEGE OF OPTOMETRY

Courses offered to students in the four-year professional phase (2002) leading to the award of Doctor of Optometry (OD) without residency requirements (information was obtained from the Internet):

YEAR 1
FALL
1. Anatomy and Physiology I; 2. Biochemistry; 3. Public Health I; 4. Optics; 5. Visual Psychophysics; 6. Practices Management 1; 7. Optometric Clinical Services.

(DO: 1, 2, 4, 5, 7; P: 0)

(DO = diagnosis and optometry-related courses)

WINTER
1. Anatomy and Physiology II; 2. Ocular Anatomy; 3. Optics II; 4. Sensory Vision; 5. Professional Ethics; 6. Optometric Clinical Service.

(DO: 1, 2, 3, 4, 6; P: 0)

SPRING
1. Neurophysiology; 2. Clinical Medicine I; 3. Ophthalmic Optic I; 4. Optics of the Eye; 5. Interpersonal Communication; 6. Ocular.

(DO: 1, 2, 3, 4, 6; P: 0)

Number of pharmacy or drug treatment-related courses: zero (0) out of 19.

Number of diagnosis or optometry-related courses: 15 out of 19.

YEAR 2
FALL

1. Ocular Physiology; 2. Clinical Microbiology; 3. Clinical Medicine II; 4. Ophthalmic Optics II; 5. Ocular Motility; 6. Assessment of Binocular Vision.

(DO: 1, 2, 3, 4, 5, 6; P: 0)

WINTER

1. Pharmacology I; 2. Public Health II; 3. Ophthalmic Optic III; 4. Case Analysis and Prescribing I; 5. Ocular Health Procedures I; 6. Cornea and Contact Lenses I; 7. Optometric Clinical Services.

(DO: 3, 5, 6, 7; P: 1; DO and P: 4)

(DO and P = approximately equal proportion of diagnosis and optometry and pharmacy/drug treatment-related courses)

SPRING

1. Pharmacology II; 2. Ocular Disease Dx and Mx I; 3. Binoc Vision and Space Perception; 4. Case Analysis and Prescribing II; 5. Cornea and Contact Lenses II; 6. Vision Efficiency Therapy; 7. Optometric Clinical Services.

(DO: 2, 3, 5, 6, 7; P: 1; DO and P: 4)

Number of pharmacy or drug treatment-related courses: 2-4 out of 20.

Number of diagnosis or optometry-related courses: 15-17 out of 20.

YEAR 3
SUMMER

1. Practice Management II; 2. Optometric Clinical Services.

(DO: 2; P: 0)

FALL
1. Ocular Disease Dx and Mx II; 2. Pediatric Optometry; 3. Ocular Health Procedures II; 4. Cornea and Contact Lenses III; 5. Vision, Perception, and Learning; 6. Optometric Clinical Services.

(DO: 1, 2, 3, 4, 5, 6; P: 0)

WINTER
1. Pharmacology III; 2. Ocular Disease Dx and Mx III; 3. Research Proposal; 4. Geriatric Optometry; 5. Cornea and Contact Lenses IV; 6. Strabismus/Amblyopia Diagnosis; 7. Optometric Clinical Services.

(DO: 2, 3, 4, 5, 6, 7; P: 1)

SPRING
1. Public Health III; 2. Ocular Disease Case Management; 3. Ocular Health Procedures III; 4. Strabismus/Amblyopia Management; 5. Low-Vision Rehabilitation; 6. Practice Management III; 7. Optometric Clinical Service.

(DO: 2, 3, 4, 5, 7; P: 0)

Number of pharmacy or drug treatment-related courses: 1 out of 22.

Number of diagnosis or optometry-related courses: 18 out of 22.

YEAR 4
Rotations (4 clinical rotations—12 weeks each); seminars; research; optometric and outreach clinical services.

Number of pharmacy or drug treatment-related courses: Not delineated, but constitute an integral part of the rotations.

Number of diagnosis or optometry-related courses: Constitute a major part of the rotations.

Residency: Available as postgraduate doctoral programs.

OHIO STATE UNIVERSITY
COLLEGE OF OPTOMETRY

Courses offered to students in the four-year professional phase (2002) leading to the award of Doctor of Optometry (OD) without residency requirements (information was obtained from the Internet):

YEAR 1
AUTUMN QUARTER

1. Vision Science 531: Basic Anatomy; 2. Physiology 601; 3. Optometry 401: Survey of Optometry; 4. Vision Science 501: Geometric Optics.

(DO: 1, 2, 3, 4; P: 0)

WINTER

1. Vision Science 535: Microanatomy; 2. Physiology 602; 3. Vision Science 503: Geometrical and Optics; 4. Optometry 780.21: Practice Management; 5. Vision Science 520: Measurement Specifications for Visual Stimuli.

(DO: 1, 2, 3, 5; P: 0)

SPRING QUARTER

1. Pharmacology 680; 2. Vision Science 511: Optics of the Eye; 3. Vision Science 608: Ocular Anatomy; 4. Pathology 650; 5. Optometry 402: Rights and Responsibilities.

(DO: 2, 3, 4; P: 1)

Number of pharmacy or drug treatment-related courses: 1 out of 14.

Number of diagnosis or optometry-related courses: 11 out of 14.

YEAR 2
AUTUMN QUARTER

1. Vision Science 512: Ocular Motility; 2. Optometry 441: Theory and Techniques; 3. Vision Science 613: Monocular Section Mechanisms; 4. Optometry 431: Ophthalmic Optics; 5. Vision Science 624: Ocular Form and Function I.

(DO: 1, 2, 3, 4, 5; P: 0)

WINTER QUARTER

1. Optometry 442: Optometry Data Analysis; 2. Vision Science 716: Visual Perception; 3. Vision Science 625: Ocular Form and Function II; 4. Optometry 432: Ophthalmic Optics; 5. Optometry 711: Introduction to Ocular Disc.

(DO: 1, 2, 3, 4, 5; P: 0)

SPRING QUARTER

1. Optometry 443: Examination and Prescription; 2. Optometry 712: Introduction to Ocular Disc.; 3. Pharmacy 681; 4. Vision Science 715: Binocular Introduction; 5. Optometry 780.21: Practice Management.

(DO: 1, 2, 4; P: 3)

Number of pharmacy or drug treatment-related courses: 1 out of 15.

Number of diagnosis or optometry-related courses: 13 out of 15.

YEAR 3
SUMMER QUARTER

1. Optometry 640: Primary Care Services; 2. Optometry 645.01: Primary Care Practice; 3. Optometry 645.02: Dispensary; 4. Optometry 682: Ocular Pharmacology; 5. Optometry 702: Oculormotor Dist.; 6. Optometry 703: Visuals; 7. Vision Science 731: Environment.

(DO: 1, 2, 3, 5, 6, 7; P: 4)

AUTUMN QUARTER

1. Optometry 433: Ophthalmic Optics; 2. Optometry 641: Primary Care Services; 3. Optometry 645.01: Primary Care Practices; 4. Optometry 645.02: Dispensary; 5. Optometry 660: Advanced Ocular; 6. Optometry 780.21: Practice Management; 7. Vision Science 732: Vision of Children.

(DO: 1, 2, 3, 4, 5, 7; P: 0)

WINTER QUARTER

1. Optometry 642: Primary Care Service; 2.Optometry 671: Orthoptics; 3. Optometry 653: Basic Contact Lenses; 4. Optometry 645.01: Primary

Care Practice; 5. Optometry 645.02: Dispensary; 6. Vision Science 733: Optometrics.

(DO: 1, 2, 3, 4, 5, 6; P: 0)

SPRING QUARTER
1. Optometry 643: Advanced Procedure Seminar; 2. Optometry 645: Advanced Contact; 3. Optometry 645.01: Primary Care Practice; 4. Optometry 645.02: Dispensary; 5. Optometry 655: Anisekonia; 6. Optometry 656: Low Vision; 7. Optometry 721: Economics and Jurisprudence; 8. Optometry 672: Binocular Vision; 9. Optometry 722: Public Health.

(DO: 1, 2, 3, 4, 5, 6, 8; P: 0)

Number of pharmacy or drug treatment-related courses: 1 out of 29.

Number of diagnosis or optometry-related courses: 25 out of 29.

YEAR 4
SUMMER QUARTER
1. Optometry 741: Advanced Practice Optometry; 2. Optometry 745.01: Special Practice; 3. Optometry 745.11: External Experience.

AUTUMN QUARTER
1. Optometry 741 or 745.11; 2. Optometry 745.01-745.10.

WINTER QUARTER
1. Optometry 741 or 745.11; 2. Optometry 745.01-745.10

SPRING QUARTER
1. Optometry 741 or 745.11; 2. Optometry 745.01-745.10

Number of pharmacy or drug treatment-related courses: zero (0) but constitute an integral part of the rotations.

Number of diagnosis or optometry-related courses: Constitute a major part of the rotations.

Residency: Available as postgraduate doctoral programs.

NOVA SOUTHEASTERN UNIVERSITY COLLEGE OF OPTOMETRY

Courses offered to students in the four-year professional phase (2001-2002) leading to the award of Doctor of Optometry (OD) without residency requirements[11] (information was obtained from the catalog):

YEAR 1
FALL SEMESTER (22 CRS)

1. Histology and Embryology (1 cr); 2. Gross Anatomy/Anatomy: Head and Neck (4 crs); 3. Biochemistry (3 crs); 4. Microbiology (3 crs); 5. Geometrics Optics (4 crs); 6. Geometrical Optics Lab (1 cr); 7. Psychophysical Methodology in Vision Science (1 cr); 8. Public Health I: History of Optics (1 cr); 9. Optometric Theory and Methods I (2 crs); 10. Optometric Theory and Methods I Lab (2 crs).

(DO: 1, 2, 3, 4, 5, 6, 7, 9, 10; P: 0)

WINTER SEMESTER (23 CRS)

1.General NeuroAnatomy (2.5 crs); 2. General Physiology (4 crs); 3. Physical Optics (2 crs); 4. Physical Optics Lab (0.5 crs); 5. Visual Optics (2.5 crs); 6. Ocular Anatomy (2 crs); 7. Visual Neurophysiology (2 crs); 8. Ocular Motility (2 crs); 9. Optometric Theory and Methods II (2 crs); 10. Public Health II: Patient Comm. (2 crs).

(DO: 1, 2, 3, 4, 5, 6, 7, 8, 9; P: 0)

Number of pharmacy or drug treatment-related courses: zero (0) out of 20 or 45 crs.

Number of diagnosis or optometry-related courses: 18 out of 20 or 42 out of 45 crs.

YEAR 2
FALL SEMESTER (24.5 CRS)

1. General Pathology (3 crs); 2. Ocular Physiology (2 crs); 3. General Pharmacology I (4 crs); 4. Psychophysics/Monocular Sensory Processes (4 crs); 5. Ophthalmic Optics I (4 crs); 6. Ocular Disease I: Anterior Segment (3 crs); 7. Optometric Theory and Methods III (3.5 crs); 8. Vision Screening I (1 cr).

(DO: 1, 2, 4, 5, 6, 7, 8; P: 3)

WINTER SEMESTER (23.5 CRS)

1. General Pharmacology II (1.5 crs); 2. Ocular Pharmacology (1.5 crs); 3. Ophthalmic Optics II (4 crs); 4. Introduction to Binocular Vision (2 crs); 5. Anomalies of Binocular Vision I (4 crs); 6. Optometric Theory and Methods IV (3.5 crs); 7. Ocular Disease II: Posterior Segment (3.5 crs); 8. Public Health III: Health Care Systems and Agencies (2 crs); 9. Public Health IV: Epidemiology (1 cr); 10. Vision Screening II (1 cr).

(DO: 3, 4, 5, 6, 7, 10; P: 1, 2)

SUMMER SEMESTER (1.5 CRS)

1. Primary Care Clinic I (1.5 cr).

(DO: 1; P: 0)

Number of pharmacy or drug treatment-related courses: 3 out of 19 or 7 out of 49 crs.

Number of diagnosis or optometry-related courses: 14 out of 19 or 37 out of 49 crs.

YEAR 3
FALL SEMESTER (19.5 CRS)

1. Anomalies of Binocular Vision II (3 crs); 2. Contact Lenses I (3 crs); 3. Ocular Disease III: Ocular/System Eye Disease (3 crs); 4. Clinical Medicine/Physical Diagnosis Lab (3 crs); 5. Practice Management I (2 crs); 6. Learning Disabilities/Pediatrics (3 crs); 7. Primary Care Clinic II (2.5 crs).

(DO: 1, 2, 3, 4, 6, 7; P: 0)

WINTER SEMESTER (15.5 CRS)

1. Clinical Gerontology (1 cr); 2. Contact Lenses II (3 crs); 3. Ocular Disease IV: Neuro-optometry (3 crs); 4. Rehabilitative Optometry Low Vision (3 crs); 5. Environmental Optometry (1 cr); 6. Practice Management II (2 crs); 7. Primary Care Clinic III (2.5 crs).

(DO: 1, 2, 3, 4, 5, 7; P: 0)

Number of pharmacy or drug treatment-related courses: zero (0) out of 14 or 35 crs (constitute an integral part of clinic).

Number of diagnosis or optometry-related courses: 12 out of 14 or 31 out of 35 crs (constitutes a major part of the rotations).

YEAR 4
SUMMER, FALL, AND WINTER SEMESTERS (32 CRS)

1. Primary Care Clinical Externship (5.5 crs); 2. Cornea and Contact Lenses Externship (4 crs); 3. Pediatric and Binocular Vision Externship (4 crs); 4. Vision Rehabilitation and Geriatric Externship (2.5 crs); 5. Medical and Surgical Care Clinical Externship (8 crs); 6. Clinic Elective (8 crs).

Number of pharmacy or drug treatment-related courses: zero (0), but constitute an integral part of the externship.

Number of diagnosis or optometry-related courses: Constitute a major part of the externship.

VETERINARY MEDICINE

UNIVERSITY OF PENNSYLVANIA SCHOOL OF VETERINARY MEDICINE

Courses offered to students in the four-year professional phase (2001-2003) leading to the award of Doctor of Veterinary Medicine (VMD) without residency requirements[16] (information was obtained from the catalog):

YEAR 1
FALL SEMESTER (29 CRS)
1. Gross Anatomy (11 crs); 2. Histology (5 crs); 3. Biochemistry (10 crs); 4. Embryology (3 crs).

3RD QUARTER (13 CRS)
5. Neuroscience (4 crs); 6. Physiology (11 crs—including 4th quarter); 7. Physical Exam/Animal Management (5 crs) 8. Biostatics (2 crs).

4TH QUARTER (28 CRS)
9. Veterinary Ethic Issues (2 crs); 10. General Pathology (5 crs); 11. Principles of Medicine (5 crs); 12. Nutrition (3 crs); 13. Medical Genetics (2 crs); 14. Introduction to Radiology (2 crs).

(D: 1, 2, 3, 4, 5, 6, 7, 10, 11, 13, 14; P: 0)

Number of pharmacy or drug treatment-related courses: zero (0) out of 14 or 60 crs.

Number of diagnosis-related courses: 11 out of 14 or 53 out of 60 crs.

YEAR 2
FALL SEMESTER (35 CRS)
1. Parasitology (8 crs); 2. Systemic Pathology (12 crs); 3. Immunology (4 crs); 4. Microbiology (7 crs); 5. Surgical Principles (4 crs).

3RD QUARTER (15 CRS)
6. Pharmacology (11 crs—including 4th quarter); 7. Introduction to Poultry Medicine (2 crs); 8. Epidemiology (2 crs); 9. Clinical Lab Medicine (6 crs); 10. Orthopedics (3 crs).

4TH QUARTER (34 CRS)

11. Infectious and Metabolic Diseases (7 crs); 12. Public Health (3 crs); 13. Anesthesia (4 crs); 14. Medicine/Surgery I (9 crs).

(D: 1, 2, 3, 4, 5, 7, 8, 9, 10, 11,14; P: 6, 13)

Number of pharmacy or drug treatment-related courses: 2 out of 14 or 15 out of 84 crs (constitute an integral part of few other courses like medicine/surgery).

Number of diagnosis-related courses: 11 out of 14 or 66 out of 84 crs.

YEAR 3
1ST QUARTER (14 CRS), 2ND QUARTER (14 CRS), 3RD AND 4TH QUARTERS (25 CRS EACH)

1. Reproduction (5 crs); 2. Clinical Exercises (1 cr); 3. Medicine/Surgery II (9 crs); 3a. Electives (9 crs); 4. Dermatology (3 crs); 5. Clinical Exercises (1 cr); 6. Lab Animal Medicine (1 cr); 7. Medicine/Surgery III (9 crs); 8. Clinical Animal Behavior (1 cr); 8a. Elective (7 crs); 3rd quarter (9 wks—25 crs electives); 4th quarter (9 wks—25 crs electives).

(D: 2, 3, 4, 5, 6, 7, 8; P: 0)

Number of pharmacy or drug treatment-related courses: zero (0) out of 8 but may be taken as 1-3 out of the 46 available electives.

Number of diagnosis-related courses: 7 out of 8 plus electives or 25 out of 30 crs plus majority (43-45) of the electives.

YEAR 4
ROTATIONS

1. Quarter 0—rotations 1-8; 4. Quarter 3—rotations 17-20.

2. Quarter 1—rotations 9-12; 5. Quarter 4—rotations 21-25.

3. Quarter 2—rotations 13-16.

Foundation core rotation 36 credits—48 hrs/wk and 36 credits (first 6 rotations).

Elective rotations—18 rotations and 9 credits (44 hrs/wk).

Number of pharmacy or drug treatment-related courses: None, but constitute an integral part of the rotations.

Number of diagnosis-related courses: Constitute a major part of the rotations.

TUFTS SCHOOL OF VETERINARY MEDICINE.

Courses offered to students in the four-year professional phase (2001-2002) leading to the award of Doctor of Veterinary Medicine (DVM) without residency requirements[17] (information was obtained from the catalog and Internet):

YEAR 1 (42 CRS)
SEMESTER 1 (16 WEEKS—16 CRS)

1.Gross Anatomy I (5 crs); 2. Physiology Chemistry (4 crs); 3. Veterinary Cell and Tissue Biology (4 crs); 4. Veterinary Developmental Biology (3 crs); 5. Clinical Skills I (0 cr); 6. Human/Animal Relationship (0 cr); 7. Physiology I (0 cr); 8. PBL (0 cr—1 Lecture); 9. Adopt-a-Vet Student (0 cr); 10. Selective (0 cr—0 lectures).

(D: 1, 2, 3, 4; P: 0)

SEMESTER 2 (21 WEEKS—26 CRS)

1. Clinical Skills II (0 cr); 2. Gross Anatomy II (5 crs); 3. Feeds and Feeding (1 cr); 4. Immunology (3 crs); 5. Physiology II (7 crs); 6. General Pathology (3 crs); 7. PBL II (0 cr—0 lectures); 8. Adopt-a-Vet Student (0 cr); 9. Organology (3 crs); 10. Comparative Anatomy and Physiology (2 crs); 11. International Veterinary Medicine (2 crs); 12. Selective (0 cr); 13. Major Elective (0 cr).

(D: 2, 4, 5, 6, 9, 10, 11; P: 0)

Number of pharmacy or drug treatment-related courses: zero (0) out of 11 or 42 crs plus 23 zero-credit courses.

Number of diagnosis-related courses: 11 out of 11 or 42 out of 42 crs plus 23 zero-credit courses.

YEAR 2
SEMESTER 1 (21 WKS—23 CRS)
1. Molecular Biology and Microbial Pathogenesis (5 crs); 2. Diagnostic Microbiology (0 cr); 3. General Parasitology (3 crs); 4. Neuromuscular/Skeletal Pathobiology (4 crs); 5. Basic Pharmacology (4 crs); 6. Clinical Skills II (0 cr-3 Lectures); 7. Respiratory (3 crs); 8. Epidemiology and Biostatistics (2 crs); 9. Urinary (2 crs); 10. PBL III (0 cr—0 lectures); 11. Rotations I (0 cr—0 lectures); 12. Selective (0 cr).

(D: 1, 3, 4, 7, 8, 9; P: 5)

SEMESTER 2 (21 WEEKS—36 CRS)
1. Clinical Skills IV (0 cr); 2. Clinical Veterinary Genetics (2 crs); 3. Gastrointestinal Pathophysiology (3 crs); 4. Cardiovascular (5 crs); 5. Toxicology (2 crs); 6. Reproductive Physiology (2 crs); 7. Diagnostics Imaging (3 crs); 8. Principles of Surgery (2 crs); 9. Basic Dermatology (1 cr); 10. Reproductive Pathology (2 crs); 11. Public Health (2 crs); 12. Biotechnology (1 cr); 13. Clinical Animal Behavior (2 crs); 14. Clinical Pharmacology (2 crs); 15. Hemic Lymphatic and Clinical Pathology (5 crs); 16. PBL IV (0 cr); 17. Rotation II (0 cr); 18. Introduction to Zoological Medicine (2 crs); 19. Selectives (0 cr).

(D: 2, 3, 4, 6, 7, 8, 9, 10, 13, 15, 18; P: 5, 14)

Number of pharmacy or drug treatment-related courses: 3 out of 22 or 8 out of 59 crs plus 31 zero-credit courses.

Number of diagnosis-related courses: 17 out of 22 or 48 out of 59 crs plus 31 zero-credit courses.

YEAR 3
SEMESTER 1 (17 WEEKS—30 CRS)
1. Large Animal Medicine and Surgery I (6 crs); 2. Small Animal Medicine and Surgery I (7 crs); 3. Theriogenology (4 crs); 4. Jurisprudence and Ethics (3 crs); 5. Anesthesiology (2 crs); 6. International Veterinary Medicine (2 crs); 7. Small Animal Procedures Laboratory (0 cr); 8. Small Animal Spay Clinic (0 cr); 9. Clinical Dermatology (2 crs); 10. Comparative Medicine (4 crs); 11. Selectives (0 cr).

(D: 1, 2, 3, 6, 9, 10; P: 5)

SEMESTER 2 (9 WEEKS—12 CRS)

1. Large Animal Medicine and Surgery II (4 crs); 2. Small Animal Medicine and Surgery II (4 crs); 3. Veterinary Business Practices and Economics (1 cr); 4. Ophthalmology (3 crs); 5. Large Animal Clinical Anatomy (0 cr); 6. Standardized Client (0 cr); 7. Small Animal Spay Clinic (0 cr); 8. Bovine Procedures Laboratory (0 cr); 9. Elective Large Animal Surgery Laboratory (0 cr—0 labs); 10. Elective Small Orthopedic Surgery Laboratory (0 cr).

(D: 1, 2, 4; P: 0)

Number of pharmacy or drug treatment-related courses: 1 out of 12 or 2 out of 42 crs plus 21 zero-credit courses (constitute an integral part of some other courses such as comparative medicine).

Number of diagnosis-related courses: 9 out of 12 or 36 out of 42 crs plus 21 zero-credit courses.

YEAR 4 (INCLUDING LATE THIRD YEAR)
CORE ROTATION (31 CREDITS)

1. Small Animal Medicine (3 crs-3 wks); 2. Small Animal Surgery (4 crs-3 wks); 3. Large Animal Medicine (3 crs-2 wks); 4. Large Animal Surgery (3 cr-2 wks); 5. Ambulatory Medicine (4 crs-4 wks); 6. Practice Environments (0 cr-2 wks); 7. Wildlife Clinic (2 crs-2 wks); 8. Radiology (3 crs-3 wks); 9. Anatomical and Clinical Pathology (3 crs-3 wks); 10. Small Animal Critical Care (3 crs-3 wks); 11. Anesthesiology (3 crs-3 wks); 12. Ophthalmology (0 cr-1 wk); 13. Ethics Seminar (0 cr-2 hrs); 14. Subspecialty Service Rotation (0 cr); 15. Required Selectives (0 cr-8 wks); 16. Required Electives (0 cr-18 wks); 17. Vacation (3 wks).

Number of pharmacy or drug treatment-related courses: 1 out of 10 or 3 out of 31 crs plus integral part of rotations.

Number of diagnosis-related courses: 9 out of 10 or 28 out of 31 crs plus major part of rotations.

UNIVERSITY OF WISCONSIN SCHOOL OF VETERINARY MEDICINE

Courses offered to students in the four-year professional phase (2002) leading to the award of Doctor of Veterinary Medicine (DVM) without residency requirements (information was obtained from the Internet):

YEAR 1
SEMESTER 1 (18-19 CRS)

1. Fundamental Principles of Veterinary Anatomy (5 crs); 2. Veterinary Histology (5 crs); 3. Veterinary Developmental Anatomy (2 crs); 4. Veterinary Physiology A (4 crs); 5. Radiolograghic Anatomy of the Dog and Cat (1 cr); 6. Health, History, Physical Exam (0 cr); 7. Introduction to the VMTH I (1 cr); 8. Elective: Small Animal Critical Care (1 cr).

(D: 1, 2, 3, 4, 5, 7, 8; P: 0)

SEMESTER 2 (15-20 CRS)

1. Nutrition (1 cr); 2. Veterinary Biochemistry (3 crs); 3. Veterinary NeuroAnatomy and Neurophysiology (3 crs); 4. Veterinary B (4 crs); 5. Veterinary Pharmacology (2 crs); 6. Anatomy of Large Domestic Animals (1-3 crs); 7. Large Animal Radiology Elective (1 cr); 8. Health, History, Physical Exam (0 cr); 9. Elective: Large Animal Supportive Care (1 cr); 10. Elective: Small Animal Critical Care (1 cr).

(D: 2, 3, 4, 6, 7, 9, 10; P: 5)

Number of pharmacy or drug treatment-related courses: 1 out of 16 or 2 out of 33-39 crs plus 18 zero-credit courses.

Number of diagnosis-related courses: 14 out of 16 or 30-36 out of 33-39 crs plus 18 zero-credit courses.

YEAR 2
SEMESTER 1 (17-18 CRS)

1. Veterinary Immunology (3 crs); 2. Veterinary Bacteriology/Mycology (5 crs); 3. Recitation in Infectious Disease (0 cr); 4. Veterinary Epidemiology (2 crs); 5. Veterinary Virology (2 crs); 6. General Pathology (2 crs); 7. Veterinary

Systemic Pathology I (2 crs); 8. Introduction to the VMTH II (1 cr); 9. Elective: Small Animal Critical Care (1 cr).

(D: 1, 2, 4, 5, 6, 7, 8, 9; P: 0)

SEMESTER 2 (20-22 CRS)

1. Veterinary Parasitology (3 crs); 2. Recitation in Infectious Disease (1 cr); 3. Veterinary Systemic Pathology (4 crs); 4. Veterinary Clinical Pathology (4 crs); 5. Veterinary Toxicology (2 crs); 6. Surgery Fundamentals (2 crs); 7. Fundamentals of Anesthesiology I (1 cr); 8. Basic and Clinical Therapeutics (3 crs); 9. Elective: Large Animal Supportive Care (1 cr); 10. Elective: Small Animal Critical Care (1 cr).

(D: 1, 2, 3, 4, 6, 9, 10; P: 5, 7, 8)

Number of pharmacy or drug treatment-related courses: 3 out of 18 or 6 out of 33-40 crs plus 19 zero-credit courses.

Number of diagnosis-related courses: 15 out of 18 or 27-34 out of 33-40 crs plus 31 zero-credit courses.

YEAR 3
SEMESTER 1 (17-18 CRS)

1. Veterinary Medicine I (6 crs); 2. Theriogenology (3 crs); 3. Veterinary Diagnostic and Therapeutic Techniques (0 cr); 4. Veterinary Clinical Nutrition (1 cr); 5. Small Animal Surgery (4 crs); 6. Small Animal Surgery Lab (0 cr); 7. Small Animal Anesthesia Lab (0 cr); 8. Veterinary Preventive Medicine (1 cr); 9. Veterinary Ophthalmology (2 crs); 10. Elective: Small Animal Critical Care (1 cr).

(D: 1, 2, 5, 9, 10; P: 0)

SEMESTER 2 (22-24 CRS)

1. Veterinary Medicine II (6 crs); 2. Veterinary Diagnostic and Therapeutic Techniques (1 cr); 3. Regulatory Veterinary Medicine and Public Health (2 crs); 4. Fundamentals of Anesthesiology II (1 cr); 5. Large Animal Surgery (4 crs); 6. Small Animal Surgery Lab (2 crs); 7. Small Animal Anesthesia Lab (1 cr); 8. Veterinary Radiology (2 crs); 9. Special Species Medicine (2 crs); 10. Elective: Advanced Dentistry (1 cr); 11. Elective: Bovine Surgery Lab (1

cr); 12. Elective: Large Animal Supportive Care (1 cr); 13. Elective: Small Animal Critical Care (1 cr).

(D: 1, 2, 5, 6, 8, 9, 11, 12, 13; P: 4, 7)

Number of pharmacy or drug treatment-related courses: 2 (plus 5 zero-credit courses) out of 20 or 2 out of 38-42 crs plus 23 zero-credit courses.

Number of diagnosis-related courses: 14 (plus 16 zero-credit courses) out of 20 or 35-39 out of 38-42 crs plus 23 zero-credit courses.

YEAR 4 (47 CRS-48 WKS)

Each fourth-year student designs his/her fourth-year schedule to meet their personal career goals.

SPECIAL ROTATIONS

1. Equine Lameness; 2. Food Animal Surgery; 3. Clinical Pathology; 4. Clinical Reasoning; 5. Clinical Parasitology.

OTHERS

1. Senior Rotation in Large Animal Medicine Service; 2. Small Animal Neurology; 3. Small Animal Dermatology; 4. Small Animal Cardiology; 5. Small Animal Internal Medicine; 6. Small Animal Oncology; 7. Senior Rotation in Theriogenology Service; 8. Senior Rotation in Ambulatory Service; 9. Veterinary Necropsy Rotation; 10. Radiology Clinics; 11. Large Animal Surgery: Clinical Rotation; 12. Clinics: Small Animal Orthopedic Surgery; 13. Senior Rotation in Small Animal General Surgery; 14. Veterinary Anesthesiology: Clinical Rotation; 15. Clinical Ophthalmology Rotation; 16. Swine Medicine Service/Community Practice/Urgent Care/Preventative Medicine; 17. Production Medicine I: Herd Health Management; 18. Production Medicine II: Quality Milk Production Enhancement; 19. Production Medicine III: Applied Ruminant Nutrition; 20. Production Medicine IV: Economic and Farm Finance; 21. Veterinary Oncology Research; 22. Veterinary Necropsy Rotation; 23. Pathobiological Sciences Research Rotation; 24. Epidemiology (medical school); 25. Special Species; 26. Radiology Clinic Elective; 27. Advanced Anesthesiology/Critical Care Medicine; 28. Business Management; 29. Exotic Animal Medicine; 30.

Llama and Small Ruminant Medicine; 31. Restraint and Anesthesia of Exotic Animals; 32. Small Animal Orthopedics; 33. Veterinary Dentistry; 34. Small Animal Electrocardiology; 35. Pharmaceuticals; 36. Constrast Radiology; 37. Small Animal Ethology; 38. Small Animal Emergency Medicine; 39. Clinical Pathology.

Number of pharmacy or drug treatment-related courses: 1 out of 44 available courses, but constitute an integral part of the rotation.

Number of diagnosis-related courses: Most of the available courses and it constitutes major part of the rotations.

OHIO STATE UNIVERSITY COLLEGE OF VETERINARY MEDICINE.

Courses offered to students in the four-year professional phase (2002) leading to the award of Doctor of Veterinary Medicine (DVM) without residency requirements (information was obtained from the Internet):

YEAR 1
AUTUMN QUARTER

1. Principles of Epidemiology; 2. Topographic Anatomy; 3. Introduction to Radiology I; 4. Microscopic and Development Anatomy I; 5. Structure and Function of Cells; 6. Ethics and Jurisprudence I.

(D: 1, 2, 3, 4, 5; P: 0)

WINTER QUARTER

1. Topographic Anatomy (equine); 2. Introduction to Radiology II; 3. Microscopic and Developmental Anatomy II; 4. Comparative Biology of Disease I; 5. Comparative Biology Disease II; 6. Ethics and Jurisprudence II.

(D: 1, 2, 3, 4, 5; P: 0)

SPRING QUARTER

1. Topograghic Anatomy (food animals); 2. Pharmacology; 3. Neurobiology; 4. Endocrine System; 4a. Electives.

(D: 1, 3, 4; P: 2)

Number of pharmacy or drug treatment-related courses: 1 out of 16.

Number of diagnosis-related courses: 13 out of 16.

YEAR 2
AUTUMN QUARTER
1. Cardiovascular System; 2. Respiratory System; 3. Hemic-lymphatic System; 4. Population Medicine II; 4a. Electives.

(D: 1, 2, 3, 4; P: 0)

WINTER QUARTER
1. Urinary System; 2. Musculo-skeletal System; 3. Digestive System; 4. Fluid Therapy; 4a. Electives.

(D: 1, 2, 3; P: 4)

SPRING QUARTER
1. Introduction to Anesthesiology; 2. Introduction to Surgery; 3. Reproduction System; 4. Integumentary System; 5. Principles of Nonmammalian Species; 6. Parasite Control; 6a. Elective.

(D: 2, 3, 4, 6; P: 1)

Number of pharmacy or drug treatment-related courses: 1 or 2 out of 14.

Number of diagnosis-related courses: 11 out of 14.

YEAR 3
AUTUMN QUARTER
1. Introduction to Veterinary Ophthalmology; 2. Small Animal Medicine and Surgical Techniques, or 616: Food Animal Medicine and Techniques and Equine Medicine and Techniques; 3. Veterinary Toxicology; 4. Surgery quarter (recommended electives); 5. Techniques quarter (recommended electives).

(D: 1, 2, 4; P: 3)

WINTER QUARTER
1. Pharmacology II; 2. Veterinary Preventive Medicine; 3. Small Animal Medicine and Techniques or Food Animal Medicine and Techniques and Equine Medicine and Techniques; 4. Surgery quarter (recommended electives); 5. Techniques quarter (recommended electives).

(D: 3, 4; P: 1)

Number of pharmacy or drug treatment-related courses: 2 out of 10.

Number of diagnosis-related courses: 5 out of 10.

YEAR 4 AND YEAR 3 SPRING QUARTER
ROTATION CLINIC I
1. Small Animal Medicine; 2. Small Animal Surgery; 3. Radiology; 4. Ophthalmology; 5. Dermatology; 6. Electives.

CLINIC II
1. General Practice; 2. Food Animal Medicine and Surgery; 3. Equine Medicine and Surgery; 4. Anesthesiology; 5. Electives.

CLINIC III
1. Equine Outpatient Clinic; 2. Preventive Medicine; 3. Large Animal Ambulatory Clinics; 4. Small Animal Emergency/Critical Care; 5. Applied Pathology; 6. Equine Emergency/Critical Care; 7. Electives; 8. Elective quarter.

Number of pharmacy or drug treatment-related courses: Constitute an integral part of the clinic.

Number of diagnosis-related courses: Constitute a major part of the clinic.

Residency: Available as graduate or postgraduate program.

PHYSICIAN ASSISTANT

THE UNIVERSITY OF IOWA COLLEGE OF MEDICINE PHYSICIAN ASSISTANT PROGRAM

Courses offered to students in the two-year (twenty-five-month) professional phase leading to the award of Master of Physician Assistant Studies (MPAS) without residency requirements[7] (information was obtained from the catalog):

YEAR 1 (PHASE I)
SUMMER AND FALL (SH = SEMESTER HOUR)

1. Foundation of Clinical Practice for Physician Assistants (5 sh); 2. Gross Human Anatomy for Physician Assistant Students (6 sh); 3. Principles of Infectious Diseases for Physician Assistant Students (4 sh); 4. Introduction to Human Pathology (4 sh); 5. Pharmacology for Health Sciences (6 sh); 6. Human Physiology for Physician Assistant Students (4 sh); 7. Introduction to Medical History and Physical Examination for Physician Assistant Students (3 sh); 8. Introduction to Research Design and Methodology (1 sh); 9. Interpretation of Medical Literature (1 sh).

(D: 1, 2, 3, 4, 6, 7; P: 5)

SPRING

1. Foundations of Clinical Practice IV for Physician Assistant Students (15 sh); 2. Health Law (1 sh); 3. Seminar for Physician Assistant Students (1 sh).

(D: 1; P: 0)

YEAR 2 (PHASE II)

1. Clinical Laboratory Medicine for Physician Assistant Students (1 sh); 2. Introduction to Clinical Skills (1 sh).

(D: 1. 2; P: 0)

Number of pharmacy or drug treatment-related courses: 1 out of 14 or 6 out of 54 sh.

Number of diagnosis-related courses: 9 out of 14 or 42 out of 54 sh.

CLINICAL ROTATIONS

1. Gynecology for Physician Assistant Students (4 sh); 2. Pediatrics for Physician Assistant Students (6 sh); 3. Psychiatry for Physician Assistant Students (4 sh); 4. Emergency Room Elective for Physician Assistant Students (4 sh); 5. General Surgery for Physician Assistant Students (6 sh); 6. Internal Medicine for Physician Assistant Students (6 sh); 7. Family Practice I for Physician Assistant Students (6 sh); 8. Family Practice II for Physician Assistant Students (6 sh); 9. Independent Study (1 sh); 10. Elective Clinical Rotations (23 options to chose from—no pharmacy course).

Number of pharmacy or drug treatment-related courses: None, but constitute an integral or minor part of the rotations.

Number of diagnosis-related courses: Constitute a major part of the rotations.

NOVA SOUTHEASTERN UNIVERSITY COLLEGE OF ALLIED HEALTH DUAL ADMISSIONS PROGRAM-- PHYSICIAN ASSISTANT PROGRAM (BS/MPH)

Courses offered to students in the 2.5-year (twenty-nine-month) professional phase leading to the award of Bachelor of Science in physician assistant and a Master of Public Health (B.S/M.P.H) without residency requirements[11] (information were obtained from the catalog):

YEAR 1 (15 MONTHS)
1ST SEMESTER (20 CRS)

1. Anatomy (5 crs); 2. Physiology (3 crs); 3. Clinical Pathophysiology (4 crs); 4. Physical Diagnosis I (3 crs); 5. Medical Terminology (1 cr); 6. Biomedical Principles (1 cr); 7. Introduction to the Physician Assistant Profession (1 cr); 8. Rural and Underserved Medicine (1 cr); 9. Culture, Ethnicity, and Health (1 cr).

(D: 1, 2, 3, 4, 6, 8; P: 0)

SEMESTER 2: FALL 1 (SEPTEMBER-DECEMBER—21 CRS)

1. Microbiology (3 crs); 2. Legal and Ethical Issues in Public Health (3 crs); 3. Physical Diagnosis II (2 crs); 4. Pharmacology I (2 crs); 5. Clinical

Medicine and Surgery I (6 crs); 6. Clinical Laboratory Medicine (2 crs); 7. Epidemiology (3 crs).

(D: 1, 3, 5, 6, 7; P: 4)

YEAR 2 (TILL END OF PROGRAM)
SEMESTER 3: WINTER 1:1 (JANUARY-MARCH—17 CRS)

1. Biostatistics (3 crs); 2. Physical Diagnosis III (3 crs); 3. Clinical Medicine and Surgery II (6 crs); 4. Children's Health (1 cr); 5. Pharmacology II (4 crs).

(D: 2, 3, 4; P: 5)

SEMESTER 3: WINTER 1: 11 (MARCH-MAY—15 CRS)

1. Clinical Problem Solving (3 crs); 2. Social and Behavior Sciences Applied to Health (3 crs); 3. Electrocardiology (2 crs); 4. Women's Health (1 cr); 5. Clinical Psychiatry (1 cr); 6. Clinical Medicine and Surgery III (6 crs).

(D: 1, 2, 3, 4, 5, 6; P: 0)

SEMESTER 4: SUMMER 2 (JUNE-AUGUST—17 CRS)

1. Life Support Procedures and Skills (1 cr); 2. Clinical Procedures and Surgical Skills (3 crs); 3. Health Policy, Planning, and Management (3 crs); 4. Health Promotion and Disease Prevention (1 cr); 5. Health Care Delivery System (1 cr); 6. Environmental and Occupational Health (3 crs); 7. Publication Skills (2 crs).

(D: 2, 4; P: 0)

Number of pharmacy or drug treatment-related courses: 2 out of 34 or 6 out of 90 crs.

Number of diagnosis-related courses: 22 out of 34 or 63 out of 90 crs.

CLINICAL YEAR CURRICULUM: FALL 2; WINTER 2; SUMMER 3 (SEPTEMBER-AUGUST—52 CRS)

1. Obstetrics and Gynecology (6 crs); 2. Internal Medicine (6 crs); 3. Surgery (6 crs); 4. Emergency Medicine (6 crs); 5. Pediatrics; (6 crs); 6. Family Medicine (6 crs); 7. Elective I (6 crs); 8. Primary Care Internship (6 crs); 9. Alternative and Complementary Medicine (1 cr); 10. Health care Nutrition (2 crs); 11. Physician Assistant Professional Issues (1 cr); 12. Public Health Practicum (34 crs). (Note 6 crs = 6 wk courses)

Number of pharmacy or drug treatment-related courses: Constitute an integral part of the rotations.

Number of diagnosis-related courses: Constitute a major part of the rotations.

UNIVERSITY OF FLORIDA PHYSICIAN ASSISTANT PROGRAM

Courses offered to students in the two-year professional phase leading to the award of Master of Physician Assistant Studies (MPAS) without residency requirements (information was obtained from the Internet):

YEAR 1 (40 CRS)
SEMESTER 1: SUMMER B

1. Gross and Radiologic Anatomy (4 crs); 2. Medical Communications (2 crs).

(D: 1, P: 0)

SEMESTER 2: FALL

1. Introduction to Medicine (6 crs); 2. Behavioral and Community Medicine (1 cr); 3. Human Physiology (4 crs); 4. Physical Diagnosis.

(D: 1, 2, 3, 4; P: 0)

SEMESTER 3: SPRING

1. Introduction to Medicine II (6 crs); 2. Behavioral and Community Medicine II (1 cr); 3. Pharmacotherapeutics (4 crs); 4. Patient Evaluation and Hospital Practicum (2 crs); 5. Clinical Problem Solving and Differential Diagnosis (1 cr); 6. Clinical Procedures (1 cr); 7. EKG and ACLS (1 cr).

(D: 1, 2, 4, 5, 6, 7; P: 3)

SEMESTER 4: SUMMER A

1. Evidence-based Medicine for Physicians Assistants (3 crs); 2. Advanced Clinical Practicum (2 crs).

(D: 1, 2; P: 0)

Number of pharmacy or drug treatment-related courses: 1 out of 15 or 4 out of 40 crs.

Number of diagnosis-related courses: 13 out of 15 or 34 out of 40 crs.

YEAR 2 (40 CRS)

Semester 5 (Summer B): Two rotations (3 crs each—6 crs); special topics (1 cr).

Semester 6 (Fall): Four rotations (3 crs each—12 crs); special topics (1 cr).

Semester 7 (Spring): Four rotations (3 crs each—12 crs); special topics (1 cr).

Semester 8 (Summer A): Two rotations (3 crs each—6 crs); special topics (1 cr).

Required Clinical Rotations are: 1. Emergency Medicine (1 month); 2. Family Medicine (2 months); 3. General Surgery (1 month); 4. Geriatrics (1 month); 5. Internal Medicine (2 months); 6. Obstetrics-Gynecology (1 month).

Number of pharmacy or drug treatment-related courses: Constitute an integral part of the rotations.

Number of diagnosis-related courses: Constitute a major part of the rotations.

UNIVERSITY OF WISCONSIN PHYSICIAN ASSISTANT PROGRAM

Courses offered to students in the two-year professional phase (2001) leading to the award of Master of Physician Assistant Studies (MPAS) without residency requirements (information was obtained from the Internet):

YEAR 1
SUMMER I (6 CRS)

1. Anatomy; 2. History and Physical Examination for Physician Assistants
(D: 1, 2; P: 0)

FALL SEMESTER (15 CRS)

1. Pharmacology; 2. Medical Microbiology; 3. Theories and Practice in Emergency Care; 4. Clinical Medicine for Physician Assistants I; 5. Pediatrics for Physician Assistants I; 6. Advanced Patient Evaluation in the Primary Care Setting I; 7. Obstetrics and Gynecology for Physician Assistants.
(D: 2, 3, 4, 5, 6, 7; P: 1)

SPRING SEMESTER (15 CRS)

1. Clinical Medicine for Physician Assistants II; 2. Pediatrics for Physician Assistants II; 3. Issues in Professional Practice for Physician Assistants; 4. Advanced Patient Evaluation in the Primary Care Setting II; 5. Laboratory Medicine for Physician Assistants; 6. A Team Approach to Emergency Care.

(D: 1, 2, 4, 5, 6; P: 0)

YEAR 2
SUMMER II (5 CRS)

1. Pharmacy Practice; 2. Field Experience in Patient Assessment; 3. Surgical Principles and Procedures.

(D: 2. 3; P: 1)

Number of pharmacy or drug treatment-related courses: 2 out of 18.

Number of diagnosis-related courses: 15 out of 18.

Fall and Spring Semesters

1. Surgery Preceptorship; 2. Primary Care Preceptorship I; 3. Primary Care Preceptorship II; 4. Internal Medicine Preceptorship.

Number of pharmacy or drug treatment-related courses: Constitute an integral part of the rotations or Preceptorship.

Number of diagnosis-related courses: Constitute a major part of the rotations or Preceptorship.

NURSING PROGRAM

Registered nurse (RN) is an associate program, which is less than a first-degree program in nursing. Licensed practicing nurse (LPN) is more or less like a cram program, which is less than the registered nurse program in duration of school training. All nursing programs (LPN, RN, and BSC) require a high school diploma as an entry-level prerequisite. Throughout this chapter, the entry level for all aspects of medicine is higher than a high school diploma. The first degree, a baccalaureate degree (BSc or BA), is the entry level for all branches of medicine except pharmacy, which presently requires an associate degree or two years of college work as entry level. (This is bound to change and level up with other branches of medicine in the future as the demand for pharmacy increases with greater responsibility and remuneration for cognitive functions.) The nursing program in this chapter will be focused on first degree—the four-year baccalaureate degree in nursing (BSN)—and the higher degree—a master's degree in nursing as a certified nurse practitioner (CNP). The four-year nursing curriculum involves two years of a pre-professional phase and two years of a professional phase leading to the award of a BSN nursing degree.

CREIGHTON UNIVERSITY SCHOOL OF NURSING

Courses offered to students in the two-year pre-professional and professional phases (total of 4 years as of 2001) leading to the award of Bachelor of Science in nursing (BSN) (information was obtained from the Internet):

YEAR 1 (34 SH)
FALL SEMESTER (17 HRS)

1. Basic Anatomy (4 hrs); 2. Seminar in Professional Nursing (1 hr); 3. Introductory Psychology (3 hrs); 4. SOC 101 or ANT 111 (3 hrs); 5. Fundamentals of General Chemistry (3 hrs); 6. Skills (ENG 150 required if ENG ACT score below 22—3 hrs).

(DN: 1, 2; P: 0)

(DN = diagnosis and nursing-related courses)

SPRING SEMESTER (17 HRS)

1. Fundamentals of Biological Chemistry/Practicum (4 hrs); 2. History (3 hrs); 3. Physiology (4 hrs); 4. World Literature I (3 crs); 5. Christianity in Context (3 hrs).

(DN: 1, 3; P: 0)

Number of pharmacy or drug treatment-related courses: zero (0) out of 11 or 34 hrs.

Number of diagnosis and nursing-related courses: 3 out of 11 or 9 out of 34 hrs.

YEAR 2 (33 HRS)
FALL SEMESTER (15 HRS)

1. Health Assessment (2 hrs); 2. Health Assessment Practicum (1 hr); 3. Lifespan Development (3 hrs); 4. Microbiology (4 hrs); 5. Skills Course (2 crs); 6. Crypt and History Introduction to Philosophy (3 hrs).

(DN: 1, 2, 4; P: 0)

Spring Semester (18 hrs)
1. Human Pathphysiology (3 hrs); 2. Human Pathophysiology Practicum (1 hr); 3. Nutrition (2 hrs); 4. THL 200 level (3 hrs); 5. Ethics (3 hrs); 5a. Elective (3 hrs); 6. World Literature II (3 hrs).

(DN: 1, 2; P: 0)

Number of pharmacy or drug treatment-related courses: zero (0) out of 12 or 33 hrs.

Number of diagnosis and nursing-related courses: 5 out of 12 or 11 out of 33 hrs.

Year 3 (33 hrs)
Fall Semester (18 hrs)
1. Informatics in Health Care (2 hrs); 2. Informatics in Health Care Practicum (1 hr); 3. Care Management Concepts for Health Promotion Maintenance and Restoration (5 crs); 4. Care Management Practicum I (4 hrs); 5. Nursing Management of Pharmacy Therapy (3 hrs); 6. Research for Health Professionals (3 hrs).

(DN: 1, 2, 3, 4, 6; P: 5)

Spring Semester (15 hrs)
1. Principles of Population-based Health Care (3 hrs); 2. Care Management Processes for Episodic and Chronic Health Alterations I (5 hrs); 3. Care Management Practicum II (5 hrs); 4. Introduction to Power, Politics, and Policy in Health Care (2 hrs).

(DN: 1, 2, 3; P: 0)

Number of pharmacy or drug treatment-related courses: 1 out of 10 or 3 out of 33 hrs.

Number of diagnosis and nursing-related courses: 8 out of 10 or 28 out of 33 hrs.

YEAR 4 (28 HRS)
FALL SEMESTER (15 HRS)
1. Care Management Processes for Episodic and Chronic Health Alterations II (5 hrs); 2. Care Management Practicum III (5 hrs); 3. Leadership for Care Management (2 hrs); 4. Applied Ethics (3 hrs).

(DN: 1, 2, 3; P: 0)

SPRING SEMESTER (13 HRS)
1. Senior Seminar in Professional Nursing (3 hrs); 2. Senior Preceptorship (10 hrs)

(DN: 1, 2; P: 0)

Number of pharmacy or drug treatment-related courses: zero (0) out of 6 or 28 hrs, but constitute an integral part of preceptorship.

Number of diagnosis and nursing-related courses: 5 out of 6 or 28 hrs and it constitute majority of the preceptorship.

UNIVERSITY OF TEXAS-AUSTIN SCHOOL OF NURSING

Courses offered to students in the two-year pre-professional and professional phases (total of 4 years as of 2001) leading to the award of Bachelor of Science in nursing (BSN) (information was obtained from the Internet):

YEAR 1 TO 2 (PRE-PROFESSIONAL SEQUENCE—72 OR 73 HRS)
1. Anatomy and Physiology: Zoology (7 hrs); 2. Biology (6 hrs); 3. Chemistry (8 hrs); 4. Mathematics (3 or 4 hrs); 5. Nutrition (3 hrs); 6. Rhetoric and Composition 306, English 316k (6 hrs); 7. American Government (6 hrs); 8. Human Development and Family Sciences (3 hrs); 9. American History (6 hrs); 10. Psychology (3 hrs); 11. Fine Arts Elective (3 hrs); 12. Health Promotion (3 hrs); 13. Communication in Health Care Settings (3 hrs); 14. Ethics of Health Care I (3 hrs); 15. Introductory Statistics (3 hrs); 16. Pharmacy (3 hrs).

(DN: 1, 2, 8, 12; P: 16)

Number of pharmacy or drug treatment-related courses: 1 out of 15 or 3 out of 73 hrs.

Number of diagnosis and nursing-related courses: 4 out of 15 or 13 out of 73 hrs.

YEAR 3
Fall Semester (14 hrs)
1. Health Assessment Skills (2 hrs); 2. Adult Health Nursing I (3 hrs); 3. Adult Health Nursing I (practicum) (4 hrs); 4. Conceptual and Applied Basis of Mental Health Nursing (2 hrs); 5. Conceptual Basis of Aging (2 hrs); 6. Clinical and Applied Skills I (practicum) (1 hr).

(DN: 1, 2, 3, 4, 5, 6; P: 0)

Spring Semester (16 hrs)
1. Adult Health Nursing II (4 hrs); 2. Adult Health Nursing II (practicum) (4 hrs); 3. Conceptual Basis of Mental Health Problems (3 hrs); 4. Problems in Mental Health Nursing (practicum) (4 hrs); 5. Clinical Nursing Skills II (practicum) (1 hr).

(DN: 1, 2, 3, 4, 5; P: 0)

Number of pharmacy or drug treatment-related courses: zero (0) out of 11 or 30 hrs may constitute an integral part of few courses.

Number of diagnosis and nursing-related courses: 11 out of 11 or 30 out of 30 hrs.

YEAR 4
Fall Semester (15 hrs)
1. Nursing Research (2 hrs); 2. Care of Childbearing Families (2 hrs); 3. Nursing Care of Childbearing Families (practicum) (4 hrs); 4. Nursing Care of Children and Their Families (2 hrs); 5. Nursing Care of Children and Their Families (practicum) (4 hrs); 6. Clinical Nursing Skills III (practicum) (1 hr).

(DN: 1, 2, 3, 4, 5, 6; P: 0)

SPRING SEMESTER (16 HRS)
1. Community Health Nursing (2 hrs); 2. Community Health Nursing (practicum) (4 hrs); 3. Management of Nursing Care (3 hrs); 4. Clinical Management (practicum) II (4 hrs); 5. Synthesis of Nursing Knowledge 2 (2 hrs); 6. Clinical Nursing Skills IV (practicum) (1 hr).

(DN: 1, 2, 3, 4, 5, 6; P: 0)

Number of pharmacy or drug treatment-related courses: zero (0) out of 12 or 31 hrs.

Number of diagnosis and nursing-related courses: 12 out of 12 or 31 out of 31 hrs.

UNIVERSITY OF KENTUCKY COLLEGE OF NURSING, AUSTIN

Courses offered to students in the two-year pre-professional and professional phases (a total of 4 years as of 2002) leading to the award of Bachelor of Science in nursing (BSN) (information was obtained from the Internet):

YEAR 1 (PRE-NURSING)
FALL SEMESTER (14 CRS)
1. Principles of Human Anatomy (3 crs); 2. Introductory General Chemistry (3 crs); 3. Presentational Communication Skills (1 cr); 4. Writing (3 crs); 5. Introduction to Psychology (4 crs).

(DN: 1; P: 0)

SPRING SEMESTER (16 CRS)
1. Introduction to Organic, Inorganic, and Biochemistry (4 crs); 2. Writing II (3 crs); 3. Elementary Physiology (3 crs); 4. Social Science (3 crs); 5. USP (3 crs).

(DN: 3; P: 0)

Number of pharmacy or drug treatment-related courses: zero (0) out of 10 or 30 crs.

Number of diagnosis and nursing-related courses: 2 out of 10 or 6 out of 30 crs.

YEAR 2 (PROFESSIONAL CURRICULUM)
FALL SEMESTER (16 CRS)

1. Introductory Nutrition (3 crs); 2. Principles of Microbiology (3 crs); 3. Foundations for Professional Nursing (2 crs); 4. Family Health Promotion and Communication across the Lifespan (8 crs).

(DN: 2, 3, 4; P: 0)

SPRING SEMESTER (14 CRS)

1. Pharmacology (3 crs); 2. Professional Nursing Care across the Lifespan (8 crs); 3. Statistics: A Force in Human Judgment or Health and Medical Care Delivery Systems (3 crs); 4. USP (social science—3 crs).

(DN: 2, 3; P: 1)

Number of pharmacy or drug treatment-related courses: 1 out of 8 or 3 out of 30 crs.

Number of diagnosis- and nursing-related courses: 5 out of 8 or 24 out of 30 crs.

YEAR 3
FALL SEMESTER (13 CRS)

1. Pathophysiology (3 crs); 2. Family-centered Care of Adults with Common Health Problems (7 crs); 3. Statistics: A Force in Human Judgment or Health and Medical Care Delivery Systems (3 crs).

(DN: 1, 2, 3; P: 0)

SPRING SEMESTER (16 CRS)

1. Clinical Reasoning: Quantitative, Qualitative, and Epidemiological Approaches (3 crs); 2. Nursing Care of Childbearing and Childrearing Families (7 crs); 3. USP (6 crs).

(DN: 1, 2; P: 0)

Number of pharmacy or drug treatment-related courses: zero (0) out of 6 or 29 crs.

Number of diagnosis and nursing-related courses: 5 out of 6 or 23 out of 29 crs.

YEAR 4
FALL SEMESTER (16 CRS)
1. Leadership/Management in Nursing Care Delivery (3 crs); 2. Psychiatric/Mental Health Nursing (5 crs); 3. Public Health Nursing (5 crs); 3a. Elective (3 crs).

(DN: 1, 2, 3; P: 0)

SPRING SEMESTER (13 CRS)
1. Career Management in Nursing (2 crs); 2. High Acuity Nursing (5 crs); 3. Synthesis of Clinical Knowledge for Nursing Practice (6 crs).

(DN: 1, 2, 3; P: 0)

Number of pharmacy or drug treatment-related courses: zero (0) out of 6 or 29 crs.

Number of diagnosis and nursing-related courses: 6 out of 6 or 26 out of 29 crs.

OREGON HEALTH SCIENCE UNIVERSITY SCHOOL OF NURSING

Courses offered to students in the two-year pre-professional and professional phases (a total of 4 years as of 2002) leading to the award of Bachelor of Science in nursing (BSN) (information was obtained from the Internet):

YEAR 1 AND 2
(LOWER-DIVISION REQUIREMENTS—PRE-PROFESSIONAL—91 CRS)

Natural Sciences

1. Human Anatomy and Physiology (12 crs); 2. Microbiology (4 crs); 3. Chemistry/Biochemistry (12 crs); 4. College Algebra (3 crs); 5. Statistics (3 crs); 6. Nutrition (3 crs).

Arts and Letters and Humanities

7. Literature (3 crs); 8. English (9 crs); 9. Communication (6 crs); 10. Arts and Letters and Humanities Electives (12 crs).

Social Sciences

11. Psychology (3 crs); 12. Sociology (3 crs); 13. Human Development (3 crs); 14. Social Sciences Electives (3 crs); 14a. Electives (9 crs).

(DN: 1, 2, 13; P: 0)

Number of pharmacy or drug treatment-related courses: zero (0) out of 14 or 82 crs.

Number of diagnosis and nursing-related courses: 3 out of 14 or 16 out of 82 crs.

YEAR 3
(JUNIOR YEAR—48 TO 49 CRS)

1. Foundations for Nursing Practice (2 crs); 2. Health Assessment (5 crs); 3. Pathophysiological Process (3 crs); 4. Introduction to Clinical Nursing (5 crs); 5. Clinical Pharmacology (3 crs); 6. Clinical Decision Making in Nursing Practice (2-3 crs); 7. Ethical Issues and Legal Aspects for Nursing and Health Care (3 crs); 8. Family Nursing (3 crs); 9. Gerontological Nursing (3 crs); 10. Nursing Care of Adult with Physiological Alterations (4 crs); 11. Nursing Care of Adults with Physiological Alterations Practicum (7 crs); 12. Nursing Care

of Families during Health and Illness (3 crs); 13. Nursing Care of Families during Health and Illness Practicum (5 crs).

(DN: 1, 2, 3, 4, 6, 8, 9, 10, 11, 12, 13; P: 5)

Number of pharmacy or drug treatment-related courses: 1 out of 13 or 3 out of 48-49 crs.

Number of diagnosis and nursing-related courses: 11 out of 13 or 42-43 out of 48-49 crs.

YEAR 4
(SENIOR YEAR—44 TO 49 CRS)

1. Research in Nursing Practice (3 crs); 2. Clinical Focus (5-7 crs); 3. Leadership and Management in Nursing (3 crs); 4. Health Policy in Nursing (3 crs); 5. Mental Health Nursing (4 crs); 6. Mental Health Nursing Practicum (6 crs); 7. Community Health Nursing (4 crs); 8. Community Health Nursing Practicum (6 crs); 9. Reflective Practice Theory (2 crs); 10. Reflective Practice Practicum (7 crs); 10a. Elective (1-4 crs).

Number of pharmacy or drug treatment-related courses: zero (0) out of 10 or 43-45 crs but constitute an integral part of practicum.

Number of diagnosis and nursing-related courses: 10 out of 10 or 43-45 out of 43-45 crs.

CERTIFIED NURSE PRACTITIONER PROGRAM

Certified nurse practitioners are nurses that are allowed by law to prescribe drugs, as noted previously. It is a two-year graduate or postgraduate program (after the baccalaureate degree [BSN]) leading to the award of Master of Science in nursing (MSN). The program is designed specifically for each specialty within nursing such as family, neonatal, acute care, parent-child, primary care, psychiatric/mental health, public health, and adult nurse practitioner.

CREIGHTON UNIVERSITY SCHOOL OF NURSING

Courses offered by students in the two-year postgraduate professional phase (2001) leading to the award of Master of Science in nursing (MSN) (information was obtained from the Internet):

FAMILY NURSE PRACTITIONER (49 CRS)
YEAR 1
FALL SEMESTER (9 CRS)

1. Epidemiological Principles Applied to Health Promotion and Disease Prevention (2 crs); 2. Advanced Pathophysiology (3 crs); 3. Informatics in Advanced Nursing Practices (2 crs); 4. Theoretical Foundations of Advance Nursing Practice (2 crs).

(DN: 1, 2, 3, 4; P: 0)

SPRING SEMESTER (11 CRS)

1. Bioethics and Nursing (2 crs); 2. Advanced Health Assessment and Diagnostic Reasoning (2/2-4 crs); 3. Research Design and Statistical Reasoning (3 crs); 4. Health Care Policy, Organization, and Financing I (2 crs).

(DN: 1. 2; P: 0)

SUMMER SESSION (10 CRS)

1. Advanced Pharmacology (3 crs); 2. Adult Primary Care I (3/2-5 crs); 3. Health Care Policy, Organization, and Financing II (2 crs).

(DN: 2; P: 1)

Number of pharmacy or drug treatment-related courses: 1 out of 11 or 3 out of 30 crs.

Number of diagnosis and nursing-related courses: 7 out of 11 or 21 out of 30 crs.

YEAR 2
FALL SEMESTER (10 CRS)

1. Research Utilization (3 crs); 2. Human Diversity and Social Issues in Health Care (2 crs); 3. Adult Primary Care II (3/2-5 crs).

(DN: 3; P: 0)

SPRING SEMESTER (9 CRS)

1. Maternal/Child Care Management (3/2-5 crs); 2. FNP Practicum (4 crs).

(DN: 1, 2; P: 0)

Number of pharmacy or drug treatment-related courses: zero (0) out of 5 or 19 crs.

Number of diagnosis and nursing-related courses: 3 out of 5 or 14 out of 19 crs.

ADULT NURSE PRACTITIONER
YEAR 1
FALL SEMESTER (9 CRS)

1. Epidemiological Principles Applied to Health Promotion and Disease Prevention (2 crs); 2. Advanced Pathophysiology (3 crs); 3. Informatics in Advance Nursing Practice (2 crs); 4. Theoretical Foundations of Advanced Nursing Practice (2 crs).

(DN: 1, 2, 3, 4; P: 0)

SPRING SEMESTER (11 CRS)

1. Bioethics and Nursing (2 crs); 2. Advanced Health Assessment and Diagnostic Reasoning (2/2-4 crs); 3. Research Design and Statistical Reasoning (3 crs); 4. Health Care Policy, Organization, and Financing I (2 crs).

(DN: 1. 2; P: 0)

SUMMER SESSION (10 CRS)
1. Advanced Pharmacology (3 crs); 2. Adult Primary Care I (3/2-5 crs); 3. Health Care Policy, Organization, and Financing II (2 crs).

(DN: 2; P: 1)

Number of pharmacy or drug treatment-related courses: 1 out of 11 or 3 out of 30 crs.

Number of diagnosis and nursing-related courses: 7 out of 11 or 21 out of 30 crs.

YEAR 2
FALL SEMESTER (10 CRS)
1. Research Utilization (3 crs); 2. Human Diversity and Social Issues in Health Care (2 crs); 3. Adult Primary Care II (3/2-5 crs).

(DN: 3; P: 0)

SPRING SEMESTER
1. ANP Practicum (6 crs).

(DN: 1; P: 0)

Number of pharmacy or drug treatment-related courses: zero (0) out of 4 or 16 crs.

Number of diagnosis and nursing-related courses: 2 out of 4 or 14 out of 16 crs.

UNIVERSITY OF KENTUCKY COLLEGE OF NURSING

Courses offered to students in the two-year postgraduate professional phase (2002) leading to the award of Master of Science in nursing (MSN) (information was obtained from the Internet):

ACUTE CARE NURSE PRACTITIONER (44 CRS)
YEAR 1
FALL SEMESTER (10 CRS)

1. Theoretical Basis for Advanced Practice Nursing (2 crs); 2. Primary Care Advanced Practice Seminar (3 crs); 3. Advanced Health Assessment (2 crs); 4. Pathophysiology (3 crs).

(DN: 1, 2, 3, 4; P: 0)

SPRING SEMESTER (10 CRS)

1. Clinical Reasoning in Advanced Practice Nursing (3 crs); 2. Applications of Advanced Health Assessment (2 crs); 3. Advanced Practice Nursing Care of Acutely Ill Adults (2 crs); 4. Pharmacology (3 crs).

(DN: 1, 2, 3; P: 4)

SUMMER (2 CRS)

1. Comprehensive Patient Management I (2 crs).

(DN: 1; P: 0)

Number of pharmacy or drug treatment-related courses: 1 out of 9 or 3 out of 22 crs.

Number of diagnosis and nursing-related courses: 8 out of 9 or 19 out of 22 crs.

YEAR 2
FALL SEMESTER (12 CRS)

1. Research Methods in Advanced Practice Nursing (3 crs); 2. Advanced Practice Nursing Care of Critically Ill Adults (6 crs); 3. Leadership in Advanced Practice Nursing (3 crs).

(DN: 2, 3; P: 0)

SPRING SEMESTER (10 CRS)

1. Evidence-based Nursing Practice (3 crs); 2. Comprehensive Patient Management II (4 crs); 2a. Elective (3 crs).

(DN: 1, 2; P: 0)

Number of pharmacy or drug treatment-related courses: zero (0) out of 5 or 19 crs.

Number of diagnosis and nursing-related courses: 4 out of 5 or 16 out of 19 crs.

PARENT-CHILD SPECIALTY (PRACTITIONER)
YEAR 1
FALL SEMESTER (10 CRS)

1. Theoretical Basis for Advanced Practice Nursing (2 crs); 2. Research Methods in Advanced Practice Nursing (3 crs); 3. Advanced Health Assessment (2 crs); 4. Pathophysiology (3 crs).

(DN: 1, 3, 4; P: 0)

SPRING SEMESTER

1. Clinical Reasoning in Advanced Practice Nursing (3 crs); 2. Applications of Advanced Health Assessment (2 crs); 3. Advance Parent-Child Nursing Seminar (3 crs); 4. Pharmacology (3 crs).

(DN: 1, 2, 3; P: 4)

SUMMER (2 CRS)

1. Comprehensive Patient Management I (2 crs).

(DN: 1; P: 0)

Number of pharmacy or drug treatment-related courses: 1 out of 9 or 3 out of 23 crs.

Number of diagnosis and nursing-related courses: 7 out of 9 or 17 out of 23 crs.

YEAR 2
FALL SEMESTER (9 CRS)

1. Advanced Nursing Care for Families Pre-conception through Adolescence I (6 crs); 2. Leadership in Advanced Practice Nursing (3 crs).

(DN: 1, 2; P: 0)

SPRING SEMESTER (10-12 CRS)
1. Evidence-based Nursing Practice (3 crs); 2. Advanced Nursing Care for Families Pre-conception through Adolescence II (4 crs); 3. Comprehensive Patient Management II (2 crs); 3a. Elective (3 crs).

(DN: 1, 2, 3; P: 0)

Number of pharmacy or drug treatment-related courses: zero (0) out of 5 or 16-18 crs.

Number of diagnosis and nursing-related courses: 5 out of 5 or 16-18 out of 16-18 crs.

UNIVERSITY OF IOWA COLLEGE OF NURSING

Courses offered to students in the two-year post graduate professional phase (2002) leading to the award of Master of Science in nursing (MSN)[18] (not included in data analysis):

NURSE PRACTITIONER
Consist of 46-52 semester hours with 12 semester hours from:

1. Leadership in Nursing (3 shrs); 2. Research Application (3 shrs); 3. Health Policy and Economics (3 shrs); 4. Nursing Informatics and Technology (3 shrs).

(DN: 1, 4; P: 0)

Others are clinical core in advanced: 1. Physiology; 2. Pharmacology; 3. Health Assessment; 4. Health Promotion; 5. A professional role course.

(DN: 1, 3, 4, 5; P: 2)

The course outline detail is not available from the catalogs but would be similar to Creighton University and University of Kentucky College of Nursing

OREGON HEALTH SCIENCE UNIVERSITY SCHOOL OF NURSING

Courses offered to students in the two-year postgraduate professional phase (2002) leading to the award of Master of Science in nursing (MSN) (information was obtained from the Internet):

Core Courses (15 crs)

For Certified Nurse Practitioner and Midwifery
1. Evidence-based Decision Making in Advanced Practice Nursing (3 crs); 2. Design, Conduct, and Analysis of Population-based Research I (3 crs); 3. Design, Conduct, and Analysis of Population-based Research II (3 crs); 4. Human Diversity and Social Issues (3 crs); 5. Policy, Organization, and Financing of Health Care (3 crs).

(DN: 1; P: 0)

ADULT NURSE PRACTITIONER (53 + 15 = 68 CRS)
1. Practicum in Primary Care Management I (2 crs); 2. Practicum in Primary Care Management II (4 crs); 3. Practicum in Primary Care Management III (3 crs); 4. Practicum in Primary Care Management IV (8 crs); 5. Health Promotion and Health Protection (3 crs); 6. Regulatory Physiology and Pathophysiology (5 crs); 7. Health Assessment for Advanced Practice Nursing (4 crs); 8. Reproductive Health Care Management (3 crs); 9. Applied Pharmacology I (2 crs); 10. Introduction to Primary Care Management (3 crs); 11. Adult Primary Care Management I (3 crs); 12. Adult Primary Care Management II (3 crs); 13. Professional Issues for Nurse Practitioners (3 crs); 14. Advanced Primary Care Management II (3 crs).

(DN: 1, 2, 3, 4, 5, 6, 7, 8, 10, 11, 12, 13, 14; P: 9)

Number of pharmacy or drug treatment-related courses: 1 out of 19 or 2 out of 68 crs.

Number of diagnosis and nursing-related courses: 14 out of 19 or 56 out of 68 crs.

NURSE MIDWIFERY PROGRAM
NURSE MIDWIFERY (65 + 15 = 80 CRS)

1. Practicum in Antepartum and Postpartum Management (2 crs); 2. Practicum in Nurse-Midwifery, Management of the Intrapartum Period (3 crs); 3. Practicum in Nurse-Midwifery Management I (3 crs); 4. Practicum in Advanced Women's health care Management (2 crs); 5. Practicum in Nurse-Midwifery Management II (4 crs); 6. Advanced Practicum in Nurse-Midwifery (8 crs); 7. Health Promotion and Health Protection (3 crs); 8. Regulatory Physiology and Pathophysiology (5 crs); 9. Health Assessment for Advanced Practice Nursing (4 crs); 10. Reproductive Health Care Management (3 crs); 11. Applied Pharmacology I (2 crs); 12. Applied Pharmacology II (2 crs); 13. Introduction to Primary Care Management (3 crs); 14. Adult Primary Care Management I (1 cr); 15. Adult Primary Care Management II (1 cr); 16. Professional Issues for Nurse Practitioners (3 crs); 17. Nurse-Midwifery Management of the Intrapartum Period (3 crs); 18. Management of the Newborn (3 crs); 19. Professional Issues in Nurse-Midwifery (1 cr); 20. Psychological, Cultural, and Social Context of Women's Health Care (3 crs); 21. Antepartum and Postpartum Management (4 crs); 22. Advanced Women's Health Care Management (2 crs).

(DN: 1, 2, 3, 4, 5, 6, 7, 8, 9, 10, 13, 14, 15, 16, 17, 18, 19, 21, 22; P: 11, 12)

Number of pharmacy or drug treatment-related courses: 2 out of 27 or 4 out of 80 crs

Number of diagnosis and nursing/midwifery-related courses: 20 out of 27 or 67 out of 80 crs.

SEATTLE MIDWIFERY SCHOOL

Courses offered to students in the two-year postgraduate professional phase (2002) (information was obtained from the Internet):

FIRST QUARTER (14.5 CRS)

1. Orientation (1 cr); 2. Well Women Health and Assessment (3.5 crs); 3. Midwifery Care I: Introduction to Midwifery (4 crs); 4. Education and Counseling for Midwives (2 crs); 5. Basic Nutrition (2.5 crs); 6. Midwifery/Nursing Skills I (1.5 crs).

(DN: 2, 3, 6; P: 0)

Second Quarter (12 crs)
1. Midwifery Care II: Pregnancy and Prenatal Care (4 crs); 2. Prenatal Nutrition (2 crs); 3. Midwifery/Nursing Skills II (1.5 crs); 4. Gynecology (4.5 crs).

(DN: 1, 3, 4; P: 0)

Third Quarter (9.5 crs)
1. Midwifery III: Advanced Pregnancy and Prenatal Care B (4.5 crs); 2. Introduction to Pharmacology/Treatments (2 crs); 3. Professional Issues Seminar I: History of Midwifery/Medicine (3 crs); 4. Perinatal Epidemiology (1 cr).

(DN: 1, 4; P: 2)

Fourth Quarter (8.5 crs)
1. Midwifery Care IV: Labor and Birth (5.5 crs); 2. Professional Issues Seminar II: The Rise of the Modern Midwife in North America (2 crs); 3. Perinatal Epidemiology II (1 cr).

(DN: 1, 3; P: 0)

Fifth Quarter (8.5 crs)
1. Midwifery Care V: Labor and Birth (5.5 crs); 2. Professional Issues Seminar III: The Rise of Modern Midwife in North America (2 crs); 3. Perinatal Epidemiology 2 (1 cr).

(DN: 1, 3; P: 0)

Six Quarter (6.5 crs)
1. Midwifery Care VI: Challenges in Practice (4 crs); 2. Professional Issues Seminar IV: Cross-cultural Perspectives (1.5 crs).

(DN: 1; P: 0)

Seventh Quarter (5 crs)
1.Midwifery Care VII: Complications (3 crs); 2. Professional Issues Seminar V: Health Care Systems and Health Policy (2 crs).

(DN: 1, 2; P: 0)

Eighth Quarter (65.5 crs)
1. Professional Issues Seminar VI: The Business of Midwifery (2 crs); 2. Basic and Advance Clinical Seminars (13.5 crs); 3. Basic and Advanced Practica (50 crs).

(DN: 2, 3; P: 0)

Number of pharmacy or drug treatment-related courses: 1 out of 27 or 2 out of 130 crs.

Number of diagnosis and nursing/midwifery-related courses: 17 out of 27 or 110 out of 130 crs.

SCHOOLS OF PHARMACY DOCTOR OF PHARMACY DEGREE PROGRAM

The 1997 *U.S. News & World Report* rating for Doctor of Pharmacy programs obtained from the Internet in March 2001 will be use as a guide here. The rating is based on the average reputation score of 5 as the highest point, and it is used as a modality for choosing the top three schools. The three middle and bottom schools are a conglomeration of this rating, and the popular general school ratings, obtained from *U.S. News & World Report*, for undergraduate, master's, and PhD programs. (SP = school of pharmacy; GS = general schools.)

#	TOP-RANKING SCHOOLS	SP	GS
1.	University of California, San Francisco	4.5	Top 50
2.	University of Texas, Austin	4.2	Top 50
3.	University of Kentucky	4.0	2nd Tier

#	MIDDLE-RANKING SCHOOLS	SP	GS
1.	St. Louis University	2.9	2nd Tier
2.	Auburn University	2.8	2nd Tier
3.	University of Missouri	2.8	3rd Tier

#	LOW-RANKING SCHOOLS	SP	GS
1.	University of Colorado	None Top	4th Tier
2.	University of Montana	None Top	4th Tier
3.	Texas Southern University, Houston	None Top	4th Tier

UNIVERSITY OF CALIFORNIA-SAN FRANCISCO, SCHOOL OF PHARMACY

Courses offered to students in the four-year professional phase leading to the award of Doctor of Pharmacy degree (PharmD) without residency requirement (information obtained from the Internet):

YEAR 1
FALL QUARTER (16 CRS)

1. Pharmacy Practice I (4 crs); 2. Biopharmaceutics (3.5 crs); 3. Thermodynamics (4 crs); 4. Biostatics (2.5 crs); 5. Elective: Pathway Introductions (2 crs).

(D: 0; P: 1, 2, 3, 4)

WINTER QUARTER (17 CRS)

1. Pharmacy Practice II (4 crs); 2. Biochemistry (4 crs); 3. Advanced Organic Chemistry (3 crs); 4. Histology (2 crs); 5. Chemical Kinetics (2 crs); 6. Study Design (2 crs).

(D: 2, 4; P: 1, 5, 6)

SPRING QUARTER (17 CRS)

1. Pharmacy Practice III (3 crs); 2. Gross Anatomy (3 crs); 3. Biopharmaceutics (3 crs); 4. Drug Metabolism (3 crs); 5. Introduction to Health Care Informatics (3 crs); 5a. Electives (2 crs).

(D: 2; P: 1, 3, 4)

Number of pharmacy or drug treatment-related courses: 10 out of 15 or 31 out of 46 crs plus a major part of rotations, otherwise tagged pathway.

Number of diagnosis-related courses: 3 out of 15 or 9 out of 46 crs plus an integral part of rotations, otherwise tagged pathway.

YEAR 2
FALL QUARTER (17 CRS)

1. Immunology (3 crs); 2. Pharmaceutical Chemistry/Pharmacology (5 crs); 3. Physiology (5 crs); 4. Pharmacokinetics (4 crs)

(D: 1, 3; P: 2, 4)

WINTER QUARTER (17 CRS)
1. Health Policy (3 crs); 2. Pharmaceutical Chemistry/Pharmacology (5 crs); 3. Physiology (3 crs); 4. Pharmacokinetics (3 crs); 5. Law and Ethics (3 crs).

(D: 3; P: 2, 4)

SPRING QUARTER (17-18 CRS)
1. Therapeutics (6 crs); 2. Pharmaceutical Chemistry/Pharmacology (5 crs); 3. Microbiology (4 crs); 3a. Elective (2-3 crs).

(D: 3; P: 1, 2)

Number of pharmacy or drug treatment-related courses: 6 out of 12 or 29 out of 49 crs.

Number of diagnosis-related courses: 4 out of 12 or 15 out of 49 crs.

YEAR 3
FALL QUARTER (17 CRS)
1. Therapeutics (6 crs); 2. Pharmaceutical Chemistry/Pharmacology (4 crs); 3. Pathology (3 crs); 4. Drug Information (2 crs); 5. Elective/Pathway (2 crs).

(D: 3; P: 1, 2, 4)

WINTER QUARTER (17 CRS)
1. Therapeutics (6 crs); 2. Management (2 crs); 3. Health Economics (2 crs); 4. Elective/Pathway (7 crs).

(D: 0; P: 1, 3)

Number of pharmacy or drug treatment-related courses without pathway: 5 out of 7 or 20 out of 25 crs plus a major part of rotations or pathway.

Number of diagnosis-related courses without pathway: 1 out of 7 or 3 out of 25 crs plus an integral part of rotations, otherwise tagged pathway.

SPRING QUARTER (12-15 CRS)
1. Clerkship (0 or 12 crs); 2. Elective/Pathway (0 or 15 crs).

The PharmD program has three pathway curricula that are introduced in the first year and begin in third year:

1. Pharmaceutical Care; 2. Pharmaceutical Health Policy and Management; 3. Pharmaceutical Sciences.

Pharmaceutical care sample schedule is given below:

YEAR	FALL	WINTER	SPRING	SUMMER
3	CORE COURSES CP 130 (6 crs) CP 135A (1.5 crs) Path 135 (3 crs) PC/Pcol 131 (4 crs)	CORE COURSES CP 131 (6 crs) CP 133 (2 crs) CP 134 (2 crs) CP 135B (0.5 crs) Pathway courses CP 137 (3) Electives as needed	PATHWAY COURSES Elective appes (12 crs)	PATHWAY COURSES CP 148A (6 crs) CP 148C (2 crs) CP 148B (6 crs) CP 148D (2 crs)
4	PATHWAY COURSES CP 149A (6 crs) CP 149C (2 crs) CP 149B (6 crs) CP 149D (2 crs)	PATHWAY COURSES Elective appes (2 crs) CP 150 (2 crs) Electives as needed	Electives as needed to full graduation requirements.	

Some of the available CP courses are:

CP 137—Advanced Topics in Clinical Care (3 crs).

CP 148 A & B—Acute Care: Advanced Practice Experience (6 crs).

CP 148 C & D—Acute Care Supplemental Advanced Practice Experience (2 crs).

CP 149 A & B—Advanced Pharmacy Practice Experience in Ambulatory and Long-term Care (6 crs).

CP 149 C & D—Supplemental Advanced Pharmacy Practice Experience in Ambulatory and Long-term Care (6 crs).

CP 170s 180s—Elective Advanced Pharmacy Practice Experience.

CP 150—Pharmaceutical Care Pathway Project (2 crs).

Number of pharmacy or drug treatment-related courses: Constitute a major part of the rotations or clerkship, otherwise tagged pathway.

Number of diagnosis-related courses: Constitute an integral part of the rotations or clerkship, otherwise tagged pathway.

Residency: Available as postgraduate program.

UNIVERSITY OF TEXAS, AUSTIN, COLLEGE OF PHARMACY

Courses offered to students in the four-year professional phase leading to the award of Doctor of Pharmacy degree (PharmD) without residency requirement (information obtained from the Internet, 2001):

YEAR 1
FALL SEMESTER (16 CRS)

1. Pharmaceutical Biochemistry (3 crs); 2. Physical and Chemical Principles of Drugs (3 crs); 3. Physical and Chemical Principles of Drugs Laboratory (1 crs); 4. Function and Anatomy of Human Systems I (3 crs); 5. Basic Medicinal Chemistry Principles (1 cr); 6. Basic Medicinal Chemistry Principles Laboratory (1 cr); 7. Pharmacy Administration I (2 crs); 8. Pharmacy Administration Laboratory (1 cr); 9. Introduction to Pharmacy (1 cr).
(D: 1, 4; P: 2, 3, 5, 6, 9)

SPRING SEMESTER (16 CRS)

1. Introduction to Pharmacy (1 cr); 2. Macromolecular Chemistry and Biotechnology (2 crs); 3. Biopharmaceutics and Pharmacokinetics (3 crs); 4. Biopharmaceutics and Pharmacokinetics Laboratory (1 cr); 5. Function and

Anatomy of Human Systems II (2 crs); 6. Principles of General Pathology (2 crs); 7. Basic Pharmacology Principles (1 cr); 8. Pharmaceutics I (3 crs); 9. Pharmaceutics I Laboratory (1 cr)

(D: 5, 6; P: 1, 2, 3, 4, 7, 8, 9)

Number of pharmacy or drug treatment-related courses: 12 out of 18 or 19 out of 36 crs.

Number of diagnosis-related courses: 4 out of 18 or 10 out of 36 crs.

YEAR 2
FALL SEMESTER (13 CRS)

1. Introduction to Drug Information (1 cr); 2. Pharmacotherapeutics IA (3 crs); 3. Pharmacotherapeutics IB (5 crs); 4. Pharmacotherapeutics I Laboratory (1 cr); 5. Pharmacy Ethics and Professional Communications (3 crs).

(D: 0; P: 1, 2, 3, 4)

SPRING SEMESTER (13 CRS)

1. Pharmacy Administration II (3 crs); 2. Pharmacotherapeutics IIA (3 crs); 3. Pharmacotherapeutics IIB (2 crs); 4. Pharmacotherapeutics IIC (3 crs); 5. Pharmacotherapeutic II Laboratory (1 cr); 6. Experimental Pharmacy Practice and Patient Counseling (1 cr).

(D: 0; P: 2, 3, 4, 5, 6)

SUMMER SESSION (6 CRS)

1. Pharmacotherapeutics IIIA (3 crs); 2. Pharmacotherapeutics IIIB (2 crs); 3. Pharmacotherapeutic III Laboratory: Bacterial Infectious Diseases (1 cr).

(D: 0; P: 1, 2, 3)

Number of pharmacy or drug treatment-related courses: 12 out of 14 or 29 out of 32 crs.

Number of diagnosis-related courses: zero (0) out of 14 or 32 crs.

YEAR 3
FALL SEMESTER (7 CRS)
1. Basic Intravenous Admixtures (1 cr); 2. Basic Intravenous Admixtures Laboratory (1 cr); 3. Pharmacy Law (2 crs); 4. Nonprescription Drug Products (3 crs); 4a. Professional Elective (2-3 crs).

(D: 0; P: 1, 2, 4)

SPRING SEMESTER (17 CRS)
1. Applied Pharmacokinetics (3 crs); 2. Patient Assessment Skills Laboratory (3 crs); 3. Pharmacoeconomics (3 crs); 4. Drug Literature Evaluation and Biostatistics (3 crs); 5. Advanced Pharmacotherapy (3 crs); 6. Advanced Pharmacotherapy Laboratory (2 crs).

(D: 2; P: 1, 3, 4, 5, 6)

Number of pharmacy or drug treatment-related courses: 8 out of 10 or 19 out of 24 crs.

Number of diagnosis-related courses: 1 out of 10 or 3 out of 24 crs.

YEAR 4
Summer Session (6 crs)—Rotations (internships)

1. Acute Care Pharmacy Practice (6 crs).

FALL SEMESTER (18 CRS)
1. Pharmacy Practice I Elective (6 crs); 2. Institutional Pharmacy Practice (6 crs); 3. Ambulatory Care Pharmacy Practice (6 crs).

SPRING SEMESTER (18 CRS)
1. Selective in Pharmacy Practice I (6 crs); 2. Acute Care Pharmacy Practice II (6 crs); 3. Elective in Pharmacy Practice II (6 crs).

Number of pharmacy or drug treatment-related courses: Constitute a major part of the rotations.

Number of diagnosis-related courses: Constitute an integral part of the rotations.

UNIVERSITY OF KENTUCKY COLLEGE OF PHARMACY

Courses offered to students in the four-year professional phase leading to the award of Doctor of Pharmacy degree (PharmD) without residency requirement (information obtained from the Internet, 2001):

YEAR 1
FALL SEMESTER (19 CRS)

1. Physiological Basis for Therapeutics I (4 crs); 2. Physiological Chemistry and Molecular Biology I (3 crs); 3. Pharmacological Basis of Therapeutics: Antibiotics (3 crs); 4. Basic Principles of Pharmaceutical Science: Drug Design (3 crs); 5. Nonprescription Pharmaceuticals and Supplies I (2 crs); 6. Contemporary Aspects of Pharmacy Practice I (4 crs).

(D: 2; P: 1, 3, 4, 5, 6)

SPRING SEMESTER (20 CRS)

1. Physiological Basis for Therapeutics II (4 crs); 2. Physiological Chemistry and Molecular Biology II (3 crs); 3. Pharmacological Basis of Therapeutics: Nutrition, Health Promotions (3 crs); 4. Basic Principles of Pharmaceutical Science: Drug Form Design (3 crs); 5. Nonprescription Pharmaceuticals and Supplies II (2 crs); 6. Early Pharmacy Practice Experience (4 crs); 7. Contemporary Aspects of Pharmacy Practice II (4 crs).

(D: 2; P: 1, 3, 4, 5, 6, 7)

Number of pharmacy or drug treatment-related courses: 11 out of 13 or 31out of 39 crs.

Number of diagnosis-related courses: 2 out of 13 or 8 out of 39 crs.

YEAR 2
FALL SEMESTER (17 CRS)

1. Pharmacological Basis for Therapeutics: Nervous System (5 crs); 2. Pharmacological Basis for Therapeutics: Immunology/Biotechnology (3 crs); 3. Pharmacological Basis for Therapeutics: Endocrine Systems (3 crs); 4. Contemporary Aspects of Pharmacy Practice III (6 crs).

(D: 0; P: 1, 2, 3, 4)

Spring Semester (17 crs)
1. Pharmacological Basis for Therapeutics: Cardiopulmonary and Renal System (5 crs); 2. Basic Pharmaceutical Science: New/Novel Dosage Forms (3 crs); 3. Applied Biopharmaceutics and Pharmacokinetics (4 crs); 4. Contemporary Aspects of Pharmacy Practice IV (5 crs).

(D: 0; P: 1, 2, 3, 4)

Number of pharmacy or drug treatment-related courses: 8 out of 8 or 34 out of 34 crs.

Number of diagnosis-related courses: zero (0) out of 8 or 34 crs.

YEAR 3
Fall Semester (17 crs)
1. Integrated Therapeutics I (7 crs); 2. Disease Processes I (3 crs); 3. Contemporary Aspects of Pharmacy Practice V (7 crs).

(D: 2; P: 1, 3)

Spring Semester (17 crs)
1. Integrated Therapeutics II (7 crs); 2. Disease Processes II (3 crs); 3. Contemporary Aspects of Pharmacy Practice VI (7 crs).

(D: 2; P: 1, 3)

Number of pharmacy or drug treatment-related courses: 4 out of 6 or 28 out of 34 crs.

Number of diagnosis-related courses: 2 out of 6 or 6 out of 34 crs.

YEAR 4
Clerkship
1. Pharmacy Practice Clerkship (4 crs), repeated up to a maximum of 44 credits and 40 or more laboratory hours per week. Rotation varies in content and requirements.

Number of pharmacy or drug treatment-related courses: Constitute a major part of the clerkship.

Number of diagnosis-related courses: Constitute an integral part of the clerkship.

Residency: Optional.

ST. LOUIS COLLEGE OF PHARMACY

This is the only university with a pharmacy program that admits students directly with high school diploma into the Bachelor of Science degree program in pharmacy (BS Pharm), then students are given the option of switching to the Doctor of Pharmacy degree (PharmD) in the ninth semester, fifth year. Thus, the tenth semester is used to either complete the BSc or continue with the PharmD program followed by a nine-month clerkship or externship in the sixth year. This school was excluded from data analysis because of inadequate information about individual courses. Courses offered to students in the six-year pre-professional and professional phase leading to the award of Doctor of Pharmacy degree (PharmD) without residency requirement[19] (information obtained from the catalog, 2001):

Semester hours required for entry-level degrees

COURSES	BSc	PharmD
Liberal arts studies, which include the social sciences and 10 or 12 hours of electives	22	24
Written and oral communication Skills	9	9
Mathematics and statistics	6	6
Biological sciences	31	31
Chemical and physical sciences	31	31
Law and management	9	9
Pharmaceutics and dispensing	15	15
Therapeutics, drug information, and advanced pharmacy practice topics	14	25
Clerkships and externships	12	32

COURSES	BSc	PharmD
Professional electives	7	9
Unspecified electives	6	6
Seminars	1	3
Total	163	200

Number of pharmacy or drug treatment-related courses: about 95 -126 out of 200 including clerkship for PharmD and 80 out of 163 for BSc.

Number of diagnosis-related courses: about 31 out of 200 for PharmD and 163 for BSc.

Residency: Optional.

AUBURN UNIVERSITY SCHOOL OF PHARMACY

Courses offered to students in the four-year professional phase leading to the award of Doctor of Pharmacy degree (PharmD) without residency requirement (information obtained from the Internet, 2001):

YEAR 1
FALL SEMESTER (17 CRS)

1. Mammalian Physiology (6 crs); 2. Biochemistry; 3. Pharmaceutics I (2 crs); 4. Pharmaceutics I Lab (1 cr); 5. Pharmacy Care System I (3 crs); 6. Patient Assessment (1 cr); 7. Pharmacy Practice Experience I (1 cr).

(D: 1, 2, 6; P: 3, 4, 5, 7)

SPRING SEMESTER (18 CRS)

1. Biochemistry II (3 crs); 2. Principles of Drug Action I (4 crs); 3. Drug Literature I (2 crs); 4. Pharmacy Care System II (3 crs); 5. Pharmaceutics II (2 crs); 6. Pharmaceutics II Lab (1 cr); 7. Biopharmaceutics (2 crs); 8. Pharmacy Practice Experience II (1 cr).

(D: 1; P: 2, 3, 4, 5, 6, 7, 8)

Number of pharmacy or drug treatment-related courses: 11 out of 15 or 22 out of 35 crs.

Number of diagnosis-related courses: 4 out of 15 or 13 out of 35 crs.

YEAR 2
FALL SEMESTER (19 CRS)

1. Human Pathology (3 crs); 2. General Microbiology (4 crs); 3. Principles of Drug Action II (4 crs); 4. Principles of Pharmacokinetics (3 crs); 5. Pharmacy Care System III (2 crs); 6. Drug Literature II (2 crs); 7. Pharmacy Practice Experience III (1 cr).

(D: 1, 2; P: 3, 4, 5, 6, 7)

SPRING SEMESTER (18 CRS)

1. Patient Assessment II (2 crs); 2. Principles of Antimicrobial Therapy (3 crs); 3. Pharmaceutical Biotechnology (2 crs); 4. Pharmacy Care System IV (2 crs); 5. Pharmacotherapy I (3 crs); 6. Pharmacotherapy II (3 crs); 7. Pharmacy Practice Experience IV (1 cr); 7a. Professional Electives (2 crs)

(D: 1; P: 2, 3, 4, 5, 6, 7)

Number of pharmacy or drug treatment-related courses: 11 out of 14 or 26 out of 37 crs.

Number of diagnosis-related courses: 3 out of 14 or 9 out of 35 crs.

YEAR 3
FALL SEMESTER (17 CRS)

1. Pharmacotherapy III (3 crs); 2. Pharmacotherapy IV (3 crs); 3. Pharmacotherapy V (3 crs); 4. Pharmacotherapy VI (3 crs); 5. Pharmacy Practice Experience V (1 cr); 5a. Professional Elective (4 crs).

(D: 0; P: 1, 2, 3, 4, 5)

Spring Semester (17 crs)
1. Drug-induced Disease (2 crs); 2. Pharmacotherapy VII (3 crs); 3. Pharmacotherapy VIII (3 crs); 4. Pharmacotherapy IX (3 crs); 5. Pharmacotherapy X (3 crs); 6. Pharmacy Practice Experience VI (1 cr); 6a. Professional Elective (2 crs).

(D: 0; P: 1, 2, 3, 4, 5, 6)

Number of pharmacy or drug treatment-related courses: 11 out of 11 or 28 out of 28 crs.

Number of diagnosis-related courses: zero (0) out of 13 or 28 crs.

Year 4
Fall and Spring Semesters (15 & 17 crs)
1. Drug Information (3 crs); 2. Community Pharmaceutical Care (3 crs); 3. Internal Medicine (3 crs); 4. Medical Specialties (3 crs); 5. Primary/Ambulatory Care I (3 crs); 6. Primary/Ambulatory Care II (3 crs); 7. Primary/Ambulatory Care III (3 crs); 8. Clerkship Elective (9 crs); 9. Clinical Seminar (2 crs); 10. Longitudinal Pharmacy Services (0 cr).

Number of pharmacy or drug treatment-related courses: Constitute a major part of the clerkships/rotations.

Number of diagnosis-related courses: Constitute an integral part of the clerkships/rotations.

Residency: Optional.

UNIVERSITY OF MISSOURI, KANSAS CITY, COLLEGE OF PHARMACY

Courses offered to students in the four-year professional phase leading to the award of Doctor of Pharmacy degree (PharmD) without residency requirement (information obtained from the Internet, 2001):

YEAR 1
FALL SEMESTER (16 CRS)

1. Medicinal Chemistry I (3 crs); 2. Pharmaceutical I (4 crs); 3. Human Biochemistry I (3 crs); 4. Pharmacy Physiology I (3 crs); 4a. General Elective (3 crs).

(D: 3, 4; P: 1, 2)

SPRING SEMESTER (19 CRS)

1. Pharmaceutical II (4 crs); 2. Medicinal Chemistry II (3 crs); 3. Human Biochemistry II (3 crs); 4. Pharmacy Physiology II (3 crs); 5. Personal Communications in Pharmacy (3 crs); 6. Completion of sequence one of top 200 drugs: General Elective (3 crs).

(D: 3, 4; P: 1, 2, 6A)

Number of pharmacy or drug treatment-related courses: 5 out of 10 or 17 out of 32 crs.

Number of diagnosis-related courses: 4 out of 10 or 12 out of 32 crs.

YEAR 2
FALL SEMESTER (17 CRS)

1. Pharmacology I (4 crs); 2. Disease Processes for Pharmacy (6 crs); 3. Pharmacokinetics and Biopharmaceutics (4 crs); 4. Business Selective (3 crs).

(D: 2; P: 1, 3)

SPRING SEMESTER (16 CRS)

1. Pharmacology II (5 crs); 2. Therapeutics I (3 crs); 3. Toxicology (2 crs); 4. Clinical Kinetics (4 crs); 5A. Completion of sequence two of top 200 drugs: General Elective (3 crs).

(D: 0; P: 1, 2, 3, 4, 5A)

Number of pharmacy or drug treatment-related courses: 7 out of 9 or 28 out of 34 crs.

Number of diagnosis-related courses: 1 out of 9 or 34 crs.

YEAR 3
FALL SEMESTER (18 CRS)

1. Evidence-based Medicine I (3 crs); 2. Pharmacy Law and Ethics (2 crs); 3. Clinical Practice I (1 cr); 4. Therapeutics II (5 crs); 4a. Professional Electives (4 crs); 5. Health Assessment (3 crs).

(D: 5; P: 1, 3, 4)

SPRING SEMESTER (18 CRS)

1. Therapeutics III (5 crs); 2. Evidence-based Medicine II (3 crs); 3. Clinical Practice I (1 cr); 3a. General Elective (3 crs); 3b. Professional Electives (6 crs).

(D: 0; P: 1, 2, 3)

Number of pharmacy or drug treatment-related courses: 6 out of 8 or 18 out of 23 crs.

Number of diagnosis-related courses: 1 out of 8 or 3 out of 23 crs.

YEAR 4
Fall Semester (16 crs)

Four 4-credit-hour pharmacy clerkships.

SPRING SEMESTER (20 CRS)

Five 4-credit-hour-pharmacy clerkships.

Available clerkships:

1. Drug Information Clerkship; 2. Emergency Medicine Clerkship (elective); 3. Adult Patient Care Clerkship I; 4. Ambulatory Care Clerkship; 5. Psychopharmacy Clerkship; 6. Hospital Pharmacy Practice Externship (selective); 7. Adult Patient Care Clerkship; 8. Community Pharmacy Practice Externship (selective); 9. Pediatric Care Clerkship (elective); 10. Directed Individual Rotations in Pharmacy Practice I (elective); 11. Directed Individual Rotations in Pharmacy Practice II (elective).

Number of pharmacy or drug treatment-related courses: Constitute a major part of the clerkship.

Number of diagnosis-related courses: Constitute an integral part of the clerkship.

Residency: Optional.

UNIVERSITY OF COLORADO, DENVER, SCHOOL OF PHARMACY

Courses offered to students in the four-year professional phase leading to the award of Doctor of Pharmacy degree (PharmD) without residency requirement (information obtained from the Internet, 2001):

YEAR 1
FALL SEMESTER (18 CRS)

1. Professional Skills I (3 crs); 2. Seminar on Pharmacy Issues I (1 cr); 3. Experiential Practice (1 cr); 4. Pharmacy and Health Care I: Drug Information (1 cr); 5. Pharmacy and Health Care II: Health Care Economics (1 cr); 6. Pharmacy Law (2 crs); 7. Science Foundations 1: Chemistry and Pharmaceutics (3 crs); 8. Science Foundations II: Biochemistry and Cell Function (4 crs).

(D: 8; P: 1, 2, 3, 4, 5, 7)

SPRING SEMESTER (18.3 CRS)

1. Professional Skills II (3 crs); 2. Seminar on Pharmacy Issues II (1 cr); 3. Experiential Practice II (1 cr); 4. Pharmacy and Health Care II: U.S. Health Care System (2 crs); 5. Health Care Ethics (1.3 crs); 6. Principles of Drug Action (3 crs); 7. Integrated Organ System I: Physiology (4 crs); 8. Integrated Organ System II: Autonomics Autoloids (3 crs).

(D: 7, 8; P: 1, 2, 3, 6)

Number of pharmacy or drug treatment-related courses: 10 out of 16 or 20 out of 36.3 crs.

Number of diagnosis-related courses: 3 out of 16 or 8 out of 36.3 crs.

YEAR 2
FALL SEMESTER (19 CRS)

1. Professional Skills III (3 crs); 2. Seminar on Pharmacy Issues III (1 cr); 3. Experiential Practice III (1 cr); 4. Pharmacy and Health Care III: Evidence-based Practice (2 crs); 5. Clinical Science Foundations (3 crs); 6. Integrated Organ System III: F/E, A/B, and Renal (2 crs); 7. Integrated Organ System IV: Cardiovascular (3 crs); 8. Integrated Organ System V: Cardio-pulmonary (4 crs).

(D: 6, 7, 8; P: 1, 2, 3, 4, 5)

SPRING SEMESTER (19 CRS)

1. Professional Skills IV (3 crs); 2. Seminar on Pharmacy Issues IV (1 cr); 3. Experiential Practice IV (2 cr); 4. Pharmacy and Health Care IV: Informatics—Humanistic Issues (2 crs); 5. Integrated Organ System VI: Immunology (3 crs); 6. Integrated Organ System VII: GI, Nutrition (4 crs); 7. Integrated Organ System VIII: CNS (4 crs).

(D: 5, 6, 7; P: 1, 2, 3, 4)

Number of pharmacy or drug treatment-related courses: 9 out of 15 or 18 out of 38 crs.

Number of diagnosis-related courses: 6 out of 15 or 20 out of 38 crs.

YEAR 3
FALL SEMESTER (18 CRS)

1. Professional Skills V (3 crs); 2. Seminar on Pharmacy Issues V (1 cr); 3. Experiential Practice V (2 cr); 4. Pharmacy and Health Care V: Population Base Practice (2 crs); 5. Integrated Organ System IX: Infectious Diseases (3 crs); 6. Integrated Organ System X: Endocrine, Rheum, Other (4 crs); 6a. Elective (2 crs).

(D: 5, 6; P: 1, 2, 3, 4)

SPRING SEMESTER (18 CRS)

1. Professional Skills VI (3 crs); 2. Seminar on Pharmacy Issues VI (1 cr); 3. Experiential Practice VI (2 cr); 4. Comprehensive Patient Care (8 crs); 4a. Elective (2 crs); 4b. Elective (2 crs).

(D: 0; P: 1, 2, 3, 4)

Number of pharmacy or drug treatment-related courses: 8 out of 10 or 22 out of 30 crs.

Number of diagnosis-related courses: 2 out of 10 or 7 out of 30 crs.

YEAR 4 (42 CRS)
SUMMER SESSION (6 CRS)
1. Clerkship (6 crs).

FALL SEMESTER (18 CRS)
1. Three 6-credit-hour clerkships.

SPRING SEMESTER (18 CRS)
1. Three 6-credit-hour clerkships.

Number of pharmacy or drug treatment-related courses: Constitute a major part of the clerkship.

Number of diagnosis-related courses: Constitute an integral part of the clerkship.

Residency: Optional.

UNIVERSITY OF MONTANA SCHOOL OF PHARMACY

Courses offered to students in the four-year professional phase leading to the award of Doctor of Pharmacy degree (PharmD) without residency requirement (information obtained from the Internet, 2001):

YEAR 1
AUTUMN SEMESTER (17 CRS)
1. Biochemistry (4 crs); 2. Medical Microbiology (3 crs); 3. Microbiology Lab (1 cr); 4. Anatomy and Physiology (4 crs); 5. Pharmaceutical Sciences Lab I (1 cr); 6. Integrated Studies I (1 cr); 7. Pharmacy Practices I (3 crs).

(D: 1, 2, 3, 4; P: 5, 6, 7)

Springer Semester (16 crs)
1. Pharmacy Practice II (3 crs); 2. Antimicrobial Agents (3 crs); 3. Pharmaceutics (4 crs); 4. Physiology/Immunology (4 crs); 5. Pharmaceutical Sciences Lab II (1 cr); 6. Integrated Studies II (1 cr).

(D: 4; P: 1, 2, 3, 5, 6)

Number of pharmacy or drug treatment-related courses: 8 out of 13 or 17 out of 33 crs.

Number of diagnosis-related courses: 5 out of 13 or 16 out of 33 crs.

Year 2
Autumn/Spring Intersession
1. Community Externship (4 crs).

Autumn Semester (17 crs)
1. Pharmaceutics II (3 crs); 2. Medicinal Chemistry (3 crs); 3. Chemo Agents (3 crs); 4. Pharmacology (4 crs); 5. Therapeutics I (3 crs); 6. Integrated Studies III (1 cr).

(D: 0; P: 1, 2, 3, 4, 5, 6)

Spring Semester (15 crs)
1. Pharmacy Relations (3 crs); 2. Medicinal Chemistry (3 crs); 3. Pharmacology/Toxicology (4 crs); 4. Therapeutics II (3 crs); 5. Integrated Studies IV (1 cr); 5a. Elective (1 cr).

(D: 0; P: 2, 3, 4, 5)

Number of pharmacy or drug treatment-related courses: 10 out of 11 or 28 out of 31 crs.

Number of diagnosis-related courses: zero (0) out of 11 or 31 crs.

Autumn/Spring Intersession
1. Hospital Externship (4 crs).

YEAR 3
AUTUMN SEMESTER (15 CRS)
1. Pharmacy Care (4 crs); 2. Drug Literature Evaluation (3 crs); 3. Therapeutics III (4 crs); 4. Public Health in Pharmacy (2 crs); 5. Integrated Studies V (1 cr); 5a. Elective (1 cr).

(D: 0; P: 1, 2, 3, 5)

SPRING SEMESTER (16 CRS)
1. Pharmacoeconomics (3 crs); 2. Pharmacy Ethics (3 crs); 3. Therapeutics IV (4 crs); 4. Physical Assessment (2 crs); 5. Integrated Studies VI (1 cr); 5a. Elective (3 crs).

(D: 4; P: 1, 3, 5)

Number of pharmacy or drug treatment-related courses: 7 out of 10 or 20 out of 31 crs.

Number of diagnosis-related courses: 1 out of 10 or 2 out of 31 crs.

YEAR 4
AUTUMN SEMESTER (16 CRS)
1. Inpatient Clerkship (8 crs); 2. Pharmacy Elective Clerkship (8 crs).

SPRING SEMESTER (16 CRS)
1. Ambulatory Care Clerkship (8 crs); 2. Pharmacy Elective Clerkship (8 crs).

Number of pharmacy or drug treatment-related courses: Constitute a major part of the externship and clerkship.

Number of diagnosis-related courses: Constitute an integral part of the externship and clerkship.

Residency: Optional.

TEXAS SOUTHERN UNIVERSITY, HOUSTON, COLLEGE OF PHARMACY

Courses offered to students in the four-year professional phase leading to the award of Doctor of Pharmacy degree (PharmD) without residency requirement[20] (information obtained from the catalog):

YEAR 1
FALL SEMESTER (17 CRS)

1. Pharmaceutical Chemistry I (3 crs); 2. PHCH 411 Lab (1 cr); 3. Pharmaceutics I (3 crs); 4. PHAR 413 Lab (1 cr); 5. Pathophysiology I (4 crs); 6. PAS 415 (1 cr); 7. Pharmacy Health Care Systems (3 crs); 8. Computer Applications (2 crs).

(D: 5; P: 1, 2, 3, 4)

SPRING SEMESTER (18 CRS)

1. Pharmaceutical Chemistry II (3 crs); 2. PHCH 412 Lab (1 cr); 3. Pharmaceutics II (3 crs); 4. PHAR 414 Lab (1 cr); 5. Pathophysiology II (3 crs); 6. Principles of Pharmacotherapy (1 cr); 7. Biostatistics (2 crs); 8. Microbiology I Lab (4 cr).

(D: 5, 8; P: 1, 2, 3, 4, 6, 7)

Number of pharmacy or drug treatment-related courses: 10 out of 16 or 19 out of 35 crs.

Number of diagnosis-related courses: 3 out of 16 or 10 out of 35 crs.

YEAR 2
FALL SEMESTER (18 CRS)

1. Pharmaceutical Chemistry III (3 crs); 2. Pharmaceutics III (3 crs); 3. PHAR 513 Lab (1 cr); 4. Pharmacology/Toxicology I (3 crs); 5. PAS 517 (1 cr); 6. Pathophysiology III (2 crs); 7. Ethics in Pharmacy Practice (3 crs); 8. Nonprescription Products (2 crs).

(D: 6; P: 1, 2, 3, 4, 8)

Spring Semester (18 crs)

1. Pharmaceutical Chemistry IV (3 crs); 2. Pharmaceutics IV (3 crs); 3. PHAR 514 Lab (1 cr); 4. Patient Assessment phy. DX (3 crs); 5. Chemotherapeutics (3 crs); 6. Pharmacology/Toxicology II (4 crs); 7. Pharmacy Seminar (1 cr).

(D: 4; P: 1, 2, 3, 5, 6, 7)

Number of pharmacy or drug treatment-related courses: 11 out of 15 or 25 out of 36 crs.

Number of diagnosis-related courses: 2 out of 15 or 5 out of 36 crs.

YEAR 3
Fall Semester (16 crs)

1. Pharmaceutics V (3 crs); 2. PHAR 614 Lab (1 cr); 3. Drug Information, Literature Evaluation, and Res. Methods (3 crs); 4. Pharmacotherapeutics I (3 crs); 5. Professional Communications/Counseling (3 crs); 6. Pharmacy Management (3 crs).

(D: 0; P: 1, 2, 3, 4, 5)

Spring Semester (18 crs)

1. Applied Pharmacokinetics (3 crs); 2. PHAR 616 Lab (1 cr); 3. Prescription Practice (3 crs); 4. PHAR 625 Lab (2 crs); 5. Pharmacotherapeutics II 93 crs); 6. Strategic Management in Health Care (3 crs); 7. Jurisprudence (3 crs).

(D: 0; P: 1, 2, 3, 4, 5)

Number of pharmacy or drug treatment-related courses: 10 out of 13 or 25 out of 34 crs.

Number of diagnosis-related courses: zero (0) out of 13 or 34 crs.

YEAR 4
Summer Session (8 crs)

1. Two pharmaceutical care clerkships (4 crs each—8 crs).

Fall Semester (12 crs)

1. Three pharmaceutical care clerkships (4 crs each—12 crs).

Spring Semester (12 crs)
1. Three pharmaceutical care clerkships (4 crs each—12 crs).

Number of pharmacy or drug treatment-related courses: Constitute a major part of the clerkships/rotations.

Number of diagnosis-related courses: Constitute an integral part of the clerkships/rotations.

BACHELOR OF SCIENCE DEGREE PROGRAM IN PHARMACY

Some schools with the three-year professional phase program will be discussed below. The two-year pre-professional phase program is not included in this study.

LONG ISLAND UNIVERSITY, BROOKLYN CAMPUS, COLLEGE OF PHARMACY

Courses offered to students in the three-year professional phase leading to the award of Bachelor of Science degree (BSc Pharm) in pharmacy without residency requirement (information obtained from the 1995-96 schedule):

YEAR 1
Fall Semester (18 crs)
1. Biochemical Foundations of Therapy (4 crs); 2. Physiological Foundations of Therapy (4 crs); 3. Public Health I (Microbiology—3 crs); 4. Basic Concepts of Pharmaceutical Science (4 crs); 4a. Elective (3 crs).
(D: 2, 3; P: 1, 4)

Spring Semester (16 crs)
1. Medicinal Chemistry (4 crs); 2. Pharmacy Techniques I (4 crs); 3. Pharmacy Techniques I Lab (0 cr); 4. Experiemental Pharmacy Lab (2 crs); 5. Pharmacology (4 crs); 6. Clinical Pharmacy I (2 crs).

(D: 0; P: 1, 2, 4, 5, 6)

Number of pharmacy or drug treatment-related courses: 7 out of 9 or 24 out of 31 crs plus 1 zero-credit course.

Number of diagnosis-related courses: 2 out of 9 or 7 out of 31 crs.

YEAR 2
FALL SEMESTER (18 CRS)

1. Pharmacy Techniques II (4 crs); 2. Pharmacy Techniques II Lab (0 cr); 3. Pharmacology II (4 crs); 4. Clinical Pharmacy II (4 crs); 5. Pharmaceutical Law (3 crs); 5a. Elective (1 cr).

(D: 0; P: 1, 3, 4)

SPRING SEMESTER (18 CRS)

1. Biopharm and Pharmacokinetics (4 crs); 2. Toxicology (3 crs); 3. Clinical Pharmacy III (4 crs); 4. Health Care Organization (2 crs); 5. Laboratory Principles (2 crs); 6. Behavioral and Social Aspects of Pharmacy (3 crs).

(D: 0; P: 1, 2, 3, 5)

Number of pharmacy or drug treatment-related courses: 7 out of 10 or 23 out of 35 crs.

Number of diagnosis-related courses: zero (0) out of 10 or 35 crs.

YEAR 3
FALL SEMESTER (12 CRS)

1. Institution Externship (6 crs); 2. Institution Clerkship (6 crs).

SPRING SEMESTER (18 CRS)

1. Community Pharmacy Externship (6 crs); 2. Clinical Pharmacology (3 crs); 3. Elective (9 crs).

Number of pharmacy or drug treatment-related courses: Constitute a major part of the clerkship/externship/rotations.

Number of diagnosis-related courses: Constitute an integral part of the clerkship/externship/rotations.

UNIVERSITY OF MONTANA SCHOOL OF PHARMACY

Courses offered to students in the three-year professional phase leading to the award of Bachelor of Science degree (BSc Pharm) in pharmacy without residency requirement (information obtained from the Internet 2000-2001 schedule):

YEAR 1
Autumn Semester (17 crs)

1. Microbiology Lab (1 cr); 2. Biochemistry (4 crs); 3. Medical Microbiology (3 crs); 4. Pharmacy Practice I (3 crs); 5. Anatomy and Physiology I (4 crs); 6. Pharmacy Science Lab I (1 cr); 7. Integrated Studies I (1 cr).

(D: 1, 2, 3, 5; P: 4, 6, 7)

Spring Semester (16 crs)

1. Pharmacy Practice II (3 crs); 2. Antimicrobial Agents (3 crs); 3. Pharmaceutics (4 crs); 4. Anatomy and Physiology II (4 crs); 5. Pharmacy Science Lab II (1 cr); 6. Integrated Studies II (1 cr).

(D: 4; P: 1, 2, 3, 5, 6)

Number of pharmacy or drug treatment-related courses: 8 out of 13 or 17 out of 33 crs.

Number of diagnosis-related courses: 5 out of 13 or 16 out of 33 crs.

YEAR 2
Autumn Semester (17 crs)

1. Medical Chemistry I (3 crs); 2. Chemotherapeutic Agents (3 crs); 3. Biopharmaceutics/PK (3 crs); 4. Pharmacology I (4 crs); 5. Therapeutics I (3 crs); 6. Integrated Studies III (1 cr); 6a. Electives (2 crs).

(D: 0; P: 1, 2, 3, 4, 5, 6)

Spring Semester (16 crs)
1. Medical Chemistry (3 crs); 2. Pharmacy Practice III (3 crs); 3. Phamacology/Toxicology (4 crs); 4. Therapeutics II (3 crs); 5. Integrated Studies IV (1 cr); 5a. Electives (2 crs).

(D: 0; P: 1, 2, 3, 4, 5)

Number of pharmacy or drug treatment-related courses: 11 out of 11 or 31 out of 31 crs.

Number of diagnosis-related courses: zero (0) out of 11 or 31 crs.

Year 3
Autumn Semester (15 crs)
1. Pharmacy Practice IV (4 crs); 2. Pharmacy Ethics (3 crs); 3. Therapeutics III (4 crs); 4. Public Health in Pharmacy (2 crs); 5. Integrated Studies V (1 cr); 6. Pharmacy Care (1 cr).

(D: 0; P: 1, 3, 5, 6)

Spring Semester (16 crs)
1. Community Pharmacy Externship (4 crs); 2. Hospital Pharmacy Externship (4 crs); 3. Inpatient Clerkship (4 crs); 4. Elective Clerkship (4 crs).

Number of pharmacy or drug treatment-related courses: 4 out of 6 and it constitutes major part of the clerkship/externship.

Number of diagnosis-related courses: zero (0) out of 6 but constitutes an integral part of the clerkship/externship.

UNIVERSITY OF TEXAS, AUSTIN, COLLEGE OF PHARMACY

Courses offered to students in the three-year professional phase leading to the award of Bachelor of Science degree (BSc Pharm) in pharmacy without residency requirement (information obtained from the 2000-2002 schedule on the Internet):

YEAR 1
FALL SEMESTER (15 CRS)
1. Biochemistry (3 crs); 2. Pharmacy Science I (4 crs); 3. Pharmacy Science Lab I (1 cr); 4. A & P I (3 crs); 5. Pharmacy Ad I (2 crs); 6. Pharmacy Ad I Lab (1 cr); 7. Introduction to Pharmacy A (1 cr).

(D: 1; P: 2, 3, 5, 6, 7)

SPRING SEMESTER (17 CRS)
1. MM. chem./biotech (3 crs); 2. A & P II (2 cr); 3. Pharmacy Science II (4 crs); 4. Pharmacy Science Lab II (1 cr); 5. General Pathology (2 crs); 6. Pharmaceutics (3 crs); 7. Pharmaceutics Lab (1 crs); 8. Introduction to Pharmacy B (1 cr).

(D: 5; P: 1, 3, 4, 6, 7, 8)

Number of pharmacy or drug treatment-related courses: 11 out of 15 or 25 out of 32 crs.

Number of diagnosis-related courses: 2 out of 15 or 5 out of 32 crs.

YEAR 2
FALL SEMESTER (15-16 CRS)
1. Introduction to Drug Information (1 cr); 2. pharmacother Ia (3 crs); 3. pharmacother Ib (2 crs); 4. pharmacother Ic (3 crs); 5. pharmacother Lab I (1 cr); 6. pharm Practice Lab I or pharm AD II (3 crs); 6a. Elective (2-3 crs).

(D: 0; P: 1, 2, 3, 4, 5, 6)

SPRING SEMESTER (15-16 CRS)
1. Pharmacotherapy II a (3 crs); 2. Pharmacotherapy II b (2 crs); 3. Pharmacotherapy II c (3 crs); 4. Pharmacotherapy Lab II (1 cr); 5. pharm AD II pharm prac Lab I (3 crs); 6. exp. Practice (1 cr); 6a. Elective (2-3 crs).

(D: 0; P: 1, 2, 3, 4, 5, 6)

SUMMER SESSION (6 CRS)
1. Pharmacotherapy IIIa (3 crs); 2. Pharmacotherapy IIIb (2 crs); 3. Pharmacotherapy III Lab (1 cr).

Number of pharmacy or drug treatment-related courses: 15 out of 15 or 32 out of 32 crs.

Number of diagnosis-related courses: zero (0) out of 15 or 32 crs.

YEAR 3
Fall Semester (25 crs)

1. Pharmacy Law (2 crs); 2. Pharmacy Practice Lab II (2 crs); 3. Elective (2-3 crs); 4. Community Internship (6 crs); 5. Clinical Internship (6 crs); 6. Hospital Internship (6 crs).

(D: 0; P: 2)

Spring Semester (18 crs—10 rotations)

1. Community Internship (6 crs); 2. Clinical Internship (6 crs); 3. Hospital Internship (6 crs).

Number of pharmacy or drug treatment-related courses: Constitute a major part of the internship/rotations.

Number of diagnosis-related courses: Constitute an integral part of the internship/rotations.

DATA SUMMARY

MEDICINE	Schools	Year 1	Year 2	Year 3	Year 4	Total Ratio
1	HARVARD NOP NOD	1/23 (0.04) 17/23 (0.74)	1/24 (0.04) 18/24 (0.75)	IN MAJ	IN MAJ	0.040 0.745
2	JOHNS HOPKINS NOP NOD	0/5 (0) 4/5 (0.8)	— —	IN MAJ	IN MAJ	N/A
3	UNIV. OF PENN. NOP NOD	2-4/12(0.25) 8-10/12 (0.77)	0/22 (0) 18/22 (0.82)	IN MAJ	IN MAJ	0.125 0.795
4	UNIV. OF IOWA NOP NOD	0/9 (0) 9/9 (1)	2/7 (0.29) 4/7 (0.57)	IN MAJ	IN MAJ	0.145 0.785
5	UNIV. OF MIAMI NOP NOD	1/13 (0.077) 12/13 (0.92)	YR 1 & 2	IN MAJ	IN MAJ	0.077 0.92
6	UNIV. OF MARYLAND NOP NOD	0/9 (0) 8/9 (0.89)	0/3 (0) 3/3 (1)	IN MAJ	IN MAJ	0 0.95
7	UNIV. OF WISCONSIN NOP NOD	0/9 (0) 9/9 (1)	2/16 (0.13) 13/16 (0.81)	IN MAJ	IN MAJ	0.065 0.905
8	UNIV. OF LOUISVILLE NOP NOD	0/8 (0) 8/8 (1)	1/7 (0.14) 6/7 (0.86)	IN MAJ	IN MAJ	0.07 0.93

	Schools	Year 1	Year 2	Year 3	Year 4	Total Ratio
9	UNIV. OF ALABAMA NOP NOD	1/9 (0.11) 7/9 (0.78)	1/5 (0.2) 4/5 (0.8)	IN MAJ	IN MAJ	0.155 0.79
10	WRIGHT STATE UNI. NOP NOD	0/7 (0) 5/7 (0.71)	0/10 (0) 10/10 (1)	IN MAJ	IN MAJ	0 0.86
11	NOVA SOUTHEA UNIV. NOP NOD	0/22 (0) 16/22(0.73)	3/34 (0.088) 21/34 (0.62)	IN MAJ	IN MAJ	0.044 0.674
12	UNIV. OF PUERT RICO NOP NOD	0/11 (0) 8/11 (0.73)	1/10 (0.1) 6/10 (0.6)	IN MAJ	IN MAJ	0.05 0.66
13	UNIV. OF FLORIDA NOP NOD	0/13 (0) 11/13 (0.85)	0/12 (0) 9/12 (0.75)	IN MAJ	IN MAJ	0 0.798
14	STATE UNIV. OF NY. NOP NOD	0/11 (0) 9/11(0.82)	1/8 (0.125) 5/8 (0.63)	IN MAJ	IN MAJ	0.063 0.725
15	ARIZ COL OF OSTE. NOP NOD	0/24 (0) 23/24 (0.958)	3/25 (0.12) 22/25 (0.88)	IN MAJ	IN MAJ	0.06 0.92
	AVER TOTAL RATIO NOP NOD					0.063 0.82

DENTISTRY

	Schools	Year 1	Year 2	Year 3	Year 4	Total Ratio
1	HARVARD NOP NODD	1/12 (0.083) 11/12 (0.92)	0/8 (0) 8/8 (1)	0/5 (0) 5/5 (1)	IN (0/3) MAJ (3/3)	0.028 0.97
2	UNIV. OF PENN. NOP NODD	0/14 (0) 14/14 (1)	1/18 (0.056) 16/18 (0.89)	0/19 (0) 17/19 (0.895)	IN (0/13) MAJ (12/13)	0.019 0.93
3	BALTIMORE COLL NOP NODD	0/14 (0) 14/14 (1)	1/18 (0.06) 17/18 (0.95)	0/22 (0) 22/22 (1)	IN (1/5) MAJ (4/5)	0.02 0.98
4	NOVA SOUTHEA UNIV. NOP NODD	0/20 (0) 19/20 (0.95)	4/28 (0.143) 24/28 (0.86)	0/17 (0) 15/17 (0.88)	IN (0/7) MAJ (7/7)	0.05 0.897
	AVER TOTAL RATIO NOP NOD					0.029 0.945

OPTOMETRY

	Schools	Year 1	Year 2	Year 3	Year 4	Total Ratio
1	SOUTHER CAL. COL NOP NODO	0/19 (0) 15/19 (0.79)	2-4/20(0.15) 15-17/20(0.8)	1/22 (0.045) 18/22 (0.82)	IN MAJ	0.065 0.80
2	OHIO STATE UNIV. NOP NODO	1/14 (0.071) 11/14 (0.79)	1/15-(0.067) 13/15-(0.867)	1/29-(0.035) 25/29-(0.86)	IN MAJ	0.058 0.84
3	NOVA SOUTHEA UNIV. NOP NODO	0/20 (0) 18/20 (0.9)	3/19 (0.16) 14/19 (0.74)	0/14 (0) 12/14 (0.86)	IN MAJ	0.053 0.83
	AVER TOTAL RATIO NOP NODO					0.059 0.82

VETERINARY MEDICINE

	Schools	Year 1	Year 2	Year 3	Year 4	Total Ratio
1	UNIV. OF PENN. NOP NOD	0/14 (0) 11/14 (0.79)	2/14 (0.14) 11/14 (0.79)	0/8 (0) 7/8 (0.875)	IN MAJ	0.047 0.82
2	TUFT'S SCHOOL NOP NOD	0/11 (0) 11/11 (1)	3/22 (0.14) 17/22 (0.77)	1/12 (0.071) 9/12 (0.75)	IN (1/10) MAJ(9/10)	0.07 0.85
3	UNIV. OF WISCONSIN NOP NOD	1/16-(0.06) 14/16-(0.875)	3/18 (0.167) 15/18 (0.83)	2/20 (0.10) 14/20 (0.7)	IN MAJ	0.11 0.80
4	OHIO STATE UNIV. NOP NOD	1/16-(0.63) 13/16-(0.81)	1-2/14 (0.11) 11/14 (0.786)	2/10 (0.2) 5/10 (0.5)	IN MAJ	0.12 0.70
	AVER TOTAL RATIO NOP NOD					0.087 0.79

PHYSICIAN ASSISTANT

	Schools	Year 1	Year 2	Year 3	Year 4	Total Ratio
1	UNIV. OF IOWA NOP NOD	1/14 (0.071) 9/14 (0.64)	IN MAJ	— 	— 	0.071 0.64
2	NOVA SOUTHEA UNIV. NOP NOD	2/34 (0.059) 22/34 (0.65)	IN MAJ	— 	— 	0.059 0.65
3	UNIV. OF FLORIDA NOP NOD	1/15 (0.067) 13/15 (0.87)	IN MAJ	— 	— 	0.067 0.87
4	UNIV. OF WISCONSIN NOP NOD	2/18 (0.11) 15/18 (0.83)	IN MAJ	— 	— 	0.11 0.83
	AVER TOTAL RATIO NOP NOD					0.077 0.75

NURSING (BSc)

	Schools	Year 1	Year 2	Year 3	Year 4	Total Ratio
1	CREIGHTON UNIV. NOP NODN	0/11 (0) 3/11 (0.27)	0/12 (0) 5/12 (0.42)	1/10 (0.1) 8/10 (0.8)	0/6 (0) 5/6 (0.83)	0.025 0.579
2	UNIV. OF TEXAS NOP NODN	1/15 (0.067) 4/15 (0.3)	Yr 1 & 2	0/11 (0) 11/11 (1)	0/12 (0) 12/12 (1)	0.034 0.65
3	UNIV. OF KENTUCKY NOP NODN	0/10 (0) 2/10 (0.2)	1/8 (0.12) 5/8 (0.63)	0/6 (0) 5/6 (0.83)	0/6 (0) 6/6 (1)	0.03 0.67
4	OREG HLTH SCI UNIV NOP NODN	0/14 (0) 3/14 (0.2)	YR 1 & 2	1/13 (0.077) 11/13 (0.85)	0/10 (0) 10/10 (1)	0.02 0.56
	AVER TOTAL RATIO NOP NODN					0.027 0.615

CERTIFIED NURSE PRACTITIONER

	Schools	Year 1	Year 2	Year 3	Year 4	Total Ratio
1	CREIGHTON UNIV.	FAMILY	NURSE	PRACT	—	0.046
	NOP	1/11 (0.091)	0/5 (0)	—		0.62
	NODN	7/11 (0.636)	3/5 (0.6)			
		ADULT	NURSE	PRACT	—	0.046
	NOP	1/11 (0.091)	0/4 (0)	—		0.57
	NODN	7/11 (0.636)	2/4 (0.5)			
2	UNIV. OF KENTUCKY	ACUTE	CARE	NURSE	PRACT	0.055
	NOP	1/9 (0.11)	0/5 (0)	—	—	0.85
	NODN	8/9 (0.89)	4/5 (0.80)			
		PARENT	CHILD	SPECIALTY	—	0.055
	NOP	1/9 (0.11)	0/5 (0)	—		0.89
	NODN	7/9 (0.78)	5/5 (1)			
3	UNIV. OF IOWA		SAME	AS	ABOVE	
4	OREG HLTH SCI UNIV	ADULT	NURSE	PRACT	—	0.053
	NOP	1/19 (0.053)	YR 1 & 2	—		0.74
	NODN	14/19 (0.74)				

PHARMACY IN BONDAGE   327

MIDWIFERY

	Schools	Year 1	Year 2	Year 3	Year 4	Total Ratio
1	OREG HLTH SCI UNIV					
	NOP	2/27 (0.074)	YR 1 & 2	—	—	0.074
	NODN	20/27 (0.74)				0.74
2	SEATT MIDWIF SCH					
	NOP	1/27 (0.04)	YR 1 & 2	—	—	0.04
	NOD	17/27 (0.63)				0.63
	AVER TOTAL RATIO					
	NOP					0.053
	NODN					0.72

PHARMACY   BACHELOR OF SCIENCE

	Schools	Year 1	Year 2	Year 3	Year 4	Total Ratio
1	LONG ISLAND UNIV.					
	NOP	7/9 (0.78)	7/10 (0.70)	MAJ (5/5)	—	0.74
	NOD	2/9 (0.22)	0/10 (0)	IN (0/5)		0.11
2	UNIV. OF MONTANA					
	NOP	8/13 (0.62)	11/11 (1)	MAJ (3/6)	—	0.81
	NOD	5/13 (0.39)	0/11 (0)	IN (0/6)		0.19
3	UNIV. OF TEXAS					
	NOP	11/15 (0.73)	15/15 (1)	MAJ (1/3)	—	0.87
	NOD	2/15 (0.13)	0/15 (0)	IN (0/3)		0.065
	AVER TOTAL RATIO					
	NOP					0.81
	NODN					0.12

DOCTOR OF PHARMACY

	Schools	Year 1	Year 2	Year 3	Year 4	Total Ratio
1	UINV. OF CALIF NOP NOD	10/15 (0.67) 3/15 (0.2)	6/12 (0.5) 4/12 (0.33)	MAJ (5/7–0.71) IN (1/7–0.14)	MAJ IN	0.63 0.22
2	UNIV. OF TEXAS NOP NOD	12/18 (0.67) 4/18 (0.22)	12/14 (0.89) 0/14 (0)	8/10 (0.8) 1/10 (0.1)	MAJ IN	0.79 0.11
3	UNIV. OF KENTUCKY NOP NOD	11/13 (0.85) 2/13 (0.15)	8/8 (1) 0/8 (0)	4/6 (0.67) 2/6 (0.33)	MAJ IN	0.84 0.16
4	AUBURN UNIV. NOP NOD	11/15 (0.73) 4/15 (0.27)	11/14 (0.79) 3/14 (0.21)	11/11 (1) 0/11 (0)	MAJ IN	0.84 0.16
5	UNIV. OF MISSOURI NOP NOD	5/10 (0.5) 4/10 (0.4)	7/9 (0.78) 1/9 (0.11)	6/8 (0.75) 1/8 (0.13)	MAJ IN	0.68 0.21
6	UNIV. OF COLORADO NOP NOD	10/16 (0.63) 3/16 (0.19)	9/15 (0.6) 6/15 (0.4)	8/10 (0.8) 2/10 (0.2)	MAJ IN	0.68 0.26
7	UNIV. OF MONTANA NOP NOD	8/13 (0.62) 5/13 (0.39)	10/11 (0.91) 0/11 (0)	7/10 (0.7) 1/10 (0.1)	MAJ IN	0.74 0.16
	Schools	Year 1	Year 2	Year 3	Year 4	Total Ratio

8	TEXAS SO. UNIV. NOP NOD	10/16 (0.63) 3/16 (0.19)	11/15 (0.73) 2/15 (0.13)	10/13 (0.77) 0/13 (0)	MAJ IN	0.71 0.11
	AVER TOTAL RATIO NOP NOD					0.74 0.17

IN = Integral part of rotation/clerkship.

MAJ = Major part of rotation/clerkship.

NOD = Number of diagnosis-related courses.

NOP = Number of pharmacy- or drug treatment-related courses.

NODD = Number of diagnosis- and dental-related courses.

NODO = Number of diagnosis- and optometry-related courses.

NODN = Number of diagnosis- and nursing-related courses.

AVER = Average

DATA ANALYSIS

Data analysis of the above school courses/programs takes into consideration the fact that the criteria used in setting school credits, courses, and standards are individualized and independent. Thus, one school might choose to condense its program by assigning five to ten courses consisting of 0 to 10 credit hours (0 credits were ignored because the author assumed that the school authorities did not consider the course important enough to merit one credit) per semester, while another school will spread out the same content in about 25 to 30 or more courses consisting of 5 or more credit hours. For example, the University of Pennsylvania School of Veterinary Medicine has a pathology course for 12 credits a semester, and twice that number of credits (total 24 crs) in another school with a condensed curriculum is enough to complete the semester requirement. Final analysis is such that all school programs are leveled and equalized with national board examinations, which spells out the basic entry requirements and skills for all professions. Despite the diversity of schools' programs and assigned credit hours, it is possible to compare various programs and courses offered by different schools by weighing individual courses against the overall program in a particular school, then comparing the resultant ratio with that obtained from another school. Be that as it may, what is in an optometry school curriculum/program that would convince an optometrist to coat himself with an inferiority complex in presence of an ophthalmologist, at the same time allows him to address himself as an optometry physician because he is qualified to do so in all respects. Ironically the same optometrist will question the rationale behind a clinical pharmacist with a Doctor of Pharmacy degree addressing himself as a therapeutic physician without good reasons. He knows that he spent the same number of years—four years in school training as the clinical pharmacists—but cannot come to terms with the fact that both of them are qualified to use the same title. The fact remains that this optometrist has been indoctrinated with societal norms and pharmacists' acceptance of their bondage within the medical community. In an attempt to coat himself with a superiority complex in the presence of a clinical pharmacist, he forgets about the fact that the clinical pharmacists is just beginning to confront the same system that derogates him as an optometry physician and holds him in contempt; consequently, he has no alternative but to fight against the system. All branches of medicine, including ophthalmology in its infancy in the early 1920s, can relate to this phenomenon because it takes time for them to gain recognition of the public and general practitioners. General practitioners suffered the same fate, as noted earlier, when specialization became the norm and others cast aspersions on them until they became family practice physician specialists.

Human and animal ailments border on two major issues, and they are "diagnosis and treatment." All other issues are either irrelevant or trivial to these two major issues. Analysis of various schools' curricula based on detailed outlines in this chapter reveal how various schools/branches of medicine deal with these two major issues. The 14 sampled medical schools execute four years of coursework leading to the award of MD and DO (Doctor of Medicine and Doctor of Osteopathic) degree before residency. Residency eventually leads to specialization in various areas such as allergy and immunology, anesthesiology, dermatology, emergency medicine, family practice, internal medicine, genetics, neurology, nuclear medicine, obstetrics and gynecology, ophthalmology/otolaryngology, pathology, pediatrics, physical medicine and rehabilitation, psychiatry, preventive medicine, radiology, surgery, and urology. The four years coursework comprises of two phases, which are pre-clinical and clinical phases with two years duration each.

PRE-CLINICAL PHASE

The first two pre-clinical years set the precedence by laying the ground work/foundation upon which the entire career is based. In most cases, pre-clinical years academic work are the only didactic/classroom experience the students will be exposed to in their entire career. Students' exposure to the two major issues of medicine—diagnosis and treatment—varies from school to school according to the available data.

DIAGNOSIS-RELATED COURSES: Judging by the ratio of the number of diagnosis-related courses to the overall coursework in the 14 sampled medical schools (excluding Johns Hopkins Medical School), the university with the lowest average ratio in the first two pre-clinical years is the University of Puerto Rico with 8 out of 11 courses in the first year (ratio of 0.73) and 6 out of 10 courses in the second year (ratio of 0.6), making a total average ratio of 0.66 or 66%. The university with the closest average ratio to 0.82 or 82% is the University of Florida with 11 out of 13 courses in the first year (ratio of 0.85) and 9 out of 12 courses in the second year (ratio of 0.75), making a total average ratio of 0.798 or 79.8%. The university with the highest average ratio is the University of Maryland with 8 out 9 courses in the first year (ratio of 0.89) and 3 out of 3 courses in the second year (ratio of 1), making a total average ratio of 0.95 or 95%. On the whole, using these data it can be estimated that medical doctors or students in the U.S. are exposed to an average of 0.798 (79.8%), which is approximately 80% or 8 out of every 10, courses that are diagnosis related in the two-year pre-clinical phase.

LIMITATIONS: Johns Hopkins School of Medicine data were excluded from data analysis because of inadequate information about second-year courses. Some of the courses with diagnosis component constituting major part of the course content and treatment component constituting minor part were considered to be diagnosis-related courses even though there were some elements of treatment in them. Human behavior courses were considered diagnosis related because of the vital role it plays in diagnosing brain diseases such as anxiety, depression, psychosis, etc. Data from the State University of New York Health Science 1995-1996 are out of sequence because most of the data used were obtained around the year 2000. Excluding this data made no difference to the outcome/results; consequently, it was included to show that contemporary data have little or no difference from previous years.

DRUG TREATMENT OR PHARMACY-RELATED COURSES: Using the same criteria as in diagnosis, coincidentally there were three universities with the lowest average ratio of zero (0) among the 14 sampled medical schools during the two-year pre-clinical phase. These three universities are the University of Maryland, Wright State University, and the University of Florida. They have no pharmacy or drug-treatment courses in the two-year pre-clinical phase. The university with the closest average ratio to 0.063 is State University of New York Health Science Center at Brooklyn with zero (0) out of 11 courses in the first year (ratio of 0) and 1 out of 8 courses in the second year (ratio of 0.125), making a total average ratio of 0.063 or 6.3%. The university with the highest average ratio among the 14 is the University of Alabama with 1 out of 9 courses in the first year (ratio of 0.11) and 1 out of 5 courses the second year (ratio of 0.2), making a total average ratio of 0.155 or 15.5% (i.e., approximately 16%, which is 16 out of every 100 courses or 1.6 out of every 10 courses). On the whole, using these data, it can be estimated that medical doctors or students in the U.S. are exposed to an average number of 0.063 or 6.3%, which is approximately 6% or 6 out of every 100 courses (3 out of every 50 courses or 1 out every 17 courses) in drug treatment or pharmacy-related courses during the two-year pre-clinical phase.

LIMITATIONS: Same as in diagnosis.

CLINICAL PHASE

The two-year clinical phase comprises of rotations or clerkships, which are meant to build on the foundation laid by the two-year pre-clinical phase/didactic class work. The modalities for the clinical phase do not change dramatically as to reverse treatment for diagnosis and vice versa; rather, the status quo remain the same because the clinical phase serves to entrench and inculcate the values/knowledge gained during the pre-clinical didactic classroom work. This explains why doctors spend hours diagnosing cases but few minutes or seconds assigning drugs/treatment on the basis of pharmacodynamics without regards to other aspects of drug treatment. The data presented here showed that majority of the course content during rotations is diagnosis related, while an integral part of it is assigned to pharmacy or drug treatment. The transition from the pre-clinical phase to the clinical phase or rotations can be used to generalize the fact that 80% of rotations coursework is diagnosis related, while 15 percent are pharmacy or drug-treatment related. As seen in the two-year pre-clinical phase, ascribing a maximum of 15% to pharmacy is generous. The remaining aspect of 5% can be ascribed to other issues dealing with human and animal ailment that do not include diagnosis and drug treatment. It is fair to say that treatment does not always entail usage of drug or pharmacy products in healing ailments, but more than 80% of any treatment at any give time involved chemicals/drugs or pharmacy products. Surgery is an alternative means of treatment but the operation involves usage of drugs to enhance patient's compliance, reduce pain, and speed up the recovery/healing process. At the end of the two-year clinical phase or rotations, students graduate with an MD or DO degree. However, instead of going straight to work like the engineer, dentist, optometrist, veterinary doctor, teacher, microbiologist, and others he goes into residence program, which varies in years. Most graduates spend three years while some spend 4 to 5 years before going into practice.

RESIDENCY

Residency is the twin brother of rotation/clerkship that occurs during the last two years of study in medical school (see clinical phase above). Residency is the final stage of training that leads to various specialties listed above. Residency is the stage where graduates start putting into use knowledge acquired over the years in the pre-clinical and clinical phases with some degree of independence. Although clinical practice (putting acquired knowledge into use) is alive throughout the four years especially in the clinical phase, the supervisory role of the clinical director begins to degenerate during residence. Graduates begin to perfect their knowledge and skills, handle patients independently, teach or assist students in the four-year program, and assist young residents at the final year of their residence. All schools handle residency programs in a different manner just like the school curriculum. Harvard University, for example, considered the first year of residency as internship, the second year as junior residency, and the third year as senior residency. Residency is another transitional phase of the two-year clinical phase before graduation.

As a transitional phase, residency is very much modeled after the two-year didactic class work (pre-clinical phase) and the two-year clinical phase in terms of course content or job assignments. However, it is fair to say that priority given to drug treatment or pharmacy products increases slightly to around 20-30% because of the necessities, assignments, personal challenge to find answer to any given situation (you are alone without help from anyone), and the desire to satisfy patients. On the whole, it can reasonably be argued that unlike engineering, mathematics, physics, microbiology, chemistry, biology, and others the only college didactic class work the physicians are exposed to at the professional level is the two-year pre-clinical phase and some part of the last two-year clinical phase. In relation to pharmacy or drug treatment, these two years plus didactic class work or coursework are like the availability of mathematics courses in a physicist's curriculum and vice versa, or the availability of chemistry courses in the engineering curriculum and vice versa, or the availability of history or biology in a pharmacy curriculum. All colleges have interdisciplinary courses, and this does not warrant our calling a physicist a mathematician and vice versa, or a chemist a biologists and vice versa; nor non-major course graduates taken over the role of major course graduates in daily life tasks or job activities (i.e., a mathematician doing the job of a physicist, thinking that he can do a better job than the original specialists, the physicist, and vice versa). As noted earlier, no matter how well we think we trained our physicians to be smart and responsive to all situations, they can never do a better job than the engineers in the engineering field. No matter the number of years they spent in engineering rotation/residency, without the deep-rooted four to five-year college didactic class work or former education in engineering they cannot do a better job than an engineer in constructing bridges, roads, houses, airplanes, rockets, cars, computers, trucks, etc. Moreover, residency and clinical phase rotations are very much like the nineteenth-century apprenticeship, in which an apprentice (in most cases young men) spent certain number of years with the master to learn an art or trade until his skills are perfect enough to be on his own. At the turn of the twentieth century (around 1900), apprenticeship was the modus operandi for training physicians. These physicians were not college educated and there was huge/wide outcry by the media, government, and well-meaning citizens about the substandard nature of physicians' education (non-formal education). Although no one is saying that residency and clinical rotations are substandard these days but the operation and existence of such program without deep-rooted college didactic class work in relation to pharmacy or drug treatment is questionable. Today, we learn from experience that professionals such as engineers, teachers, lawyers, mathematicians, physicists, optometrists, dentists, veterinary medical doctors, microbiologists, chemists, and many others except some branches of medicine can survive, strive very well, and improve the lot of the society without residency and not the reverse. That is to say, professionals can survive with certain number of years of college training based on didactic class work (formal education) without residence. None of these professions has been known to survive currently with residency alone without college training or formal education, which is the same as the outdated apprenticeship. It is difficult to imagine how contemporary society can survive with residence or apprenticeship alone. That is to say, young, aspiring teachers will rely on old teachers to teach them how to teach in the classroom; an engineer will become a roadside mechanic that relies on his master to teach him the skills of the trade; young, aspiring lawyers on old lawyers; and so on and so forth. The situation will be chaotic, and that is like setting back the hands of the clock in human development and technological advancement. In the final analysis, most physicians probably have discovered that, in sharp contrast to the medical school training, pharmacy or drug treatment actually make more demands on their talents and skills than the diagnosis they spent so many years learning. It is unrealistic to expect medical school curriculum to change overnight or incorporate pharmacy school, dentistry school, optometry school, veterinary school, and other curricula. This view in itself is retrogressive because it kills specialization and sets back the hands of the clock probably to the nineteenth century—an era in which medical doctors were jacks-of-all-trades, masters of none. There is no room for such expansion because students are already overwhelmed with their current curriculum, coursework, or school load in all branches of medicine. Moreover, the law of comparative advantages stresses the need for division of labor, and for everyone to perfect his skills in his area of specialization so that the society can gain tremendously by advancing well into the future.

OTHER BRANCHES OF MEDICINE

Other branches of medicine and allied health that are associated with prescription-writing authority are dentistry, optometry, veterinary medicine, physician assistant, certified nurse practitioner, and midwifery. Fewer schools were sampled here because of the need to avoid monotony or turning the book into school catalog.

DENTISTRY

Four schools/colleges of dentistry were sampled. These schools have no residency requirements after the four years coursework leading to the award of DDS or DMD or DDM. Residency program is optional as a postgraduate course for interested graduates. The four years coursework comprises of two phases, which are three years didactic class work/experience, otherwise tagged as pre-clinical phase in previous analysis; and one-year rotation or clerkship, otherwise tagged as clinical phase in previous analysis. Using the same criteria, the number of diagnosis and dentistry-related courses and pharmacy or drug-treatment related courses available to the students during these years can be assessed.

PRE-CLINICAL PHASE

DIAGNOSIS- AND DENTISTRY-RELATED COURSES: In terms of diagnosis and dentistry-related courses, the university with the lowest average ratio among the four is Nova Southeastern University with 19 out of 20 courses in the first year, 24 out of 28 courses in the second year, and 15 out of 17 courses in the third, making a total average ratio of 0.897. The closest average ratio to 0.945 is the University of Pennsylvania with 14 out of 14 courses in the first year, 16 out of 18 courses in the second year, and 17 out of 19 courses in the third year, making a total average ratio of 0.93 or 93%. The university with highest average ratio is Baltimore College of Dental School with 14 out of 14 courses in the first year, 17 out of 18 courses in the second year, and 22 out of 22 in the third year, making a total average ratio of 0.98 or 98%. On the whole, it can be estimated that dentists/dentistry students in the U.S. are exposed to an average number of 0.93 or 93%, which is approximately 90% or 9 out of every 10 courses in diagnosis and dental-related courses, during the three-year pre-clinical phase.

LIMITATIONS: The number of schools sampled is small compared to the total number of dentistry schools in the nation. However small it may be, it is a reflection of the broad dental school perspective, because graduates from these schools are not only qualified but board-certified dentists from high-ranking schools like Harvard. Other limitations involved some schools like Harvard and Nova Southeastern with third-year rotations, of which diagnosis and dental-related coursework constitute major part, and drug treatment or pharmacy-related courses constitute an integral part of the rotations.

DRUG TREATMENT OR PHARMACY-REALTED COURSES: Using same criteria to judge the number of pharmacy or drug-treatment courses available to dentists/dentistry students, the university with the lowest average ratio is the University of Pennsylvania with zero (0) out of 14 courses in the first year, 1 out of 18 courses in the second year, and zero (0) out of 19 courses in the third year, making a total average ratio of 0.019 or 1.9 %. The university with the closest average ratio to 0.029 is the Harvard School of Dental Medicine with 1 out of 12 courses in the first year, zero (0) out of 8 courses in the second year, and zero (0) out of 5 courses in the third year, making a total average ratio of 0.028 or 2.8%. The university with the highest average ratio is Nova Southeastern University with zero (0) of 20 courses in the first year, 4 out of 28 courses in the second year, and zero (0) of 17 courses in the third year, making a total average ratio of 0.05 or 5%. On the whole, using the above data, it can be estimated that the average number of drug treatment or pharmacy-related courses that qualify a dentist to write a prescription is 0.028 or 2.8 %, which is approximately 3%, and that is 3 out of every 100 courses or 1 out of every 33 courses during the three-year pre-clinical phase.

LIMITATIONS: The same as in diagnosis.

CLINICAL PHASE

The one-year clinical phase comprises of rotations or clerkships, which is meant to build on the foundation laid by the three-year pre-clinical phase didactic/class work. Like in previous clinical phase analyses, the status quo remain the same because the rotations serve to entrench and inculcate knowledge gained during didactic class work. The rotations are made of diagnosis and dental-related coursework as a major component and pharmacy or drug treatment-related coursework as a minor component. As a transition phase of pre-clinical years, it can be estimated that rotation is made up of 90% diagnosis and dental-related coursework, 5 percent pharmacy or drug treatment, and 5% for other aspects of dentistry. After graduation, the dentist goes to practice and discovers that drug treatment at work deserves greater attention than their level of exposure during college class work. Consequently, necessities, personal challenges, and the desire to satisfy patients galvanizes them into action and prompts their curiosity as well as ingenuity to increase drug knowledge to about 10 to 15% depending on their practice setting and commitment.

OPTOMETRY

Three schools of optometry were sampled. Like dentistry, optometry has no residency requirement after the four-year coursework leading to the award of

OD. It is equally optional as a postgraduate course for interested graduates. The four-year coursework comprises of two phases: the pre-clinical phase with three years didactic class work and the clinical phase with one-year rotation or clerkship. The number of diagnosis and optometry-related courses and pharmacy or drug treatment-related courses available to students during the four years are assessed below using same criteria.

PRE-CLINICAL PHASE

DIAGNOSIS AND OPTOMETRY-RELATED COURSES: In relation to these courses, the university with the lowest average ratio is Southern California College of Optometry with 15 out of 19 courses in the first year, 15 to 17 out of 20 courses in the second year, and 18 out of 22 courses in the third year, making a total average ratio of 0.80 or 80%. The university with the closest average ratio to 0.82 is Nova Southeastern University with 18 out of 20 courses in the first year, 14 out of 19 courses in the second year, and 12 out of 14 courses in the third year, making a total average ratio of 0.83 or 83%. The university with the highest average ratio is Ohio State University with 11 out of 14 courses in the first year, 13 out of 15 courses in the second year, and 25 out of 29 courses in the third year, making a total average ratio of 0.84 or 84%. On the whole, using this data, it can be estimated that the optometrist graduates in the U.S. are exposed to an average number of 0.83 or 83%, which is approximately 80% or 8 out of every 10 diagnosis and optometry-related courses during the three-year pre-clinical phase.

LIMITATIONS: The number of schools sampled is small compared to the total number of optometry schools in the nation. However small it may be, it is a reflection of the broad optometry school perspective because graduates from these schools are not only qualified but also board-certified optometrists from high-ranking schools like the University of Southern California College of Optometry. Other limitations involve Nova Southeastern with third-year rotations, of which diagnosis and optometry-related coursework constitute a major part, and drug treatment or pharmacy-related courses constitute an integral part of the rotations.

DRUG TREATMENT OR PHARMACY-REALTED COURSES: Using same criteria for pharmacy or drug-treatment courses available to the optometrist students, the university with the lowest average ratio is Nova Southeastern University with zero (0) out of 20 courses in the first year, 3 out of 19 courses in the second year, and zero (0) out of 14 courses in the third year, making a total average ratio of 0.053 or 5.3%. The university with the closest average ratio to 0.059 is Ohio State University with 1 out of 14 courses in the first year, 1 out of 15 courses in the second year, and 1 out of 29 courses in the third year, making a total average ratio of 0.058

or 5.8%. The university with the highest average ratio is Southern California College of Optometry, which has zero (0) out of 19 courses in the first year, 2 to 4 out of 20 courses in the second year, and 1 out of 22 courses in the third year, making a total average ratio of 0.065 or 6.5%. On the whole, using this data, it can be estimated that the average number of drug treatment or pharmacy-related courses that qualify an optometrist to write a prescription is 0.058 or 5.8%, which is approximately 6% or 6 out of every 100, or 1 out of every 17 courses during the three-year pre-clinical phase.

LIMITATIONS: Same as in diagnosis.

CLINICAL PHASE

Same as in dentistry.

VETERINARY MEDICINE

Four schools of veterinary medicine were sampled. Like dentistry and optometry, veterinary medicine has no residence requirement after the four years coursework leading to the award of DVM. The four years coursework comprises of two phases, which are pre-clinical, with three years didactic class work; and the clinical phase, with one-year rotation or clerkship. Residency is optional and available as a postgraduate program for interested candidates. Similar criteria are used to assess the four years coursework below.

PRE-CLINICAL PHASE

DIAGNOSIS-RELATED COURSES: As far as diagnosis-related courses are concerned, the university with the lowest average ratio is Ohio State University with 13 out of 16 courses in the first year, 11 out of 14 courses in the second year, and 5 out of 10 courses in the third year, making a total average ratio of 0.70 or 70%. Two universities with closest average ratio to 0.79 or 79% are the University of Wisconsin with 14 out of 16 courses in the first year, 15 out of 18 courses in the second year, and 15 out of 20 courses in the third year, making a total average ratio of 0.82 or 82%; and the University of Pennsylvania with 11 out of 14 courses in the first and second year, and 7 out of 8 courses in the third year, making a total average ratio of 0.82 or 82%. The university with the highest average ratio is Tufts School of Veterinary Medicine with 11 out of 11 courses in the first year, 17 out of 22 courses in the second year, and

9 out of 12 courses in the third year, making a total average ratio of 0.85 or 85%. On the whole, using this data, it can be estimated that the veterinary medical doctors/students in the U.S. are exposed to an average number of 0.82 or 82%, which is approximately 80% or 8 out of every 10, courses that are diagnosis related in veterinary medicine during the three-year pre-clinical phase.

LIMITATIONS: The number of schools sampled is small compared to the total number of veterinary medical schools in the nation. However small it may be, it is a reflection of the broad veterinary medical school perspective because graduates from these schools are not only qualified but board-certified veterinary medical doctors from high-ranking schools like the University of Pennsylvania. Other limitations involve the Tufts School of Veterinary Medicine, which has few courses that integrate diagnosis-related coursework as a major component and drug treatment or pharmacy-related courses as integral component of the course content.

DRUG TREATMENT OR PHARMACY-REALTED COURSES: Using same criteria, the university with the lowest average ratio in relation to pharmacy or drug-treatment courses available to veterinary medical doctors/students is the University of Pennsylvania with zero (0) out of 14 courses in the first year, 2 out of 14 courses in the second year, and zero (0) out of 8 courses in the third year, making a total average ratio of 0.047 or 4.7%. Two universities with the closest average ratio to 0.087 are Tufts School of Veterinary Medicine with zero (0) of 11 courses in the first year, 3 out of 22 courses in the second year, and 1 out of 12 courses in the third year, making a total average ratio of 0.07 or 7%; and University of Wisconsin with 1 out of 16 courses in the first year, 3 out of 18 courses in the second year, and 2 out of 20 courses in the third year, making a total average ratio of 0.11 or 11%. The University with the highest average ratio is Ohio State University with 1 out of 16 courses in the first year, 1 to 2 out of 14 courses in the second year, and 2 out of 10 courses in the third year, making a total average ratio of 0.12 or 12%. On the whole, it can be estimated that the average number of drug treatment or pharmacy-related courses that qualify the veterinary medical doctor to prescribe drug is 0.087 or 8.7%, which is approximately 9% or 9 out of every 100, or 1 out of every 11 courses during the three-year pre-clinical phase.

LIMITATIONS: Same as in diagnosis.

CLINICAL PHASE

Same as in dentistry.

PHYSICIAN ASSISTANT

Four schools were sampled. The two years coursework leading to the award of Master of Physician Assistant Studies degree comprises of one year in pre-clinical and clinical phase each. There is no residency in any form in the physician assistant program. Using the same criteria to analyze the number of diagnosis-related courses and pharmacy or drug treatment-related courses available to physician assistant students during the two-year program, the above data revealed:

PRE-CLINICAL PHASE

DIAGNOSIS-RELATED COURSES: The one-year didactic class work for diagnosis-related courses shows the university with the lowest ratio as the University of Iowa with 9 out of 14 courses, making a ratio of 0.64 or 64%. Two universities with the closest average ratio to 0.75 are Nova Southeastern University with a course content of 22 out of 34 courses, making a ratio of 0.65 or 65% in approximately 1.5 years because of the combined programs; and the University of Florida with 13 out of 15 courses, making a ratio of 0.87. The university with the highest ratio is University of Wisconsin with 15 out of 18 courses, making a ratio of 0.83 or 83%. Although no one expects the course content of PA courses to be the same as the prevailing courses in medical schools, even if they bear the same title, it is important to note that the PA has only one year didactic class work except Nova Southeastern University, as noted above, which has a dual-degree program, and none of them have a residency requirement. On the whole, the average number of diagnosis-related courses that the physician assistants/students are exposed to in the U.S. is 0.75 or 75%, which is approximately 80% or 8 out of every 10 courses during the one year didactic class work.

LIMITATIONS: The number of schools sampled is small compared to the total number of physician assistant schools in the nation. However small it may be, it is a reflection of the broad physician assistant school perspective because graduates from these schools are not only qualified but board-certified physician assistants from high or average-ranking schools like the University of Iowa. Other limitations involve Nova Southeastern University as the only school with a two and a half-year program because of the combined/dual-degree program.

DRUG TREATMENT- OR PHARMACY-REALTED COURSES: The university with the lowest ratio in terms of pharmacy or drug-treatment courses is Nova Southeastern University with 2 out of 34 courses making a ratio of 0.059 or 5.9%. The university with closest average ratio to 0.077 is the University of Iowa with 1 out of 14 courses making a ratio of 0.071 or 7.1%. The university with the highest ratio is the University of Wisconsin with 2 out of 18 courses, making a ratio of 0.11 or 11%. On the whole, the average number of drug-treatment or pharmacy courses that qualify the physician assistant to write more prescriptions than the clinical pharmacist is 0.071 or 7%, which is 7 out of every 100 courses, or 1 out of every 14 courses in one-year didactic class work. One course in a year laid the basic foundation upon which the whole career including rotations is based. The course content of this one pharmacy course (or far-reaching/embracing nature) is anyone's guess.

LIMITATIONS: Same as in diagnosis.

CLINICAL PHASE

The one-year clinical phase comprises of rotations that are meant to build on the foundation laid by the one-year didactic class work. As a transitional phase, rotations are tailored after the one-year class work in terms of content and expectations. Thus, it is not out of place to say that as a major part of the rotation, diagnosis takes 80% while drug treatment or pharmacy takes about 10 to 15%. The other 5 to 10% is devoted to other aspects of PA job expectations. At the end of the two-year course the PA graduates goes into practice under the supervision of a physician. In most offices, the phrase "supervision" is a theoretical, meaningless phrase, thereby leaving the PA with a wide range of choices as an independent diagnostician and prescriber, throwing pills at patients like candy bars. The physicians in these offices thus become administrators or colleagues because of an overwhelming situation with patients' influx or tied schedule. Little wonder why the nation is spending $177 billion, the year 2000 dollars adjustment of Johnson and Bootman's 1995 estimate of a $76.6 billion annual expenditure on drug-related morbidity and mortality.

CERTIFIED NURSE PRACTITONER

In order to get the overall view of certified nurse practitioner course content, we start with the first degree, Bachelor of Science (BSc) in nursing, and three schools were sampled for the program. As noted earlier, BSc nursing is of a higher status than the registered nurse (RN), which is equally higher than the licensed practicing nurse (LPN). The four years coursework leading to the award of Bachelor of Science (BSc) in nursing is analyzed below using same criteria for diagnosis and nursing-related courses and pharmacy or drug-treatment courses. Two years out of the four-year program are devoted to pre-nursing program because this is the only program here that allows admission direct from high school.

NURSE

DIAGNOSIS AND NURSING-RELATED COURSES: The university with the lowest average ratio in terms of diagnosis and nursing-related courses is Oregon Health Science University with 3 out of 14 courses in the first and second year, 11 out of 13 courses in the third year, and 10 out of 10 courses in the fourth year, making a total ratio of 0.56 or 56%. The university with the closest average ratio to 0.615 is the University of Texas with 4 out of 15 courses in the first and second year, 11 out of 11 courses in the third, and 12 out of 12 courses in the fourth year, making a total average ratio of 0.65 or 65 percent. The university with the highest average ratio is the University of Kentucky with 2 out of 10 courses in the first year, 5 out of 8 courses in the second year, 5 out of 6 courses in the third year, and 6 out of 6 courses in the fourth year, making a total average ratio of 0.67 or 67%. On the whole, it can be estimated that the average number of diagnosis and nursing-related courses that the nurses are exposed in the U.S. is 0.65 or 65%, which is 6.5 out of every 10 courses in nursing school during the four years coursework.

LIMITATIONS: The number of schools sampled is small compared to the total number of nursing schools in the nation. However small it may be, it is a reflection of the broad nursing school perspective because graduates from these schools are not only qualified but board-certified nurses from high or average-ranking schools like the University of Texas. Other limitations involve Creighton University with a fourth-year preceptorship, of which diagnosis and nursing-related courses constitute a major portion, while drug administration or pharmacy-related courses constitute an integral part of the program.

DRUG TREATMENT OR PHARMACY-REALTED COURSES: In relation to pharmacy or drug-treatment courses, the university with the lowest average ratio is Oregon Health Science University with zero (0) out of 14 courses in the first and second year, 1 out of 13 courses in the third year, and zero (0) out of 10 courses in the fourth year, making a total average ratio of 0.02 or 2%. The university with the closest average ratio to 0.027 is Creighton University with zero (0) out of 11 courses in the first year, zero (0) out of 12 courses in the second year, 1 out of 10 courses in the third year, and zero (0) out of 6 courses in the fourth year, making a total average ratio of 0.025. The university with the highest average ratio is the University of Texas with 1 out of 15 courses in the first and second year, zero (0) of 11 courses in the third year, and zero (0) out of 12 courses in the fourth year, making a total ratio of 0.034 or 3.4%. On the whole, it can be estimated that the average number of drug treatment or pharmacy-related courses that the nurses are exposed to in the U.S. is 0.025 or 2.5% which is one fourth out of every 10 courses or 1 out of every 40 courses.

LIMITATIONS: Same as in diagnosis.

The certified nurse practitioner and midwife require two-year postgraduate courses after the four-year Bachelor of Science degree in nursing. Three schools with five, certified nurse practitioner specialties and two school of midwifery programs were sampled using same criteria.

NURSE PRACTITIONER

DIAGNOSIS AND NURSING-RELATED COURSES: The school with the lowest average ratio is Creighton University with 7 out of 11 courses in the first year and 2 out of 4 courses in the second year for adult nurse practitioner, making a total average ratio of 0.57 or 57%. The university with the closest average ratio to 0.72 is Oregon Health Science University with 14 out of 19 courses in the first and second year, making a total average ratio of 0.74. The university with the highest average ratio is the University of Kentucky with 7 out of 9 courses in the first year and 5 out 5 courses in the second year for parent-child nurse practitioner, making a total ratio of 0.89 or 89%.

DRUG TREATMENT OR PHARMACY-REALTED COURSES: The school with the lowest average ratio here is Creighton University with 1 out of 11 courses in the first year and zero (0) of 5 courses in second year for adult and family nurse practitioners, making a total average ratio of 0.046 or 4.6%. The university with the closest average ratio to 0.053 is Oregon Health Science University with 1 out of 19 courses in the first and second year, making a total average ratio of 0.053 or 5.3%. The university with the highest average ratio is the University of Kentucky with 1 out of 9 courses in the first year and zero (0) out of 5 courses in the second year for parent-child and acute care nurse practitioners, making a total average ratio of 0.055 or 5.5%

MIDWIFEFRY

DIAGNOSIS AND NURSING-RELATED COURSES: The lowest average ratio school is Seattle Midwifery School with 17 out of 27 courses in the first and second year (8 quarters), making a total ratio of 0.63 or 63%. The university with the highest average ratio is Oregon Health Science University with 20 out of 27 courses in the first and second year, making a total average ratio of 0.74 or 74%. The average of these two schools gives 0.69, and that is approximately 0.7 or 70% in terms of number of diagnosis and nursing-related courses.

DRUG TREATMENT OR PHARMACY-REALTED COURSES: The school with the lowest average ratio is Seattle Midwifery School with 1 out of 27 courses in the first and second year (8 quarters), making a total ratio of 0.04 or 4%. The university with the highest average ratio is Oregon Health Science University with 2 out of 27 courses in the first and second year, making a total average ratio of 0.074 or 7.4%. The average of these two schools gives 0.057 or 5.7%, which is approximately 0.06 or 6% in terms of the number of pharmacy or drug-treatment courses.

COMBINED ANALYSIS

A combination of the first degree (BSc) and postgraduate degree in certified nurse practitioner and midwifery determines the total number of courses for nurse practitioners and midwifery. What follows is a two-way analysis using overall average scores and average scores for the schools involved (that is, Creighton University, University of Kentucky, and Oregon Health Science University).

Nurse Practitioner

1. Overall average scores

c. DIAGNOSIS AND NURSING-RELATED COURSES:

$$\frac{\text{Average of BSc (0.61)} + \text{Average of certified nurse practitioner (0.72)}}{2}$$

= (0.61 + 0.72) / 2 = 0.665 or 0.67 (67%)

d. DRUG TREATMENT OR PHARMACY-REALTED COURSES:

$$\frac{\text{Average of BSc (0.0273)} + \text{Average of certified nurse practitioner (0.053)}}{2}$$

= (0.0273 + 0.053) / 2 = 0.04 (4%)

2. Average scores for the three schools

a. Creighton University

> DIAGNOSIS AND NURSING-RELATED COURSES:
> (0.27 + 0.39 + 0.8 + 0.83 + 0.64 + 0.6) / 6 = 3.53 / 6 = 0.59 (59 percent)
>
> DRUG TREATMENT OR PHARMACY-REALTED COURSES:
> (0 + 0 + 0.1 + 0 + 0.091 + 0) / 6 = 0.032 (3.2%)

b. University of Kentucky

> DIAGNOSIS AND NURSING-RELATED COURSES:
> (0.2 + 0.63 + 0.83 + 1 + 0.89 + 0.80) / 6 = 0.73 (73%)
>
> DRUG TREATMENT OR PHARMACY-REALTED COURSES:
> (0 + 0.125 + 0 + 0 + 0.11 + 0) / 6 = 0.0392 or 0.04 (4%)

c. Oregon Health Science University

> DIAGNOSIS AND NURSING-RELATED COURSES:
> (0.2 + 0.2 + 0.85 + 1 + 0.74 + 0.74) / 6 = 0.62 (62%)
>
> DRUG TREATMENT OR PHARMACY-REALTED COURSES:
> (0 + 0 + 0.077 + 0 + 0.053 + 0.053) / 6 = 0.031 (31%)

Total average of a, b, and c.

> DIAGNOSIS AND NURSING-RELATED COURSES:
> (0.59 + 0.73 + 0.62) / 3 = 0.65 (65%)
>
> DRUG TREATMENT OR PHARMACY-REALTED COURSES:
> (0.032 + 0.04 + 0.031) / 3 = 0.034 (3%)

MIDWIFERY
Oregon Health Science University (only available data)

1. Overall average scores

e. DIAGNOSIS AND NURSE-RELATED COURSES:

$$\frac{\text{Average of BSc (0.56)} + \text{average of certified nurse practitioner (0.74)}}{2}$$

= (0.56 + 0.74) / 2 = 0.65 (65%)

f. DRUG TREATMENT OR PHARMACY-REALTED COURSES:

$$\frac{\text{Average of BSc (0.02)} + \text{average of certified nurse practitioner (0.074)}}{2}$$

= (0.02 + 0.053) / 2 = 0.047 (4.7%)

The results of the two-way analysis are almost similar with the number of diagnosis and nursing-related courses as 0.67 (overall average score) and 0.65 (three schools' average scores), and the number of pharmacy or drug treatment-related courses as 0.04 (overall average score) and 0.034 (three schools' average score); consequently, the overall average scores, which are the highest with more inclusive average data, will be used. On the whole, it can be estimated that a certified nurse practitioner is exposed to 0.67 or 67%, which is approximately 70% or 7 out of every 10, diagnosis and nursing-related courses. In relation to pharmacy or drug treatment-related courses that qualify the certified nurse practitioner to prescribe far more drugs than the clinical pharmacists, it can be estimated that the certified nurse practitioner is exposed to an average number of 0.04 or 4%, which is 4 out of every 100 or 1 out of every 25 courses. The certified nurse practitioners in most cases have greater liberty, freedom, and independence than the physician assistants in diagnosing and prescribing drugs or running physicians' offices/independent offices.

LIMITATIONS: The number of schools sampled is small compared to the total number of certified nurse practitioner schools in the nation. However small it may be, it is a reflection of the broad certified nurse practitioner school perspective because graduates from these schools are not only qualified but board-certified nurse practitioners from high-ranking schools like Oregon Health Science University. Other limitations involve the exclusion of the

University of Iowa because of inadequate data. Similar deductions can be made for certified nurse midwifery using Oregon Health Science University's overall average scores, which are similar to the certified nurse practitioner. Lack of data for the Bachelor of Science in nursing in Seattle Midwifery School created a vacuum in the data analysis. However, the Oregon Health Science University fills the vacuum with statistics from BSc and midwifery courses. The two midwifery schools have a two-year average duration of study and this statistic matches those for BSc and certified nurse practitioners.

PHARMACY

Eight schools were sampled for Doctor of Pharmacy degree programs and three schools for first degree or Bachelor of Science degree in pharmacy programs. Like dentistry, optometry, and veterinary medicine, pharmacy programs have no residency requirements; it is optional as a postgraduate program for interested graduates. The Doctor of Pharmacy is a four years coursework leading to the award of PharmD, while the Bachelor of Science degree program that is now on the path of dinosaur is a three years coursework leading to the award of BSc in pharmacy. Both programs comprises of two phases, which are pre-clinical and clinical phases. The number of diagnosis-related courses and pharmacy or drug treatment-related courses available to students in both programs can be assessed using same criteria below.

BACHELOR OF SCIENCE DEGREE PROGRAM

The program is made up of two-year pre-clinical and one-year clinical phases.

PRE-CLINICAL PHASE

DIAGNOSIS-RELATED COURSES: The university with the lowest average ratio is the University of Texas with 2 out of 15 courses in the first year and zero (0) out of 15 courses in the second year, making a total average ratio of 0.065 or 6.5%. The university with the closest average ratio to 0.12 is Long Island University with 2 out of 9 courses in the first year and zero (0) out of 10 courses in the second year, making a total average ratio of 0.11 or 11%. The university with the highest average ratio is the University of Montana with 5 out of 13 courses in the first year and zero (0) out of 11 courses in the second year, making a total average ratio of 0.19 of 19%. On the whole, it can be estimated that pharmacy students/pharmacists with Bachelor of Science degree program in the U.S. are exposed to an average of 0.11 courses, which is approximately 10% or 1 out of every 10 courses in diagnosis-related courses.

LIMITATIONS: The number of schools sampled is small compared to the total number of pharmacy schools in the nation. However small it may be, it is a reflection of the broad pharmacy school perspective because graduates from these schools are not only qualified but board-certified pharmacists from high-ranking schools like the University of Texas. Other limitations involve few courses that are offered during the clinical year (rotations). These courses were excluded and considered as part of clinical year courses. Data from Long Island University College of Pharmacy 1995-1996 are out of sequence because most of the data used were obtained around the year 2000. This data was included to show that contemporary data for the first degree (BSc) in pharmacy have little or no difference from previous years.

DRUG TREATMENT OR PHARMACY-REALTED COURSES: The university with the lowest average ratio here is Long Island University with 7 out of 9 courses in the first year and 7 out of 10 courses in the second year, making a total average ratio of 0.74 or 74%. The university with the closest average ratio 0.81 is the University of Montana with 8 out of 13 courses in the first year and 11 out of 11 courses in the second year, making a total average ratio of 0.81 or 81%. The university with the highest average ratio is the University of Texas with 11 out of 15 courses in the first year and 15 out of 15 courses in the second year, making a total average ratio of 0.87 or 87%. On the whole, it can be estimated that the average number of pharmacy or drug treatment-related courses to which Bachelor of Science degree program holders are exposed in the U.S. is 0.81 or 81%, which is approximately 80% and that is 8 out of every 10 courses during the two-year didactic class work (pre-clinical phase).

LIMITATIONS: Same as in diagnosis.

CLINICAL PHASE

For the Bachelor of Science degree program in pharmacy, the one-year clinical phase comprises of rotations, otherwise tagged externship and internship. These rotations are meant to build on the foundation laid by the two-year pre-clinical phase didactic class work. It further entrenches the knowledge gained from the classroom by helping students to put into practice most of the learned theories. Unlike other branches of medicine, there is a reverse proceeding in terms of course content during pharmacy rotations. Pharmacy or drug treatment constitutes major part of the rotations, while diagnosis constitutes minor part of the rotations. As a pre-clinical phase transition, rotations can be said to be a direct reflection of the classroom work, with about 80 % pharmacy or drug treatment, about 10 to 15% diagnosis, and 5% for the rest of the pharmacy requirements. After graduation, the pharmacist goes to practice and discovers that the dispensing role does not merit the number of years training in school. Instead of facing a challenging situation that demands more of their expertise, knowledge, and talents from school, they are meant to throw pills from bottle to bottle and fill the role of the "Seinfeld Pharmacist." Except for self-motivation, personal challenges, and clinical demands for those in a clinical setting, the knowledge dwindles and goes downhill.

Presently, there are postgraduate Doctor of Pharmacy degree programs designed to assist pharmacy first-degree holders who wish to upgrade their professional status to doctorate level. It is a two-year program that is composed of one-year pre-clinical and clinical phases each. Many schools of pharmacy operate the program as a temporary means of bridging the gap. The program will be phased out with a first-degree program in U.S. as the market diminishes to the point of no return. Postgraduate Doctor of Pharmacy degree program was not considered in this chapter because it is not the modus operandi for training future pharmacists. However, Nova Southeastern University is one of the schools of pharmacy that operates the program, with 8 courses in the first-year pre-clinical phase (6 pharmacy or drug treatment-related courses and one diagnosis-related course) and 6 clinical rotations in the second-year clinical phase. 47 credits is the minimum number required for graduation. Thus, a clinical pharmacist that goes through first-degree and doctoral degree programs separately requires five years for graduation, while those that go into Doctor of Pharmacy degree programs directly require four years for graduation after the initial entry requirements.

DOCTOR OF PHARMACY DEGREE PROGRAM

The Doctor of Pharmacy degree program is made up of a three-year pre-clinical phase and a one-year clinical phase.

PRE-CLINICAL PHASE

DIAGNOSIS-RELATED COURSES: The two universities with the lowest average ratio among the 8 sampled schools are the University of Texas with 4 out of 18 courses in the first year, zero (0) out of 14 courses in the second year, and 1 out of 10 courses in the third year, making a total average ratio of 0.11 or 11%; and Texas Southern University with 3 out of 16 courses in the first year, 2 out of 15 courses in the second year, and zero (0) out of 13 courses in the third year, making a total average ratio of 0.11 or 11%. Three universities with the closest average ratio to 0.17 are the University of Kentucky with 2 out of 13 courses in the first year, zero (0) out of 8 courses in the second year, and 2 out of 6 courses in the third year, making a total average ratio of 0.16 or 16%; Auburn University with 4 out of 15 courses in the first year, 3 out of 14 courses in the second year, and zero (0) out of 11 courses in the third year, making a total average ratio of 0.16 or 16%; and the University of Montana with 5 out of 13 courses in the first year, zero (0) out of 11 courses in the second year, and 1 out of 10 courses in the third year, making a total average ratio of 0.16 or 16%. The university with the highest average ratio is the University of Colorado with 3 out of 16 courses in the first year, 6 out of 15 courses in the second year, and 2 out of 10 courses in the third year, making a total average ratio of 0.26 or 26%. On the whole, using these data, it can be estimated that the clinical pharmacists with Doctor of Pharmacy degrees in the U.S. are exposed to an average of 0.16 (16%), which is approximately 20% and that is 2 out of every 10, courses in diagnosis during the three years didactic classwork, or pre-clinical phase.

LIMITATIONS: The number of schools sampled is small compared to the total number of pharmacy schools in the nation. However small it may be, it is a reflection of the broad pharmacy school perspective because graduates from these schools are not only qualified but board-certified pharmacists from high-ranking schools like the University of California, San Francisco. Other limitations involve few courses with drug treatment or pharmacy-related courses as a major component and diagnosis-related courses as a minor component of the course content. Like in medicine and other programs, these courses were considered to be drug treatment or pharmacy-related courses (the major component) even though they contained some element of diagnosis. Some schools like the University of California have third-year clinical rotations that belong to the clinical-phase program, of which diagnosis-related courses constitute an integral part and pharmacy or drug treatment-related courses constitute a major part of the rotations. St. Louis College of Pharmacy data were excluded from data analysis because of its deviation from other schools' curricula.

DRUG TREATMENT OR PHARMACY-REALTED COURSES: The university with the lowest average ratio is the University of California with 10 out of 15 courses in the first year, 6 out of 12 courses in the second year, and 5 out of 7 courses in the third year, making a total average ratio of 0.63 or 63%. The university with the closest average ratio to 0.74 is the University of Montana with 8 out of 13 courses in the first year, 10 out of 11 courses in the second year, and 7 out of 10 courses in the third year, making a total average ratio of 0.74 or 74%. Two highest average ratio universities are the University of Kentucky with 11 out of 13 courses in the first year, 8 out of 8 courses in the second year, and 4 out of 6 courses in the third year, making a total average ratio of 0.84 or 84%; and Auburn University with 11 out of 15 courses in the first year, 11 out of 14 courses in the second year, and 11 out of 11 in the third year, making a total average ratio of 0.84 or 84%. On the whole, using these data it can be estimated that clinical pharmacists with Doctor of Pharmacy degrees in the U.S. are exposed to an average number of 0.74 or 74%, which is approximately 70% or 7 out of every 10, pharmacy or drug treatment-related courses during the three years didactic classwork or pre-clinical phase.

LIMITATIONS: Same as in diagnosis.

CLINICAL PHASE

The one-year clinical phase comprises of rotations or clerkships, which is meant to build on the foundation laid by the three-year pre-clinical phase didactic class work. Unlike other branches of medicine, there is a reversed order of proceedings even though the status quo remain the same as transition of the pre-clinical phase. Pharmacy or drug treatment constitutes a major part of the rotations, while diagnosis constitutes a minor part of the rotations. Rotations serve to entrench and inculcate the knowledge gained during the pre-clinical phase didactic classwork; consequently, about 70-80% of the rotation coursework is pharmacy or drug treatment-related, 15-25% is diagnosis related, and 5-10% to other forms of treatment such as nutrition (total parenteral nutrition or TPN) and non-drug treatment. In comparism to the first degree BSc, the Doctor of Pharmacy degree has more years in training, emphasis on clinical pharmacy, and greater clinical impact. However, after graduation the majority of the Doctor of Pharmacy degree holders face the same dilemma as the first-degree holders. Many will discover that the extra years in training are meaningless while few others face challenging situations in clinical settings. This deplorable situation is bound to continue until we as a society are prepared to call "a spade a spade" by tapping the clinical pharmacists' ingenuity and knowledge to better our understanding of drug and drug treatment, thereby reducing the astronomical waste in manpower, economics, and life resulting from drug-related morbidity and mortality. EXPERTS ARE BETTER AT WORK THAN NON-EXPERTS.

GENERAL LIMITATIONS: The general limitations involve elective courses—except specific electives with elucidated course outlines, health system courses, liberal acts, basic sciences, laws requiring courses for various programs, administrative courses, veterinary courses relating to nutrition-reproduction, etc., and few other courses were excluded from the subject matter because they were neither specific nor did they relate directly to diagnosis or pharmacy/drug treatment-related courses, which was the subject matter of the study/research. Unspecified pre-clinical phase's electives with credits or hours were assigned number with suffix alphabet (e.g. 10a) and excluded from data analysis. The same is true of clinical/rotation's phase or zero credits electives even though they were assigned numbers.

CONCLUSION

In conclusion, there is nothing wrong or unusual with pharmacy courses in relation to other courses such as engineering, dentistry, optometry, veterinary medicine, physics, mathematics, microbiology, and other branches of medicine. However, there is something wrong in a situation where an optometrist is meant to act like a dentist and vice versa and pharmacists, especially clinical pharmacists with Doctor of Pharmacy degrees, are relegated to the background and prevented from exhibiting their talents in their own jurisdiction while the following situations prevail in the U.S.:

a. A physician assistant with just one pharmacy or drug treatment-related course out of every 14 courses in just one year (maximum of 2 courses, and that is if the school offers 28 courses in one year) is authorized to prescribe a wide range of drugs that are out of reach of the pharmacist with no residency requirement.

b. A certified nurse practitioner or midwife with just one pharmacy or drug treatment-related course out of every 25 courses in two years (maximum of 1.5 in 2 years, and that is if the school offers about 38 courses in 2 years) is authorized to prescribed drugs that are not only out of the pharmacist's reach but are unimaginable to the pharmacist with no residence requirement. There are low probabilities of taking more than 25 courses in two years, yet some CNPs operate as independent providers/prescribers all over the nation.

c. A dentist with just one pharmacy or drug treatment-related course out of every 33 courses in three years (maximum of 3 courses in 3 years, and that is if the school offers 33 courses per year) can prescribe drugs that the pharmacist can not even dream of. Yet they spent the same number of years in school training as a clinical pharmacist with no residence requirement.

d. An optometrist with one pharmacy or drug-treatment course out of every 17 courses in three years (maximum of 4 courses in 3 years, and that is if the school offers 22 courses per year) can prescribe drugs (e.g., all eye drops such as alphagan, azopt, ciloxan, tobradex, or any antibiotics, etc.) that are by far out of reach of the pharmacist. Yet they spent same number of years in school training as a clinical pharmacist with no residence requirement.

e. A veterinary medical doctor with one pharmacy or drug treatment-related course out of every 11 courses in three years (maximum of 6 courses in 3 years, and that is if the school offers 22 courses per year) can prescribe any type of drugs for the pharmacist to dispense, yet they spent same number of years in school training as a clinical pharmacist with no residence requirement.

f. All other branches of medicine and osteopathic medical doctors with one pharmacy or drug treatment-related course out of every 17 courses in two years (the only classroom didactic work—a maximum of 4 courses in two years, and that is if the school offers 34 courses per year—without the clinical/residency phase) can prescribe any type of drugs for the pharmacist to dispense.

g. The clinical pharmacist with 7 pharmacy or drug treatment-related courses out of every 10 courses in three years (maximum of 42 courses in three years and that is if the school offers 20 course per year) can not prescribe any drugs for anyone to dispense (the course content is the same for first-degree holders in pharmacy except that the clinical pharmacist spent more years in school training and has more clinical training than the first-degree holders). Some will say that there are few allowable drugs on the pharmacists' formulary depending on the state—these few drugs are mostly over-the-counter (OTC) drugs and probably a few drugs that are one step above OTC. Pharmacists quite often resist the temptation to prescribe these drugs, because in an attempt to do so they are readily pushed beyond the boundary to break the law by pressurizing patients. Moreover, most insurance companies or third-party payers do not recognize pharmacists as prescribers, so whatever services or drugs they prescribe are not paid for. By and large we discovered that the pharmacists' formulary is as good as null and void.

The school of thought that designed medicine with all its branches was meant to create a super-diagnostician as a specialist with the concomitant effect of drug-treatment deficiency. This deficiency in drug treatment was expected to be overcome with rotations/clinical clerkships and residency, which in a nutshell is as good as the outdated apprenticeship mode of training physicians. Contemporary society can survive and flourish with professionals such as engineers going through standard training in formal education rather than residency or apprenticeship, because the resultant consequences of relying on the latter as a means of training younger generation is a chaotic society. It is not only out of place but also improper to blame the pioneers of medicine as originators of this problem, because medicine at the beginning was practiced as a whole model. However, pharmacy and surgery crept into medicine as specialties at the earliest stage and practitioners didn't take pharmacy as serious as surgery. This view was carried forward to the early twentieth century; the era of specialties and pioneers of various specialties concentrated on diagnosis because it is the first phase of human ailment (patients have to know the root cause of their ailments before treatment can proceed). Today's reality is different from those days; if anyone thinks in a similar fashion to those pioneers, one would be tempted to ask an obvious question, which is if we believe that the traditional medical doctors can overcome drug-treatment deficiency with clinical clerkships/rotations and residency, what makes us think that the clinical pharmacists cannot overcome similar deficiencies in diagnosis with clinical clerkships/rotations and residency? Moreover, it has been noted that many programs/professions survive (and not the opposite) without residency. Apparently there is nothing wrong with pharmacy curriculum in relation to others; even if we notice any deficiency in the program/profession, it is our responsibility to correct the deficiency, strengthen the program/profession, and allow it to take its proper role as a branch of medicine instead of being subservient to it. Pharmacists currently take more courses in diagnosis than the traditional medical doctors take pharmacy or drug-treatment courses. The current practice of violating pharmacy and holding the profession in contempt by robbing it to pay other branches of medicine (robbing Peter to pay Paul) is not in the best interest of humanity. Humanity makes great strides when we correct anomalies of the past and centuries-old injustices of the depraved voiceless people in our society. Good enough pharmacy program has clinical clerkships/rotations. Some clinical pharmacists have taking the initiative to go through a residency program in the past, while young graduates from pharmacy schools see residency programs as an attractive force today. These clinical clerkships/rotations and residency need modification, if need be, and we need to strengthen the role of drug treatment for pharmacists and diagnosis for other branches of medicine rather than weaken them. CLINICAL PHARMACISTS ARE TRAINED THERAPEUTICIANS OR THERAPEUTIC PHYSICIANS, WHILE THE MAJORITY OF PRACTITIONERS IN OTHER BRANCHES OF MEDICINE ARE TRAINED DIAGNOSICIANS. After all said and done, it is important to note that the existence of pediatricians has not stopped other doctors from attending to children; neither has the existence of dentists stopped other doctors from attending to patients' dental problems. All branches of medicine serve their jurisdiction by emphasizing their area of specialty and complementing each other at the long run. And so THE LIBERATION OF PHARMACY AS AN INDEPENDENT BRANCH OF MEDICINE IS NOT THE END OF MEDICINE, AS MANY PROPHETS OF DOOM WILL MAKE US BELIEVE, BUT A GREAT ADVENTURE THAT WILL PROTECT HUMANTIY AND SAVE MANY HUMAN LIVES. PHARMACY IS A BRANCH OF MEDICINE AND NOT AN ERAND BOY OF MEDICINE.

REFERENCES

1. Graham, A. E., and R. J. Morse. How *U.S. News* ranks colleges: America's best colleges, *U.S. News and World Report*, June 1, 2000: 26-29.

2. Best national universities: America's best colleges, *U.S. News and World Report* (1 June 2000): 30-34.

3. Morse, R. J., and S. M. Flanigan. How we rank the colleges, special report: America's best colleges, *U.S. News and World Report* (11 September 2000): 104-105.

4. Best national universities, special report: America's best colleges, *U.S. News and World Report* (11 September 2001): 106-110.

5. Schools of medicine: America's best graduate schools, *U.S. News and World Report* (9 April 2001): 88-92.

6. University of Pennsylvania School of Medicine brochure: Applicant information and curriculum, 2000-2002.

7. University of Iowa College of Medicine catalog, 2000-2002.

8. University of Maryland School of Medicine catalog, 2002-2004

9. Wright State University School of Medicine catalog.

10. University of Miami School of Medicine catalog. Admission information.

11. Nova Southeastern University (NSU) Health Professions Division catalog, 2001-2002.

12. State University of New York Health Science Center at Brooklyn, New York, 1995-1996, information for medical school applicants.

13. Baltimore College of Dental Surgery and Dental School, University of Maryland, 2000-2002 catalog.

14. Harvard School of Dental Medicine catalog.

15. University of Pennsylvania School of Dental medicine, 2001-2002.

16. University of Pennsylvania School of Veterinary Medicine admission catalog, 2001-2003.

17. Tufts School of Veterinary Medicine, Bulletin of Tufts University, 2001-2002/2002-2003.

18. University of Iowa College of Nursing catalog, 2000-2002, and master's program in nursing.

19. St. Louis College of Pharmacy catalog, 1996/97.

20. Texas Southern University College of Pharmacy catalog, 2002-2003.

CHAPTER SIX

WORLDWIDE STUDY OF MEDICAL SCHOOLS' CURRICULA IN COMPARISM TO SCHOOLS OF PHARMACY

A worldwide study of medical schools and schools of pharmacy curricula took the investigator to six habitable continents of the world, namely Africa, Asia, Australia, Europe, North America, and South America. It started in Africa then went to Europe, North America, Asia, Australia, and South America. The investigator's choice to start the study in what he believed was the greatest institution of higher leaning in the world, which he attended, is a monumental decision based on unique experience. See the appendix for the investigator's unique experience.

SCHOOL CURRICULUM

This study by its very nature is limited in scope by funding; consequently, one or two schools might be used as case example(s) for each continent. The choice of one school per continent is a necessary tool to prevent the reader's boredom. This is not a school catalog or prospectus but a book or study that is meant to drive home one message about the pharmacy program in relation to other branches of medicine. These schools might not be the best in each sampled continent but they have one thing in common, and that is they are the microcosm, or representative, of what is obtainable in the vast continent in which they dwell. If paradventure any of the selected sampled schools falls into the worst category, people can be rest assured that the affected school is in existence and permitted to operate and produce graduates in accordance with rules and regulations of the respective country and government. Moreover, graduates from these schools do not only meet the standard of professional practice in their respective country or countries but can survive their professional practice anywhere in the world. That is to say these graduates (with the exception of China—because of the mixture of Western medicine and Chinese traditional medicine in their educational system) are second to none in their professional practice around the world besides linguistic barrier and various government regulatory policies. They can practice anywhere in the world, be it Brazil, Australia, Morocco, the United States, Spain, and others notwithstanding the linguistic barrier and various government regulatory policies.

AFRICA

Africa is the second largest continent in the world, with 11.6 million square miles and a population of 600 million people as of 1990. It is the traditional home of blacks. Naturally there are two sets of human beings that make up humanity's two great races. Irrespective of what we do to segregate, divide, and rule the world, these two races are blacks and whites. Like the over 1.2 billion Chinese in Asia, no human study can be said to be complete without taking into consideration the interest of blacks in the world. The University of Ife, now Obafemi Awolowo University, is used as a case example of higher institutions in Africa.

UNIVERSITY OF IFE

The entry level for medical school is the same for the university: a secondary school/high school certificate, otherwise tagged West Africa school certificate (WASC), or ordinary and advanced-level passes in general certificate of education (GCE); successfully passing the joint admission matriculation board (JAMB) examination, and a personal interview. The only exception is that admission into the medical school has top-level cutoff and all students have a high level of academic excellence in sciences (physics, chemistry, biology or zoology, and mathematics). The medical school program was previously a seven-year program, but major changes in 1978 reduced it to six years and students are awarded the MBCh.B degree at the end of the program. The six-year program comprises of pre-professional year 1 program as phase P, years 2 and 3 as phase I, and year 4 as phase II, and year 5 and 6 as phase III.[1] The award of an MBCh.B degree and board certification qualifies graduates to practice medicine as medical doctors in gynecology and obstetrics, pediatrics, anesthesia, orthopedics, internal medicine, mental health, community health, ophthalmology, otorhinolarhyngology, dermatology and venerology, forensic medicine, ambulatory care, radiology, and surgery. The clinical years in phase III enable students to exploit their area of interest and specialize in any of the above. The fact that the course outline for 1988-90 is used to show what is obtainable in the university in 2000-2001 is not absurd because the courses are still the same with little or no modification. Any modification was reflected with handwriting and crossover, which were taken into consideration. Moreover, comparison of courses occurs simultaneously within the same period; as a result there is no discrepancy.

Course Outline (1988-90)

Pre-Professional Phase (Phase P: "Preliminary" Year)

Year 1
Harmattan Semester (20 Units)

1. Introductory Chemistry I (5 u); 2. Form and Function in Plants (4 u); 3. Physics for Biological Science I (5 u); 4. Man in his Social Environment (4 u); 5. Use of English (2 u).

(D: 0; P: 0)

Rain Semester (19 units)

1. Introductory Chemistry II (5 u); 2. Introductory Zoology (4 u); 3. Physics for Biological Science II (5 u); 4. Man in his Social Environment (3 u); 5. Use of English (2 u)

(D: 2; P: 0)

Number of pharmacy or drug treatment-related courses: zero (0) out of 10 or 39 units.

Number of diagnosis-related courses: 1 out of 10 or 4 out of 39 units.

Phase I
Year 2 (800 hrs + 1 Month Community Health)

1. Human Anatomy (360 hrs); 2. Medical Biochemistry (120 hrs); 3. Physiology (220 hrs); 4. Biostatistics (20 hrs); 5. Introduction to Community Health (month of July); 6. Behavioral Sciences (80 hrs).

(D: 1, 2, 3, 6; P: 0)

Number of pharmacy or drug treatment-related courses: zero (0) out of 6 or 800 hrs.

Number of diagnosis-related courses: 4 out of 6 or 780 out of 800 hrs.

YEAR 3 (800 HRS)
1. Human Anatomy (300 hrs); 2. Medical Biochemistry (120 hrs); 3. Physiology and Pharmacology (220 hrs); 4. Preceptorship in Clinics (100 hrs).
(D: 1, 2; P: 0; D & P: 3, 4)

Number of pharmacy or drug treatment-related courses: 1 out of 4 or 110 out of 800 hrs.

Number of diagnosis-related courses: 3 out of 4 or 690 out of 800 hrs.

PHASE II
YEAR 4
1. Integrated Lecture Series (200 hrs); 2. Introduction to the Principles of Medical Practices (internal medicine junior posting—8 wks, surgery junior posting—8 wks, primary care—4 wks); 3. Human Pathology (introductory posting—4 wks, morbid anatomy—8 wks, chemical pathology—4 wks, hematology and blood banking—4 wks, medical microbiology and parasitology—4 wks); 4. Hematology and Blood Banking (10 wks); 5. General and Systemic Pathology (30 wks); 6. Microbiology (16 wks); 7. Parasitology (10 wks); 8. Clinical Pharmacology (13 wks); 9. Community Health (30 wks); 10. Principles of Nursing (10 wks).
(D: 1, 3, 4, 5, 6, 7, 9; P: 8)

Number of pharmacy or drug treatment-related courses: 1 out of 8 or constitute an integral part of clerkship/medical practices.

Number of diagnosis-related courses: 7 out of 8 or constitute a major part of clerkship/medical practices.

PHASE III
YEAR 5 (CLERKSHIP/CLINICAL ROTATIONS: 51 WEEKS)
1. Gynecology and Obstetrics (16 wks); 2. Pediatrics (13 wks); 3. Anesthesia (2 wks); 4. Orthopedics (45 wks); 5. Ear, Nose, and Throat (2 wks); 6.

Ophthalmology (2 wks); 7. Radiology (2 wks); 8. Mental Health (6 wks); 9. Dermatology and Venerology (4 wks).

Number of pharmacy or drug treatment-related courses: constitute an integral part of clerkship.

Number of diagnosis-related courses: constitute a major part of clerkship.

YEAR 6 (80 WEEKS—SOME OVERLAP)
1. Community Health and Rural Posting (8 wks); 2. Internal Medicine (12 wks); 3. Surgery (12 wks); 4. General Outpatients (4 wks); 5. Elective (4 wks); 6. Forensic Medicine (4 wks).

Number of pharmacy or drug treatment-related courses: constitute an integral part of clerkship.
Number of diagnosis-related courses: constitute a major part of clerkship.

Total of Phase I and II
Before clerkship (phase III) without phase P
Number of pharmacy or drug treatment-related courses: 2 out of 18.
Number of diagnosis-related courses: 14 out of 18.
(D = 0.78 & P = 0.1)

DENTISTRY

Like the medical schools, the department of restorative dentistry has same admission protocol and number of years (six) in school training leading to award of B.CH.D. The phase program is also similar to the above except that the courses are different.[1]

Course Outline (1988-90)
Pre-Professional Phase (Phase P: "Preliminary" Year)
Year 1
Harmattan Semester (19 Units)

1. Introductory Chemistry I (5 u); 2. Form and Function in Plants (4 u); 3. Physics for Biological Science I (5 u); 4. Man in his Social Environment (3 u); 5. Use of English (2 u).
(DD: 0; P: 0)

Rain Semester (16 Units)
1. Introductory Chemistry II (5 u); 2. Introductory Zoology (4 u); 3. Physics for Biological Science II (5 u); 4. Use of English (2 u).
(DD: 2; P: 0)
Number of pharmacy or drug treatment-related courses: zero (0) out of 9 or 35 units.

Number of diagnosis and dental-related courses: 1 out of 9 or 4 out of 35 units.

Phase I
Year 2 and Half of Year 3 (18 Months)
1. Human Anatomy (36 wks); 2. Medical Biochemistry (36 wks); 3. Physiology (36 wks); 4. Biostatistics (20 wks); 5. Introduction to History of Dentistry (4 wks); 6. Behavior Sciences.
(DD: 1, 2, 3, 6, 7; P: 0)
Number of pharmacy or drug treatment-related courses: zero (0) out of 6 or 172 wks.

Number of diagnosis and dental-related courses: 5 out of 6 or 112 out of 172 wks.

Year 3 (Last Half)
1. Human Anatomy (36 wks); 2. Medical Biochemistry (36 wks); 3. Physiology including Pharmacology (36 wks); 4. Principles of Dental Practice (3 months).
(DD: 1, 2, 4; DD & P: 3)
Number of pharmacy or drug treatment-related courses: 0.5 out of 4.

Number of diagnosis and dental-related courses: 3.5-4 out of 4.

PHASE II
YEAR 4 (9-MONTH CLERKSHIP)

1. Human Pathology; 2. Principles of General Surgery, General Medicine: Pediatrics, General Anesthesia, and Radiology; 3. Oral Diagnosis, Medicine, and Radiology; 4. Principles of Dental Practices; 5. Introduction to Oral Surgery; 6. Oral Pathology.
  (DD: 1, 2, 3, 4, 5, 6; P: 0; DD & P: 2)
Number of pharmacy or drug treatment-related courses: 0.5 out of 6 or 9 months but constitute an integral part of the clerkship.

Number of diagnosis and dental-related courses: 5.5 out of 6 or 9 out of 9 months but constitute a major part of clerkship

PHASE III (24 MONTHS)
YEAR 5 AND 6: CLERKSHIP

1. Oral Medicine and Radiology II; 2. Oral Surgery II; 3. Restorative Dentistry; 4. Paedodontics; 5. Orthodontics; 6. Peridontology; 7. Preventive and Community Dentistry; 8. Forensic Dentistry and Professional Ethics; 9. Junior Internship Dental Practice.
  (DD: 1, 2, 3, 4, 5, 6, 7, 8; P: 0)
Number of pharmacy or drug treatment-related courses: zero (0) out of 9 but constitute an integral part of the clerkship.

Number of diagnosis and dental-related courses: 8 out of 9 but constitute a major part of clerkship.

Total of Phase I to III
Number of pharmacy or drug treatment-related courses: 1 out of 25.
Number of diagnosis and dental-related courses: 22.5 out of 25.
  (DD = 0.90 & P = 0.04)

NURSING

The department of nursing operates a five-year program leading to the award of Bachelor of Nursing Science degree (B.N.Sc). The admissions requirement is the same as the medical school admission except that the required passing levels in the JAMB examination and WASC/GCE are lower.[1]

Course Outline (1988-90)

YEAR 1
Harmattan Semester
1. Botany (2 u); 2. Chemistry (3 u); 3. Physics (3 u); 4. Mathematics (4 u); 5. Use of English (2 u).
(DN: 0; P: 0)

Rain Semester
1. Zoology (3 u); 2. Chemistry (3 u); 3. Social Science (2 u); 4. Use of English (2 u); 5. Introduction to Professional Nursing (6 wks).
(DN: 1, 4; P: 0)

Number of pharmacy or drug treatment-related courses: zero (0) out of 10.

Number of diagnosis and nursing-related courses: 2 out of 10.

YEAR 2
1. Foundations of Professional Nursing (12 wks); 2. Introduction to Biostatistics (10 wks); 3. Physiological and Pathological Chemistry I (12 wks); 4. Medical Microbiology and Parasitology (10 wks); 5. Human Anatomy (12 wks); 6. Human Physiology (12 wks); 7. African History and Culture.
(DN: 1, 3, 4, 5, 6; P: 0)

Rain Semester
1. Foundations of Professional Nursing (12 wks); 2. Psychology Applied to Nursing (12 wks); 3. Physiological and Pathological Chemistry II (12 wks); 4. General and Cellular Pathology (12 wks); 5. Human Anatomy II (12 wks); 6. Human Physiology II (12 wks); 7. African History and Culture; 8. Foundation Nursing Practice (6 wks—concentrated clinical practice).
(DN: 1, 2, 3, 4, 5, 6, 8; P: 0)
Number of pharmacy or drug treatment-related courses: zero (0) out of 15.

Number of diagnosis and nursing-related courses: 12 out of 15.

YEAR 3
HARMATTAN SEMESTER

1. Epidemiology (8 wks); 2. Man and His Family in the Community (12 wks); 3. Medical-Surgical Nursing I (12 wks); 4. Environmental Health (12 wks); 5. Pharmacodynamics I (0 wk); 6. Introduction to Sociology I (0 wk); 7. Man and Nature: The Scientific Adventure.
(DN: 1, 3; P: 5)

RAIN SEMESTER

1. Community Health Nursing (16 wks); 2. Medical-Surgical Nursing II (12 wks); 3. Pharmacodynamics II: Chemotherapy; 4. Medical Ethics; 5. Introduction to Sociology; 6. Man and Nature: The Scientific Adventure; 7. Community Health Nursing (3 wks—conc clinical practice); 8. Medical-Surgical Nursing (3 wks—conc clinical practice).
(DN: 1, 2, 7, 8; P: 3)

Number of pharmacy or drug treatment-related courses: 2 out of 15 plus an integral part of rotation.

Number of diagnosis and nursing-related courses: 6 out of 15 plus a major part of rotations.

YEAR 4
HARMATTAN SEMESTER

1. Mental Health Nursing (12 wks); 2. Maternal and Child Health Nursing I (12 wks); 3. Advanced Medical-Surgical Nursing I (12 wks); 4. Curriculum Development and Teaching Methodology (12 wks).
(DN: 1, 2, 3; P: 0)

RAIN SEMESTER

1. Maternal and Child Health Nursing II (12 wks); 2. Advanced Medical-Surgical Nursing II (12 wks); 3. Research Method in Nursing (12 wks); 4. Management of Nursing Care Services (12 wks); 5. Teaching/Management Practice (12 wks); 6. Maternal and Child Health Nursing (3 wks—conc. clinical practice); 7. Medical-Surgical Nursing (3 wks—conc. clinical practice).
(DN: 1, 2, 4, 6, 7; P: 0)

Number of pharmacy or drug treatment-related courses: zero (0) out of 11 but constitute an integral part of rotation.

Number of diagnosis and nursing-related courses: 8 out of 11 constitute a major part of rotation.

YEAR 5
HARMATTAN SEMESTER

1. Advanced Community Health Nursing I (12 wks); 2. Advanced Maternal and Child Health Nursing (16 wks); 3. Research Project and Special Topics Seminar I (12 wks); 4. Pediatric Nursing or Occupational Health Nursing as Elective (8 wks).

(DN: 1, 2, 4; P: 0)

RAIN SEMESTER

1. Advanced Community Health Nursing II (12 wks); 2. Advanced Psychiatric Nursing (12 wks); 3. Research Project and Special Topics Seminar II (12 wks); 4. Intensive Care Nursing or Primary Care Nursing as Elective (8 wks).

(DN: 1, 2, 4; P: 0)

Number of pharmacy or drug treatment-related courses: zero (0) out of 8 but constitute an integral part of rotation.

Number of diagnosis and nursing-related courses: 6 out of 8 constitute a major part of rotation.

Total of Year 2 to 5

Number of pharmacy or drug treatment-related courses: 2 out of 49.
Number of diagnosis and dental-related courses: 32 out of 49.

(DN = 0.65 & P = 0.041)

FACULTY OF PHARMACY

The faculty of pharmacy operates independently of the faculties of science and health science. The faculty runs a five-year program leading to the award of a Bachelor of Pharmacy (B.Pharm) degree. The admissions requirement is the same as the medical school requirements except that physics and mathematics or biology and agricultural science can be substituted for each other within the science core courses.[2]

Course Outline (1987-90)

Year 1 (Pre-professional Phase)
Harmattan Semester (21 units)
1. Elementary Mathematics (5 u); 2. Physics for Biological Science I (4 u); 3. Experimental Physics I (1 u); 4. Introductory Chemistry I (5 u); 5. Forms and Function in Plants I (4 u); 6. Use of English (2 u).
(D: 0; P: 0)

Rain Semester (21 units)
Harmattan Semester (21 units)
1. Elementary Mathematics I (5 u); 2. Physics for Biological Science II (4 u); 3. Experimental Physics II (1 u); 4. Introductory Chemistry II (5 u); 5. Introductory Zoology (4 u); 6. Use of English (2 u).
(D: 5; P: 0)

Number of pharmacy or drug treatment-related courses: zero (0) out of 12 or 42 units.

Number of diagnosis-related courses: 1 out of 12 or 4 out of 42 units.

Year 2
Harmattan Semester (19.5 units)
1. Introduction to Pharmaceutics (2 u); 2. Introductory Pharmaceutical Microbiology (1.5 u); 3. Practical Pharmaceutics I (1 u); 4. Introduction to Pharmacognosy and Organized Vegetable Drugs (3 u); 5. Anatomy and Physiology of Essential Organs I (5 u); 6. Pharmaceutical Inorganic and Physical Chemistry (2 u); 7. Pharmaceutical Organic Chemistry (2 u); 8. Practical Pharmaceutical Chemistry I (1 u); 9. Use of English (2 u).
(D: 2, 5; P: 1, 3, 4, 6, 7, 8;)

Rain Semester (17.5 units)
1. Introduction to Pharmaceutics (1 u); 2. Introductory Pharmaceutical Microbiology (1.5 u); 3. Practical Pharmaceutics I (1 u); 4. Unorganized Drugs (2 u); 5. Anatomy and Physiology of Essential Organs II (3 u); 6. Pharmaceutical Inorganic and Physical Chemistry (3 u); 7. Pharmaceutical Organic Chemistry (3 u); 8. Practical Pharmaceutical Chemistry I (1 u); 9. Use of English (2 u).
(D: 2, 5; P: 1, 3, 4, 6, 7, 8;)

Number of pharmacy or drug treatment-related courses: 12 out of 18 or 22 out of 37 units.

Number of diagnosis-related courses: 4 out of 18 or 11 out of 37 units.

YEAR 3
HARMATTAN SEMESTER (19.5 UNITS)

1. Liquid and Semi-solid Dosage Forms (2 u); 2. Applied Pharmaceutical Microbiology I (2.5 u); 3. Dispensing (1 u); 4. Separation Techniques in Pharmacy (1 u); 5. Drugs of Biological Origin I (3 u); 6. General Pharmacology I (3 u); 7. Radiopharmacy and Selected Physico-chemical Methods of Analysis (1 u); 8. Introductory Biochemistry (4 u); 9. Use of English (2 u).
(D: 2, 8; P: 1, 3, 4, 5, 6, 7)

RAIN SEMESTER (17.5 UNITS)

1. Liquid and Semi-solid Dosage Forms (2 u); 2. Dispensing (1 u); 3. Applied Pharmaceutical Microbiology II (1.5 u); 4. Drugs of Biological Origin II (3 u); 5. General Pharmacology II (3 u); 6. Radiopharmacy and Selected Physico-chemical Methods of Analysis (1 u); 7. Principles of Diseases and Pathology (2 u); 8. Use of English (2).
(D: 3, 7; P: 1, 2, 4, 5, 6)

Number of pharmacy or drug treatment-related courses: 11 out of 17 or 23 out of 37 units.

Number of diagnosis-related courses: 4 out of 17 or 10 out of 37 units.

YEAR 4
HARMATTAN SEMESTER (12.5 UNITS)

1. Liquid and Semi-solid Dosage Forms (2 u); 2. Applied Pharmaceutical Microbiology III (1.5 u); 3. Herbal Remedies in Traditional Medicine (1 u); 4. General Pharmacology III (0 u); 5. Chemotherapy (1 u); 6. Medicinal Chemistry I (3 u); 7. Forensic Pharmacy and Pharmacy Ethics (1 u); 8. Pharmacy Management and Administration I (2 u); 9. Biopharmaceutics and Pharmacokinetics (1 u).
(D: 2; P: 1, 3, 5, 6, 7, 9)

Rain Semester (15 units)
1. Liquid and Semi-solid Dosage Forms (1.5 u); 2. Applied Pharmaceutical Microbiology III (1.5 u); 3. Nigerian Medicinal Plants (2 u); 4. Chemotherapy (2 u); 5. Medicinal Chemistry II (3 u); 6. Forensic Pharmacy and Pharmacy Ethics (1 u); 7. Pharmacy Management and Administration II (2 u); 8. Biopharmaceutics and Pharmacokinetics (2 u).
(D: 2; P: 1, 3, 4, 5, 6, 8)
Number of pharmacy or drug treatment-related courses: 13 out of 17 or 20.5 out of 27.5 units.

Number of diagnosis-related courses: 2 out of 17 or 3 out of 27.5 units.

YEAR 5
Harmattan Semester (18 units)
1. Pharmaceutical Industrial Development and Processing (3 u); 2. Herbicides, Pesticides, and Molluscides (1 u); 3. Toxicology (1 u); 4. Principles of Drug Development and Design (IV); 5. Pharmaceutical Analysis and Drug Quality Control (3 u); 6. Clinical Pharmacokinetics (1 u); 7. Drug Information Evaluation and Communication Skill (2 u); 8. Clinical Pharmacy Clerkship (2 u); 9. Clinical Pharmacology (2 u); 10. Project (2 u).
(D: 0; P: 1, 2, 3, 4, 5, 6, 7, 9)

Rain Semester (11 units)
1. Applied Pharmaceutical Microbiology IV (2 u); 2. Developments in Dosage Forms Design (IV); 3. Toxicology (2 u); 4. Pharmaceutical Analysis and Drug Quality Control (1 u); 5. Clinical Pharmacy Clerkship (3 u); 6. Project (2 u).
(D: 1; P: 2, 3, 4)
Number of pharmacy or drug treatment-related courses: 11 out of 16 or 19 out of 29 units plus a major part of clerkship.

Number of diagnosis-related courses: 1 out of 16 or 2 out of 29 units plus an integral part of clerkship.

Total of Year 2 to 5
Number of pharmacy or drug treatment-related courses: 46 out of 68.
Number of diagnosis-related courses: 11 out of 68.
(D = 0.16 & P = 0.68)

UNVERISTY OF BENIN

The University of Benin is about 300 miles from the University of Ife. As of January 2001, the Faculty of Health/Department of Medicine has no faculty handbook because they were awaiting the release of newly updated handbook. However, the faculty of pharmacy had only one faculty office updated copy in February 2001, and the investigator had to pay for photocopies of a copied handbook also. As the most current handbook, the course outline is given below. The faculty of pharmacy runs a five-year program leading to the award of a Bachelor of Pharmacy (B Pharm) degree. The admissions requirement is the same as that of the University of Ife.[3]

YEAR 1
1ST SEMESTER

1. Mechanics, Thermal Physics, and Properties of Matter; 2. Vibrations, Waves, and Optics; 3. General Chemistry I; 4. Organic Chemistry I; 5. Diversity of Organisms; 6. Introductory Ecology, Genetics, and Evolution; 7. Use of English I; 8. Philosophy and Logic; 9. Practical Physics.
(D: 0; P: 0)

2ND SEMESTER

1. Practical Physics; 2. Electromagnetism and Modern Physics; 3. General Chemistry II; 4. Organic Chemistry II; 5. Plant Forms and Functions; 6. Diversity of Animals History and Embryology; 7. Use of English II; 8. Nigeria's People and Culture; 9. Everyday Technology.

(D: 0; P: 0)

Number of pharmacy or drug treatment-related courses: zero (0) out of 18.

Number of diagnosis-related courses: zero (0) out of 18.

YEAR 2
1ST SEMESTER (19 CREDITS)

1. Introductory Physiology (2 crs); 2. Cardiovascular/Respiratory Physiology (2 crs); 3. Subsidiary Mathematics I (3 crs); 4. Biochemistry Theory/Practice (4 crs); 5. General Pharmacognosy (2 crs); 6. Basic Dispensing Procedures and Phase Equilibria (2 crs); 7. General Pharmaceutical Microbiology (2 crs); 8. General and Pharmaceutical Inorganic Chemistry (2 crs).
(D: 1, 2, 4, 7; P: 5, 6, 8)

2ND SEMESTER (19 CREDITS)
1. Anatomy (3 crs); 2. Gastrointestinal/Endocrine Physiology (2 crs); 3. Neurophysiology and Special Sense (2 crs); 4. Practical Physiology (1 cr); 5. Biochemistry theory II (2 crs); 6. Subsidiary Mathematics II (3 crs); 7. Physical Pharmaceutical Chemistry and Introductory Radio Pharmacy (2 crs); 8. Pharmaceutical Chemistry Practical (1 cr); 9. Practical Pharmaceutical Microbiology (1 cr); 10. Practical Pharmaceutics (dispensing) I (2 crs).
(D: 1, 2, 3, 4, 5, 9; P: 7, 8, 10)

Number of pharmacy or drug treatment-related courses: 6 out of 18 or 11 out of 38 credits.

Number of diagnosis-related courses: 10 out of 18 or 21 out of 38 credits.

YEAR 3
1ST SEMESTER (18 CREDITS)
1. Chemical Disinfection: Microbiology of Air (2 crs); 2. Pharmaceutical Organic Chemistry I (3 crs); 3. Surface and Interfacial Phenomena (4 crs); 4. General Pharmacology (2 crs); 5. Autonomic/Neuropharmacology (2 crs); 6. Practical Pharmacognosy (1 cr); 7. Vegetable Drugs (3 crs).
(D: 0; P: 1, 2, 3, 4, 5, 6, 7)

2ND SEMESTER (23 CREDITS)
1. Practical Pharmaceutical Microbiology (1 cr); 2. General Principles of Sterilization and Their Applications (2 crs); 3. Pharmaceutical Organic Chemistry II (3 cr); 4. Pharmaceutical Chemistry Practice (1 cr); 5. pharmacy Management (3 crs); 6. Chemistry of drugs of natural origin (2 crs); 7. Practical Phytochemistry (1 cr); 8. Practical Pharmaceutics (dispensing) II (2 crs); 9. Pharmaceutical unit operations I (4 crs); 10. systemic Pharmacology (3 crs); 11. Practical Pharmacology (1 cr)
(D: 1; P: 2,3,4,6,7,8,9,10,11)

Number of pharmacy or drug treatment-related courses: 16 out of 18 or 37 out of 41 credits

Number of diagnosis-related courses: 1 out of 18 or 1 out of 41 credits

YEAR 4
1ST SEMESTER (14 CREDITS)
1. Medicinal Chemistry I (3 crs); 2. Pharmacy Law (2 crs); 3. Pharmaceutics unit operations II (3 crs); 4. industrial training (6 crs)
(D: 0; P: 1,3)

2ND SEMESTER (20 CREDITS)
1. Practical Pharmaceutics (dispensing -1 cr); 2. CNS Pharmacology (3 crs); 3. chemotherapy (3 crs); 4. Practical Pharmaceutical (1 cr); 5. Practical Pharmaceutics Microbiology (1 cr); 6. sterile products & pathogenic Microbiology (3 crs); 7. Nigerian medicinal and techniques in pharmacognosy (4 crs); 8. Pharmaceutical Chemistry Practice (1 cr); 9. Pharmaceutical analysis (3 crs)
(D: 5; P: 1, 2, 3, 4, 6, 7, 8, 9)

Number of pharmacy or drug treatment-related courses: 10 out of 13 or 25 out of 34 credits plus a major part of clerkship (individual training).

Number of diagnosis-related courses: 1 out of 13 or 34 credits plus an integral part of clerkship (individual training).

YEAR 5
1ST SEMESTER (21 CREDITS)
1. Pathophysiology and Applied Therapeutics (3 crs); 2. Principles of Pharmacy Practices (3 crs); 3. Endocrine Pharmacology (2 crs); 4. Hemopoietic/Biochemical Pharmacology (2 crs); 5. Biogenesis and Special Classes of Natural Products (2 crs); 6. Chemotherapy and Bacteria Genetics/Resistance (2 crs); 7. Disintegration and Dissolution of Solid Dosage Forms (3 crs); 8. Analysis of Pharmaceutical Dosage (1 cr); 9. Medicinal Chemistry II (3 crs).
(D: 1; P: 2, 3, 4, 5, 6, 7, 8, 9)

2ND SEMESTER (19 CREDITS)
1. Dispensing of Prescription and nonprescription Products (1 cr); 2. Principles and Applied Clinical Pharmacokinetics (3 crs); 3. Pharmacy Clerkship/Externship (3 crs); 4. Toxicology/Drug Interaction (2 crs); 5. Microbial Contaminants and Preservation against Biodeterioration, Disease States (2 crs); 6. Drug Stability and Pharmaceutical Packaging (2 crs); 7. Pharmaceutical Analysis I (2 crs); 8. Project (4 crs).
(D: 5; P: 1, 2, 4, 6, 7)

Number of pharmacy or drug treatment-related courses: 13 out of 17 or 29 out of 40 credits plus a major part of clerkship/externship.

Number of diagnosis-related courses: 2 out of 17 or 5 out of 40 credits plus an integral part of clerkship/externship.

Total of Year 2 to 5
Number of pharmacy or drug treatment-related courses: 45 out of 66.
Number of diagnosis-related courses: 14 out of 66.
(D = 0.212 & P = 0.68)

COMMENTS

As at January 2001, plans where in advanced stages at the University of Ife and the University of Benin for the implementation of the Doctor of Pharmacy degree or clinical pharmacy program. The implementation of a Doctor of Pharmacy degree or clinical pharmacy program in Africa would hopefully level pharmacy program with other branches of medicine as a six-year program and eventually results in production of therapeutician/therapeutic physician or clinical pharmacists. There is no doubt about the fact that such program will eliminates some current courses in pharmacognosy, dosage preparation and others which have been taken over by the manufacturing industries or pharmaceutical companies in modern societies. Clinical application of pharmacy directly to patients will replace these courses, as it is currently Practice in USA. According to Dr. G.E. Erhabor, head of department of medicine at the University of Ife, clinical pharmacy separated from the faculty of health science and department of medicine and became an integral part of pharmacy at the faculty of pharmacy in 1995. Dr. Erhabor went further to assert that the only two available pharmacy courses which are pre-clinical year clinical Pharmacology and final year clinical Pharmacology & Therapeutics are given by faculty of pharmacy to medical students.

DATA ANALYSIS

Data analysis of the course outline above shows that, on the whole, it can be estimated that medical doctors/students in Africa are exposed to an average number of 0.78 or 78%, which is approximately 80%, and that is 8 out of every 10 courses in diagnosis-related courses in the pre-clinical years (didactic class work); and 0.11 or 11%, which is approximately 10%, and that is 1 out of every 10 courses in medical school that are pharmacy or drug-treatment related courses in the pre-clinical years (didactic class work). Study limitations involved the fact that one school is used as a case study for hundreds of schools in the continent, and the year 4, phase II program was considered part of the didactic/class work years even though it is composed of pre-clinical and clinical courses as an intermediary phase between didactic/class work and the clinical years. Few courses that are composed of diagnosis and pharmacy or drug-treatment courses were considered to be one or the other depending on course information in the handbook. The dentistry school curriculum showed that the dentists/students are exposed to an estimated average number of 0.90 or 90%, which is approximately 9 out of every 10 courses in diagnosis and dental-related courses; and 0.04 or 4 %, which is 4 out of every 100 courses or 1 out of every 25 courses in pharmacy or drug-treatment courses. The nurse program, on the other hand, showed that nurses/students are exposed to an estimated average number of 0.65 or 65% , which is approximately 70% or 7 out of every 10 courses in diagnosis and nursing-related courses; and 0.04 or 4%, which is 4 out of every 100 courses or 1 out of every 25 courses in pharmacy or drug treatment-related courses. Course outline data analysis for faculty of pharmacy showed a similar trend in the two schools, which are the University of Ife and the University of Benin. The University of Ife faculty of pharmacy's statistics that are used as a case example showed that the pharmacists/students are exposed to an estimated average number of 0.16 or 16% , which is approximately 20% or 2 out of every 10 courses in diagnosis-related courses; and 0.68 or 68% , which is approximately 70 or 7 out of every 10 courses in pharmacy or drug-treatment courses. The University of Benin showed 0.212 or 20% number of diagnosis related; and 0.68 or 68%, which is approximately the same as the University of Ife.

In a nutshell, 1 out of every 10 courses in medical school is pharmacy or drug-treatment related. This amounted to two pharmacy or drug-treatment courses in the pre-clinical phase and an additional clinical program, which incorporated pharmacy as an integral or minor part of clinical experience, as the basic qualification for prescribing drugs as a medical doctor in Africa. The dentists' exposure, on the other hand, is 1 out of 25 courses, which qualifies them to prescribe any drug for the pharmacists to dispense. The pharmacists' exposure to 7 out of every 10 courses in the faculty of pharmacy or drug treatment does not qualify a pharmacist to prescribe drugs even for animals in Africa. There are no certified nurse practitioners or physician assistants in nearly all parts of Africa. Nurses cannot prescribe drugs in Africa. Comparative analysis of African school statistics and North American school statistics using the U.S. data as above showed no major difference in course outline analysis. For example, medical students in the U.S. are exposed to average number of 0.798 or 79.8% (about 80%) diagnosis-related courses, and 0.063 or 6.3% (about 6%) pharmacy or drug treatment-related courses; and in Africa they are exposed to an average number of 0.78 or 78% (about 80%) diagnosis-related courses and 0.11 or 11% (about 10%) pharmacy or drug-treatment courses in medical schools' pre-clinical years. The pre-clinical years lay the basic foundation upon which the clinical years and practice are built. The dentistry schools showed a similar trend of 0.93 or 93% (about 90%) diagnosis and dental-related courses and 0.028 or 2.8% (about 3%) pharmacy or drug treatment-related courses in the U.S., and 0.90 or 90 % diagnosis and dental-related courses and 0.04 or 4% pharmacy or drug treatment-related courses in Africa. The first-degree program, Bachelor of Science degree in pharmacy, is facing extinction in the U.S. because of the clinical pharmacy or Doctor of Pharmacy degree (PharmD) program. However, the first degree is a five-year program in both continents, and in the U.S. pharmacists/students are exposed to 0.11 or 11% (about 10%) diagnosis-related courses and 0.81 or 81% (about 80) pharmacy or drug treatment-related courses. Same pharmacists/students are exposed to 0.16 or 16% (about 20%) diagnosis-related courses and 0.68 or 68% (about 70%) pharmacy or drug-treatment courses in Africa.

ASIA

Asia is the largest continent in the world, with an area of 17.6 million square miles and a population of 2.693 billion people as of 1990. The largest country in Asia is China, and China is home to one fifth of the human population, an average of about 1.2 to 1.4 billion people. Like blacks, no human study can be said to be complete without taking into consideration the interest of these 1.2 billion people in China. Medical education and the practice of medicine in China are a little bit different from the rest of the world, owing largely to its adherence to traditional Chinese medicine (TCM). Today, the world is moving at a fast pace towards a global village. One of the key elements of the global village is that anywhere there is an existing phenomenon, a new discovery and a nearly perfect condition excels by superseding every other thing around it. The news spreads readily around the world and everybody adopts it. For example, airplanes, which were invented in 1903, are the fastest means of traveling around the world today. If by tomorrow, South Africans invent something new that supersedes the airplane in all ways, be it vincible or invincible. Such a discovery would readily spread around and replace the airplane provided the science and technology can be duplicated. The airplane will become obsolete and gradually peter out of human existence. The same is true of Western education, which has its root in the old civilizations of Egypt, Mesopotamia, and the Greek and Roman empires. Western education has spread so much throughout the globe that it has become the modus operandi for teaching younger generations and educating the society at large. Even in different parts of the world such as Africa, Asia, and South America where people struggle to retain their traditional values (i.e., African and Chinese traditional medicine), Western civilization and education have superseded and taken over everything.

In China, people's desire to retain their traditional medicine is strong, but the practice of medicine and its settings are very much westernized. For instance, pharmacy is full of Western-oriented drugs, and medical education is a conglomeration of Chinese traditional medicine and Western medicine. The only danger in such a move is that the society is not benefiting from the exploration of each phenomenon to its zenith by mixing or blending both together. Thus, it will be difficult for a Chinese medical doctor to challenge or come up with a Western medical discovery that supersedes those in purely Western-oriented societies. Unlike China, Western medicine and traditional medicine are very much separated in most parts of the world such as in Africa, South America, and other parts of Asia. Europe, Australia, and most parts of North America are purely Western-oriented societies.

China Medical University was established in 1931 and Beijing University of Chinese Medicine was founded in 1956. There are no dentists, physician assistants, or certified nurse practitioners in China. Beijing College of Acupuncture and Moxibution was officially merged with Beijing University of Chinese Medicine in July 2000. The university now consists of 7 schools, which are the School of Pre-clinical Medicine, the School of Acupuncture/Tuina, the School of Chinese Pharmacy, the International School of Clinical Medicine, the School of Administration, and the School of E-learning. Students' entry requirement into medical school is high school or its equivalence. The Chinese medicine program is a 5-year course leading to the award of Bachelor of Science in Chinese medicine (BS) or acupuncture (BS), and a four-year course leading to the award of Bachelor of Science in Chinese pharmacology (BS), Bachelor of Engineering in Chinese pharmaceutical processing (BE), and Bachelor of Science in Chinese medicine nursing (BS).[4]

INTERNATIONAL SCHOOL, BEIJING UNIVERSITY OF CHINESE MEDICINE AND PHARMACOLOGY COURSE OUTLINE (2002)

Chinese Medicine (BS): Ancient Chinese Medical Language; Basic Theories of Traditional Chinese Medicine (TCM); Traditional Chinese Diagnostics; Study of Chinese Medical Formulae; Selection of Chinese Medical Classics; Traditional Chinese Internal Medicine; Chinese Gynecology; Chinese Pediatrics; Acupuncture and Moxibustion; Basic Western Diagnosis; Western Internal Medicine; Western Surgery.

Acupuncture (BS): Basic Theories of Chinese Medicine; Chinese Pharmacology; Study of Chinese Medical Formulae; Human Anatomy; Physiology; Chinese Internal Medicine; Classics on Acupuncture; Study of Meridians; Study of Acupoints; Acupuncture Therapy; Tuina and Experimental Acupuncture.

Chinese Pharmacology (BS): Basic Theories of Chinese Medicine; Chinese Pharmacology; Inorganic Chemistry; Organic Chemistry; Analytical Chemistry; Physical Chemistry; Computer Medicine Physics; Higher Mathematics; Chinese Herb Processing Science; Chinese Herb Preparation Science; Chinese Pharmacology; Medicinal Botany.

Chinese Pharmaceutical Processing: Basic Theories of Chinese Medicine; Chinese Pharmacology; Study of Chinese Medical Formulae; Physical Chemistry; The Science of Chinese Herb Preparation; Biochemistry; Chinese Pharmacology; Chinese Pharmaceutics; Chinese Herb Chemistry; Chinese Pharmaceutical Equipment and Technology.

Chinese Medicine Nursing: Basic Theories of Chinese Medicine; Chinese Pharmacology; Study of Chinese Medical Formulae; Human Anatomy; Physiology; Pathology; Nursing Psychology; Nursing Ethics; Basic Theories of Chinese Nursing; Study of Internal Medical Nursing; Study of Surgical Nursing.[4]

The university objective for students in each program shows that Chinese medical students are expected to master research theory and the principles of differential diagnosis in traditional Chinese medicine as well as basic Western medical theories and techniques of diagnosis and treatment; acupuncture students are expected to master basic theories of Chinese medicine, acupuncture, moxibustion, tuina, differentiation of syndromes, and needling technique; Chinese pharmacology students are expected to master identification, the active principles of medicinal herbs, the chemical composition of medicinal herbs, and the preparation of Chinese herbs; and Chinese medicinal nursing students are expected to master basic theories of Chinese medicine, clinical medicine, and nursing science as well as the principles of nursing and emergency case techniques.[4] Numerous attempts were made at getting a yearly or semester breakdown of courses for the medical students but all efforts yielded no dividends. A yearly or semester breakdown of courses would have enabled the investigator to make an effective comparison of various programs as well as an intercontinental comparison. However, course outlines and university objectives are good to some extent in making the deduction that there is a correlation between Africa, North America, and Chinese study, which indicates that traditional medical doctors are expected to concentrate heavily on diagnosis and minimally on treatment as an integral part of didactic coursework, while pharmacists are expected to concentrate heavily on pharmacy or drug treatment and minimally on diagnosis as an integral part of didactic coursework.

Unlike the rest of the world, pharmacists, otherwise know as Yaodian, function as general practitioners in China. Thus, a patient can walk into the pharmacy in China and explain his or her medical problem to the Yaodian, who prescribes and dispenses the appropriate drug to the patient. The pharmacist or Yaodian operates as an autonomous medical practitioner in China; hence, a lot of the medical problems such as high demand, insufficient number of medical doctors to meet the demand, patient financial problems without insurance coverage, and others that dominate Western-oriented societies are reduced to minimal level in China. As seen above, pharmacists undergo medical training similar to that of other branches of medicine in China. After graduation and licensure, physicians including pharmacists have the option of going into the advanced training program for clinical studies, which is one year for basic theories of Chinese medicine, one year for acupuncture and moxibustion, one year for Chinese pharmacology, and one to two years for Chinese internal medicine, Chinese surgery, Chinese gynecology, Chinese pediatrics, Chinese dermatology, Chinese orthopedics, and traumatology. This advanced training program leads to specialization in China. An alternative to the advanced training program is available in the form of a short-term training program, which lasts from one week to six months.

Pharmacists or Yaodian might be autonomous in China, but pharmacy practice is not the ideal direction of change that clinical pharmacists want for the profession in the U.S. Clinical pharmacists or pharmacy originated in the United States and it is spreading fast to other parts of the world. Though not autonomous, clinical pharmacists in America function like every other specialist with the aim of using their great knowledge of drugs, drug/drug interactions, drug/food interactions, drug/disease interactions, laboratory values, adverse drug reactions, etc., to impact patient therapeutic outcomes as trained therapeuticians/drug specialists/disease-state managers.

One of the key elements in disease-state management is patients' privacy and documentation, which is paramount to the clinical pharmacist. The Chinese government probably needs to demand more from their Yaodian by requesting patients' privacy, and documentation of all encounters for effective patient follow-up and disease-state management.

JAPAN

Japan, the world's second largest economy, is in Asia. Schools in Japan offer another opportunity for understanding medical, dental, and pharmacy schools' curricula as well as graduates' exposure to diagnosis- and drug treatment or pharmacy-related courses. Akita University School of Medicine offers a six-year undergraduate program that leads to the award of a Medical Doctor degree and medical practice of medicine in Japan. Admission criteria is 12 years of standard school education outside Japan, or 18 years of age during admission, possession of an international baccalaureate certified by Japan's Ministry of Education, and university entrance examinations test scores. Akita University was founded as Akita Prefectural Women's Medical College in 1945. The school of medicine with various departments started as the first national postwar medical school in Japan in 1970 and continued until the establishment of a cardiovascular surgery department in 1991. During the first year, courses are offered in liberal arts with fundamental medical seminars on the Tegata campus, and in the second to third year courses are offered in basic medicine, while the fourth through sixth-year courses are offered as clinical rotations all at the Hondo campus. Successful graduates take the national examination for medical license and start practicing medicine or proceed further to graduate school.[20]

Akita University School of Medicine Course Outline (2002)

Pre-clinical Years
Year 2 & 3 (Basic Medicine)

1. Anatomy I; 2. Anatomy II; 3. Pathology I; 4. Pathology II; 5. Pharmacology; 6. Physiology I; 7. Physiology II; 8. Biochemistry I; 9. Biochemistry II; 10. Microbiology; 11. Hygiene; 12. Public Health; 13. Parasitology; 14. Forensic Medicine.

(D: 1, 2, 3, 6, 7, 8, 9, 10, 13, 14; P: 5)

Number of pharmacy or drug treatment-related courses: 1 out of 14.

Number of diagnosis-related courses: 10 out of 14.

(D = 0.71 & P = 0.071)

Clinical Years
Year 4-6 (Rotations)

1. Internal Medicine I; 2. Internal Medicine II; 3. Internal Medicine III; 4. Psychiatry; 5. Surgery I; 6. Surgery II; 7. Cardiovascular Surgery; 8. Neurosurgery; 9. Orthopedic Surgery; 10. Dermatology; 11. Urology; 12. Pediatrics; 13. Obstetrics and Gynecology; 14. Ophthmology; 15. Oto-Rhino-Laryngology; 16. Anesthesiology; 17. Radiology; 18. Laboratory Medicine; 19. Emergency and Critical Care Medicine; 20. Clinical Pharmacology and Therapeutics; 21. Dentistry and Oral and Maxillofacial Surgery.

Number of pharmacy or drug treatment-related courses: Constitute an integral part of the clinical rotations.

Number of diagnosis-related courses: Constitute a major part of the clinical rotations.

Dentistry

Dentistry like medicine is a six-year program in Japan. Kagoshima University is one of the universities in Japan that produces dentists through a dental school. The dental school of Kagoshima University was established in May 1976 and now accommodates eight departments, which are Oral Anatomy II,

Oral Microbiology and Immunology, Dental Pharmacology, Peridodontology, Prosthetic Dentistry I, Prosthetic Dentistry II, Oral and Maxillofacial Surgery II, and Pediatric Dentistry.[21]

KAGOSHIMA UNIVERSITY DENTAL SCHOOL COURSE OUTLINE (2002)

PRE-CLINICAL YEARS
YEAR 2 & 3 (BASIC DENTAL SCIENCE)

1. Anatomy for Dental Science I; 2. Anatomy for Dental Science II; 3. Oral Physiology; 4. Biochemistry; 5. Oral Pathology; 6. Oral Microbiology and Immunology; 7. Dental Pharmacology; 8. Biomaterials; 9. Dental Humanities.

(DD: 1, 2, 3, 4, 5, 6, 9; P: 7)

Number of pharmacy or drug treatment-related courses: 1 out of 9.

Number of diagnosis and dental-related courses: 7 out of 9.
(DD = 0.78 & P = 0.11)

CLINICAL YEARS
YEAR 4-6 (CLINICAL DENTAL SCIENCE)

1. Preventive Dentistry; 2. Operative Dentistry and Endodotology; 3. Periodontology; 4. Prosthetic Dentistry I; 5. Prosthetic Dentistry 2; 6. Oral and Maxillofacial Surgery I; 7. Oral and Maxillofacial Surgery 2; 8. Orthodontics; 9. Pediatric Dentistry; 10. Dental Radiology.

Number of pharmacy or drug treatment-related courses: Constitute an integral part of the clinical rotations.

Number of diagnosis and dental-related courses: Constitute a major part of the clinical rotations.

Veterinary Medicine

The University of Tokyo School of Veterinary Medicine offers a program that produces veterinary medical doctors. The program consists of basic animal medicine and clinical medicine.[22]

University of Tokyo School of Veterinary Medicine Course Outline (2002)

Pre-Clinical Years (Basic Animal Medicine)

1. Animal Breeding; 2. Veterinary Anatomy; 3. Veterinary Physiology; 4. Veterinary Pharmacology; 5. Veterinary Microbiology; 6. Veterinary Public Health; 7. Cellular Biochemistry; 8. Veterinary Ethology; 9. Reproductive and Developmental Biology; 10. Developmental Genetics; 11. Laboratory of Experimental Animal Resource Science.

(D: 2, 3, 5, 7, 9, 10, 11; P: 4)

Number of pharmacy or drug treatment-related courses: 1 out of 11.

Number of diagnosis-related courses: 7 out of 11.

(D = 0.64 & P = 0.091)

Clinical Years (Clinical Medicine)

1. Comparative Pathophysiology; 2. Veterinary Pathology; 3. Veterinary Internal Medicine; 4. Veterinary Surgery and Obstetrics; 5. Biomedical Science; 6. Veterinary Clinical Pathobiology.

Number of pharmacy or drug treatment-related courses: Constitute an integral part of the clinical years.

Number of diagnosis-related courses: Constitute a major part of the clinical years.

Pharmacy

Pharmacy is a four-year program in Japan, and Okayama University is one of the schools that offer such program. In Okayama University, the department of pharmaceutical sciences (DPS) and pharmaceutical technology (DPT) were established in 1969 and 1975, respectively, as branches of medicine in the medical school. The two departments separated from the medical school to become separate entities as faculty of pharmaceutical sciences (FPS) in 1976. Pharmaceutical science is of paramount interest to the Japanese. Many schools and institutes in Japan choose pharmaceutical sciences as way of identifying pharmacy. A pharmaceutical science is a broad-based approach used to identify the well-rounded pharmacists, researchers, and technologists. It was designed to repudiate the traditional "school of pharmacy," which is often correlated with graduating dispensers (people who administer medical treatment).[23]

Okayama University
Faculty of Pharmaceutical Sciences
Course Outline (2002)

YEAR 1 TO 4

1. Introduction to Clinical Medicine (2 crs); 2. Organic Chemistry (2 crs); 3. Physical Chemistry (2 crs); 4. Cell Biology (2 crs); 5. Pharmaceutical Sciences (2 crs); 6. Biochemistry I (2 crs); 7. Physiology Anatomy (2 crs); 8. Biological Assay (2 crs); 9. Organic Pharmaceutical Chemistry I (2 crs); 10. Organic Pharmaceutical Chemistry II (2 crs); 11. Organic Pharmaceutical Chemistry III (2 crs); 12. Biochemistry II (2 crs); 13. Biochemistry III (2 crs); 14. Pharmacognosy I (2 crs); 15. Pharmacognosy II (2 crs); 16. Natural Products Chemistry (2 crs); 17. Pharmacology I (2 crs); 18. Pharmacology II (2 crs); 19. Pharmacology III (2 crs); 20. Health Chemistry I (2 crs); 21. Health Chemistry II (2 crs); 22. Health Chemistry III (2 crs); 23. Bio-organic Chemistry I (2 crs); 24. Bio-organic Chemistry II (2 crs); 25. Pharmacogeneomics (2 crs); 26. Pharmaceutics I (2 crs); 27. Biopharmaceutics (2 crs); 28. Pharmaceutics II (2 crs); 29. Pharmaceutical Analytical Sciences I (2 crs); 30. Pharmaceutical Analytical Sciences II (2 crs); 31. Analytical Chemistry for Vital Materials (2 crs); 31. Pharmaceutical Physical Chemistry I (2 crs); 32. Pharmaceutical Physical Chemistry II (2 crs); 34. Biophysical Chemistry (2 crs); 35. Microbiology (2 crs); 36. Microbiology I (2 crs); 37. Applied Genetics (2

crs); 38. Immunochemistry II (2 crs); 39. Immunotherapeutics (2 crs); 40. Immunochemistry I (Introduction to Immunology—2 crs); 41. Cell-signaling Network (2 crs); 42. Synthetic and Medicinal Chemistry I (2 crs); 43. Synthetic and Medicinal Chemistry II (2 crs); 44. Synthetic and Medicinal Chemistry (2 crs); 45. Radiopharmaceuticals (2 crs); 46. Environmental Hygienic Chemistry (2 crs); 47. Public Health; 48. Medical Botany (2 crs); 49. Inorganic Pharmaceutical Chemistry (2 crs); 50. Pharmaceutical Laws (2 crs); 51. Pathology (2 crs); 52. Computer Chemistry (2 crs); 53. Hospital Pharmacy (2 crs); 54. Pharmacoepia (2 crs); 55. Drug Informatics (2 crs); 56. Diagnostics and Therapeutics (2 crs); 57. Pharmaceutical Manufacturing Sciences (2 crs); 58. clinical Pharmaceutical sciences I (2 crs); 59. clinical Pharmaceutical II (2 crs); 60. Clinical Pharmaceutical III (2 crs); 61. Guidance for Pharmaceutical Sciences (2 crs); 62. Introduction to Information Processing (2 crs); 63. Introduction to Information Processing I (2 crs); 64. Introduction to Drug Research (2 crs); 65. Practice in Hospital Pharmacy (2 crs); 66. Practice in Fundamental Pharmaceutical Sciences I (1.5 crs); 67. Practice in Fundamental Pharmaceutical Sciences II (3 crs); 68. Practice in Fundamental Pharmaceutical Sciences III (1 cr); 69. Practice in Hygienic Pharmaceutical Sciences (3 crs); 70. Practice in Clinical and Biopharmaceutical Sciences I (1 cr); 71. Practice in Clinical and Biopharmaceutical Sciences II (1 cr); 72. Practice in Clinical and Biopharmaceutical Sciences III (1.5 crs).[23]

(D: 4, 6, 7, 8, 12, 13, 35, 36, 37, 38, 40, 41, 51; P: 5, 9, 10, 11, 14, 15, 16, 17, 18, 19, 20, 21, 22, 25, 26, 27, 28, 29, 30, 31, 32, 39, 41, 42, 43, 44, 45, 48, 49, 53, 54, 55, 57, 58, 59, 60, 61, 64)

Number of pharmacy or drug treatment-related courses: 38.5 out of 64 plus a major part of clinical rotations or practices.\

Number of diagnosis-related courses: 13.5 out of 64 plus an integral part of clinical rotations or practices.
(D = 0.21 & P = 0.60)

INDIA

India, the world largest democracy, is also in Asia. Schools in Japan and India offer good opportunities to understand medical, dental, and pharmacy schools' curricula in Asia and the subsequent exposure of their graduates to diagnosis- and drug/pharmacy-related courses. The modus operandi for these curricula in China differs from the rest of the world because of adherence to its traditional medicine. Manipal Academy of Higher Education provides great information for these curricula in India. Manipal College of Medical Sciences, Nepal, is one of the schools that offers a 5.5-year program leading to the award of Bachelor of Medicine and Bachelor of Surgery (MBBS). Admission criteria are the same for medical, dental, and pharmacy schools and it entails a passing grade on Indian national testing; pass in 10 + 2, A level, IB; American twelfth grade (high school and college grades) or equivalent in physics, chemistry, biology, and English and 50% in physics, chemistry, and mathematics or biology; and study of classes 11 and 12 in India plus entrance test merit. Foreign nationals: pass in 10 + 2 (CBSE, A level, IB, STPM, SAM, SPU, PUC, ISC, or equivalent) with 60% mark in physics, chemistry, biology, and English (PCBE). For American students, one year of college with C grade in PCB, or high school with AP courses in PCB with C or above, plus qualifying examination merit.[25]

By the year 2002, the medical school curriculum consists of two years of didactic class work, two and a half years of clinical rotations, and a one-year residential internship.

MANIPAL COLLEGE OF MEDICAL SCIENCES COURSE OUTLINE (2002)

PRE-CLINICAL YEARS
YEAR 1 & 2

1. Anatomy; 2. Physiology; 3. Biochemistry; 4. Pathology; 5. Microbiology; 6. Pharmacology; 7. Community Medicine.

(D: 1, 2, 3, 4, 5; P: 6 D & P: 7)

Number of pharmacy or drug treatment-related courses: 1.5 out of 7.

Number of diagnosis-related courses: 5.5 out of 7.

(D = 0.79 & P = 0.21)

CLINICAL YEARS
YEAR 3-4.5 (ROTATIONS)

1. General Medicine; 2. General Obstetrics and Gynecology; 3. Forensics Medicine; 4. Community Medicine Pediatrics; 5. Otorhinolaryngology; 6. Ophthalmology; 7. Orthopedics; 8. Dentistry; 9. Psychiatry; 10. Dermatology;

11. Radiology; 12. Anesthesiology; 13. Emergency 14. Medicine; 15. Surgical Specialties and Subspecialties.

Number of pharmacy or drug treatment-related courses: Constitute an integral part of the clinical rotations.

Number of diagnosis-related courses: Constitute a major part of the clinical rotations.

Dentistry

Dentistry is a four-year program plus a one-year internship in India. Graduates receive a Bachelor of Dental Surgery (BDS) degree after the entire coursework, obtain their license, and start practicing as a dentist. The college of dental surgery was established at Manipal in 1965 and Mangalore in 1987. Both schools offer similar programs, which provide an insight into dentistry in India. The two schools equally offer postgraduate courses in various dental specialties.[25]

Course Outline (2002)

Pre-clinical Years

1. Human Anatomy; 2. Human Physiology and Biochemistry; 3. Oral Anatomy; 4. Histology and Physiology; 5. Dental Materials; 6. Pre-clinical Prosthetics Dentistry; 7. General and Dental Pharmacology; 8. General Pathology; 9. Microbiology.
 (DD: 1, 2, 3, 4, 5, 6, 8, 9; P: 7)
Number of pharmacy or drug treatment-related courses: 1 out of 9.

Number of diagnosis and dental-related courses: 8 out of 9.
 (DD = 0.88 & P = 0.11)

Clinical Years

1. Prosthetic and Conservative Dentistry; 2. General Medicine and Surgery; 3. Dental and Oral Pathology and Microbiology; 4. Oral Diagnosis and

Radiology; 5. Orthodontics; 6. Pedodontia and Preventive Dentistry; 7. Oral Surgery; 8. Anaesthesia; 9. Conservative Dentistry and Endodontics; 10. Prosthodontics; 11. Periodontia and Oral Medicine.

Number of pharmacy or drug treatment-related courses: Constitute an integral part of the clinical rotations.

Number of diagnosis and dental-related courses: Constitute a major part of the clinical rotations.

PHARMACY

Pharmacy is a four-year program in India. The College of Pharmaceutical Sciences, Manipal, was established in 1963 and offers courses leading to the award of B Pharm, M Pharm, and PhD. The admission criteria are the same as that of the medical school, as noted earlier. The program consists of some months of practical training in a hospital or pharmaceutical manufacturing house.[25]

COURSE OUTLINE (2002)

YEAR 1

1. Mathematics/Biology; 2. Anatomy and Physiology; 3. Biochemistry; 4. Pharmaceutical Inorganic Chemistry; 5. Pharmaceutical Organic Chemistry; 6. Computer Science and Statistics.

(D: 2, 3; P: 4, 5)

Number of pharmacy or drug treatment-related courses: 2 out of 6.

Number of diagnosis-related courses: 2 out of 6.

YEAR 2

1. Phathophysiology; 2. Pharmaceutical Microbiology, 3. Pharmaceutical Technology; 4. Pharmaceutical Chemistry; 5. Pharmaceutical Analysis; 6. Pharmacognosy I.

(D: 1, 2; P: 3, 4, 5, 6)

Number of pharmacy or drug treatment-related courses: 4 out of 6.

Number of diagnosis-related courses: 2 out of 6.

YEAR 3

1. Hospital and Community Pharmacy; 2. Pharmaceutical Biotechnology; 3. Physical Pharmaceutics and Biopharmaceutics; 4. Medicinal Chemistry I; 5. Pharmacology I; 6. Pharmacognosy II; 7. Pharmaceutical Jurisprudence.
(D: 0; P: 1, 2, 3, 4, 5, 6)

Number of pharmacy or drug treatment-related courses: 6 out of 7.

Number of diagnosis-related courses: 0 out of 7.

YEAR 4

1. Clinical Pharmacy and Therapeutics; 2. Instrumental and Biomedical Analysis; 3. Industrial Pharmacy; 4. Medicinal Chemistry II; 5. Pharmacology II; 6. Pharmacognosy III; 7. Pharmaceutical Management
(D: 0; P: 1, 2, 4, 5, 6)

Number of pharmacy or drug treatment-related courses: 6 out of 7 plus a major part of clerkship (industrial training).

Number of diagnosis-related courses: 0 out of 7 plus an integral part of clerkship (industrial training).

Total of Years 1 to 4

Number of pharmacy or drug treatment-related courses: 18 out of 26.

Number of diagnosis-related courses: 4 out of 26.
(D = 0.15 & P = 0.69)

DATA ANALYSIS

India and Japan in Asia provide a good analogy for curricula and students' exposure to diagnosis-related courses and pharmacy or drug treatment-related courses in medical schools, dentistry schools, veterinary medical schools, and pharmacy schools. Average results of the chosen schools in the two countries will be stated, and the highest will be used as an estimate for the continent. Using the results above, medical doctors/students are exposed to an average number of 0.79 or 79%, which is approximately 80% in India, and 0.71 or 71%, which is approximately 70 percent in Japan in diagnosis-related courses. It can therefore be estimated that medical doctors/students in Asia are exposed to an average number of 0.80 or 80%, which is 8 out of every 10 courses in diagnosis-related courses in the pre-clinical years (didactic class work). Same medical doctors/students are exposed to an average number of 0.21 or 21% in India, and 0.071 or 7%, which is approximately 10% in Japan in pharmacy or drug treatment-related courses. Consequently, it can be estimated that medical students in Asia are exposed to 0.2 or 20%, which is 2 out of every 10 courses in pharmacy or drug-treatment courses in the pre-clinical years (didactic class work). Study limitations involved the fact that one or two schools are used as a case study for hundreds of schools on the continent. Few courses are composed of diagnosis and pharmacy or drug treatment but were considered one or the other depending on which constituted a majority.

The dentistry school curriculum results showed that students are exposed to an average number of 0.88 or 88%, which is approximately 90% in India, and 0.78 or 78%, which is approximately 80 percent in Japan in diagnosis and dental-related courses. Therefore, it can be estimated that dentists/students in Asia are exposed to an average number of 90 percent, which is 9 out of every 10 courses in diagnosis and dental-related courses. The same students are exposed to an average number of 0.11 or 11%, which is approximately 10% in India and Japan in pharmacy or drug treatment-related courses; hence, it can be estimated that dentists/students in Asia are exposed to 0.10 or 10%, which is 1 out of every 10 courses in pharmacy or drug treatment-related courses. These courses are taken in the pre-clinical years. Veterinary medical doctors/students, on the other hand, are exposed to an average number of 0.64 or 64%, which is approximately 60% or 6 out of every 10 courses in diagnosis-related courses; and 0.091 or 9.1%, which is approximately 9% or 1 out of every 11 courses in pharmacy or drug-treatment related courses during the pre-clinical years. As in other continents, the modus operandi for course outlines in pre-clinical years is the same as that of the clinical years. Data analysis of pharmacy course outlines showed that pharmacists/pharmacy students are exposed to an average number of 0.21 or 21%, which is approximately 20% in Japan, and 0.15 or 15% in India in diagnosis-related courses. Therefore, it can be estimated that pharmacy students in Asia are exposed to 20%, which is 2 out of every 10 courses in diagnosis. The same pharmacists/pharmacy students are exposed to an average number of 0.69 or 69%, which is approximately 70% in India, and 0.60 or 60% in Japan in pharmacy or drug-treatment related courses. Consequently, it can be estimated that pharmacy students in Asia are exposed to 70% or 7 out of every

10 courses in pharmacy or drug treatment-related courses. Study limitations are the same as above.

In a nutshell, 2 out of every 10 courses in pharmacy or drug treatment-related courses in pre-clinical years and pharmacy or drug treatment as an integral part of clinical rotations/internships qualifies the medical doctor to prescribe any drugs for the pharmacist to dispense. The same explanation goes for the veterinary medical doctors and dentists, whose exposure to approximately 1 out of every 11 courses and 1 out of every 10 courses in pharmacy or drug treatment, respectively, qualifies them to write any prescription for the pharmacist to dispense. The pharmacists' exposure to 7 out of every 10 courses in pharmacy or drug treatment does not qualify them to write prescriptions for any clinical condition.

AUSTRALIA

Australia is the smallest habitable continent of the world (area of 2.271 million square miles and population of 16.072 million people as of 1990). It is a penal colony like Ghana in Africa and others that were formed by British Empire to house criminals or convicts of the Empire. Australia, home of the kangaroo, black aborigines, and white convicts from the British Empire, has become one of the most developed continents/countries in the world. Medical education and practice in Australia is very much westernized and modeled after the United States's system. Australia has about fourteen universities, and the oldest one is the University of Sydney founded in 1850. There are no physician assistants or certified nurse practitioners in Australia. Like the U.S., admission criteria into medical schools in Australia are based on three requirements, which are: 1. first (bachelor) degree in any discipline at credit level, 2. graduation from Australian medical school admission test (GAMSAT), and 3. personal interview by medical school. Medical school training in Australia is a four-year (192 credits) program leading to the award of Bachelor of Medicine and Bachelor of Surgery (MBBS) with a one-year internship program. After one year of internship, graduates are eligible for practice provided they complete the registration requirements by the medical board of New South Wales.[5,6] The four-year program is divided into two sections. The first section is made up of years 1 and 2 and it's the bulk of the didactic class work experience/learning. These first two years lay the foundation or rudiments upon which the second section, which is made up of years 3 and 4, is based. Years 3 and 4 are basically the clinical attachment/rotation years.

The first two years are made up of blocks learning of basic and clinical science, community and doctor, patient and doctor, and personal and professional development in and outside the campus. The students spend one day per week for patient and doctor sessions in the clinical schools. These four parts of basic and clinical science constitute 12 credits per semester for the first three years and are incorporated into study in the fourth year; community and doctor constitute 3 credits per semester for the first three years and are incorporated into study in the fourth year; patient and doctor constitute 6 credits per semester for the first three years and are incorporated into study in the fourth year; and the personal and professional development constitute 3 credits per semester for the first three years and are incorporated into study in the fourth year. The four parts are made of blocks learning which comprises of the following[6]:

YEAR 1
BLOCK 1: Introduction Lifespan and Lifestyle; BLOCK 2: Musculoskeletal; BLOCK 3: Haematology; BLOCK 4: Cardiovascular; BLOCK 5: Respiratory.

First Semester: Foundation Studies, Musculoskeletal Sciences, Drugs and Alcohol.

Second Semester: Respiratory Science, Haemtology, Cardiovascular Sciences.

YEAR 2
BLOCK 6: Neuroscience, Vision, and Behavior; BLOCK 7: Endocrine, Nutrition, and Gastroenterological; BLOCK 8: Renal, Reproduction, and Sexual Health; BLOCK 9: Cancer Palliation.

First Semester: Neuroscience, Vision, Behavior, Endocrinology, Nutrition, and Gastroenterology.

Second Semester: Renal sciences, Reproduction, Sexual Health, Cancer Services, and Palliative Care.[6]

UNIVERSITY OF SYDNEY
COURSE OUTLINE (2002)

YEAR 1 & 2
SEMESTER 1

1. Anatomy and Histology (4 crs); 2. Microscopy and Histochemistry (12 crs); 3. Forensic Osteology (6 crs); 4. Visceral Anatomy (6 crs); 5. Immunology (4 crs); 6. Cell Pathology A (12 crs); 7. Pharmacology Fundamentals (4 crs); 8. Pharmacology 2A (2 crs); 9. Molecular Pharmacology and Toxicology (12 crs); 10. Pharmacology 3A (6 crs); 11. Advanced Molecular Pharmacology and Toxicology (12 crs); 12. Pharmacology A (Advanced—10 crs); 13. Cells and Cell Communication (6 crs); 14. Genes and Genetic Engineering (6 crs); 15. Regulation of the Internal Environment (8 crs); 16. Introduction Physiology A (4 crs); 17. Physiology A (8 crs); 18. Physiology 2A (3 crs); 19. Neuroscience (12 crs); 20. Human Cellular Physiology (12 crs); 21. Neuroscience (Advanced—12 crs); 22. Human Cellular Physiology (Advanced—12 crs).
(D: 1, 2, 3, 4, 5, 6, 13, 14, 15, 16, 17, 18, 19, 20, 21, 22; P: 7, 8, 9, 10, 11, 12)

SEMESTER 2

1. Anatomy and Histology (4 crs); 2. Concepts in Neuroanatomy (4 crs); 3. Principles of Development (94 crs); 4. Cells and Development (12 crs); 5. Cranial and Cervical Anatomy (6 crs); 6. Topographical Anatomy (12 crs); 7. Musculoskeletal Anatomy (6 crs); 8. Immunology (12 crs); 9. Pathological Basis of Human Disease (12 crs); 10. Bioinformatics Project (4 crs); 11. Introduction to Pharmacology: Drugs and People (4 crs); 12. Pharmacology: Drugs and Society (8 crs); 13. Pharmacology 2B (2 crs); 14. Neuro and Cardiovascular Pharmacology (12 crs); 15. Pharmacology 3B (2 crs); 16. Neuro and Cardiovascular Pharmacology (Advanced—12 crs); 17. Pharmacology B (Advanced—10 crs); 18. Introductory Physiology B (4 crs); 19. Physiology B (8 crs); 20. Physiology 2B (8 crs); 21. Neuroscience: Cellular and Integrative (12 crs); 22. Heart and Circulation (12 crs); 23. Neuroscience: Cellular and Integrative (Advanced—12 crs); 24. Heart and Circulation (Advanced—12 crs).
(D: 1, 2, 3, 4, 5, 6, 7, 8, 9, 18, 19, 20, 21, 22, 23, 24; P: 11, 12, 13, 14, 15, 16, 17)

TOTAL OF YEAR 1 & 2

Number of pharmacy or drug treatment-related courses: 13 out of 46 or 96 out of 371 credits.

Number of diagnosis-related courses: 32 out of 46 or 96 out of 371 credits. (D = 0.70 & P = 0.28)

YEAR 3

Composed of 4 sections of integrated attachment and 1 rotating, practicing placement. The integrated clinical attachment is a transitional phase where frequency and the number of formal teaching sessions are reduced from the third year to none in the last phase of the fourth year (the pre-internship year). Students are clinically attached to the main medical and surgical wards as well as associate ambulatory clinics in teaching hospitals in the third year.[8]

YEAR 4

Composed of 3 sections of rotating practice placement and 1 section of pre-internship. Like years 1 to 3, the four main parts or blocks in the fourth year comprises of Child and Adolescent Health (10 crs); Perinatal and Women's Health (10 crs); Community Practice (10 crs); and psychological Medicine/Drugs and Alcohol (10 crs), plus an elective term (4 crs). As noted before, the four main parts of years 1 to 3 are incorporated in the fourth-year curriculum.[8]

SUMMARY OF YEAR 3 & 4

Number of pharmacy or drug treatment-related courses: Constitute an integral part of integrated clinical attachment, rotations, and pre-internship.

Number of diagnosis-related courses: Constitute a major part of the integrated clinical attachment, rotations, and pre-internship.

INTERNSHIP (1-YEAR POSTGRADUATE PROGRAM)

Mostly rotations, modeled after the American system.

SPECIALTY IN AUSTRALIA

Medical specialty (specialist) training in Australia is not the responsibility of any university, including the University of Sydney. However, there is a program arranged by one of the recognized professional colleges such as the Royal Australasian's college of physicians or surgeons or dermatologists, radiologists, obstetricians and gynecologist, etc. Majority of the program occurs in the teaching hospitals with the assistance of university staff. Teaching hospitals normally select and place medical specialist aspirants in training positions with the consent of the state health departments and colleges to some extent. All aspirants are medical practitioners who are licensed to practice medicine in the country, and detailed information about the various specialty programs is available at the various colleges.[7]

Besides the specialty programs, there are various postgraduate programs leading to the award of degrees such as Doctor of Philosophy (PhD), Master of Medicine, Master of Surgery, and others available as graduate programs in medicine at the University of Sydney in Australia. The duration of training varies from 1 to 3 years or 3 to 5 or 6 years depending on the course; MBBS degree or medical practice are not prerequisites for these courses but can be used for admission requirements. That is to say, you can get into the graduate programs without being a medical doctor or practitioner.[7]

DENTISTRY

Dentistry at the University of Sydney, Australia, changed its program from a five-year course to a four-year Bachelor of Dentistry (B Dent) course in 2001. The Bachelor of Dentistry course is a four-year program, which follows the same protocol as the medical school in terms of admission and the first two years (year 1 and 2) in school. The only exception in the first two years is that one day a week is required for patient and doctor sessions and any clinical requirements are fulfilled as a dentistry clinical practice component or as foundations of total patient care. The curriculum is made up of three major parts, which are total patient care, personal and professional development/dentist and community and life sciences.[8] Year 3 is made up of clinical placement with supervision at United Dental Hospital and Westmead Center for Oral Health, while year 4 is made up of community placement and specialization such as pediatric dentistry, orthodontics, and elective subspecialty. Year 1 and 2 prepares students and it is the solid-rock of foundation upon which students' clinical experience of later years (3 and 4) is based. Teaching sessions decrease while clinical work experience increases from the third to the fourth year. Entrance into the fourth year automatically qualifies students for registration with the New South Wales Dental Board.[8] Summary of year 3 and 4 is the same for medicine except that clinical rotations and pre-internships are purely dentistry.

VETERINARY SCIENCE

The veterinary science program at the University of Sydney is a five-year course with admission requirements of a high school certificate (examination performance ranked on aggregate universities' admission index—UAI—scale) or a university student with a minimum of one year of full-time study, a good GPA, special tertiary admission test (STAT), and commitment to veterinary science. Students are awarded a Bachelor of Veterinary Science (BVSC) degree at the completion of the program.[9]

COURSE OUTLINE (2001/2002)

YEAR 1
SEMESTER 1 (24 CREDITS)
1. Animal Husbandry IA (5 crs); 2. Cell Biology IA (4 crs); 3. Chemistry (6 crs); 4. Veterinary Anatomy and Physiology IA (6 crs); 5. Professional Practice IA (3 crs).
(D: 2, 4; P: 0)

SEMESTER 2 (24 CREDITS)
1. Professional Practice IB (3 crs); 2. Cell Biology IB (6 crs); 3. Animal Husbandry IB (7 crs); 4. Veterinary Anatomy and Physiology IB (8 crs).
(D: 2, 4; P: 0)

Number of pharmacy or drug treatment-related courses: zero (0) out of 9 or 48 credits.

Number of diagnosis-related courses: 4 out of 9 or 24 out of 48 credits.

YEAR 2
SEMESTER 1 (24 CREDITS)

1. Professional Practice 2 (4 crs); 2. Genetics and Biometry (6 crs); 3. Animal Digestion and Nutrition (7 crs); 4. Veterinary Anatomy and Physiology 2A (7 crs).

(D: 2, 4; P: 0)

SEMESTER 2 (24 CREDITS)

1. Equine Anatomy (4 crs); 2. Principles of Disease (8 crs); 3. Veterinary Conservation Biology (4 crs); 4. Veterinary Anatomy and Physiology 2B (8 crs).

(D: 1, 2, 4; P: 0)

Number of pharmacy or drug treatment-related courses: zero (0) out of 8 or 48 credits.

Number of diagnosis-related courses: 5 out of 8 or 33 out of 48 credits.

YEAR 3
SEMESTER 1 (24 CREDITS)

1. Veterinary Pathology (8 crs); 2. Veterinary Pharmacology and Toxicology (3 crs); 3. Animal Behavior and Welfare Science (3 crs); 4. Professional Practice 3A (2 crs); 5. Veterinary Parasitology (4 crs); 6. Veterinary Microbiology (4 crs).

(D: 1, 3, 5, 6; P: 2)

SEMESTER 2 (24 CREDITS)

1. Animal Disease (11 crs); 2. Public Health (4 crs); 3. Veterinary Clinical Sciences (7 crs); 4. Professional Practice 3B (2 crs).

(D: 1, 3; P: 0)

Number of pharmacy or drug treatment-related courses: 1 out of 10 or 3 out of 48 credits plus an integral part of one or two other courses.

Number of diagnosis-related courses: 6 out of 10 or 37 out of 48 credits plus a major part of one or two other courses.

YEAR 4
SEMESTER 1 (24 CREDITS)
1. Animal Husbandry Practice Report (6 crs); 2. Applied Veterinary Anatomy (2 crs); 3. Clinical Practice 4A (3 crs); 4. Veterinary Anaesthesia 4A (2 crs); 5. Veterinary Medicine 4A (3 crs); 6. Veterinary Radiology 4A (3 crs); 7. Veterinary Surgery 4A (3 crs); 8. Veterinary Clinical Pathology A (2 crs).
(D: 2, 5, 6, 7, 8; P: 4)

SEMESTER 2 (25 CREDITS)
1. Animal Nutrition 4 (3 crs); 2. Applied Reproduction and Obstetrics (3 crs); 3. Clinical Practice 4B (2 crs); 4. Veterinary Anaesthesia 4B (2 crs); 5. Veterinary Clinical Pathology (3 crs); 6. Veterinary Medicine 4B (3 crs); 7. Veterinary Parasitology 4 (4 crs); 8. Veterinary Radiology 4B (2 crs); 9. Veterinary Surgery 4B (3 crs).
(D: 5, 6, 7, 8, 9; P: 4)

Number of pharmacy or drug treatment-related courses: 2 out of 17 or 4 out of 49 credits plus an integral part of two or three other courses.

Number of diagnosis-related courses: 10 out of 17 or 28 out of 49 credits plus a major part of two or three other courses.

YEAR 5
SEMESTER 1 (CLINICAL ROTATIONS)
1. Bird Health and Production; 2. Clinical Practice 5A; 3. Equine Medicine and Surgery 5A; 4. Essay; 5. Pig Health and Production; 6. Veterinary Public Health.

SEMESTER 2
1. Cattle Health and Production; 2. Clinical Practice 5B; 3. Equine Medicine and Surgery; 4. Sheep Health and Production; 5. Special Medicine.

Number of pharmacy or drug treatment-related courses: Constitute an integral part of the rotations.

Number of diagnosis-related courses: Constitute a major part of the rotations.

TOTAL OF YEAR 2 TO 4 (Core Courses)
Number of pharmacy or drug treatment-related courses: 3 out of 35 or 7 out of 145 credits.

Number of diagnosis-related courses: 21 out of 35 or 98 out of 145 credits.
(D = 0.60 & P = 0.086)

OPTOMETRY

University of Sydney has no optometry school, but the University of Melbourne does have a Department of Optometry and Vision Science. The University of Melbourne offers five years of coursework leading to the award of Bachelor of Optometry. The program consists of one year (or first-year) pre-optometry coursework and four years of coursework in optometry. The program was recently expanded to five years to incorporate therapeutic treatment of ocular disease with S4 drugs. The entry requirements for optometry are same as those for veterinary science at the University of Sydney. These requirements are either a high school certificate, or a university student who has completed one year of coursework with a good GPA.[10]

UNIVERSITY OF MELBOURNE
COURSE OUTLINE (2002)

YEAR 1 (PRE-OPTOMETRY YEAR)

1. Biology of Cells and Organisms; 2. Genetics and the Evolution of Life; 3. Chemistry A; 4. Chemistry B; 5. Vision; 6. How the Eye Sees the World; 7. Experimental Design and Data Analysis; 8. Physics A; 9. Physics B.
(DO: 1, 2, 5; P: 0)
Number of pharmacy or drug treatment-related courses: zero (0) out of 9.

Number of diagnosis and optical-related courses: 3 out of 9.

YEAR 2

1. Anatomy and Histology of the Eye; 2. Physiology; 3. Biochemistry and the Eye; 4. Human Visual Functions; 5. Basic Principles of Pathology-Optometry; 6. Visual Processing and Control; 7. Optical Systems; 8. Structure and Function of the Brain.
(DO: 1, 2, 3, 4, 5, 6, 7, 8; P: 0)
Number of pharmacy or drug treatment-related courses: zero (0) out of 8.

Number of diagnosis and optical-related courses: 8 out of 8.

YEAR 3
1. Visual Physiology and Perception; 2. Ocular Pharmacology; 3. Optical Design and Ophthalmic Metrology; 4. Functional Disorders of Vision; 5. Ocular Histopathologgy; 6. Ophthalmic Prosthetics I; 7. Microbiology and Immunology (optometry).
(DO: 1, 3, 4, 5, 6, 7; P: 2)
Number of pharmacy or drug treatment-related courses: 1 out of 7.

Number of diagnosis and optical-related courses: 6 out of 7.

YEAR 4
1. Fundamentals of Ocular Disease Management; 2. Diseases of the Eye; 3. Ophthalmic Prosthetics II; 4. Clinical Optometry Practice; 5. Clinical Ocular Therapeutics; 6. Occupational Optometry and Visual Standards.
(DO: 2, 3, 4, 6; P: 5; DO & P: 1)
Number of pharmacy or drug treatment–related courses: 1.5 out of 6 may constitute an integral part of one or two other courses.

Number of diagnosis and optical-related courses: 4.5 out of 6 may constitute major part of one or two other courses.

YEAR 5
1. General Optometry Practice; 2. Contact Lenses; 3. Pediatric and Low-Vision Practice; 4. Ocular-Disease Management; 5. Project Studies in Vision Sciences.
(DO: 1, 2, 3; P: 0; DO & P: 4)
Number of pharmacy or drug treatment–related courses: 0.5 out of 5

Number of diagnosis and optical-related courses: 3.5 out of 5.

TOTAL OF YEARS 2–5 (Core Courses)
Number of pharmacy or drug treatment–related courses: 3 out of 26.

Number of diagnosis and optical-related courses: 22 out of 26.
(DO = 0.85 and P = 0.12)

PHARMACY

University of Sydney offers four years of coursework leading to the award of bachelor's degree in pharmacy. Admission requirements for pharmacy are the same as veterinary science and optometry requirements. That is, a high school certificate examination ranked on the basis of aggregate university admission index (UAI—94.00 in 2002) and a successful special tertiary admission test (STAT), or at least a one-year full-time superior tertiary record at bachelor's-degree level and a successful STAT. There are no doctor of pharmacy degree program neither are there plans for its implementation in the near future. However, like veterinary sciences, medicine, dentistry, and optometry, there are graduate programs leading to the award of certificate in clinical pharmacy (Grad Cert. Clin Pharm), master of pharmacy (M Pharm), master of pharmacy (clinical—M Pharm 'clin'), and doctor of philosophy (PhD).[11]

UNIVERSITY OF SYDNEY COURSE OUTLINE (2002)

YEAR 1
SEMESTER 1 (24 CREDITS)

1. Concepts in Biology (6 crs); 2. Chemistry A (6 crs); 3. Concepts in Pharmacy (3 crs); 4. Introductory Psychology (6 crs); 5. Statistics (3 crs)

(D: 0; P: 3)

SEMESTER 2 (24 CREDITS)

1. Human Biology (6 crs); 2. Chemistry B (6 crs); 3. Calculus (3 crs); 4. Introductory Pharmaceutical Science (4 crs); 5. Social, Behavior, and Professional pharm (5 crs).

(D: 0; P: 4, 5)

Number of pharmacy or drug treatment–related courses: 3 out of 10 or 12 out of 48credits.

Number of diagnosis-related courses: zero (0) out of 10 or 48 credits.

YEAR 2
SEMESTER 1 (24 CREDITS)

1. Protein, Enzymes, and Metabolism (3 crs); 2. Microbiology (3 crs); 3. Pharmacology 2A (2 crs); 4. Medicinal Chemistry 2A (6 crs); 5. Pharmacy Practice 2A (2 crs); 6. Physical Pharmaceutics 2A (5 crs); 7. Physiology 2A (3 crs).

(D: 2, 7; P: 1, 3, 4, 6)

SEMESTER 2 (24 CREDITS)

1. Metabolism 2 and Genes (3 crs); 2. Pharmacology 2B (2 crs); 3. Pharmaceutical Microbiology (4 crs); 4. Medicinal Chemistry 2B (4 crs); 5. Pharmacy Practice 2B (4 crs); 6. Physical Pharmaceutical 2B (5 crs); 7. Physiology 2B (3 crs).

(D: 3, 7; P: 1, 2, 4, 6)

Number of pharmacy or drug treatment–related courses: 8 out of 14 or 30 out of 48 credits.

Number of diagnosis-related courses: 4 out of 14 or 13 out of 48 credits.

YEAR 3
SEMESTER 1 (24 CREDITS)

1. Pharmacology 3A (6 crs); 2. Formulation A (3 crs); 3. Medicinal Chemistry 3A (6 crs); 4. Pharmacokinetics (3 crs); 5. Pharmacy Practice 3A (6 crs).

(D: 0; P: 1, 2, 3, 4)

SEMESTER 2 (24 CREDITS)

1. Pharmacology 3B (2 crs); 2. Dispensing (4 crs); 3. Formulation B (2 crs); 4. Medicinal Chemistry 3B (6 crs); 5. Pharmacokinetics B (3 crs); 6. Pharmacy Practice 3B (7 crs).

(D: 0; P: 1, 2, 3, 4, 5)

Number of pharmacy or drug treatment–related courses: 9 out of 11 or 35 out of 48 credits plus major part of pharmacy practice.

Number of diagnosis-related courses: zero (0) out of 11 or 48 credits, but this constitutes an integral part of pharmacy practice.

YEAR 4
SEMESTER 1 (24 CREDITS)

1. Integrated Dispensing (4 crs); 2. New Drug Technologies (4 crs); 3. Pharmaceutics Workshop (4 crs); 4. Clinical Pathology A (2 crs); 5. Pharmacotherapeutics (5 crs); 6. Clinical Practice A (5 crs); [7. Pharmaceutics A (Advanced—10 crs); 8. Pharmaceutical Chemistry A (Advanced—10 crs); 9. Pharmacy Practice A (Advance—10 crs); 10. Pharmacology A (Advanced—10 crs)].

(D: 4; P: 1, 2, 3, 4 [7, 8, 10])

All advanced courses, in bracket [ ], require high WAM and invitation or permission for enrollment.

SEMESTER 2 (24 CREDITS)

1. Clinical Pathology B (2 crs); 2. Clinical Information Technology (2 crs); 3. Pharmacotherapeutics B (4 crs); 4. Clinical Practice B (10 crs); 5. Ethics and History of Pharmacy (2 crs); 6. Pharmaceutical Management (4 crs); [7. Pharmaceutics B (Advanced—10 crs); 8. Pharmaceutical Chemistry B (Advanced—10 crs); 9. Pharmacy Practice B (Advanced—10 crs); 10. Pharmacology B (Advanced—10 crs)].

(D: 1; P: 2, 3, 6 [7, 8, 10])

All advanced courses, in bracket [ ], require high WAM and invitation or permission for enrollment.

Number of pharmacy or drug treatment–related courses: 7 out of 12 or 27 out of 48 credits plus major part of clinical practice and workshop.

Number of diagnosis-related courses: 2 out of 12 or 4 out of 48 credits plus an integral part of clinical practice and workshop.

TOTAL OF YEAR 2 TO 4 (Core Courses)

Number of pharmacy or drug treatment–related courses: 24 out of 37 courses.

Number of diagnosis-related courses: 6 out of 37.

(D = 0.16 & P = 0.65)

CLINICAL PHARMACY

Clinical pharmacy is available as a postgraduate program leading to the award of master of pharmacy (clinical) or a graduate diploma and graduate diploma and graduate certificate in clinical pharmacy at the University of Sydney. Entry requirements are a minimum of a pharmacy degree plus a minimum of three years experience as a pharmacist or an honors pharmacy degree for masters. The master program is a one-year full-time study comprised of two semesters of 24 credits of coursework and 24 credits of research project offered simultaneously, making a total of 48 credits. The graduate diploma program is offered in a similar manner with 36 credits placement. The master and diploma can also be completed on a part-time basis within 3 and 2 years, respectively. The certificate program is available only as a part-time program to be completed in eighteen months.[12]

COURSE OUTLINE (2002)
Semester 1

1. Medication review; 2. Drug Information; 3. Advanced Therapeutics A.
(D: 0; P: 1, 2, 3)

Semester 2

1. Scientific Presentation; 2. Advanced Therapeutics B; 3. Clinical Pharmacokinetics; 4. Pharmacoeconomics.
(D: 0; P: 1, 2, 3, 4)

Semester 3

(For part-time and 1 year for full-time students)
1. Statistics; 2. Research Methods; 3. Pharmacoepidermiology; 4. Advanced Therapeutics B.
(D: 3; P: 4)

Number of pharmacy or drug treatment–related courses: 7 out of 10 courses plus major part of some courses and clinical placement.
Number of diagnosis-related courses: 1 out of 10 courses plus an integral part of some courses and clinical placement.

DATA ANALYSIS

Data analysis of the above course outline showed that in summary, it can be estimated that medical and dentistry school graduates in Australia are exposed to an average number of 0.70 or 70%, which is 7 out of every 10, diagnosis-related courses in pre-clinical years (didactic class work) and 0.28 or 28%, which is approximately 3 out of every 10, pharmacy or drug treatment–related courses in pre-clinical years (didactic class work). As in the U.S., the two pre-clinical years lay the foundation upon which the last 2 clinical years and one-year internship are based. The clinical rotations and internship adhere to the format of course outline in the pre-clinical years; hence, it can be concluded that diagnosis or diagnosis and dental-related courses constitute about 70% (majority) of the rotation and pharmacy or drug treatment–related courses constitute about 30% (integral part or minority) of the rotation. Study limitation involve the usage of one school as case example and the possibilities that few courses might contain both diagnosis and pharmacy or drug treatment, of which the affected course(s) was classified as one with majority of the content.

The veterinary science graduates in Australia are estimated to be exposed to an average number of 0.60 or 60% which is 6 out of every 10, courses that are diagnosis related during the pre-clinical years, and 0.086 or 8.6%, which is approximately 9 percent, and that is 9 out of every 100 or 1 out of every 11, pharmacy or drug treatment–related courses during the four pre-clinical years. The optometrists, on the other hand, are estimated to be exposed to an average number of 0.85 or 85%, which is approximately 90% or 9 out of every 10, diagnosis and optical-related courses, and 0.12 or 12% which is approximately 10% or 1 out of every 10, pharmacy or drug treatment–related courses during the program. The limitations are the same as above.

Data analysis of the pharmacy course outline showed that pharmacy graduates are exposed to an average number of 0.16 or 16% which is approximately 20% or 2 out of every 10, diagnosis-related courses, and 0.65 or 65% which is approximately 7 out of every 10, pharmacy or drug-treatment courses during the program. In a nutshell, 3 out of every 10 courses in pharmacy or drug treatment in the pre-clinical years and pharmacy or drug treatment as an integral part of clinical rotation/internship qualifies the medical doctors and dentists in Australia to prescribe any drugs for the pharmacist to dispense. The same is true of a veterinary medical doctor, whose exposure to approximately 1 out of every 11 courses, and an optometrist, whose exposure to approximately 1 out of every 10 courses in pharmacy or drug treatment, qualifies him to write any prescription for S4 drugs in case of optometrists for the pharmacists to dispense to animals and people.

The pharmacist, on the other hand, are exposed to approximately 7 out of every 10 courses in pharmacy or drug-treatment related courses during the program and the clinical pharmacists are, in addition to the 7 out of every 10 courses, well rounded in clinical experience with greater didactic class work in pharmacy or drug-treatment courses, yet they cannot prescribe any drugs for animals in Australia. There are no certified nurse practitioners or physician assistants in Australia. The only healthcare practitioners that are allowed to prescribe drugs in Australia are traditional medical doctors, dentists, veterinary medical doctors, and optometrists, to some extent.

NEW ZEALAND

New Zealand and Australia have a lot in common in terms of culture, education, immigration policies, and other areas. These two countries act like one country, and New Zealand is part of the Australian continent. Medical practitioners from any of the two countries who wish to practice medicine in any of the two countries are treated like indigenes, unlike other practitioners from other parts of the world. However, medical studies in both countries differ to some extent in terms of entry requirements and number of years in training. The University of Auckland in New Zealand has a six-year medical program leading to the award of bachelor of human biology/bachelor of medicine, bachelor of surgery.[13] The six-year program comprises of first three years, which leads to the award of bachelor of human biology, and the second or last three years, which leads to the award of bachelor of medicine, bachelor of surgery (MBchB). At the end of the six years, graduates go into seventh or intern year in the hospital, after which he is free to register as a practicing doctor. The new graduate can go into any area of practice; however, specialist registration and further training is required in general practice, general medicine, psychiatry, public health, neurology, surgery, obstetrics and gynecology, immunology, geriatric medicine, pediatrics, dermatology, oncology, radiology, and pathology. The entry requirements are open for school-leavers who are secondary school (high school) graduates with a score of 386 or more in the 2001 NZUEB examinations (BURSARY); or those who have completed part 1 or a full course of a first-degree program or Maori and Pacific program admission scheme (MAPAS). The bachelor of pharmacy program (B Pharm) at the University of Auckland is a four-year program followed by one-year pre-registration training (intern year). The entry requirements are the same as for medicine, with a selection process involving interviews. The course outline for medicine, pharmacy, and other branches of medicine in relation to diagnosis and pharmacy or drug-treatment related courses are similar to the analysis obtained in Australia and other continents.[13]

EUROPE

Europe is the fifth largest continent in the world, with 3.8 million square miles areas and a population of 683 million people, as of 1990. Europe is home to three big powers (France, Britain, and Russia) out of five United Nation Security Council members and it is the powerhouse that once colonized the world and set in motion a realistic Tower of Babel for humanity—a global village that is nurtured by people's ability to speak common languages like English, Spanish, French, and others across continents. Europe is the second smallest habitable continent of the world, yet it was able to preserve human civilization that started in Egypt in Africa, then Babylon (Mesopotamia—present-day Iraq) in Asia, Greek and Roman empires in Europe, and later came to Britain, Spain, France, Germany, and Portugal, all in Europe. Europe has successfully passed the torchlight to United States of America in North America for onward transmission to unknown destinations by future generations. By and large, all those who have succeeded in preserving human civilization and transforming it to greater heights deserve kudos and lots of commendations for their brilliant performance/work. Today the idea of humanity living on the moon and other planets besides Earth, such as Mars, is becoming a reality rather than a fiction. The moon and other planets were once considered heavenly bodies beyond man's reach (by our forefathers in yesteryears) but now they are becoming Earth's backyard. The Bible speaks of the construction of Tower of Babel to reach heaven but was destroyed by God who caused the builders to speak a multitude of different languages. Let's us hope, by God's grace, that humanity/Earth will never again experience asteroid destruction (which caused the extinction of the dinosaurs) or any other seen/unseen/unpredictable destruction that will set back the hands of the clock and plunge humanity into darkness.

THE SPACE PROGRAM IS THE FUTURE OF HUMANITY/MANKIND.

Medical schools in Europe have a lot in common, and United Kingdom or Britain is a case example. The medical program in United Kingdom is a six-year course that is comprised of three years pre-clinical coursework leading to the award of honors degree (BA) in physiological sciences, and three years of clinical coursework leading to the award of BM, Bch in some schools, and six years straight of coursework in other schools. Entry requirements are three different levels, which are: 1. Advanced Level GCE (General Certificate of Education), SCE or IB (International Baccalaureate) with at least credit (grade C) in math, biology, and physics for pre-clinical study; 2. BA physiological sciences honor degree in pre-clinical study from other schools; and 3. graduate study for bioscience graduates.[14] Advanced-level entry students spend six years to obtain a medical degree before registering to practice medicine, while honors graduates spend four years to obtain the same thing through an accelerated program in the United Kingdom. Oxford University is one of the oldest universities in the world and is used as a case example in the United Kingdom. There is information from other universities such as the University of Cambridge, University College of London, and others in reference to other branches of medicine. Like other schools above, the course outline for Oxford Medical School is the summary of the broad subject/courses, as in some other places.

OXFORD UNIVERSITY COURSE OUTLINE (2002)

YEAR 1 (FIRST BM PART I)
1. Organization of the Body; 2. Physiology and Pharmacology; 3. Biochemistry and Medical Genetics; 4. Medical Sociology.

(Plus sessions twice a term of a patient and doctor course as clinical experience—Approach to Medical Sociology—examination at the end of first BM part I.)

(D: 1, 3, 4; P: 0 D & P: 2)

Number of pharmacy or drug treatment–related courses: 0.5 out of 4 plus an integral part of medical sociology.

Number of diagnosis-related courses: 3.5 out of 4.

YEAR 2 (FIRST BM PART II)
1. Integrative Systems of the Body; 2. The Nervous System; 3. General Pathology and Microbiology; 4. Psychology for Medicine.

(Plus sessions twice a term of patient and doctor course as clinical experience—examination at the end of fifth BM part II.)
(D: 2, 3, 4; P: 1)
Number of pharmacy or drug treatment–related courses: 1 out of 4 plus an integral part of few others.

Number of diagnosis-related courses: 3 out of 4 plus an integral part of integrative system of the body.

YEAR 3 (FINAL HONOR SCHOOL)
1. Biochemistry: Molecular Mechanisms of Disease; 2. Neurosciences I (Cellular); 3. Neurosciences II (Systems); 4. Circulation; 5. Respiration; 6. Physiology of Epithelia; 7. Endocrinology; 8. Cell Biology; 9. Immunology; 10. Pharmacology; 11. Development biology; 12, Cellular Physiology; 13. Physiological Sciences.

(Plus dissertation [aka project in U.S.] and two sets of practical classes. Examination is six three-hour written examinations on six out of thirteen options or courses.)
(D: 1, 2, 3, 4, 5, 6, 7, 8, 9, 11, 12, 13; P: 10)
Number of pharmacy or drug treatment–related courses: 1 out of 13, but constitutes an integral part of some other courses.

Number of diagnosis-related courses: 12 out of 13.

Breakdown of two courses in part II is giving as follows:
1. INTEGRATIVE SYSTEMS OF THE BODY: A. BREATHING AND CIRCULATION: 1. Respiratory Pharmacology; 2. Regulation of the Cardiovascular System; 4. Exercise Physiology; B. BODY FLUID: 4. Regulation of Body Fluid Volume and Composition; 5. Acid-Base Balance; C. ENDOCRINOLOGY: 6. Regulation of Calcium, Phosphate, and Bone; 7. Pharmacological Aspects of the Female Sex Hormones; 8.

Endocrine Regulation of Growth and Metabolism; D. INTEGRATIVE ROLE OF THE HYPOTHALAMUS: 9. Functions of Hypothalamus; 10. Physiological Response to Stress; 11. Control of Appetite; E. RESPONSE TO ENVIRONMENTAL STRESS: 12. Body-Temperature Regulation; 13. Life at High Altitude; F. BODY SYSTEMS IN GENERAL ANESTHESIA.

2. THE NERVOUS SYSTEM: A. HEAD AND NECK: 1. Osteology; 2. Blood Supply; 3. Special Areas; B. EMBRYONIC DEVELOPMENT: 4. Development of the CNS; C. CNS MORPHOLOGY: 5. CNS Compartments; 6. Neuroanatomy; D. PRINCIPLES OF NEURONAL FUNCTION: 7. Method of Study of the Nervous System; 8. Structure and Function of Neurons and Glia; 9. Neuronal Degeneration; 10. Neuronal Repair and Regeneration; 11. Synaptic Transmission; 12. Epileptic Discharges; E. SENSORY SYSTEMS: 13. Somatosensory Pathways; 14. Pain; 15. Vision; 16. Audition; 17. Vestibular System; 18. Smell and Taste; 19. Sensory Integration; F. MOTOR SYSTEM: 20. Lower Motor Neuron Pools; 21. Muscle Stretch Reflex; 22. Upper Motor Neurons; 23. Basal Ganglia; 24. Cerebellum; 25. Locomotion; 26. Eye-Movement Control and Papillary Reflexes; G. CRANIAL NERVES: 27. Specific Cranial Nerves; H. THALAMUS AND HYPOTHALAMUS: 28. Thalamus; 29. Hypothalamus; 30. Epithalamus; I. HIGHER CEREBRAL FUNCTIONS: 31. Consciousness; 32. Sleep; 33. Components and Connections of the Limbic System; 34. Functions of the Limbic System; 35. Memory; 36. Neuronal Plasticity; 37. Development and Aging; J. PSYCHOPHARMACOLOGY: 38. Depression; 39. Schizophrenia; 40. Social Drugs and Addiction.

TOTAL OF YEAR 1 TO 3 (Pre-clinical Years)
Number of pharmacy or drug treatment–related courses: 2.5 out of 21.
Number of diagnosis-related courses: 18.5 out of 21.
$(D = 0.88 \text{ \& } P = 0.12)$

CLINICAL YEARS
YEAR 4

1. Foundation Course (5 wks); 2. General Practice (2 wks); 3. Laboratory Medicine (8 wks); 4. Surgery including Anesthetics (8 wks); 5. Medicine (8 wks); 6. District General Hospital (DGH) Attachment in Medicine and Surgery (4 wks); 7. Special Study Module (4 wks); 8. Thread Courses: Evidence-Based Medicine and Information Skills, Medical Ethics and Law, Communication Skills and Human Sexuality, Clinical Pharmacology, Radiology, Oncology.

Number of pharmacy or drug treatment–related courses: Constitutes an integral part of the clinical rotations.\

Number of diagnosis-related courses: Constitutes major part of the clinical rotations.

YEAR 5 (6–8 WK BLOCKS)

Block 1: Neurology and Neurosurgery, ENT, Ophthalmology; Block 2: Psychiatry; Block 3: Clinical Gerontology, Primary Healthcare, Public Health Medicine, Palliative Care; Block 4: Obstetrics and Gynecology, Genitourinary Medicine; Block 5: Accident and Emergency, Orthopedic Surgery and Musculoskeletal Medicine; Block 6: Pediatrics.

Number of pharmacy or drug treatment–related courses: Constitutes an integral part of the clinical rotations.

Number of diagnosis-related courses: Constitutes major part of the clinical rotations.

YEAR 6

1. Medical Firm, including Clinical Pharmacology and Radiology (5 wks); 2. Surgical Firm, including Radiology (5 wks); 3. Clinical Attachment in a DGH (6 wks); 4. Dermatology (2 wks); 5. Clinical Options and Special Study Modules (12 wks); 6. Elective (10 wks); 7. Preparing for Practice as a Doctor Module (2 wks), including Advanced Life Support and ALERT (Medical Emergencies Course); 8. PRHO Shadowing (2 wks); 9. Revision Course (3 wks of ward-based teaching and lectures).

Number of pharmacy or drug treatment–related courses: Constitutes an integral part of the clinical rotations.

Number of diagnosis-related courses: Constitutes major part of the clinical rotations.

UNIVERSITY OF CAMBRIDGE

The University of Cambridge clinical or medical school has the same protocol as Oxford University. The clinical course is comprised of an introductory course, Phase I—Basic Skills and Knowledge, Pathology Block course, Radiology and Nuclear Medicine, Rheumatology, Phase II—The Specialties, Final MB Part I and II, Elective, Phase II—Senior Attachments, Final MB Part III, Pre-Registration House Officer Posts and Clinical Course Summary Diagram.

Like the year-five block rotations in Oxford University, Phase II is the specialties year at the University of Cambridge. The specialties year is the period when medical student learn much about specialties, develop their interest, intensify their interest with electives by choice, and expand their specialties knowledge during practice. Further specialties learning is available as a postgraduate program. The specialties in Phase II at the University of Cambridge are comprised of Ear, Nose, and Throat (ENT—2 wks); Cardiology and Respiratory Medicine (2 wks); Dermatology, Genito-Urinary Medicine, Plastic Surgery, and Urology (5 wks); General Practice (2 wks); Clinical Neurosciences and Rehabilitation, and Ophthalmology (7 wks); Orthopedics (3 wks); Psychiatry (7 wks); Obstetrics and Gynecology (7 wks); and Pediatrics (7 wks).

At the end of the course, students must complete one year of supervised service in an approved pre-registration post combination before the university presents them to the General Medical Council (GMC) as full graduates for certification and subsequent practice as medical doctors.[15]

DENTISTRY

Dentistry in the United Kingdom is a five-year program leading to the award of bachelor of dentistry (BDS). University of London or King's College, London, is one of the universities that offer dentistry. The first three years is the pre-clinical program, which is devoted to didactic class work, and the last two years are the clinical program, which serves to entrench various aspects of dental care with didactic experience in a clinical setting. Students are given the option of taking intercalated BSc degree in subjects of their choice at the end of the second year. Admission into the dentistry program is coordinated through universities and college admissions service (UCAS). A small number of the applicants are science graduates, while others are General Certificate of Education Advanced level (GCE A-level) holders or its equivalent. Specialist programs like MSc periodontology are available as postgraduate courses.[16]

KING'S COLLEGE COURSE OUTLINE (2002)

YEAR 1

1. Biomedical Sciences Delivered in Systems-Based Courses; 2. Introduction to Applied Dental Science

(DD: 1, 2; P: 0)

Number of pharmacy or drug treatment–related courses: zero (0) out of 2.

Number of diagnosis and dental-related courses: 2 out of 2.

YEAR 2

1. Introduction to Clinical Dentistry of Dentate Patient; 2. Neuroscience; 3. Oral Biology; 4. Pathology.

(DD: 1, 2, 3, 4; P: 0)

Number of pharmacy or drug treatment–related courses: zero (0) out of 4, but constitutes an integral part of clinical dentistry.

Number of diagnosis and dental-related courses: 4 out of 4.

YEAR 3

1. Clinical Dentistry of the Partially Dentate Patient; 2. Dental Materials Science; 3. Human Disease.

Intercalated year probably in anatomy, biochemistry, materials science, molecular biology, psychology, physiology and pathology.

(DD: 1, 2, 3; P: 0)

Number of pharmacy or drug treatment–related courses: zero (0) out of 3, but constitutes an integral part of 1 or 2 courses.

Number of diagnosis and dental-related courses: 3 out of 3.

YEAR 4 (CLINICAL ROTATIONS)

1. Full Range of Clinical Dentistry for Adults and Children; 2. Dental Public Health.

Number of pharmacy or drug treatment–related courses: Constitutes an integral part of clinical rotations.

Number of diagnosis- and dental-related courses: Constitutes major part of clinical rotations.

YEAR 5 (CLINICAL ROTATIONS)
1. Integrated Clinical Dentistry; 2. Development of Year-Four Topics to include Oral Disease; 3. Elective Study.

Number of pharmacy or drug treatment–related courses: Constitutes an integral part of clinical rotations.

Number of diagnosis- and dental-related courses: Constitutes a major part of clinical rotations.

TOTAL OF YEAR 1 TO 3
Number of pharmacy or drug treatment–related courses: zero (0) out of 9 courses.

Number of diagnosis- and dental-related courses: 9 out of 9 courses.
$(D = 1 \& P = 0)$

VETERINARY MEDICINE

Veterinary science in the United Kingdom is a six-year program that consists of a five-year BVSC program and D100 courses. University of Liverpool is reputed to be the first British veterinary school founded in 1904. The faculty of veterinary science offers the BSc/BVSC bachelor of veterinary science with intercalated honors year. The first three years are the pre-clinical phase of didactic class work, which lays the groundwork for the clinical phase in the fourth and final years. Students have the option of taking an intercalated BSc degree in subjects of their choice at the end of the second or third year. Admission protocol is the same as the dentistry school at the University of London, and it is coordinated through UCAS.[17]

UNIVERSITY OF LIVERPOOL COURSE OUTLINE (2002)

YEAR 1
SEMESTER 1
1. Concepts in Cell Biology, Molecular Biology, and Pharmacology; 2. Introduction to Systems Physiology—Cellular Support; 3. Basic Tissues, Embryology, and Cardiovascular System; 4. Animals in Their Environment.
(D: 2, 3; P: 0 D & P: 1)

SEMESTER 2
1. Genetics DNA/RNA, Prokaryotic and Eukaryotic Genomes, and Genetics; 2. Limbs; 3. Respiration, Thorax, and Excretory Systems; 4. Whole-Animal Design and Function

HACS (MB) & Pre-Clinical EMS (DARD) thru year 1.
(D: 1, 2, 3, 4; P: 0)
Number of pharmacy or drug treatment–related courses: 0.5 out of 8.

Number of diagnosis-related courses: 6.5 out of 8.

YEAR 2
SEMESTER 1
1. Molecular and Cellular Basis of Disease (includes Immunology); 2. Gastrointestinal Tract Physiology; 3. Gastrointestinal Tract, Head Anatomy; 4. Reproduction.
(D: 1, 2, 3; P: 0)

SEMESTER 2
1. Integrated and Applied Veterinary Biology; 2. Systems: Neuroscience and Neuropharmacology; 3. Biodiversity including Elective Posters; 4. Animal Maintenance.
(D: 1, 3; P: 0 P & D: 2)
Pre-Clinical EMS (DARD) through year 2

Number of pharmacy or drug treatment–related courses: 0.5 out of 8

Number of diagnosis-related courses: 5.5 out of 8.

YEAR 3
SEMESTER 1

1. Infectious Disease I; 2. Veterinary Parasitology and Public Health; 3. Introduction to Pathology; 4. Veterinary Epidemiology and Public Health I
(D: 1, 2, 3, 4; P: 0)

SEMESTER 2

1. Applied Infectious and Parasitic Disease; 2. Project Module; 3. Systemic Pathology; 4. Veterinary Epidemiology and Public Health II.
(D: 1, 3, 4; P: 0)

Number of pharmacy or drug treatment–related courses: zero (0) out of 8.

Number of diagnosis-related courses: 7 out of 8.

CLINICAL YEARS (4 AND 5)
VETERINARY ROTATIONS

Number of pharmacy or drug treatment–related courses: Constitutes an integral part of clinical rotations.

Number of diagnosis-related courses: Constitutes a major part of clinical rotations.

TOTAL OF YEAR 1 TO 3 (Pre-Clinical Years)
Number of pharmacy or drug treatment–related courses: 1 out of 24 courses.

Number of diagnosis-related courses: 19 out of 24 courses.
(D = 0.79 & P = 0.042)

OPTOMETRY

Optometry in the United Kingdom is an allied profession of medicine that is ascribed the functions of detection, diagnosis, and "non-medical treatment of eye and vision problems". It is a three-year full-time course leading to the award of Bachelor of Science (BSc) degree in optometry. The University of Bradford Optometry Department is one of the largest in the United Kingdom. Admission criteria are the same as for dentistry and veterinary science, and it is coordinated through UCAS.[18]

UNIVERSITY OF BRADFORD
COURSE OUTLINE (2002)

YEAR 1
SEMESTER 1

1. Clinical Optometry I; 2. Pure and Visual Optics; 3. General Anatomy and Physiology; 4. Ocular Anatomy and Physiology; 5. Learning and Key Skills Development; 6. Physiology of Vision and Perception I.

(DO: 1, 2, 3, 4, 6; P: 0)

SEMESTER 2

1. Clinical Optometry; 2. Pure and Visual Optics; 3. General Anatomy and Physiology; 4. Ocular Anatomy and Physiology; 5. Ophthalmic Lenses and Dispensing; 6. Biochemistry.

(DO: 1, 2, 3, 4, 5, 6; P: 0)

Number of pharmacy or drug treatment–related courses: zero (0) out of 12.

Number of diagnosis- and optometry-related courses: 11 out of 12.

YEAR 2
SEMESTER 1

1. Clinical Optometry II; 2. Ophthalmic Lenses and Dispensing II; 3. General and Ocular Pharmacology; 4. Visual and Ocular Assessment; 5. Assessment of Binocular Vision; 6. Physiology of Vision & Perception II.

(DO: 1, 2, 4, 5, 6; P: 3)

SEMESTER 2

1. Clinical Optometry II; 2. Contact Lens Practice I; 3. General and Ocular Pharmacology; 4. Ocular Pathology and Microbiology; 5. Clinical Methodology and Statistics; 6. Low Vision and Aging.

(DO: 1, 2, 4, 5, 6; P: 3)

Number of pharmacy or drug treatment–related courses: 2 out of 12.

Number of diagnosis and optometry-related courses: 10 out of 12.

YEAR 3
SEMESTER 1

1. Abnormal Ocular Conditions; 2. General Clinical Practice; 3. Advanced Clinical Practice; 4. Research Project; 5. Binocular Vision and Orthoptics; 6. Contact Lens Practice II.

(DO: 1, 5, 6; P: 0)

SEMESTER 2

1. Abnormal Ocular Conditions; 2. General Clinical Practice; 3. Advanced Clinical Practice; 4. Research Project; 5. Visual Ergonomics; 6. Law and Optometric Management.

(DO: 1, 5; P: 0)

Number of pharmacy or drug treatment–related courses: zero (0) out of 12 plus an integral part of clinical practice.

Number of diagnosis and optometry-related courses: 5 out of 12 plus a major part of clinical practice.

TOTAL OF YEAR 1 TO 3

Number of pharmacy or drug treatment–related courses: 2 out of 36 courses.

Number of diagnosis and optometry-related courses: 26 out of 36 courses.
(DO = 0.72 & P = 0.056)

PHARMACY

Pharmacy in the United Kingdom is a five-year program with a foundation year and/or four years of direct program leading to the award of an M Pharm degree. The foundation year is meant for mature candidates older than twenty-one years but who do not have the necessary qualifications to guarantee them a place in the first year. Aston University, Birmingham, is one of the universities in the United Kingdom that offer a pharmacy program through a school of pharmacy. Admissions requirement is the same as the entry level for medical school except that three A levels also are needed including chemistry at a minimum of BBB and graduates may not have special entry-level privileges. Course outlines are summarized in a manner similar to the medical school's curriculum.[19]

ASTON UNIVERSITY
COURSE OUTLINE (2000)

YEAR 1
1. Cell and Molecular Biology (10 crs); 2. Medicinal Chemistry (30 crs); 3. Medical Microbiology (10 crs); 4. Pharmaceutics (30 crs); 5. Physiology (20 crs); 6. Pharmacy Practice (20 crs).

(D: 1, 3, 5; P: 2, 4, 6)

Number of pharmacy or drug treatment–related courses: 3 out of 6 plus major part of

Number of diagnosis-related courses: 3 out of 6.

YEAR 2
1. Essential Skills (10 crs); 2. Medicinal Chemistry (30 crs); 3. Pharmaceutical Microbiology (10 crs); 4. Pharmaceutics (30 crs); 5. Pharmacology (30 crs); 6. Pharmacy Practice (10 crs).

(D: 3; P: 1, 2, 4, 5, 6)

Number of pharmacy or drug treatment–related courses: 5 out of 6

Number of diagnosis-related courses: 1 out of 6.

YEAR 3
1. Essential Skills (10 crs); 2. Applied Pharmacology and Therapeutics (20 crs); 3. Chemotherapy and Molecular Biology (10 crs); 4. Medicinal Chemistry (20 crs); 5. Pharmaceutics (30 crs); 6. Pharmacy Practice (30 crs)

(D: 0; P: 1, 2, 3, 4, 5, 6)

Number of pharmacy or drug treatment–related courses: 6 out of 6.

Number of diagnosis-related courses: zero (0) out of 6.

YEAR 4
1. Applied Pharmacology and Therapeutics (20 crs); 2. Pharmaceutics in Practices (10 crs); 3. Clinical Pharmacy; 4. Pharmacy Practice; 5. Evidence

Based Pharmacotherapy (10 crs); 6. Optional Studies (10 crs); 7. Research Project (40 crs).

(D: 0; P: 1, 2, 4, 5)

Number of pharmacy or drug treatment–related courses: 4 out of 7 plus major part of clinical pharmacy.

Number of diagnosis-related courses: 0 out of 7 plus integral part of clinical pharmacy.

INFORMATION ABOUT THREE COURSES IS AS FOLLOWS:

Clinical Pharmacy: Includes the study of rational selection and the use and effects of drugs for individual patients and patient groups. You will be introduced to quantitative clinical data and the way it is used to optimize drug therapy. The course will involve clinical case discussions and visits to hospitals and medical practices to study the clinical role of pharmacists.

Chemotherapy and Molecular Biology: Examines the use of drugs as a chemotherapeutic agent in the treatment of infectious diseases and cancer. The course also introduces you to genetic engineering and its impact on the design and production of therapeutic agents and diagnosis of disease.

Pharmacology: The study of drug action on living organisms. The course examines the molecular basis of drug action, the pharmacology of groups of drugs, the way they work, and their effects on the human system (systemic pharmacology). You will also be introduced to immunology.[19]

TOTAL OF YEAR 1 TO 4

Number of pharmacy or drug treatment–related courses: 18 out of 25 courses.

Number of diagnosis-related courses: 4 out of 25 courses.

(D = 0.16 & P = 0.72)

CLINICAL PHARMACY

Clinical pharmacy is available as a postgraduate diploma course in the United Kingdom. The course consists of six modules, which are Introduction, Gastroenterology and Endocrinology, Cardiovascular, Respiratory and

Infections, Rheumatology and Disorders of the Central Nervous System, and Research Methodology. Students' assessments are based on complete assignment at work or placement in GP surgery, nursing or residential home, as well as examination. Tutors are predominantly practicing pharmacists who are either clinicians or clinical pharmacists or academic researchers or others. Students have the option of proceeding to obtain their MSc (masters) on a part-time basis with the addition of a year, provided they complete their research project.[19] No matter the degree/depth of pharmacists' drug knowledge, clinical experience/orientation, and therapeutic expertise, they cannot prescribe drugs for patients in the United Kingdom. Their drug knowledge and clinical experience might be greater than the recent medical school graduate's, yet they are limited by law not to display their talents openly for the benefit of patients. There is no doctor of pharmacy degree program in the United Kingdom.

COMMENTS

A telephone conversation with Dr. Allen Prince of clinical pharmacology (part of the medicine or medical school) at Oxford University, sometime in May 2001, confirmed the paucity of pharmacy courses in the medical school as noted above. He reiterated the availability of pharmacology—0.5 units in the first year, 4 units in the second year, and clinical pharmacy examination in the third year. There are no physician assistants or certified nurse practitioners in the United Kingdom.

DATA ANALYSIS

Using the above data, analysis of the course outline in Europe shows that it can be estimated that medical school graduates in Europe are exposed to an average number of 0.88 or 88% which is approximately 90% or 9 out of every 10, diagnosis-related courses in pre-clinical years (didactic class work) and 0.12 or 12% which is approximately 10% or 1 out of every 10, pharmacy or drug treatment–related courses in the pre-clinical years. As in other continents, the three pre-clinical years in Europe lay the foundation upon which the last three clinical years are based. The clinical rotations adhere to the course outline format of the pre-clinical years; consequently it can be estimated that diagnosis-related issues constitute about 70 to 90% of the rotations, which is a majority, and pharmacy or drug treatment–related issues constitute about 10 to 30% of the rotations, which is a minority or integral part of the program. The study limitations are the same as in Australia.

The dentistry school graduates, on the other hand, are estimated to be exposed to an average number of 1 or 100%, which is approximately 10 out of 10, diagnosis and dental-related courses and zero (0) out of every 10 courses in pharmacy or drug treatment during the three pre-clinical years. Pharmacy or drug treatment is a minute part of the major course work in dentistry. The veterinary medical doctors in the United Kingdom are exposed to an estimated average number of 79% or 80%, which is approximately 8 out of every 10, courses in diagnosis and 0.042 or 4.2% which is approximately 4% or 4 out of every 100 or 1 out of every 25, pharmacy or drug-treatment courses during the three pre-clinical years. The optometrists are estimated to be exposed to an average number of 0.72 or 72% which is approximately 70% or 7 out of every 10, courses in diagnosis and optometry and 0.056 or 5.6% which is approximately 6% or 1 out of every 17, courses in pharmacy or drug treatment during the three-year, full-time program. The pharmacists are estimated to be exposed to an average number of 0.16 or 16% which is approximately 20% or 2 out of every 10, courses in diagnosis and 72% or 72% which is approximately 70% and that is 7 out of every 10, courses in pharmacy or drug treatment during the four-year, full-time program.

In summary, 1 out of every 10 courses in pharmacy or drug treatment during the pre-clinical years and pharmacy or drug treatment as integral part of clinical rotations/internships qualifies a medical doctor to prescribe any drugs for the pharmacist to dispense in Europe. The same is true of the dentists, whose exposure to pharmacy or drug-treatment courses as a minute part of the major program (not even a whole number in any given year—0%) qualifies them to write any prescription for the pharmacists to dispense. The veterinary medical doctors' exposure to 1 out of every 25 courses in pharmacy or drug treatment in pre-clinical years and as an integral part of clinical rotations qualifies them to write any prescriptions for the pharmacists to dispense to the animals. The medical doctors, dentists, and veterinary medical doctors have clinical experience that differentiates them from optometrists in Europe. This clinical experience limits optometrists' ability to prescribe certain drugs in Europe. However, optometrists' exposure to 1 out of every 17 courses in pharmacy or drug treatment qualifies them to write some prescriptions for the pharmacists to dispense. The pharmacists' exposure to 7 out of every 10 courses in pharmacy or drug treatment does not qualify them to prescribe any drugs for any persons or animals in Europe. This is irrespective of the pharmacists' clinical experience, clinical practice, and number of postgraduate degrees in clinical pharmacy.

SOUTH AMERICA

South America is the fourth largest continent (7.035 million square miles) and Brazil, a Portuguese-speaking country, is the largest country on the continent, with 3.288 million square miles and a population of 150 million as of 1990. Medical education and practice in Brazil is Westernized and much of it has a lot in common with the United States and Europe. Brazil has about twenty-five universities and there are no physician assistants or certified nurse practitioners. There also is no doctor of pharmacy degree program; however, clinical analysis is available as an option for interested pharmacy students. Clinical analysis may one day in the future metamorphose into a clinical pharmacy or doctor of pharmacy degree program in Brazil. Admission into medical schools, schools of dentistry, veterinary medicine, pharmacy, and others is based on successful completion of high school with good results and few other criteria. Medical school training in Brazil is a six-year program that qualifies graduates for licensing exams before practicing medicine. Specialization or training in the various branches of medicine (specialties) is a postgraduate program offered in medical schools. Federal University of Rio de Janeiro (Universida De Federal Do Rio de Janeiro) is one of the universities that offer medical school training through a center of health sciences. The program consists of four and a half-year didactic class work, one-year rotation, and a half-year internship.[24]

FEDERAL UNIVERSITY OF RIO DE JANEIRO (UNIVERSIDA DE FEDERAL DO RIO DE JANEIRO) COURSE OUTLINE (2002)

YEAR 1
1ST PERIOD (27 CREDITS)

1. Anatomy (6 crs); 2. Basic Histology and Embryology (8crs); 3. Biophysics (6 crs); 4. Biochemistry (7 crs).

(D: 1, 3, 4; P: 0)

2ND PERIOD (24 CREDITS);

1. Respiratory and Cardiovascular Systems (11 crs); 2. Nervous System (11 crs); 3. Genetics and Evolution for Medicine (2 crs).

(D: 1, 2, 3; P: 0)

Number of pharmacy or drug treatment–related courses: zero (0) out of 7 or 51 credits.

Number of diagnosis-related courses: 6 out of 7 or 45 out of 51 credits.

YEAR 2
3ʳᴰ PERIOD (28 CREDITS)

1. Urinary System (6 crs); 2. Gastrointestinal System (6 crs); 3. Reproductive and Endocrine System (9 crs); 4. Health (7 crs).
(D: 1, 2, 3; P: 0)

4ᵀᴴ PERIOD (27 CREDITS)

1. Microbiology and Immunology (10 crs); 2. Parasitology (3 crs); 3. Clinical Propaedeutical (Prosthetics --- 7 crs); 4. General Pathology (7 crs).
(D: 1, 2, 4; P: 0)

Number of pharmacy or drug treatment–related courses: zero (0) out of 8 or 55 credits.

Number of diagnosis-related courses: 6 out of 8 or 41 out of 55 credits.

YEAR 3
5ᵀᴴ PERIOD (27 CREDITS)

1. Internal Medicine I (16 crs); 2. Pharmacology (5 crs); 3. Epidemiology (6 crs).
(D: 3; P: 2 D & P: 1)

6ᵀᴴ PERIOD (27 CREDITS)

1. Internal Medicine II (16 crs); 2. Pharmacology II (5 crs); 3. Labor and Health (3 crs); 4. Medical Psychology (3 crs).
(D: 4; P: 2 D & P: 1)

Number of pharmacy or drug treatment–related courses: 3 out of 7 or 26 out of 54 credits.

Number of diagnosis-related courses: 3 out of 7 or 25 out of 54 credits.

YEAR 4
7TH PERIOD (25 CREDITS)
1. Internal Medicine III (17 crs); 2. Clinical Pediatric (7 crs); 3. Forensic Pathology (1 cr).

(D: 3; P: 0; D & P: 1, 2)

8TH PERIOD (27 CREDITS)
1. Health and Administration (2 crs); 2. Surgery (11 crs); 3. Gynecology (5 crs); 4. Orthopedics and Traumatology (3 crs); 5. Ophthalmology (3 crs); 6. Otorhinolaryngology (3 crs).

(D: 2, 3, 4, 5, 6; P: 0)

Number of pharmacy or drug treatment–related courses: 1 out of 9 or 12 out of 52 credits.

Number of diagnosis-related courses: 7 out of 9 or 34 out of 52 credits.

YEAR 5
9TH PERIOD (26 CREDITS—HALF A YEAR)
1. Clinical Pediatric II (7 crs); 2. Mental Health and Psychiatry (5 crs); 3. Legal Medicine (2 crs); 4. Obstetrics (5 crs); 5. Infectious and Parasitology Diseases (7 crs).

(D: 2, 4, 5; P: 3; D & P: 1)

Number of pharmacy or drug treatment–related courses: 1.5 out of 5 or 5.5 out of 26 credits.

Number of diagnosis-related courses: 3.5 out of 5 or 20.5 out of 26 credits.

10TH PERIOD (65 CREDITS—ROTATIONS—HALF A YEAR)
1. Rotation A (Medical Clinic—13 crs); 2. Rotation B (Surgery—13 crs); 3. Rotation C (Pediatrics—13 crs); 4. Rotation D (Obstetrics/Gynecology—13 crs).

YEAR 6
11TH PERIOD (65 CREDITS—ROTATIONS—HALF A YEAR)
1. Rotation A (Medical Clinic—13 crs); 2. Rotation B (Surgery—13 crs); 3. Rotation C (Pediatrics—13 crs); 4. Rotation D (Obstetrics/Gynecology—13 crs).

Number of pharmacy or drug treatment–related courses: Constitutes an integral part of the rotations.

Number of diagnosis and dental-related courses: Constitutes a major part of the rotations.

12ᵀᴴ PERIOD (80 CREDITS)
1. Internship in Medical Clinic (20 crs); 2. Internship in Surgery (20 crs); 3. Internship in Pediatrics (20 crs); 4. Internship in Gynecology/Obstetrics (20 crs).

Number of pharmacy or drug treatment–related courses: Constitutes an integral part of the internship.

Number of diagnosis and dental-related courses: Constitutes major part of the internship.

TOTAL OF YEAR 2 TO 4½
Number of pharmacy or drug treatment–related courses: 5.5 out of 29 courses.

Number of diagnosis-related courses: 19.5 out of 29 courses.
(D = 0.67 & P = 0.19)

DENTISTRY

Dentistry is a four-year program after high school in Brazil. Federal University of Rio de Janerio is one of the universities that offer dentistry as ODONTOLOGY through the college of dental medicine.[24]

COURSE OUTLINE (2002)

YEAR 1
1ˢᵀ PERIOD (23 CREDITS)
1. Anatomy I (5 crs); 2. Histology I (5 crs); 3. Embryology I (1 crs); 4. Biochemistry I (4 crs); 5. Sociology and Anthropology (2 crs); 6. Genetics

Evolution Odontology (2 crs); 7. Psychology I (3 crs); 8. Community Dentistry Odontology (1 crs).

(DD: 1, 2, 3, 4, 6, 8; P: 0)

2ND PERIOD (21 CREDITS)

1. Anatomy II (5 crs); 2. Physiology (6 crs); 3. Histology II (4 crs); 4. Embryology II (1 cr); 5. Social Odontology (3 crs); 6. Morphology and Dental Restoration (2 crs).

(DD: 1, 2, 3, 4, 5, 6; P: 0)

Number of pharmacy or drug treatment–related courses: zero (0) out of 14 or 44 credits.

Number of diagnosis and dental-related courses: 12 out of 14 or 38 out of 44 credits.

YEAR 2
3RD PERIOD (26 CREDITS)

1. Pharmacology (3 crs); 2. Parasitology (2 crs); 3. General Pathology Process (2 crs); 4. Microbiology and Immunology (9crs); 5. Restorative Dental Laboratory I (5 crs); 6. Dental Material (4 crs); 7. Primary Attention to Odontology (1 cr).

(DD: 2, 3, 4, 5, 6, 7; P: 1)

4TH PERIOD (19 CREDITS)

1. Periodontology Laboratory I (2 crs); 2. Restorative Dental Laboratory II (2 crs); 3. Oral Surgery I (2 crs); 4. Oral Radiology I (3 crs); 5. Oral Diagnostics I (1 cr); 6. Oral Pathology I (3 crs); 7. Prosthetics Laboratory I (Removable—4 crs); 8. Enamel (2 crs).

(DD: 1, 2, 3, 4, 5, 6, 7, 8; P: 0)

Number of pharmacy or drug treatment–related courses: 1 out of 15 or 3 out of 45 credits.

Number of diagnosis and dental-related courses: 14 out of 15 or 42 out of 45 credits.

YEAR 3
5TH PERIOD (18 CREDITS)
1. Endodontics I (4 crs); 2. Restorative Dental III (Clinic—2 crs); 3. Therapeutic Periodontology II (2 crs); 4. Oral Surgery II (2 crs); 5. Oral Pathology II (3 crs); 6. Odontological Deontology (1 cr); 7. Prosthetics II (Removable—4 crs).

(DD: 1, 2, 4, 5, 6, 7; P: 3)

6TH PERIOD (17 CREDITS)
1. Therapeutic Endodontics II (2 crs); 2. Restorative Dental IV (Clinic—2 crs); 3. Oral and Maxillofacial Surgery (1 crs); 4. Orthodontics (5 crs); 5. Oral Diagnostics II (2 crs); 6. Preventive Odontology (3 crs); 7. Fixed Prosthetics I (17 crs).

(DD: 2, 3, 4, 5, 6, 7; P: 1)

Number of pharmacy or drug treatment–related courses: 2 out of 14 or 4 out of 35 credits.

Number of diagnosis and dental-related courses: 12 out of 14 or 31 out of 35 credits.

YEAR 4
7TH PERIOD (12 CREDITS)
1. Odontological Clinic I (5 crs); 2. Pediatric Dentistry I (3 crs); 3. Fixed Prosthetics II (4 crs).

(DD: 1, 2, 3; P: 0)

8TH PERIOD (13 CREDITS)
1. Conditional Choice of Compensation (2 crs); 2. Clinic Integrated Odontology II (5 crs); 3. Legal Odontology (2 crs); 4. Professional Orientation in Odontology (2 crs); 5. Supervised Training in Odontology (2 crs).

Number of pharmacy or drug treatment–related courses: zero (0) out of 8 or 25 credits.

Number of diagnosis and dental-related courses: 6 out of 8 or 21 out of 25 credits.

COMPLIMENTARY EDUCATION (CONDITIONAL)

1. Periodontology III (2 crs); 2. Pediatric Dentistry II (4 crs); 3. Informatics in Dentistry (2 crs); 4. Restorative Dentistry (Crown and Bridge—2 crs); 5. Restorative Dentistry.

Number of pharmacy or drug treatment–related courses: zero (0) out of 5 or 12 credits.

Number of diagnosis and dental-related courses: 5 out of 5 or 12 out of 12 credits.

TOTAL OF YEAR 2 TO 4

Number of pharmacy or drug treatment–related courses: 3 out of 37 courses.
Number of diagnosis and dental-related courses: 32 out of 37 courses.
(DD = 0.86 & P = 0.081)

VETERINARY MEDICINE

Veterinary medicine is a five-year program after high school in Brazil.

COURSE OUTLINE

YEAR 1
1ST PERIOD

1. General Ecology; 2. Computer Science; 3. Fundamental Mathematics; 4. Introduction to the College Studies; 5. General Chemistry; 6. Organic Chemistry; 7. Cytology, Histology, and General Embryology; 8. Veterinary Anatomy I.
(D: 7, 8; P: 0)

2ND PERIOD

1. Statistics; 2. Sporting Practice I; 3. Analytical Chemistry; 4. Biochemistry; 5. Veterinary Anatomy II; 6. Veterinary Histology.
(D: 4, 5, 6; P: 0)

Number of pharmacy or drug treatment–related courses: zero (0) out of 14.

Number of diagnosis-related courses: 5 out of 14.

YEAR 2
1ST PERIOD

1. Experimental Biostatistics; 2. Scientific Initiation; 3. Sporting Practice II; 4. Veterinary Physiology I; 5. Immunology; 6. Veterinary Parasitology; 7. Metabolism.

(D: 4, 5, 6, 7; P: 0)

2ND PERIOD

1. General Microbiology; 2. Genetic; 3. Veterinary Physiology II; 4. Veterinarian Pharmacology I; 5. Veterinary General Pathology; 6. Introduction to Zoo Technique.

(D: 1, 2, 3, 5; P: 4)

Number of pharmacy or drug treatment–related courses: 1 out of 13.

Number of diagnosis-related courses: 8 out of 13.

YEAR 3
1ST PERIOD

1. Rural Sociology; 2. Veterinarian Pharmacology II; 3. Veterinarian Microbiology; 4. Special Veterinarian Pathology; 5. Veterinary Epidemiology; 6. Sanitation.

(D: 3, 4, 5; P: 2)

2ND PERIOD

1. Rural Economy; 2 Semiologia; 3. Disease I; 4. Veterinarian Clinical Pathology; 5. Radio Diagnostic; 6. Food and Alimentation.

(D: 2, 3, 4; P: 0)

Number of pharmacy or drug treatment–related courses: 1 out of 12.

Number of diagnosis-related courses: 6 out of 12.

YEAR 4
1ST PERIOD
1. Rural Administration; 2. Veterinary Medical Clinic I; 3. Anesthesiology and Surgical Techniques; 4. Disease II; 5. Reproduction Physiology, Semen Technology; 6. Bovine Culture.
$$(D: 4, 5; P: 3\ D\ \&\ P: 2)$$

2ND PERIOD
1. Milk Techniques and Lactose Products Inspection; 2. Meat and Fishery Technology; 3. Veterinarian Medical Clinic II; 4. Veterinary Surgery I; 5. Disease III; 6. Production, Reproduction, and Artificial Insemination; 7. Swine and Aviculture
$$(D: 4; P: 0\ D\ \&\ P: 3)$$
Number of pharmacy or drug treatment–related courses: 2 out of 13.

Number of diagnosis-related courses: 4 out of 13.

YEAR 5
1ST PERIOD
1. Milk and Lactose Products Inspection; 2. Meat, Fishery, Eggs, and Honey Inspection; 3. Rural Extension; 4. Veterinarian Surgery II; 5. Veterinarian Obstetrical; 6. Deontology and Legal Veterinarian Medicine; 7. Veterinarian Toxicology; 8. Veterinarian Medical Clinic III.
$$(D: 4, 5; P: 7\ D\ \&\ P: 8)$$

2ND PERIOD
1. Supervised Training.

Number of pharmacy or drug treatment–related courses: 1.5 out of 8 plus integral part of supervised training.

Number of diagnosis-related courses: 2.5 out of 8 plus major part of supervised training.

TOTAL OF YEAR 2 TO 5
Number of pharmacy or drug treatment–related courses: 5.5 out of 46 courses.

Number of diagnosis-related courses: 20.5 out of 46 courses.
$$(D = 0.45\ \&\ P = 0.12)$$

PHARMACY

Pharmacy is a four-year program; however, a pharmacy program with the option of clinical analysis is a four and a half-year program. Federal University of Rio de Janeiro offers both programs.

COURSE OUTLINE

YEAR 1
1ST PERIOD (19 CREDITS)
1. Anatomy (2 crs); 2. Histology (2 crs); 3. Embryology (2 crs); 4. Physics for Biological Sciences (4 crs); 5. General Chemistry I (4 crs); 6. Pharmacy Calculations (5 crs).
(D: 1, 2, 3; P: 6)

2ND PERIOD (14 CRS)
1. Analytical Chemistry (4 crs); 2. General Chemistry II (3 crs); 3. Experimental General Chemistry II (2 crs); 4. Organic Chemistry I (3 crs); 5. Experimental Organic Chemistry I (2 crs).
(D: 0; P: 0)

Number of pharmacy or drug treatment–related courses: 1 out of 11 or 5 out of 33 credits.

Number of diagnosis-related courses: 3 out of 11 or 6 out of 33 credits.

YEAR 2
3RD PERIOD (22 CREDITS)
1. Analytical Chemistry IIA (4 crs); 2. Physical Chemistry I (4 crs); 3. Inorganic Chemistry (4 crs); 4. Organic Chemistry II (3 crs); 5. Expérimental Organic Chemistry II (3 crs); 6. Statistics (4 crs).
(D: 0; P: 0)

4TH PERIOD (18 CREDITS)
1. Biochemistry I (6 crs); 2. Organic Chemistry Druggist I (2 crs); 3. Botany Applied to Pharmacy (4 crs); 4. Physical Chemistry II (3 crs); 5. Organic Analysis I (3 crs).

(D: 1; P: 2, 3)
Number of pharmacy or drug treatment–related courses: 2 out of 11 or 6 out of 40 credits.

Number of diagnosis-related courses: 1 out of 11 or 6 out of 40 credits.

YEAR 3
5TH PERIOD (30 CREDITS)
1. Physiology I—Pharmacy (6 crs); 2. Parasitology (4 crs); 3. Biochemistry II (6 crs); 4. Organic Chemistry Druggist II (2 crs); 5. General Process of Pathology (1 cr); 6. Genetics (2 crs); 7. Microbiology and Immunology (9 crs).
(D: 1, 2, 3, 5, 6, 7; P: 4)

6TH PERIOD
1. Pharmacology I (4 crs); 2. Pharmacology Technique I (4 crs); 3. Pharmacognosy I (3 crs); 4. Economy and Business Administration of Pharmacy (4 crs); 5. Organic Analysis II (2 crs).
(D: 0; P: 1, 2, 3)

Number of pharmacy or drug treatment–related courses: 4 out of 12 or 13 out of 47 credits.
Number of diagnosis-related courses: 6 out of 12 or 28 out of 47 credits.

YEAR 4
7TH PERIOD (28 CREDITS)
1. Physiology II—Pharmacy (2 crs); 2. Pharmacology II (3 crs); 3. Druggists' Biochemistry (6 crs); 4. Social Hygiene (2 crs); 5. Supervised Training in Pharmacy (2 crs); 6. Druggist Disease and Legislation (1 crs); 7. Pharmaceutical Chemistry (3 crs); 8. Pharmacology Technique II (4 crs); 9. Pharmacognosy II (3 crs); 10, Bromatological Chemistry (Nutritional Pharmacy—2 crs).
(D: 1, 3; P: 2, 5, 7, 8, 9, 10)

8TH PERIOD (8CRS)
1. Clinical Microbiology (4 crs); 2. Clinical Immunology (4 crs).

Number of pharmacy or drug treatment–related courses: 6 out of 10 or 17 out of 36 credits plus major part of clinical rotation.

Number of diagnosis-related courses: 2 out of 10 or 9 out of 36 credits plus an integral part of clinical rotation.

TOTAL OF YEAR 2 TO 3½
Number of pharmacy or drug treatment–related courses: 12 out of 33 or 34 out of 123 credits.
Number of diagnosis-related courses: 9 out of 33 or 43 out of 123 credits.
(D = 0.27 & P = 0.364)

PHARMACY

Pharmacy is a four-year program; however, the pharmacy program with the option of clinical analysis is a four and-a-half-year program. Federal University of Rio de Janeiro offers both programs.

COURSE OUTLINE

YEAR 1
1ST PERIOD (19 CREDITS)
1. Anatomy (2 crs); 2. Histology (2 crs); 3. Embryology (2 crs); 4. Physics for Biological Sciences (4 crs); 5. General Chemistry I (4 crs); 6. Pharmacy Calculations (5 crs).
(D: 1, 2, 3; P: 6)

2ND PERIOD (14 CRS)
1. Analytical Chemistry (4 crs); 2. General Chemistry II (3 crs); 3. Experimental General Chemistry II (2 crs); 4. Organic Chemistry I (3 crs); 5. Experimental Organic Chemistry I (2 crs).
(D: 0; P: 0)
Number of pharmacy or drug treatment–related courses: 1 out of 11 or 5 out of 33 credits.

Number of diagnosis-related courses: 3 out of 11 or 6 out of 33 credits.

YEAR 2
3ʀᴅ PERIOD (22 CREDITS)

1. Analytical Chemistry IIA (4 crs); 2. Physical Chemistry I (4 crs); 3. Inorganic Chemistry (4 crs); 4. Organic Chemistry II (3 crs); 5. Experimental Organic Chemistry II (3 crs); 6. Statistics (4 crs).

(D: 0; P: 0)

4ᴛʜ PERIOD (18 CREDITS)

1. Biochemistry I (6 crs); 2. Organic Chemistry Druggist I (2 crs); 3. Botany Applied to Pharmacy (4 crs); 4. Physical Chemistry II (3 crs); 5. Organic Analysis I (3 crs).

(D: 1; P: 2, 3)

Number of pharmacy or drug treatment–related courses: 2 out of 11 or 6 out of 40 credits.

Number of diagnosis-related courses: 1 out of 11 or 6 out of 40 credits.

YEAR 3
5ᴛʜ PERIOD (30 CREDITS)

1. Physiology I—Pharmacy (6 crs); 2. Parasitology (4 crs); 3. Biochemistry II (6 crs); 4. Organic Chemistry Druggist II (2 crs); 5. General Process of Pathology (1 cr); 6. Genetics (2 crs); 7. Microbiology and Immunology (9 crs).

(D: 1, 2, 3, 5, 6, 7; P: 4)

6ᴛʜ PERIOD

1. Pharmacology I (4 crs); 2. Pharmacology Technic I (4 crs); 3. Pharmacognosy I (3 crs); 4. Economy and Business Administration of Pharmacy (4 crs); 5. Organic Analysis II (2 crs).

(D: 0; P: 1, 2, 3)

Number of pharmacy or drug treatment–related courses: 4 out of 12 or 13 out of 47 credits.

Number of diagnosis-related courses: 6 out of 12 or 28 out of 47 credits.

YEAR 4
|7ᵀᴴ PERIOD (28 CREDITS)
1. Physiology II—pharmacy (2 crs); 2. Pharmacology II (3 crs); 3. Druggists Biochemistry (6 crs); 4. Social Hygiene (2 crs); 5. Supervised Training in Pharmacy (2 crs); 6. Druggist Disease and Legislation (1 crs); 7. Pharmaceutical Chemistry (3 crs); 8. Pharmacology Technique II (4 crs); 9. Pharmacognosyn II (3 crs); 10. Bromatological Chemistry (Nutritional Pharmacy—2 crs).
(D: 1, 3; P: 2, 5, 7, 8, 9, 10)

8ᵀᴴ PERIOD (8 CRS)
1. Clinical Microbiology (4 crs); 2. Clinical Immunology (4 crs).

Number of pharmacy or drug treatment–related courses: 6 out of 10 or 17 out of 36 credits plus major part of clinical rotation.

Number of diagnosis courses: 2 out of 10 or 9 out of 36 credits plus an integral part of clinical rotation.

TOTAL OF YEAR 2 TO 3½
Number of pharmacy or drug treatment–related courses: 12 out of 33 or 34 out of 123 credits.

Number of diagnosis-related courses: 9 out of 33 or 43 out of 123 credits.
(D = 0.27 and P = 0.364)

PHARMACY
(WITH CLINICAL ANALYSIS OPTION—4½-YEAR PROGRAM)
SAME CURRICULUM TILL 7TH PERIOD
8TH PERIOD (16 CREDITS)
1. Clinical Biochemistry (4 crs); 2. Clinical Cytopathology (4 crs); 3. Clinical Microbiology (4 crs); 4. Clinical Immunology (4 crs).

9ᵀᴴ PERIOD (15 CRS)
1. Supervised Training in Clinical Analysis (4 crs); 2. Clinical Parasitology (4 crs); 3. Hematology (4 crs); 4. Toxicology I (3 crs).

Number of pharmacy or drug treatment–related courses: Constitutes major part of clinical rotations.

Number of diagnosis courses: Constitutes an integral part of clinical rotations.

DATA ANALYSIS

Using the above course outline in Brazil, data analysis showed that medical doctors in South America are exposed to an average number of 0.67 or 67% which is approximately 70% or 7 out of every 10, courses that are diagnosis-related courses in their pre-clinical years (didactic class work) and 0.19 or 19% which is approximately 20% or 2 out of every 10, pharmacy or drug treatment–related courses in pre-clinical years. The three and half (3.5) pre-clinical years lay the foundation for the last one and half clinical years. The course outline format of the pre-clinical years culminates in the clinical years; hence, it can be estimated that diagnosis-related courses constitutes about 70 to 80% of rotations (majority) and pharmacy or drug treatment–related courses constitute about 20 to 30 % (integral part) of rotations. The study limitation is same as in Australia.

Dentists, on the other hand, are estimated to be exposed to an average number of 0.86% or 86% which is approximately 90% or 9 out of every 10, diagnosis and dental-related courses and 0.081 or 8.1% which is approximately 8% and that is about 1 out of every 13, pharmacy or drug treatment–related courses during the three years course work. The veterinary medical doctors are exposed to an average number of 0.45 or 45% which is approximately 50% and that is 5 out of every 10, courses that are diagnosis related and 0.12 or 12% which is approximately 10% and that is 1 out of every 10, pharmacy or drug treatment–related courses.

The pharmacy program in Brazil, South America, appears to be a little different from the rest of the world. Chemistry courses play a major role in the pharmacy program in Brazil, while in other parts of the world these courses are left to the chemistry major program (chemists). However, based on data analysis it can be estimated that pharmacists in Brazil, South America, are exposed to an average number of 0.27 or 27% which is approximately 30% and that is 3 out of every 10, courses that are diagnosis related and 0.364 or 36.4% which is approximately 40% or 4 out of every 10, pharmacy or drug treatment–related courses during the two and half (2.5) pre-clinical years. The two and half (2.5) pre-clinical years lay the foundation for clinical experience (clinical years) in the last half year for pharmacy major and one year for a pharmacy major with a clinical-analysis option. The course out line format of the pre-clinical years predominates during the clinical years; hence, it can be estimated that diagnosis-related courses constitute about 30 to 40% of rotations (integral part) and pharmacy or drug treatment–related courses constitute about 40 to 50 % of rotations.

In summary, 2 out of every 10 courses in pharmacy or drug treatment during the pre-clinical years and pharmacy or drug treatment as an integral part of clinical rotations/internship, qualifies a medical doctor to prescribe any drugs for the pharmacist to dispense in South America. The same is true of the dentists, whose exposure to 1 out of every 13 courses in pharmacy or drug treatment during the three-year full-time program (no internship) qualifies them to write any prescription for the pharmacists to dispense. Veterinary medical doctors' exposure to 1 out of every 10 courses in pharmacy or drug treatment during the four-year full-time program (no internship) qualifies them to write any prescription for pharmacists to dispense to animals. The pharmacists' exposure to 4 out of every 10 courses in pharmacy or drug treatment during the pre-clinical years and pharmacy or drug treatment as a major part of half-year clinical rotations (1 year for pharmacists with clinical option) does not qualify pharmacists or pharmacists with the clinical option to prescribe any drugs for any person or animal in South America. The first year in all schools' programs with high school entry requirements is not considered part of the core courses or pre-clinical years.

SUMMARY

In conclusion, a comparative analysis of the statistics of the six habitable continents—Africa, Asia, Australia, Europe, North America, and South America—showed close similarity in terms of medical school and other branches of medicine curriculum/course outline. For example:

In Africa: medical doctors are exposed to approximately 78% (or 80%) diagnosis-related courses and 11% (or 10%) pharmacy or drug treatment–related courses in pre-clinical years. Dentists are exposed to approximately 90% diagnosis and dental-related courses and 4% pharmacy or drug treatment–related courses. Pharmacists are exposed to approximately 16% (or 20%) diagnosis-related courses and 68% (or 70%) pharmacy or drug treatment–related courses.

In Asia: medical doctors are exposed to approximately 79% (or 80%) diagnosis-related courses and 21% (or 20%) pharmacy or drug treatment–related courses in pre-clinical years. The dentists are exposed to approximately 88% (or 90%) diagnosis and dental-related courses and 11% (or 10%) pharmacy or drug treatment–related courses. The veterinary medical doctors are exposed to approximately 64% (or 60%) diagnosis-related courses and 9.1% (or 9%) pharmacy or drug treatment–related courses. The pharmacists are exposed to approximately 21% (or 20%) diagnosis-related courses and 69% (or 70%) pharmacy or drug treatment–related courses.

In Australia: the medical doctors and dentists are exposed to approximately 70% diagnosis-related courses and 28% (or 30%) pharmacy or drug treatment–related courses. In comparison to others, Australian medical and dentistry graduates appear to be exposed to more pharmacy or drug treatment–related courses even though it is not up to half of diagnosis-related courses. These pharmacy or drug treatment–related courses therefore fit into the category of minority or integrated part of the total program/courses. Australian medical training appears to be shorter in duration than others. The veterinary medical doctors are exposed to 60% diagnosis-related courses and 8.6% (or 9%) pharmacy or drug treatment–related courses. The optometrists are exposed to approximately 85% (or 90%) diagnosis and optical related courses and 12% (or 10%) pharmacy or drug treatment–related courses. The pharmacists are exposed to 16% (or 20%) diagnosis-related courses and 65% (or 70%) pharmacy or drug treatment–related courses.

In Europe: medical doctors are exposed to approximately 88% (or 90%) diagnosis-related courses and 12% (or 10%) pharmacy or drug treatment–related courses in pre-clinical years. The dentists are exposed to approximately 100% diagnosis and dental-related courses and no pharmacy or drug treatment–related courses (but these constitute an integral part of few courses and rotations/residency). The optometrists are exposed to approximately 72% (or 70%) diagnosis and optical-related courses and 5.6% (or 6%) pharmacy or drug-treatment courses. The veterinary medical doctors are exposed to approximately 60% diagnosis-related courses and 8.6% (or 9%) pharmacy or drug treatment–related courses. The pharmacists are exposed to approximately 16% (or 20%) diagnosis-related courses and 72% (or 70%) pharmacy or drug treatment–related courses.

In North America: medical doctors are exposed to approximately 79.8% (or 80%) diagnosis-related courses and 6.3% (or 6%) pharmacy or drug treatment–related courses in pre-clinical years. The dentists are exposed to approximately 93% (or 90%) diagnosis and dental-related courses and 2.8% (or 3%) pharmacy or drug treatment–related courses. The optometrists are exposed to approximately 83% (or 80%) diagnosis and optical-related courses and 5.8% (or 6%) pharmacy or drug-treatment courses. The veterinary medical doctors are exposed to approximately 82% (or 80%) diagnosis-related courses and 8.7% (or 9%) pharmacy or drug treatment–related courses. The physician assistants are exposed to approximately 76% (or 80%) diagnosis-related courses and 7.1 (or 7%) in pharmacy or drug treatment–related courses in just one year. The certified nurse practitioners are exposed to approximately 67% (or 70%) diagnosis and nursing related courses and 4% in pharmacy or drug treatment–related courses. The clinical pharmacists are exposed to approximately 16% (or 20%) diagnosis-related courses and 74% (or 70%) pharmacy or drug treatment–related courses.

In South America: medical doctors are exposed to approximately 67% (or 70%) diagnosis-related courses and 19% (or 20%) pharmacy or drug treatment–related courses in pre-clinical years. The dentists are exposed to approximately 86 (or 90%) diagnosis and dental-related courses and 8.1% (or 8%) pharmacy or drug treatment–related courses. The veterinary medical doctors are exposed to approximately 45% (or 50%) diagnosis-related courses and 12% (or 10%) pharmacy or drug treatment–related courses. The pharmacists are exposed to approximately 27% (or 30%) diagnosis-related courses and 36.4% (or 40%) pharmacy or drug treatment–related courses. The pharmacists in Brazil, South America, are probably exposed to more diagnosis-related courses and less pharmacy or drug treatment–related courses (much of the pharmacy or drug treatment–related courses are dominated by chemistry, which is left to chemists/chemistry major students in other places) than any other place in the world.

In all cases, the clinical years' curriculum and course composition is not different from pre-clinical years experienced because the pre-clinical years set the pace for academic rigor and the building blocks for subsequent training. In a nutshell, whatever percentage any given course has in pre-clinical years is the same or almost the same as in the clinical, internship, and residency years. There are no physician assistants and certified nurse practitioners in other parts of the world except the United States. Clinical pharmacists operate in the United States, some parts of Europe (e.g., the United Kingdom), and Australia and plans are in the advanced stage for the production of clinical pharmacists in Africa. Clinical pharmacy program started in the U.S. but the implementation in the UK and Australia is far less advanced than in the U.S. On the whole it can be summarized that medical doctors' exposure to pharmacy or drug-treatment courses ranges from a minimum of 6% (i.e., 1 out of every 17 courses) in the U.S. to a maximum of 30% (i.e., 3 out of every 10 courses) in Australia, qualifies medical doctors to write prescription drugs for the pharmacists to dispense anywhere in the world; dentists' exposure to pharmacy or drug-treatment courses ranges from a minimum of 0% (i.e., zero) in UK to a maximum of 30% (i.e., 3 out of every 10 courses) in Australia, qualifies dentists to write prescription drugs for the pharmacists to dispense anywhere in the world; optometrists' exposure to pharmacy or drug-treatment courses ranges from a minimum of 6% (i.e., 1 out of every 17 courses) in the UK and the U.S. to a maximum of 10% (i.e., 1 out of every 10 courses) in Australia, qualifies optometrists to write prescriptions for drugs to some extent for the pharmacists to dispense in various part of the world; veterinary medical doctors' exposure to pharmacy or drug-treatment courses ranges from a minimum of 4% (i.e., 1 out of every 25 courses) in the UK to a maximum of 10% (i.e., 1 out of every 10 courses) in Brazil, qualifies veterinary medical doctors to write prescriptions for drugs for the pharmacists to dispense to animals anywhere in the world; physician assistants' exposure to 7% (i.e., 1 out of every 14 courses) pharmacy or drug-treatment courses in one year qualifies them to write a lot of prescriptions for drugs for the pharmacists to dispense in U.S. only; certified nurse practitioners' exposure to 4% (i.e., 1 out of every 25 courses) pharmacy or drug-treatment courses qualifies them to write a lot of prescriptions for drugs for the pharmacists to dispense in the U.S. only; pharmacists' exposure to pharmacy or drug-treatment courses ranges from a minimum of 40% (i.e., 4 out of every 10 courses) in Brazil, to a maximum of 70% (i.e., 7 out of every 10 courses) in Nigeria, India, Australia, the UK, and the U.S. (five continents) but does not qualify pharmacists to write prescriptions for drugs for any person or animal in most parts of the world. In sharp contrast, the majority of the courses in medical schools and other branches of medicine as seen above were diagnosis- (and allied programs such as dental-) related courses.

REFERENCES

1. Obafemi Awolowo University, Ile-Ife Nigeria. *Faculty of Health Sciences Handbook 1988-90.*

2. Obafemi Awolowo University, Ile- Ife Nigeria. *Faculty of Pharmacy Handbook 1987-90.*

3. University of Benin, Benin City, Nigeria. *Faculty of Pharmacy Undergraduate Handbook.*

4. Beijing University of Chinese Medicine. *Guide for Admission of Overseas Students, International School.*

5. University of Sydney. *Studying at Sydney University, Undergraduate Courses—2003.*

6. University of Sydney. *2000 Faculty of Medicine.* Last updated April 27, 2002. Accessed July 30, 2002.

7. University of Sydney. *Medicine 2001, Graduate Programs* (brochure).

8. University of Sydney. *Dentistry 2003* (brochure).

9. University of Sydney. *Veterinary Science 2003* (brochure). Accessed October 20, 2002.

10. University of Melbourne. Information about the bachelor of optometry. Accessed October 18, 2002.

11. University of Sydney. Faculty of pharmacy handout. September 2002.

12. University of Sydney. *Pharmacy Graduate Program Handbook* or Master of Pharmacy (Clinical), Graduate Diploma and Graduate Certificate in Clinical Pharmacy (General Information Handout). September 2002.

13. University of Auckland. *Faculty of Medical and Health Sciences, 2002 Undergraduate Prospectus.*

14. Oxford University. Medical sciences information handouts, March 2001. Accessed November 2002.

15. University of Cambridge. *Clinical School Prospectus 2000.*

16. King's College, London. University of London undergraduate programme profile, Dentistry BDS. Accessed November 2002.

17. University of Liverpool. Faculty of Veterinary Science. Accessed November 2002.

18. University of Bradford. Optometry. Accessed November 2002.

19. Aston University, Birmingham. *Pharmacy Undergraduate Degree Programme, Prospectus 2000,* plus information at. Accessed May 2001.

20. Akita University, School of Medicine. Information for international students. Accessed November 2002.

21. Kagoshima University Dental School. Accessed December 2002

22. University of Tokyo. Department of Veterinary Medical Sciences. Accessed December 2002.

23. Okayama University. Faculty of Pharmaceutical Sciences. Accessed November 2002.

24. Federal University of Rio de Janeiro. *Faculty of Medicine Catalog 1997,* plus information at. Accessed September 2002.

25. Manipal Academy of Higher Education. *Manipal International Admissions 2002 Catalogue, plus at. Accessed December 2002.*

CHAPTER SEVEN

DRUG SPECIALISTS/EXPERTS AND THE MEDICAL FIELD

Humanity has strong views about phrases like "practice makes perfect" or "producer knows the ins and outs of their products." Daily duty/job entails daily practice, which enhances human skill and perfection in any art. Thus, everybody expects
* whoever produces, keeps, and maintains the airplanes to know the ins and outs, manner of operation, usage, and repair of the airplanes
* whoever produces, keeps, and maintains the space shuttle/rockets to know the ins and outs, manner of operation, usage, and repair of the shuttle/rockets;
* whoever produces, keeps, and maintains the cars/buses/trains, etc., to know the ins and outs, manner of operation, usage, and repair of them;
* whoever produces, keeps, and maintains the bombs/missiles/nuclear reactors, etc., to know the ins and outs, manner of operation, usage, and repair of them;
* whoever produces, keeps, and maintains the computers to know the ins and outs, manner of operation, usage, and repair of the computers;
* and many other phenomena/endeavors.

These people are considered experts/specialists in their respective fields/endeavors and their opinions are frequently sought first and repeatedly whenever things go wrong or information is needed in these areas. Specialists have taken over all spheres of human endeavor to the point that it is now difficult to imagine the existence of the world without specialization. As noted earlier, medicine was practiced as a holistic entity at the beginning during the Stone Age. By the fifth century before the birth of Jesus Christ, medicine went through series of reformation under the leadership of Hippocrates (c. 460-377 BC). At the tail end of the ninth century AD, medicine went through another unrecognized transformation in that Dr. Rhaze introduced the concept of specialty to medicine by creating pharmacy in Baghdad. Today, specialization is the norm of the society and by the special grace of Flexner we have discovered that humanity is capable of achieving tremendous success and miracles of biblical proportions with the aid of specialists. Rhaze created pharmacy because he felt the medical field needed specialists to compound/prepare, dispense, and advise patients about the use of drugs.[1,2]

Webster's Dictionary defines pharmacy as "the art or profession of preparing and dispensing medicinal drugs."[1,3] The president of the Florida Pharmacy Association in 2002-2003, Thomas Cuomo, found an extended meaning of pharmacy in another dictionary, and it states, "The branch of the Health Sciences dealing with the preparation, dispensing, and the PROPER UTILIZATION OF MEDICATIONS."[4] President Cuomo claims that the capitalized four words caught his attention because that is what all pharmacists go to school to learn. He then wondered why it is so difficult to convince the world about the profession and the skills the professionals learned through years of school training.[5]

By virtue of the definition of pharmacy and in whatever form we accept pharmacy as a profession, it entails the preparation, dispensing, and proper utilization of drugs. Like in the above scenarios, a pharmacist produces, keeps, and maintains drugs, and since he has acquired the much-needed knowledge about drugs in school training one would expect him to have greater knowledge of drugs (the ins and outs), manner of operation of drugs (mechanism of action), and usage of drugs to repair the body (treatment or therapeutic outcome) than other healthcare practitioners. At the beginning, pharmacy was preoccupied with the preparation and dispensing of drugs. This trend continued till the late nineteenth century when manufacturing industries/companies took over preparation of drugs (manufacturing) from the pharmacy. With the advent of clinical pharmacy in the 1930s and its propagation in 1960s, the profession began to switch gears by minimizing preparation and dispensing of drugs, thereby concentrating on greater acquisition of knowledge about the proper utilization of drugs. By and large, everything about the pharmacy profession centered on drugs, and everybody seems to acknowledge this.

In a drug manufacturers' survey, company executives acknowledge pharmacists as drug experts and the most knowledgeable professionals about drugs. The major question asked by the survey conducted by drug topics was "Which health professional has the most knowledge about your company's drug?" The executives responded by saying pharmacists (51%), physicians (39%), nurses (4%), and others (6%).[6] Abbot Laboratories in its congratulatory message to pharmacists for being the most trusted professionals according to

1992 Gallup poll, acknowledged the fact that pharmacists are medication experts. The study by Yoh et al. of Health professionals' knowledge about herbal products in terms of indications, interactions, and adverse effects placed pharmacists (78%) ahead of physicians (50%).[7] Consumer Healthcare Products Association's survey of 1,505 Americans (adults) revealed that 84% of the population agreed (50% - strongly and 34% - somewhat) that pharmacists are a good source of health information.[8] As noted earlier, a comparative study by Stimmel et al. evaluated three clinical pharmacists' and two physicians' prescriptions for inpatients in a forty-bed mental health facility in California and found that the clinical pharmacists' prescriptions in three classes of drug—neuroleptic, anticholinergic, and antidepressants—were better than the physicians' prescriptions in an overall combined six scales ($P < 0.001$).[9] A study by Thompson et al. compared the outcome of a trial with clinical pharmacists' prescribing drugs for experimental-group patients in a geriatric setting with an internist prescribing drugs for control group patients in a private-practice setting and found that the pharmacists' experimental group had significantly fewer deaths, fewer drugs, fewer hospitalization rates ($P = 0.06$), more discharges, and a savings of \$7,000 per patient more than the internist's control group. Travis Watts, a clinical pharmacist, established a community cardiovascular risk-reduction clinic and anticoagulation management service in Little Axe, Oklahoma, and succeeded in reducing heart disease and strokes, a number-one killer among the natives in this American Indian community. The clinic results revealed that 94% of the anticoagulation patients reached their goal and those on warfarin were 70% of the time within therapeutic range compared to 40% with physicians before the commencement of the clinic.

As stated in earlier chapters, numerous studies have shown the impact of clinical pharmacists on the nation's healthcare system and how they use their drug expertise to improve patients' lives/prognoses, reduce healthcare costs, and minimize morbidity and mortality resulting from adverse drug reactions. Some of these studies include Bootman a et al. study that revealed a net annual savings of about 3.6 billion dollars because of the presence of consultant pharmacists in nursing facilities across the country (U.S.)[11]; the Pathak and Nold study that revealed a biannual cost savings of \$833,723 because of clinical pharmacists' services[12]; a study by Poretz et al. that revealed a cost savings of \$432,816 for 150 patients because of pharmacists' involvement in outpatients' intravenous antibiotic therapy setting/management[13]; a study by Self et al. that projected a total cost savings of \$3 million and \$43 million in patient charges if all hospitals involved clinical pharmacists in the management of chronic obstructive pulmonary disease patients with oral theophylline[14]; and a Posey study that revealed an estimated four months cost savings of \$139,380 to $216,800 because of the activities of clinical pharmacists at Oakland Patient Clinic-Veteran Affair (VA) Northern California Healthcare Center.[15] Project Impact, which started in March 1997 in Asheville, North Carolina, involved pharmacists' clinical impact on patients. The pharmacists in the city decided to prove the worth of pharmaceutical care in improving patients' health outcome and reducing total healthcare cost for city-employed diabetic patients. In the first year, the total savings of $20,000 for forty employees was recorded and their health status improved dramatically beyond the expectation of the American Diabetic Association. For instance, the patients' average glycosylated hemoglobin A1c attenuated by 1.4% from 7.6 to 6.2%, their total cholesterol level went down by 12mg/dl from 210 to 198mg/dl, and the average LDL (bad cholesterol) level decreased by 20mg/dl from 118 to 98mg/dl. The second year showed a 78% reduction in inpatient medical costs, 30% in outpatient medical costs, 62 % increase prescription drugs, and 90% patient satisfaction compared to 59-70% baseline with physicians. The project started with diabetic patients and as early as 2001, about 365 employees from thirty-two communities were already receiving disease state management in asthma, hyperlipidemia, diabetes, and hypertension. A projected economic benefit of the program revealed initial costs of $192,000, gross savings of $287,872 per 100 people in one year, reduced absenteeism and improved productivity, decreased sick leave by 50% and a 28% decrease in per-patient overall healthcare cost. The most astonishing part of this project came from the findings of the latter studies, which showed that the pharmacist needs no additional certification (after the first degree, BSc) in order to impact patients' healthcare or outcome, and the Bond et al. study which revealed, among other things, that every time the hospital spent $320 on a pharmacist's salary, there was the saving of one life.[16,17,18,19,20]

In light of these astonishing accomplishments and the above information, one would expect the pharmacist to have a clean bill of health or free pass as drug specialist in the world's public opinion, but.... At any rate, clinical pharmacy is in its infancy in the world and the world is yet to grapple with these adroit drug experts as independent healthcare providers. Even if these drug experts are not known, why is it that pharmacy has become an exception to the rule of specialty? As a matter of fact, it might not be out of place to say that the world has unknowingly accepted pharmacy's bondage in the medical field as a norm rather than an aberration. It is important to note that the above therapeutic outcome achievements of clinical pharmacists/pharmacists is the result of a burning desire of some to make a difference/meaningful impact with their tremendous drug knowledge because there is nowhere in the world where pharmacy curriculum in schools of pharmacy encourages the act of prescribing drugs. The same laws that strangulate pharmacists and prevent them from doing their best in their own jurisdiction also prevent schools of pharmacy from teaching how to prescribe drugs because it is unlawful. At this stage, if pharmacists can function in this manner then it is safe to say that the sky is the limit when the chains that bind them in bondage are lifted and they are free to function as drug specialists/experts like other specialists in their respective field of endeavor. The desire to find out what people of the world think of drug specialists and the medical field prompted this study.

OBJECTIVES:

The purpose of the study is to find out what people think of pharmacists whenever the term drug specialist/expert is used. The study assisted us in assessing the following situations:

- The public's opinion about various healthcare practitioner's knowledge of drugs;
- The public's opinion of the most knowledgeable healthcare practitioner about drugs;
- The public's opinion of the least knowledgeable healthcare practitioner about drugs; and
- The public's opinion of pharmacists, drugs, and their usage.

The project would test two null hypotheses, which are:

1. Public opinion will reflect that pharmacists are not drug specialists; and
2. Public opinion will reflect that pharmacists have no drug knowledge.

METHODS:

The study was conducted in two phases: the United States's and the world's data collection. The United States's data collection involved a fairly large sample and it was conducted in Miami, Florida, home of the elderly and retirees. The world's data collection, on the other hand, involves a smaller sample, and it was conducted in six habitable continents of the world. A survey questionnaire with a five-level Likert scale was administered to people. The main question asked was, rate each of the healthcare practitioner (twenty-three specialties) in terms of sufficient knowledge about drug use or as a drug specialist on a scale of 1 to 5 (figure 1). Twenty-three medical specialties were obtained from the American Board of Medical Specialties (ABMS) directory (the *2000 Marquis Who's Who* publication—twenty-four specialties out of which six were subspecialties of surgery grouped as surgeon in the study), other boards not recognized by ABMS (e.g., dentistry, optometry, and veterinary medicine) but who are authorized to prescribe drugs without theoretical supervision by others, and clinical pharmacists, the supposed drug experts.[21] Respondents were asked to use drug efficacy in terms of treatment modalities, practitioner's ability to discuss drugs and their consequences with them, and any other parameters within their disposal to assess the providers. The five-level Likert scale used ranged from 1 (strongly disagree), 2 (disagree), 3 (uncertain), 4 (agree), to 5 (strongly agree). In view of the fact that clinical pharmacy is at its infancy, and most people do not know the difference between a pharmacist and clinical pharmacist, respondents were told to substitute pharmacist for clinical pharmacist. It is important to note that pharmacists in their present, limited capacity make a lot of recommendations about prescribed and non-prescribed (over-the-counter) drugs to patients and prescribers as well as discuss prescribed drugs with their patients. The international study started at Ile-Ife and Benin City, Nigeria, in Africa then moved to London, United Kingdom, in Europe; Beijing, China, in Asia; Sydney, Australia, in Australia; and Rio De Janeiro, Brazil, in South America. The questionnaire was translated into Portuguese for Brazilians, Chinese for Chinese, and the rest of the nations were English-speaking countries. A descriptive univariate analysis was performed to check the frequency distribution, means, and standard deviations of each question.

RESULTS

The results were analyzed in the following manner. Strongly disagree and disagree responses were grouped as disagree #1; uncertain #2; agree and strongly agree responses were grouped as agree #3; strongly agree #4; and no response or refused to answer the question #5. The U.S. is a case example for this project and is the major focus of attention for results analysis. Three hundred and eight questionnaires were completed by the respondents in Miami and the results are shown in table 1 and figure 2. The sum total of #1, #2, #3, and #5 makes 100%. Demographic analysis of the result shows the study consisted of 25.3% males, 60.1% females and 14.6% no response; 30.8% of the respondents were whites, 41.6% were blacks, 20.1% were Hispanics, 2.9% were others and 4.5% didn't respond to the question. The age limits range from fourteen years to eighty-six years, with a mean of 44.7 years and a standard deviation of 17.4.

The world sample as seen in table 2 and figure 3 consisted of 683 respondents with 308 (45.1%) people from Miami, US (North America); 136 (19.9%) people from Benin City and Ile-Ife, Nigeria (Africa); 31 (4.5%) people from London, UK (Europe); 71 (10.4%) people from Beijin, China (Asia); 85 (12.4%) people from Sydney, Australia (Australia); 50 (7.3%) people from Rio De Janeiro, Brazil (South America); and 2 (0.3%) people refused to answer the question. Demographic analysis for the world's results showed the study consisted of 32.4% males, 53.9% females, and 13.8% without response; 17.6% of the respondents were whites, 40% were blacks, 16.4% were Hispanics, 18% were others (mostly Asians) and 8.1% refused to answer the question. Age limits range from fourteen years to eighty-six years, with a mean of 36.4 years and a standard deviation of 16.6.

Discussion

Public opinion of the most knowledgeable healthcare practitioner about drugs agreed with other, similar studies enumerated above. In this study (U.S.), clinical pharmacists were rated as the most knowledgeable healthcare practitioner about drugs (therapeuticians), with 79.5%, and they were closely followed by family-practice physicians in second place with 76.7%; emergency physicians in third place with 64.3%; dentists in fourth place with 61.3%; internal-medicine physicians in fifth place with 57.4%; pediatricians in sixth place with 56.5%; surgeons in seventh place with 53.5%; obstetricians and gynecologists in eighth place with 52.9%; anesthesiologists in ninth place with 51.9%; preventive-medicine physicians in tenth position with 48.1%; ophthalmologist/optometrists in eleventh position with 46.7%; allergy and immunology physicians in twelfth position with 44.8%; dermatologists in thirteenth position with 43.5%; radiologists in fourteen position with 42.2%; physical medicine and rehabilitation physicians in fifteenth position with 41.9%; orthopedics physicians in sixteenth position with 38%; neurologists/psychiatrists in seventeenth position with 37.6%; urologists in eighteenth position with 37%; veterinarians in nineteenth position with 36.7%; genetics physicians in twentieth position with 34.1%; pathologist in twenty-first position with 30.2%; nuclear-medicine physicians in twenty-second position with 27.3%; and otolaryngologist in twenty-third position with 26.9%.

Using strongly agree criteria instead of agree, which combines agree and strongly agree responses together to assess the healthcare practitioners, there was little variation, and the clinical pharmacist still emerged first with 43.8%. They were followed by family-practice physicians in second place with 36.4%, ; then pediatricians in third place with 31.8%, the surgeon and dentist tied the fourth place with 28.2%; obstetricians and gynecologists in fifth place with 27.9%; and emergency physicians in sixth place with 26%. Otolaryngologist came last again with 9.7%; then pathologist with 11.4%; genetic physician with 11.7%; and nuclear-medicine physician with 12%. As reflected above, the agree criteria is used to judge the most- and least-knowledgeable healthcare practitioner about drug use. The results thus proved that clinical pharmacist, family-practice physician, and emergency physicians are the most knowledgeable, while otolargngologist, nuclear-medicine physician, and pathologist are the least-knowledgeable healthcare practitioners about drugs use.

The study results disproved and rejected the two null hypotheses that stated that pharmacists have no drug knowledge and cannot be classified as drug specialists. Public opinion overwhelmingly justified the fact that clinical pharmacists/pharmacists are relatively on top of the scale each time the term drug specialist/expert is used, and their knowledge of drugs and/or their use is greater than other healthcare practitioners'. This study coupled with others ranging from drug manufacturers' surveys to the Bond et al. study goes a long way to show that something is wrong with the system that relegates the best to the background and keeps them in bondage with others. Besides the pharmacy professional's plight, some of the results were astonishing; for example, one would have expected anesthesiologists to rate high and higher than the surgeon because of the professional propinquity to pharmacy and the aim of its creation (to handle drugs, specifically anesthetics during surgery). Anesthesiologists were ninth, while the surgeons were seventh out of twenty-three specialties. Moreover, the public might not be wrong in their perception that surgeons have more knowledge of drugs generally than anesthesiologists who concentrate on one aspect of drugs: anesthetics. Otolaryngology, on the other hand, is one of the first branches of medicine that took advantage of Flexner's publication in 1910 and was created as a specialty in 1924.[21,22] Today otolaryngology's fame and popularity is very much shrouded in its name, pronunciation, and the number of specialists operating independently as a practitioner with this title. All these factors may have played a role in participants' assessment that the otolaryngologist is the least-knowledgeable healthcare practitioner about drugs. Public opinion in this study seems to resonates well with facts and figures, because no one expected the nuclear-medicine physician (a physician that use radionuclides such as positron emission tomography (PET), radioisotopical antibody, and others to diagnose and treat diseases), in 22nd position; a pathologist (a physician that deals with causes and nature of disease-autopsy), in 21st position; or a genetics physician (a physician that use genetic composition/linkage to diagnose and treat disease), in 20th position, to have much knowledge about drug use (treatment). There is a high probability that this kind of project in other branches of medicine will produce similar results with the respective specialist on top of the scale (rating) followed by others in descending order of relevance to the branch. For example, a similar survey about children's healthcare is likely to rate pediatricians on top of the scale probably followed by family-practice physicians, emergency physicians, internists, etc. Similarly, public perception of lawyers through a Gallup poll showed low ratings in terms of trust because people are conscious of the fact that clients confessed wrongdoings to their attorneys and their attorneys pursued a different course with denial so as to remain in business. However, such a poll about upholding the laws of the land is likely is to rate them high or first in relation to other professions, because Supreme Court judges are lawyers.

The study confirmed the notion that women (60.1%) are much more likely than men are (25.3%) to seek medical care. The racial mix of participants in the survey was 30.8% whites, 41.6% blacks, 20.1% Hispanics and 2.9% other. The average age of the respondent was 44.7 years, which is approximately forty-five years. All surveys in the U.S. were conducted in some community pharmacies around Miami, and the choice of pharmacy was based on the fact that it is the most appropriate place for this kind of project. Also, other places like hospitals and universities were added to pharmacy as survey locations in other parts of the world.

The world's study showed little variation from the United States's statistics. Results, as reflected in table 2 and figure 3, revealed that clinical pharmacist or pharmacist occupied the first position with 75% of the total 683 respondents, family-practice physician came second with 61.6%, emergency physician in third position with 57.9%, surgeon in fourth position with 57.2%, pediatrician in fifth position with 56.5%, internal-medicine physician in sixth position with 55.9% and dentist in seventh position with 55.8%. However, at the end of the spectrum the least-knowledgeable healthcare practitioner about drugs was nuclear-medicine physician rated at 23rd position with 26.2%, then genetics physician in 22nd position with 27.7%, otolaryngologist in 21st position with 28.8%, pathologist in 20th position with 33.1%, radiologist in 19th position with 34.6%, orthopedic physician in 18th position with 35.7% and urologist in 17th position with 36.2%. Individual analysis of the countries' data is not shown in the results but the statistics revealed that clinical pharmacist or pharmacist was first in U.S., Nigeria, Australia, and Brazil. Pharmacists were fourth in China, where internal-medicine physicians were first, pediatricians were second, emergency physicians were third, and obstetricians and gynecologists were fifth. In London, pharmacists were fifth, while family-practice physicians and allergy and immunology physicians tied in the first position; dentist second; surgeon third; internal-medicine physician fourth; and emergency physician and preventive medicine physician tied in the sixth position.

Specialization is at a low level in China because of the nation's adherence to Chinese traditional medicine and moxibustion. Though pharmacists, otherwise known as Yaodian, operate as independent practitioners (or a branch) of medicine in China, pharmacy practice is very much like other places, with the traditional role of dispensing medication only. Pharmacy practice in China, despite its autonomy, is not surprising because much of its impact is Western oriented; hence, the dispensing-only function is a trickle-down effect of Western civilization. At any rate, this is not the ideal direction for future pharmacists as dictated by clinical pharmacy in the U.S. Pharmacists (Yaodian) in China can prescribe and dispense any medication without formalities; however, disease state management, adequate documentation, monitoring of efficacy, patient privacy, and other issues are far from the job description of the Chinese pharmacist.

LIMITATIONS

The study is generally limited in scope by the nature of its self-sponsorship and the concomitant inherent financial constraint, and inadequate access to more participants. Many will argue that the use of thirty-one respondents in London, fifty respondents in Rio de Janeiro, seventy-one respondents in Beijing, eighty-five respondents in Sydney, 136 respondents in Benin/Ife, and 308 respondents in Miami to generalize the findings of the entire general population is inadequate. This study did serve to buttress one issue and drive home the message about the public's opinion of healthcare practitioners' drugs/drug-treatment knowledge, the perception of pharmacists as healthcare providers, and its bondage among other branches of medicine. Moreover, this study gives room to others who might want to duplicate the study with a very large sample and who have the financial commitment necessary to carry out a large study.

The majority of the survey was conducted in pharmacies because that was considered the best option for this kind of research/study. The choice of location may or may not have affected few respondents, because the study in China was conducted entirely in pharmacies yet the pharmacist came fourth in the rating; in London, the study was conducted in and around Home Martin Hospital E5, and the pharmacist was fifth in the rating; in Sydney the study was conducted in some pharmacies and at the University of Sydney; and in Nigeria, the study was conducted at the University of Benin Teaching Hospital in Benin City and the University of Ife (now Obafemi

Awolowo University), Ile-Ife. There is nowhere in the world in which any study can be conducted without minimum site influence on at least a few of the respondents; hence, the problem cannot be ruled out completely. Owing largely to the fact that everything about pharmacy centered on drugs, it is reasonable to say that the best place to conduct a drug specialists' survey with minimum undue influence is the pharmacy. Homebound patients' opinion were reflected by their agents, nurses, children, and whomever they chose to represent them. These representatives may or may not reflect the direct opinion of the homebound patients; however, the fact that they have used drugs at one point or another to resolve their ailments makes them a good candidate for the survey. Other limitations are reflected in the fact that the Brazilians were classified as Hispanics or Latin Americans without regard to race (whites or blacks), markings between responses (e.g., 1 and 2) were disregarded, and few markings of two responding numbers to one question resulted in the counting of the highest response except in cases where one of the numbers is crossed out or scratched off.

Conclusion

This study revealed that respondents thought pharmacists, family-practice physicians, emergency physicians, dentists, internal-medicine physicians, and pediatricians, in sequential order, are the most knowledgeable healthcare practitioners about drugs, while the least knowledgeable healthcare practitioners about drugs are otolaryngologists followed by nuclear-medicine physicians, pathologists, genetics physicians, veterinarians, and urologists, in sequential order. The world's public opinion was in agreement with the United States's survey about healthcare practitioners' knowledge of drugs and usage. The study confirmed the views that pharmacists are drug specialist/experts with greater knowledge of drugs and their use than other healthcare practitioners.

Figure 1. Sample of the Questionnaire.

Please rate each of the healthcare practitioner below in terms of sufficient knowledge about drug use or as a drug specialist on a scale of 1 (strongly disagree) to 5 (strongly agree) by circling one number.

	Strongly Disagree	Disagree	Uncertain	Agree	Strongly Agree
1. Allergy and immunology physician	1	2	3	4	5
2. Anesthesiologist	1	2	3	4	5
3. Clinical pharmacist	1	2	3	4	5
4. Dentist	1	2	3	4	5
5. Dermatologist	1	2	3	4	5
6. Emergency physician	1	2	3	4	5
7. Family practice physician	1	2	3	4	5
8. Internal medicine physician	1	2	3	4	5
9. Genetics physician	1	2	3	4	5
10. Neurologist/Psychiatrist	1	2	3	4	5
11. Nuclear medicine physician	1	2	3	4	5
12. Obstetrician & Gynecologist	1	2	3	4	5
13. Ophthalmologist/Optometrist	1	2	3	4	5
14. Orthopedics physician	1	2	3	4	5
15. Otolaryngologist	1	2	3	4	5
16. Pathologist	1	2	3	4	5
17. Pediatrician	1	2	3	4	5
18. Physical medicine & Rehabilitation physician	1	2	3	4	5
19. Surgeon	1	2	3	4	5
20. Radiologist	1	2	3	4	5
21. Preventive medicine physician	1	2	3	4	5
22. Urologist	1	2	3	4	5
23. Veterinarian	1	2	3	4	5

Sex: M / F Age:_____ Place: _____ Race: _____

Sign: _____

Figure 2. Graphic Representation of U.S. Survey Answers—Agreement.

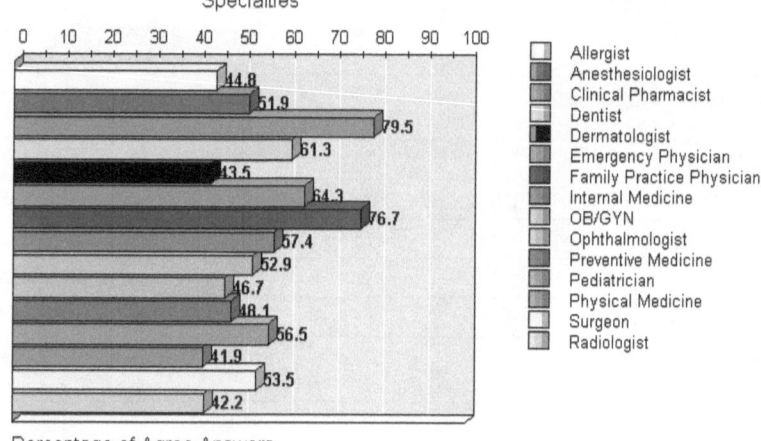

Graph shows that clinical pharmacists were the most trusted specialty, having the most medical knowledge about drugs.

Figure 3. The Fifteen Most Respected Specialties from a Survey of Six Continents.

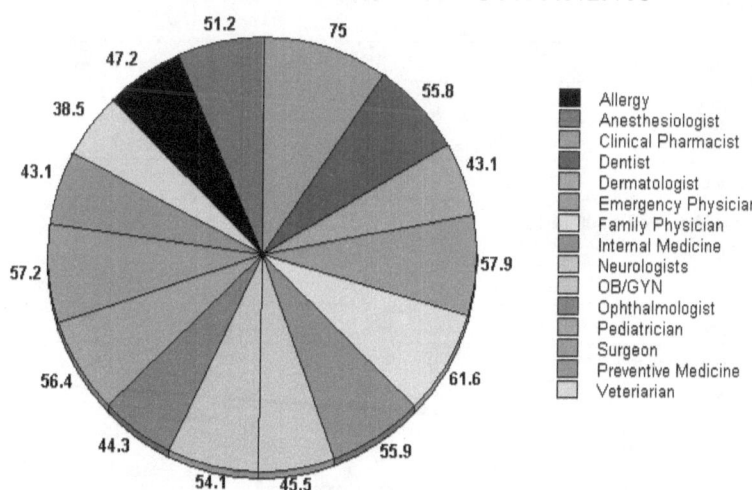

Clinical pharmacist was also number one in world survey results and therefore showed agreement with the U.S. survey.

The following tables show a breakdown of all responses in order to buttress the actual breakdown of the surveys from the United States and the world.

Table 1. Responses Reported in Percentages U.S. Survey Only.

Specialty	1. Disagree	2. Uncertain	3. Agree	4. Strongly Agree	5. No Response
Allergy and Immunology Physician	3.9	29.9	44.8	18.8	21.1
Anesthesiologist	3.2	22.4	51.9	25.0	22.4
Clinical Pharmacist	2.0	10.7	79.5	43.8	7.5
Dentist	5.8	19.5	61.3	28.2	13.3
Dermatologist	6.8	28.9	43.5	18.2	20.8
Emergency Physician	4.2	15.3	64.3	26.0	16.2
Family-Practice Physician	2.5	11.4	76.7	36.4	9.1
Internal-Medicine Physician	4.6	19.2	57.4	24	18.8
Genetics Physician	3.2	37.3	34.1	11.7	25.3
Neurologist/ Psychiatrist	4.2	33.1	37.6	14.9	25.0
Nuclear-Medicine Physician	5.8	38.5	27.3	12.0	28.2
Obstetrician and Gynecologist	5.5	19.5	52.9	27.9	22.1
Ophthalmologist/ Optometrist	5.5	28.9	46.7	22.7	18.8
Orthopedics Physician	5.2	31.2	38.0	15.9	25.6
Otolaryngo logist	4.9	38.6	26.9	9.7	29.5
Pathologist	4.8	35.7	30.2	11.4	29.2
Pediatrician	4.2	18.2	56.5	31.8	21.1
Physical Med and Rehab Physician	3.8	29.9	41.9	20.8	24.4
Surgeon	2.6	23.7	53.5	28.2	20.1
Radiologist	6.1	29.5	42.2	17.2	22.1
Preventative-Medicine Physician	3.5	24.4	48.1	20.5	24.0
Urologist	2.9	32.8	37.0	16.9	27.3
Veterinarian	5.5	29.5	36.7	15.9	28.2

Table 2. World's Public Opinion Derived from Six Countries on Six Continents, in Percentages.

Specialty	1. Disagree	2. Uncertain	3. Agree	4. Strongly Agree	5. No Response
Allergy and Immunology physician	8.5	27.2	47.2	15.7	17.0
Anesthesiologist	9.0	21.8	51.2	22.5	18.0
Clinical Pharmacist	2.9	12.2	75.0	40.0	9.8
Dentist	11.6	21.2	55.8	21.8	11.4
Dermatologist	12.9	27.5	43.1	12.9	16.5
Emergency Physician	10.7	16.5	57.9	21.4	14.9
Family-Practice Physician	9.1	17.9	61.6	25.0	11.3
Internal-Medicine Physician	7.0	21.8	55.9	19	15.2
Genetics Physician	17.1	34.6	27.7	7.8	20.6
Neurologist/Psychiatrist	8.0	26.1	45.5	13.9	20.4
Nuclear-Medicine Physician	16.1	36.0	26.2	7.8	21.7
Obstetrician and Gynecologist	9.3	17.7	54.1	22.3	18.9
Ophthalmologist/Optometrist	14.6	24.0	44.3	16.0	17.1
Orthopedics Physician	13.5	30.5	35.7	9.8	20.4
Otolaryngologist	19.0	38.7	28.8	6.7	21.5
Pathologist	13.9	31.8	33.1	11.0	21.2
Pediatrician	9.2	16.4	56.5	22.7	17.9
Physical Med and Rehab Physician	13.0	29.6	38.0	15.2	19.3
Surgeon	7.1	19.5	57.2	26.5	16.1
Radiologist	20.1	26.6	34.6	14.8	18.7
Preventive Medicine Physician	10.7	27.2	43.1	16.5	18.9
Urologist	11.6	31.5	35.2	11.3	20.8
Veterinarian	15.6	25.8	38.5	14.3	20.2

REFERENCES

1. *New Webster's comprehensive dictionary of the English language.* Deluxe Edition. Lexicon Pub. Inc., 1990.

2. Higby, G. J. Evolution of pharmacy in Remington: The science and practice of pharmacy. 19th ed. 1995, 7-28

3. New Webster's comprehensive dictionary.

4. Cuomo, T. The president's viewpoint: Pharmacy (Fahr'mah-se) n. Florida Pharmacy Today (Nov. 2002): 5.

5. Ibid.

6. Cassell, D. How manufacturers view pharmacists. Drug Topics (April 2001): 47-54.

7. Yoh, E., et al. Survey of 14 pharmacists and 33 physicians about indications, interactions, and adverse effects of some common herbal remedies. Pharmacy Today 7(8) (August 2001): 1.

8. Americans agree: Pharmacists are a good source of health information. Consumer Healthcare Products Association Self-Care in the New Millennium. Pharmacy Today 7(5) (May 2001): 1.

9. Stimmel, G. L., W. F. Mcghan, M. Z. Wincor, and D. M. Deandrea. Comparison of pharmacist and physician prescribing for psychiatric inpatients. American Journal of Hospital Pharmacy 39 (1982): 1483-86.

10. Mayer, Olivia. Travis Watts: Teacher and clinician. Community Pharmacist (Nov/Dec 2001): 14-16.

11. Bootman, J. L., D. L. Harrison, and E. Cox. The healthcare cost of drug-related morbidity and mortality in nursing facilities. Archives of Internal Medicine 157 (1997): 2089-96.

12. Pathak, D. S., and E. G. Nold. Cost-effectiveness of clinical pharmaceutical services: A follow-up report. American Journal of Hospital Pharmacy 36 (1979): 1527-29.

13. Poretz, D. M., L. J. Eron, Goldenberg et al. Intravenous antibiotic therapy in an outpatient setting. Journal of the American Medical Association 248 (1982) 336-39.

14. Self, T. H., R. F. Ellis, H. L. Davis, and M. D. Lee. Early use of oral theophylline in hospitalized chronic obstructive pulmonary disease patients: Cost-containment through medical education. Drug Intelligence and Clinical Pharmacy 19 (1985):749-53.

15. Posey, M. L. Expanding pharmacy's horizons: VA's pharmacotherapy innovations. Journal of American Pharmaceutical Association (1997): 379-82.

16. Bond, C. A., C. L. Raehl, and T. Franke. Interrelationship among mortality rates, drug costs, total cost of care, and length of stay in United States hospitals: Summary and recommendations for clinical pharmacy services and staffing. Pharmacotherapy 21(2) (2001): 129-41.

17. Jackson, M. We can improve patient outcomes. Florida Pharmacy Today 65(6) (June 2001): 7-8.

18. Bunting, B. A., J. P. Miall, D. G. Garrett et al. Providing pharmaceutical care issues, initiatives, and insights. Pharmacy Times Supplement (March 2000): 15-27.

19. Miall, John, Jr. The Asheville project: A successful model to emulate. Advanced Project Institute: Diabetes American Public Health Association publication March 2002.

20. Cranor, C. W., and D. B. Christensen. The Asheville project: short-term outcomes of community pharmacy diabetes care program. Journal of the American Pharmicists Association 43 (2003): 149-59.

21. *Marquis who's who: The official ABMS directory of board-certified medical specialists.* 32nd ed. New Jersey: A division of Reed Elsevier, Inc., 2000.

22. Tebbe, J. L. Healthcare delivery in America. In Historical and policy perspectives: Introduction to healthcare delivery by Robert L. McCarthy. An Aspen publication, 1998, 10, 63-64.

CHAPTER EIGHT

PHARMACY AS A LIFE/MONEY-SAVING PROFESSION FOR HUMANITY: UNITED STATES OF AMERICA AS A CASE EXAMPLE FOR THE WORLD

Pharmacy might be struggling to define its niche and liberate itself from perpetual domination by other branches of medicine; however, it has made an enormous impact on humanity through the ages. Pharmacy's impact stresses from its benevolence, restricted role as dispensers and providers of pharmaceutical care, disease state management/clinical pharmacy service, as well as trained therapeuticians. Pharmacists' easy access to the community, trust, and drug knowledge helped to fuel this impact. Generally people respect pharmacists for their skills and technical know-how, and the pharmacists are conscious of this; hence, they use any available opportunities to upgrade their skills and meet the ever-increasing demands of sophisticated patients/consumers. As seen in chapters 5 and 6, physicians are highly trained in diagnosis and poorly trained in drug treatments, while clinical pharmacists or pharmacists are highly trained in drug treatment and poorly trained in diagnosis. Professional practices and patients' challenges helped physicians and pharmacists to overcome this deficiency. Thus, when a patient approaches a pharmacist for probably a rash resolution, the pharmacist uses his physical-assessment skills to unravel the etiology of the rash (fungus, herpes virus, allergy, etc.) and recommends something to treat the ailment if it is within his scope. If the diagnosis is complex and beyond his scope, the pharmacist refers the patient to other specialists for a follow-up. This chapter will examine the above issue using a substantial number of studies/researches below to buttress it.

Human advancement and improvement in technology have helped to simplify diagnosis for patients and many health professionals including pharmacists. These technological advancements in the form of self-testing instruments/devices such as blood pressure meters, blood sugar

meters, blood cholesterol meters, prothrombin tests, pregnancy tests, and digitalized thermometers have helped pharmacists to assist patients in assessing their status and knowing when to seek further medical assistance. For instance, many patrons/patients ask pharmacists to interpret readings of blood pressure machines that are now common features in nearly all pharmacies in the country.[1] Ease of use of these machines coupled with confidence in data verification with pharmacists/physicians attracts patrons/patients to pharmacies with these machines/devices. Patrons/patients' confidence and reliance on pharmacists has hit the roof, plateau, and descended recently. From 1988 to 1998, a decade, pharmacists were rated as the most trusted professionals in the U.S. This high Gallup poll rating of pharmacists degenerated recently, but they are still high on the scale, within a digit in relation to other professions. In 1998, the CNN/*USA Today* Gallup poll of honesty and ethics survey of twenty-eight professions found for the tenth time that 64% of American consumers rate pharmacists very high or high. They were followed by a 59% rating for clergy, a 57% rating for medical doctors, and in 4th place a 53% rating for dentists and college teachers.

Pharmacy patrons/patients like to take advantage of pharmacists' easy access to the community to solve their ailments and prevent emergency room visits, unscheduled clinic visits, and hospitalization. There are no studies in this area to determine the impact of pharmacists; however, one study in a minority community revealed the following issues: the health issue most commonly encountered by the pharmacist in the community setting is general health problems such as common cold, headache, cough, stomachache, diarrhea, constipation, rash, and allergic reaction and they accounted for 76.7% (148 out of 182); these general health problems were followed by hypertension 8.3%, asthma 2.1%, congestive heart failure 1.6%, depression 1% and others. The pharmacist spent an average of 5.35 minutes for each consultation, with a total cost of $2.68, and his recommendations were mostly over-the-counter medications 79.8% (154 out of 179). Many patients 65.3% (126 out of 193) claimed that the pharmacist's intervention helped to improve their quality of life/clinical outcome, 23.3% (45 out of 193) of patients could not be reached for response, while 7.8% (15 out of 193) claimed that the intervention did not help them. The project was limited in scope and capacity by the pharmacist's lack of prescriptive authority for most legal drugs, and cost-benefit analysis of the study in terms of cure rate, numbers of school days/work days gained, prevention of emergency room visits, unscheduled clinic visits, hospitalization, and prevention of illness from spreading to others in the community could not be assessed.[2]

Most pharmacists are worried about the fact that charging patients for these kinds of benevolent services would backfire because patients are used to the free nature of the services. In their quest to satisfy critics and meet government, lawmaker, and third-party payers' requests, some pharmacists have begun documentation of pharmaceutical care services to justify the importance of pharmacists' consultations in reducing healthcare costs and improving patients' outcome. These pharmacists review charts, make suggestions to physicians directly or indirectly (through nurses or by leaving notes in charts), and document their findings. Some third-party payers are responding to these pharmacists' desires to provide disease state management because they realized the fact that chronic health problems are now part of daily life activities especially for elderly citizens, whose numbers are increasing because of technology and their extended life span. Elderly citizens need education and information about their health from reliable healthcare practitioners who are willing to spend time with them. One study showed how one third-party payer paid a pharmacy group $179 per patient per month to oversee their patients' healthcare and keep them out of the hospital and another paid about twenty-four pharmacies to provide health screenings for their members on a quarterly basis. Some pharmacies charge $5 to $7 for a cholesterol test or a $50 annual healthcare enrollment fee for their program.[3]

Pharmacists are readily seen now as vital healthcare practitioners that can help third-party payers, HMO, Medicaid, and large-scale employers in dealing with preventable ADR, reduce drug-related hospitalization, and improve patient compliance and clinical outcome. This was demonstrated by a joint pharmaceutical care project sponsored by the Minnesota Board of Pharmacy, the University of Minnesota College of Pharmacy, the Minnesota Pharmacy Association, and the Loch Pharmacy in Rosemount Minnesota. The study acknowledges the fact that a drug-related problem is responsible for 28% hospitalization (17 percent ADR and 11 percent noncompliance); 14 percent of patients that are forty-five years of age and older do not fill their prescription orders; 13% of patients filled but refused to use their drugs; 42% of patients failed to follow their prescription orders; and 29% of patients stopped using their medication before it was finished. It went on to highlight how pharmacists' counseling improved patients' compliance by 7% over physicians' counseling and 19% over noncompliance (i.e., pharmacist 96%, physician 89%, and noncompliance 77%); and pharmacists' intervention in changing prescription orders to therapeutically equivalent but less expensive drugs was estimated to occur more than 245,000 times every week. Three pharmacists in the study hired several pharmacy technicians to perform dispensing functions while they focused their attention on provisions of pharmaceutical care in new booths. They hoped that by documenting their interventions and clinical outcome they would force third-party payers to recognize the cost-effectiveness of the program. The study revealed that the pharmacists resolved three to five actual or potential drug-related problems in a 115-prescription volume store.[4]

In Taylorville, Chicago, Les Kazmierczak, a registered pharmacist and director of pharmacy at Suburban Heights Medical Center, set out to challenge insurance companies' views of "show us the value of your services and we will pay for it." He took a week of an intensive ambulatory care course to upgrade his clinical skills with David J. Runback's advanced program at the University of Illinois, Chicago. He then opened a pharmacist-managed clinic in combination with two clinical pharmacists at the medical center. The medical center is comprised of sixty multi-specialty physicians and 10,000 Medicare patients. The physicians referred patients who are potential candidates for high blood pressure and cardiovascular diseases to the clinic for evaluation and pharmaceutical care. Patients' blood pressures were taken and recorded on medical charts on a routine basis when they refilled their prescriptions. Clinical pharmacists suggested lifestyle changes and medication recommendations based on results of the blood pressure, and they educated/monitored patients for a meaningful clinical outcome. A pharmaceutical company gave free blood pressure machines/meters to patients and paid the pharmacists' dispensing fee to teach patients how to use the meters. Hospitalization rates for patients and patients' hospital days were drastically reduced because of pharmaceutical care services provided by pharmacists. The insurance and HMO eventually saved money and decided to pay pharmacists for the clinical/pharmaceutical care services.[5]

The leaders of National Community Pharmacists Association (NCPA), National Association of Chain Drug Stores (NACDS), and the National Association of Boards of Pharmacy (NABP) came to the aid of pharmacists in their quest to meet the demands of third-party payers, HMOs, Medicaid, and employers by implementing various certificate programs for patients' specific disease state management. NABP established protocol for the certificate examinations based on NCPA's National Institute for Pharmacist Care Outcome (NIPCO) model. NIPCO is one of the organizations that prepare pharmacists for NABP exams with patients as a major focus. The nation's largest pharmacy benefit management (PBM) company, pharmaceutical care system (PCS), now uses the NABP exam as criteria for pharmacists' acceptance in disease state management and payment of pharmaceutical care services. A National Institute for Standards in Pharmacists Credentialing (NISPC) survey of certified disease managers (Cams) found that out of 300 participating Cams/pharmacists, 57% were compensated for their services in 2003. 64% of respondents provided DSM services, 22% were compensated as individual practitioners, 42% practice in chain pharmacy, and 25% in independent pharmacy. Furthermore, 37% of the compensation came from patient/patients caregiver, 23% from private insurer, 15% from Medicare, and 12% from Medicaid. The American Pharmacists Association (AphA), NABP, NACDS, and NCPA created NISPC in 1998. DSM services involved diabetes, dyslipidemia, anticoagulation, asthma, smoking cessation, hypertension, congestive heart failure, weight management, nutrition, men's health, osteoporosis, immunizations, hormone replacement therapy, depression, and headache management. Disease state management, effective drug therapy, and provision of pharmaceutical care services demand adequate knowledge about drugs, drug choices, dosages, dosing intervals, drug usage/ benefits, adverse drug reactions, monitoring, and clarity of instructions. These criteria have been put together and used in the evaluation of medical practitioners including physicians, clinical pharmacists, nurse practitioners, and physician assistants. The end result showed that prescriptions written by clinical pharmacists are better than those written by physicians and other healthcare providers put together.[6,7,8]

Clinical pharmacists have exhibited their talents and drug expertise in various places such as India Health Services, Veteran Administration (VA), nursing home facilities, California State, and other places where they are allowed to do so. Drs. O'Neil and Poirer conducted a study to show the direct relationship between drug knowledge/perception and drug-related problems among seventy-eight patients. Pharmacists' lack of prescriptive authority limited their impact in the study; as a result their counseling made little or no difference. The study revealed the following: a strong correlation with the female gender (women were 5.2 times more likely than men to end up with unscheduled visits because of ADR); concomitant disease state (patients with three or more diseases were 3.3 times more likely to change their prescriptions because of ADR); drug knowledge (patients with drug knowledge were 0.29 times unwilling to change their prescription, while those with poor knowledge were more likely to end up in the ER—$P=0.09$); perceptions (patients with a good perception of a number of drugs were 0.0067 times less likely to end up in the ER); regimen changes (patients with four or more regimen changes had a 12.4 times higher hospitalization rate $P=0.05$); and poor collection of data by nurses and physicians resulted in a 3.08 greater chance of prescription change by patients because of ADR. Health professional-patient counseling relationships were analyzed with Wilcox on a signed rank test and results showed a rating of 39.5 for pharmacist-patient relationships against 31.5 for nurse or physician-patient relationships. Patient counseling with physicians, on the other hand, had a better rating of 48% against 37% with pharmacists, and 10% with a nurse. Twenty out of the seventy-eight patients were willing to pay $5 more for pharmacists' counseling.[8]

A clinical, controlled study published by *Journal of the American Medical Association* on July 21, 1999, drew national attention to the fact that pharmacists' participation in therapeutic decisions can "identify and prevent many potential errors in drug therapy." Dr. Lucia Leape (MD) drew national attention with the study titled "Pharmacist Participation on Physician Round and Adverse Drug Event in the Intensive Care Unit." In the study Dr. Christopher Lyman (PharmD and BCPS) made rounds with the residents, nurses, and attending staff of 17 beds intensive care unit at Massachusetts General Hospital. Dr. Lyman was always within reach for consultation and his pivotal role alone in this unit resulted in a substantial savings of $270,000 in a year. Dr. Lyman made 366 recommendations, with a 99% acceptance rate and a resultant 66% reduction in ADE (i.e., 58). He reviewed dosages, interactions, indications, drug alternatives, and detected errors before reaching prescriptions or patients. A twenty-month survey at Albany Medical Center Hospital in New York showed how Briceland and a few other pharmacists identified and prevented 1,048 errors in antibiotics prescription alone. 16% of these errors were fatal/deadly, 14% were serious, while 70% were considered significant if antibiotics had been administered. In a similar study, the researchers at the University of California, San Francisco, discovered that a prescriptions monitoring program at the medical center resulted in a 6% change in antibiotics prescription, detection of 66 antibiotics prescriptions to patients who were allergic to the medications, and 3,041 questioned prescriptions in two years because of pharmacists involvement.[9,10,12]

In September 2003, *Archives of Internal Medicine* reported two cases involving pharmacists' interventions. The first case was a controlled study in which pharmacists reduced adverse drug events (ADEs) by 78%. The study was conducted at Henry Ford Hospital in Detroit between September 5th and November 31st, 2000. The pharmacists in the interventions group rounded with a medical team, provided day discharge counseling on weekdays only, documented pharmacotherapy histories, and their interventions involved the addition of drugs to therapy (21%), removal of drug therapy (7%), laboratory monitoring/recommendations (6%), dosage or frequency adjustments (35%) and identification of therapeutic potential problems after discharge (8%). Pharmacists reviewed medication orders for expensive or medication-related problems in the control group but did not round with the medical team. Results showed that ADEs decreased by 78% from 26.5 per 1,000 hospital days for control group to 5.7 per 1,000 hospital days for intervention group. 150 documented interventions were made and 147 of them were accepted. The second case showed that interactions between pharmaceutical care practitioners (clinical pharmacists) and physicians can result in fewer medication errors, better therapeutic outcome, and satisfied patient drug needs. The study was conducted at Fairview Clinics System located in Minneapolis-St. Paul, Minnesota, with 3,000 patients over past four years. Pharmacists were required to complete a 120-hour, eight-week training program at Peters Institute of Pharmaceutical Care, University of Minnesota, in order to participate in the program. During the program, clinical pharmacists evaluated and documented drug therapeutic outcomes. Results showed that 5,810 patients' encounters occurred and about 5,900 drug therapy problems were identified and resolved. 30% of the problems needed patients' doctor's attention, 29% needed additional therapy, and 22% were subtherapeutic. Therapeutic outcomes increased from 74% with physicians before the program to 89% with clinical pharmacists. A 12-member peer-review panel consisting of pharmacists and physicians reviewed a random sample of patient records to ascertain if they agreed with the clinical pharmacists or not. Accepted cases totaled 94.2%, 3.6% cases received neutral opinions, while 2.2% were rejected. The researchers noted that the results of the study will assist healthcare providers, policymakers, and third-party payers in making well-informed decisions about pharmacists/physicians' interactions.[83,84]

In December 1995, the National Data Corporation reported the following: Nebraska's study revealed how 878 pharmacists' interventions resulted in a total savings of $752,391 ($857 per intervention); Arkansas's study revealed a cost-benefit ratio of 6.13, with 421 interventions involving thirty pharmacies, and the pharmacists were paid $2,100, for a total savings of $12,880; and Kansas's four-week study showed 681 documented pharmacists' interventions with approximately $1,669 cost savings per intervention. Collaborative practices, which limit pharmacists' prescriptive authority to physicians' permission, have been successful in various states in spite of the limitations and bondage. This practice started in Indiana Health Service in early 1970s, spread to Washington, Mississippi, and California at the latter part of the 1970s, and then to twenty-three other states by early 2001. In Washington State, the emergency contraceptive pills program (ECP) emerged as a program worthy of emulation by other states. One study showed that pharmacists charged patients an average of $35 for the ECP, and generally 92% of pharmacists and physicians expressed satisfaction with the program, while 470 patients who responded to the survey out of 7,000 patients rated the program as highly satisfactory.[11,13,14] In October 2001, Governor Gray Davis signed into law SB 1169, a bill that authorized pharmacists in California State to write prescriptions for emergency contraceptive (oral, topical, or injection) to their patients. In the latter part of 2003, clinical pharmacist practitioners (CPPs) in North Carolina and Montana gained a collaborative practice agreement to prescribe controlled substances by registering with the Drug Enforcement Agency (DEA). CPPs can now prescribe controlled drugs with a DEA number provided there is a physician agreement with the clinical pharmacists. Certified nurse practitioners and physician assistants can equally prescribe controlled drugs in these states, but unlike the CPPs their authority is limited because they have no DEA number. In North Carolina, the DEA ruling noted that pharmacists have the skills and ability to prescribe drugs because they are drug experts. The CPPs are expected to go through the North Carolina Board of Pharmacy and Medical Board's approval, while they are only expected to go through the Montana Board of Pharmacy approval in Montana. In addressing pharmacists' DEA registration in Montana in an August 28, 2003, letter to North Carolina Board of Pharmacy, the DEA noted that pharmacists have the authority to administer, initiate, and modify drug therapy in accordance with collaborative practice agreements under the state law.[85]

Smith and Christensen's six-month descriptive study of drug therapy problems involving pharmacists' interventions in Indian Health Services showed the impact of pharmacists in Aberdeen areas of Nebraska and North and South Dakota. The pharmacists' interventions resulted in 77.7% drug therapy changes and detection of fewer drug problems. Mayer evaluated the impact of clinical pharmacy services on the Indian population by examining the life career of a clinical pharmacist Dr. Travis Watts. Dr. Watts joined the Indian Health Services, a branch of Health and Human Services Department that caters to American Indians and natives of Alaska, after obtaining his bachelor of science degree in pharmacy. He later went to the University of Oklahoma for his doctor of pharmacy degree, after which he performed his residency in Veterans' Affairs. In 1996, he was stationed at the Claremore facility as lieutenant commander and later became manager of the clinic. The Claremore facility serves about 63,000 patients from twelve counties, and a year later he founded the anticoagulation management service and cardiovascular risk-reduction clinic. At that time, cardiovascular disease (heart disease) and strokes were the highest killers of American Indians in North America, and Oklahoma ranked fifth in the nation (U.S.). Six separate pharmacists' counseling rooms were set up in a manner identical to other branches of medicine (i.e., with brochures, blood pressure cuffs, patient education materials, etc.) and each of the five to six pharmacists rendered clinical services to about 15 or 20 patients as well as dispensed 700 to 1,000 medications every day. All pharmacists were involved in all clinic activities. The clinic conducted a study of its lipid and anticoagulation programs and discovered that patients reached their goals 94% and 70% respectively compared with 40% before commencement of the clinic. Dr. Watts noted the clinic's biggest challenge was physicians' hesitation in referring patients to the clinic. They overcame this obstacle by working closely with other doctors (physicians) on a one-on-one basis and proving the authenticity of the programs to them. Generally, pharmacists in Indian Health Services have been providing clinical service and patients' care with laboratory/prescribing privileges for various disease states since the early 1950s. The Claremore facility was just an extension of this gesture, and the success of the program/clinics resulted in extension of the facility because of financial grants.[18,61]

Pharmacists in the nation's Department of Veterans Affairs (VA) have expanded their role, which translates beyond collaborative functions seen in other settings. They initiate, monitor, continue, and modify drug therapy as well as order laboratory reports to correlate pharmacotherapy. The pharmacists' reputation grew within VA as a result of the 1995 document and 1996 interpretation tagged "scope of practice of clinical pharmacy specialists." The document detailed the expertise of pharmacists in comparison to nurse practitioners and physician assistants in prescription-writing skills/ability. The traditional medical doctors in these VA centers commended and expressed appreciation for the great performance of the pharmacists. Oakland Outpatient Clinic of the VA Northern California Healthcare Center is one of the VA medical centers where pharmacists made the remarkable impact with their expertise between April and August 1996. Pharmacists' interventions totaled 399, with an estimated total low-cost savings of $139,380 and high-cost savings of $216,800. The interventions included 142 lacked current indication for medications, 116 needed drug monitoring, 49 patients had compliance problems, 34 suggested better drug regimen (due to wrong medications, non-formulary drugs, and expenses), 33 incorrect dosages, 13 potential or actual drug/drug or drug/food interactions, 11 therapeutic drug duplications, and 1 ADR. Cost-saving advantages came from avoidance of physician office visits (about $3,088), emergency room visits ($14,939), hospitalization (about $161,595), long-term care (about $18,238), medication cancellations (about $10,238), urgent-care visits ($4,890), and new medications (about $3,812). Another Veteran administration–controlled study revealed that a clinic run by pharmacists/nurses can improve compliance and blood pressure control. Compliance rate was 75% for the treatment group compared to 20% for the control group, while blood pressure control was 91% for the treatment group versus 29% for the control group.[15,30]

Dillon et al. at the Veteran Administration, Northern California Healthcare System (VANCHCS), conducted a study about oxazepam cost-savings conversion rates and found a savings of $15,800, avoidance of $74,000 additional expenses, and a conversion rate of 88.6% for patients using lorazepam. Lorazepam is the generic name/drug for ativan, and producer of the hospital generic lorazepam, Mylan pharmaceutical company, decided to increase the cost of the drug by about 35% (30 - 40 fold) in January 1998. The VANCHCS pharmacy benefits management strategic health group used the 1997 lorazepam utilization analysis and discovered that the increase would result in $74,000 additional annual cost to maintain existing patients without the addition of new patients, which is a difficult task for most practitioners. At this time, the pharmacy was running a tightly constrained fiscal budget without the additional cost, which would put it in deficit. The clinical pharmacists/pharmacy went into action to excavate similarities between lorazepam and other benzodiazepines using pharmacokinetic properties and others. They discovered that on the basis of metabolism (glucuronidation), half-life, volume of distribution, clearance, and free fraction (plasma protein—unbound drug), oxazepam has properties similar to lorazepam. This data along with other benzodiazepine information and the economic impact of each drug was furnished to the providers to encourage them to switch their patients. VANCHCS operates a decentralized healthcare system with a radius of over 200 miles, and three weeks after the providers were furnished necessary information (e.g., price increase) to switch their patients in April 1998, the prescribing habits remained the same until clinical pharmacists/pharmacy intervened. The clinical pharmacists obtained oral authorization from the psychiatrists to switch patients. They educated patients about the conversion, affected drugs, and provided patients with answers to any questions by telephone. As of August 1998, the number of psychiatrists involved in the conversion went down from 33% to 16% and 88.6% of patients stopped taking lorazepam (45% oxazepam, 18.6% other benzodiazepines and 24.3% of patients were weaned off the drug). The clinical pharmacists saved VANCHCS $15,800, a cost avoidance of $74,000, because of lorazepam's price increase and the patients were happy.[33]

A four-year analysis study of the ambulatory care clinic at William S. Middleton Memorial Veterans Administration Medical Center Madison by Drs. Bond and Monson showed that a clinical pharmacist and nurse clinician can significantly improve drug documentation, patient compliance, and disease control. The aim of the study was to demonstrate the effectiveness of a clinical pharmacist and a nurse clinician in primary care ambulatory setting. The randomized study consists of 81-control group rheumatology and renal clinic patients with baseline data and 133 intervention patients in study group 1 (SG1), and 103 patients who continued with study group 2 (SG2). The patients' medical and prescription records were analyzed and reviewed at the beginning (control group baseline data), nine months later (SG1), and 4.75 years later (SG2). Prescription refill patterns were used to judge patients' compliance and statistical results of the study were analyzed with X^2

test, correlation coefficient Φ, one-tailed and two-tailed t-tests. Prescriptions documentation in medical records showed that control group patients average 4.60 prescriptions per patient, while SG1 patients average 3.91 and SG2 patients average 3.18 prescriptions per patient (SG1, P < 0.025; SG2, P < 0.001). This number of prescriptions per patient reduction from 4.6 to 3.18 translates into annual savings of $94,103.40 in prescriptions drugs for the 1,175 patients. Using 1982 data for the two clinics, clinic visits went down from 4.69 in the control group to 3.74 visits every six months in SG2 and this resulted in an annual savings of $113,969.13 for the 1,175 patients in the two clinics. Prescription duplication went down from 37% (221 out of 594) among control group patients to 28% (200 out of 712) among SG1 and 13% (49 out of 377) among SG2 patients (SG1, P < 0.001; SG2, P < 0.001). The number of same therapeutic-class duplication decreased from 12% (10) for the control group patients to 5 % (6) for SG1 and 1% (1) for SG2 patients. Compliance, on the other hand, went up in terms of the number of prescriptions filled or refilled, from 33% (80 out of 241) for the control group to 85% (211 out of 249) for SG1 and 88% (196 out of 222) for SG2 patients (P < 0.001). Blood pressure control for the hypertensive patients went up from 29 percent (13 out of 45) for the control group patients to 69 percent (40 out of 58) for SG1 and 90 percent (52 out of 58) for SG2 patients.[34]

A cost-benefit analysis study of a clinical pharmacist–managed anticoagulation clinic (AC) was undertaken by Drs. Chrétien, Gray and Garabedian-Ruffalo at Long Beach Veterans Administration Medical Center (LBVAMC). The aim of the study was to determine the effectiveness of a clinical pharmacist in anticoagulation therapy, prevention of thromboembolism or hemorrhage-precipitated hospitalizations, and cost justification. The study consisted of 26 randomized patients in control (CT) and treatment (AC) groups. Physicians referred patients to the treatment (AC) group and interviews were conducted for the treatment group patients. Prothrombin times were performed and recorded for all patients on an outpatient basis. Patients in the control group were under the management of other healthcare practitioners, specifically physicians and nurses, while treatment-group patients were under the management of clinical pharmacists. PTRs (the prothrombin time ratios) are patient time divided by control time, which is set at a therapeutic range of 1.5 - 2.5. Results were analyzed with one-tailed t-test and chi-square, and data revealed that 30.8% (269 out of 872) PTRs pre-AC and 15.5% (117 out of 753) PTRs post-AC were outside the therapeutic range for the treatment group. Out of 627 PTRs, 206 (32.6%) pre-CT and 34.7% of PTRs (188 out of 542) post-CT were outside the therapeutic range for control group. Post-AC was significantly better than post-CT (P < 0.001). Regarding hospitalization, 6 out of 26 pre-AC patients were hospitalized 8 times for a total of 215 hospital days because of hemorrhage and length of stay (LOS) ranging from 4 to 92 days. In contrast, only 1 out of 26 post-AC patients was hospitalized for a total of 3 hospital days because of hematuria (PTR on admission was 1.75). 5 out of 26 pre-CT patients were hospitalized 5 times for a total of 69 hospital days because of hemorrhage and LOS ranging from 4 to 28 days. 3 out of 26 post-CT patients were hospitalized 3 times for a total of 40 hospital days because of hemorrhage and LOS ranging from 4 to 27 days. 4 out of 26 pre-AC patients were hospitalized 5 times for a total of 63 days because of thromboembolism, with LOS ranging from 9 to 16 days. None of the patients in post-AC were hospitalized because of thromboembolism. 6 out of 26 pre-CT patients were hospitalized 7 times for a total of 115 days because of thromboembolism, LOS ranging from 9 to 30 days; 4 out of 26 post-CT patients were hospitalized 4 times for a total of 63 days because of thromboembolism, with LOS ranging from 3 to 32 days. 26 patients were maintained for 772 months in pre-AC and 745 months in post-AC on warfarin. Same maintenance took 948 months in pre-CT and post-CT patients. Studies of patients in pre-AC show that they were in therapeutic range 69.2% of the time compared with 84.5% of the time for post-AC. The 62.9% is within reported range of 55 - 70% for almost all long-term anticoagulation patients, but it is below the clinical pharmacist's achievement in this study. The net savings that resulted from decreased hospitalization was $860.88 per patient in a treatment year. Extrapolation of this result to the 246 outpatients at the medical center would result in $211,776 per year for the facility. This savings compared to the salary, $32,311 for a full-time equivalent clinical pharmacist in the facility in mid-1980s, translates into a cost-benefit ratio of 6.55.[35]

Dr. Powers's study of antimicrobial surveillance in a VAMC teaching hospital from September 1983 to June 1985 showed that clinical pharmacists can significantly impact indiscriminate use of antimicrobial agents. It has been estimated that as many as 50% prescribed antimicrobials are either unnecessary or inappropriate agents/dosages. The aim of the antimicrobial surveillance program was to promote appropriate use, safe, and effective use of the agents through education; decrease hospital cost by avoiding misuse; and prevent resistance of microorganisms. The pharmacy department is responsible for running the program in conjunction with infectious disease control unit. Clinical pharmacists intervened in 229 cases and thus save Veterans Administration Medical Centers, Memphis, Tennessee, about $65,361:60. The intervention resulted in a more cost-effective regimen such as the replacement of cefoxitin 2gm q6h ($52:40/day = $524/10 days) with cefazolin 1gm q8h ($8.28/day = $82:8/10 days), a savings of $441:20. Extensive education of other healthcare practitioners resulted in decreased frequency of administration of cefazolin from 73% of q6h (every 6-six hours) in September 1983 to 20% in June 1985, and q8h (every 8-eight hours) went up from 27% in September 1983 to 80% in June 1985.[36]

Solomon et al.'s study of 133 hypertensive patients (63 treatments and 70 controls) and 98 chronic obstructive pulmonary disease (COPD) patients (43 treatments and 55 controls) in Veterans Affairs medical centers showed drastic reduction in blood pressure and significant breath improvement. The six-month randomized clinical study involved clinical pharmacists/pharmacy residents providing pharmaceutical care to the treatment group. Results of the study were analyzed using baseline visit 1 and final visit 5. Some statistics about things like weight, respiratory rate, pulse rate, cyanosis, and cough showed little or no difference between the two groups, while others like the systolic blood pressure (SBP), diastolic blood pressure (DBP), dyspnea, clubbing of extremities, chest pain, orthopnea, compliance, global, and assessment ratings of normal activities showed significant improvement/reduction for the treatment group compared to the control group. The pharmacists identified 255 problems/needs with the hypertensive patients and 336 problems/needs with the COPD patients. Pharmacists' intervention helped to prevent hospitalization (visit 1—0.03 [0.18] to 0.02 [0.13]—visit 5) for HNT treatment group compared with control group (visit 1—0.02 [0.13] to 0.10 [0.35]—visit 5) (P = 0.043 and 0.002 one-tailed test) and COPD treatment group (visit 1—0.02 [0.16] to 0.10 [0.37]—visit 5) compared with control group (visit 1—0.02 [0.15] to 0.13 [0.35]—visit 5) (P = 0.045 one-tailed test). The same prevention occurred with emergency room visits, other healthcare providers' visits, and the number of new medications increased for the control group compared to the treatment group.[23]

Park et al.'s study of hypertenisve patients revealed similar results. The study was conducted in a chain pharmacy in Chicago, Illinois, and in Kenosha, Wisconsin (a predominantly white middle-class community of about 80,000 people). Patients were registered in the clinical, controlled/randomized study if their blood pressure was greater than or equal to 140/90 mm Hg while on antihypertensive medications and their baseline blood pressure was recorded at the beginning. Physicians were notified of their patients' participation in the program that lasted 4 months each or 7 months including planning period, etc. The pharmacy residents used patients' compliance, medication history, blood pressure, and heart rate readings to monitor drug therapy. They made necessary drug changes and dosage adjustment after consulting with physicians and provided patients in the treatment groups with drug information/education at the scheduled four visits (one visit per month) during the study. The results of the study showed that the percentage of patients with controlled blood pressure went from 17.4% at first visit to 52.2% by the fourth visit for the treatment group (P < 0.02). This represents an average systolic blood pressure decrease of 12.3 mm Hg (P < 0.05) and diastolic blood pressure decrease of 4.6 from first to fourth visit for the treatment group. The control group showed no difference from the first visit to the fourth visit. Some other statistics such as compliance and sexual dysfunction showed little or no difference, while others such as the quality of life (e.g., energy/fatigue mean score) showed significant improvement for the study group compared to the control group (P < 0.05). The physicians were generally receptive of the pharmacy residents' recommendations and the randomization process was imbalanced because of the need to assist patients with a worsening health condition. At baseline, the treatment group had 17.4% patients with controlled blood pressure and 13% more in stage III hypertension, while the control group had 26.9% patients with controlled blood pressure and none in stage III. The study confirmed the National Health and Nutrition Examination Survey (NHANES) III data, which states that only 24% of hypertensive patients who are on antihypertensive medications achieved controlled blood pressure and most chronic diseases states are 25 to 50% successfully controlled by physicians.[26,30]

Pharmacists' interventions in asthma management have also been documented in some clinics. One of the clinics where physicians and pharmacists work together to implement National Institute of Health (NIH) guidelines in the treatment of asthma patients showed how pharmacists helped to save the healthcare industry/insurer about $25,000 to $30,000 in one year with one 49 year old woman. The patient had a long-term history of asthma for about 26 years. She was treated with oral corticosteroids and theophylline for 21 years. The pharmacist's patient history revealed more than 500 emergency room visits and many hospitalizations because of asthma. 55 out of the 500 emergency room visits occurred between January and September 1996, and she was under the care of a pulmonologists, a general practitioner, a nurse visiting once a week, and a social worker. The pharmacist's interventions started in September 1996 and he noted the patient's poor inhalation technique (rapid inhalation, poor timing, and inability to hold breath), three spacer devices without use, four peak flow meters without use (she didn't know how to use them), low-dose corticosteroid inhaler (2 puffs three times daily of triamcinolone), 40mg oral daily dose of prednisone, two oral beta-agonists (terbutaline and albuterol) prescribed by two different medical doctors, and cromolyn and nedocromil therapy that she never used. The pharmacist recommended discontinuation of cromolyn, nedocromil, and oral beta-agonists. He set a goal of no emergency room visits in a month and recommended a high-dose corticosteroid inhaler (4 puffs twice daily of fluticasone 220mcg/puff), weaning the patient off prednisone, salmeterol therapy (two puffs twice daily), and staying in touch with patient. He taught the patient how to use the peak flow meter with color zone management and space device with correct inhalation technique. The patient's health dramatically improved, with peak flow meter rates going from 100 to 150 L/minutes to 360 to 400 L/minutes. The prednisone dosages went down to 12.5mg daily dose in 6 months, she begin to respond to an albuterol inhaler even in the red zone, and her emergency room visits dropped to 2 over six months. The nurse's weekly visit was eliminated, and in a year it was estimated that the pharmacist saved the insurers between $25,000 and $30,000 on the basis of six average monthly emergency room visits alone without other expenses such as the elimination of nurse's visits, unnecessary drugs, etc. The patient now sleeps through the night and gained employment for the first time after many years of debilitating asthma illness. A patient who was once crippled by asthma and forced into parasitic life as a social security disability beneficiary was brought back to a productive life with gainful employment from a near-death experience.[16]

A nationwide compliance study shows that in a year, noncompliance cost the U.S. healthcare industry over $100 billion: 11.4% hospitalization rate, 50% inappropriately used medications, 14% unfilled written prescriptions and 13% filled but unused medications. Asthma patients' statistics are worst, with about 63% partial compliance with corticosteroids therapy in severe asthma cases, 40% over usage of beta-2 agonist against medical advice (toxicity), and only 16 to 20% of patients using peak flow meters to monitor their disease state/treatment in spite of strong recommendations by the National Asthma Education Program (NAEP). Asthma in the U.S. is known to cause 470,000 hospitalizations, 5,000 deaths, $1,033 per patient's loss of adult productivity (i.e., 5-6% workforce), and cost of $6.2 billion annually. It is equally the major cause of school absenteeism among school-aged children. A study conducted by Yale-New Haven Hospital showed that pharmacists' involvement in asthma care can reduce emergency visits by 64%, hospital admissions by 63%, and create a cost savings of $172,379 per 50 high-risk patients in a year. Pharmacists' intervention/education increases patients' ability to use an inhaler correctly from 25 to 95%. Another study of a pharmacist-run emergency room asthma program shows a decrease of emergency room visits from 47 to 6, with a cost savings of $30,000 per 25 high-risk patients. The National Institutes of Health (NIH), as shown in 1995 publication 95-328030, has acknowledged the crucial roles of pharmacists in improving asthma care.[30]

Munroe et al.'s study used insurance (Blue Cross/Blue Shield [BCBS] of Virginia) claim information to evaluate two sets of patient populations, which are the intervention group (patients receiving disease state management) and the control group (patients receiving traditional pharmacy services). The two groups were matched in a compatible manner to reflect age, prescription volume, and the four targeted disease states (hypertension, diabetes, asthma, and hypercholesterolemia). Three intervention pharmacies and five control pharmacies participated in the study in Richmond, Virginia. The intervention's group was slightly more aged (67.2 years against 63.3 years) with more hypercholesterolemia problems than the control group and the study lasted for about 17 months, from September 1993 to January 1995. Results revealed an average monthly expense of $695:92 for intervention group against $839:87 for control group, a difference of $143:95 per patient. The differences increase to $206:17 ($647:08 vs $853:25) when adjustment was made for age and co-morbidity and further to $293:39 when adjustment was made for severity of disease in addition to age and co-morbidity. The insurer's (BCBS) savings per patient per month thereby varies from $143:95 to $293:39 because of pharmacists' interventions. Pharmacists' cost of providing the services is $27 per patient per month, and the intervention for each patient lasted about 15 to 20 minutes every 6 to 8 weeks. The disease state management involved physicians, patients, and pharmacists who went beyond OBRA '90-mandated counseling even though they couldn't prescribe any drug.[17]

James Waddell and others studied hematology/oncology patients at Walter Reed Army Medical Center, Washington, D.C., and found that two pharmacists, with the support of other pharmacy personnel, residents, and technicians, saved the institution about $24,000 in 7 months between October 1995 and May 1996. The $24,000 resulted from 503 interventions, which are due to less drug usage, avoidance of unnecessary non-reusable medication, and usage of less-expensive medication (cost-effectiveness-therapeutically equivalent/effective drugs but less expensive).[19]

The popular project IMPACT (Improve Persistence and Compliance with Therapy), a two-year hyperlipidemia study by the American Pharmacists Association (AphA) foundation shows the awesome impact of pharmacists on disease state management as drug specialists. Merck and Co. sponsored the project that trained 29 pharmacists to render counseling and monitoring of cholesterol to over 700 patients at high risk of cardiovascular diseases in 15 states. The 29 pharmacists have private consultation areas, effective documentation system, and enough technician support to execute the program in their respective pharmacy. The project started in January 1996 with selection of pharmacists and subsequent 3 days training, which includes antihyperlidemic therapy and use of cholestech LDX blood analyzer test for cholesterol. The patients were tested at the beginning of the program for baseline record then scheduled for follow up visits monthly for the first 3 months and quarterly (every 3 months) for the next 2 years. The test results provided basis for pharmacists' counseling, setting of goals, and recommendations, which were forwarded to physicians. Patients were encouraged by their results, pharmacists' counseling, and the degree of CHD (coronary heart disease) risk, which serves to ensure persistence (patients who remain in the program from beginning to end) and compliance (patients who didn't miss 5 days' doses or refill). As of December 1997, the persistence rate was 84%; compliance rate was 84.3% while 44.3% to 62.5% of patients achieved National Cholesterol Education Program (NCEP) lipid goals. Some individual achievement includes a 54 years year-old male whose level dropped from 270 to 190 in two months because of dietary changes and garlic; a patient whose level dropped from 350 to 170 on medication; Bergner (Minnesota) whose level dropped from 327 to 254; Phillips (Minnesota) whose level dropped from 300 to a goal of 217; and Martin (Ohio) a bypass surgery patient whose level dropped from 353 to 223. Pharmacists' charges varied according to location (some charge $20 per visit, $35 for lipid panel, etc.), and the charges were paid by patients—about 40 different third-party payers and Medicaid in some states like Wisconsin, Washington, and Mississippi that recognize and reimburse pharmacists for their cognitive services. A local employer was so much impressed with the outcome of the program that they decided to sign a contract with the pharmacist, Anderson, to provide the services to its employees. Dr. Stephanie Cook, medical director of Ohio State University's wellness program, commented about the program, noting that "pharmacists are excellent health educators, good counselors on medications and lifestyle changes." This could not have come at a better time than when America Heart Association acknowledged the fact that only 18% of congestive heart failure (CHF) patients achieve their cholesterol target goal in a society where over 500,000 people die every year because of CHD. 97 million have high cholesterol level and less than 40% of the patients take their medication over one year.[20,21,22]

Vaccinations prevent diseases and curtail subsequent morbidity and mortality that would have resulted from spread of the disease. No one can underestimate the economic benefits of vaccination in any country and pharmacists are not left out in the provision of this service. The presence of pharmacists in all localities, even where there are no other healthcare providers, has helped to spread vaccinations to people especially those that need it. The majority of the recipients are younger people, those with chronic diseases, 65 years of age or older, and others who were previously out of reach of the program. Dr. John Grabenstein of the University of North Carolina, a national immunization expert, attests to the above facts in his research study that showed how a "pharmacist can serve as educator, facilitator, and/or immunizer to ensure higher immunization rates...." The cross-sectional study of 1,730 patients who were immunized at 21 different pharmacies in 10 states revealed that all recipients were fully satisfied, and 97% of them expressed the desire to go back for a repeat episode. The pharmacists rendered 8,266 influenza vaccinations between October and December 1998. Williams et al.'s study, on the other hand, showed how pharmacists can dramatically increase immunization/vaccination and thus reduce the 10,000 -- 40,000 deaths due to influenza and 40,000 deaths due to pneumococcal every year in the U.S. The study cited the National Coalition for Adult Immunization that estimated that there are over 60,000 deaths per year from preventable infections (e.g., influenza, pneumococcal pneumonia, and diphtheria), and the Centers for Disease Control and prevention that showed a record of 10 to 42% of 2 year-old children that received complete vaccinations. In 1997, 1,000 pharmacists were involved in the vaccination program with 100,000 doses of vaccines, and two long-term care facilities in Athens, Georgia, showed how some of these pharmacists' vaccinations helped to increase vaccination rates from 4.2% to 94.4% and 1.9% to 82.8% respectively (chi-square analysis, $P \leq 0.05$).[24,79]

In 1974, indiscriminate use of medications, unwarranted and inappropriate prescription of drugs, over dosages, over usage, ADR, and other issues relating to drug use problems among nursing home residents caused Congress to enact nursing home regulations. The regulations permit pharmacists (consultants) to review each patient/resident drug regimen and report any irregularities to the nursing home medical director and administrator. Consultant pharmacists have used their drug expertise and pharmaceutical care to assist residents in dealing with their drug problems and dependence on the drugs since its inception. Bootman et al. evaluated healthcare cost of drug-related morbidity and mortality in nursing facilities across the country. The aim of the study was to estimate the cost of drug-related morbidity and mortality within nursing facilities and the impact of consultant pharmacists, experts who were mandated by the federal government to review nursing home residents' drug regimen retrospectively every month. They used decision analysis techniques and an expert panel, which consisted of fifteen consultant pharmacists and thirteen leading geriatric care physicians provided by the American Geriatric Society. The expert panel summed up the cost of drug-related problems and probabilities of therapeutic outcomes of drug therapy provided in two scenarios; 1. with consultant pharmacist and 2. without consultant pharmacist. Drug-related problems otherwise tagged as negative therapeutic outcomes and utility of healthcare facilities resulting in deaths, hospitalization ($5,415 from American Hospital Association statistics 1992), emergency room visits ($360), addition to regimen ($27 average cost), physicians' revisits ($61 Medicare reimbursement rate), other healthcare professional visits ($75 average cost for physical therapist, dietician, etc.), and laboratory and radio logic work ($100) were included in the calculations and decision analysis tree. A conservative estimate of 41 million physician visits was used, with a breakdown of 2 initial visits in a month for the 1.7 million nursing home residents. Physicians' reimbursement rate was $61, while consultant pharmacists were reimbursed $10 per healthcare encounter. Results were analyzed with a student t-test and there were some remarkable differences. Nursing home residents experienced 60% optimal therapeutic outcomes with consultant pharmacists compared with 42% without them. This difference translates into 2.9 million suboptimal outcomes (1.5 million treatment failure, 0.6 million new medical problems and 0.8 million both treatment and new medical problems). Baseline estimates of the cost of drug-related morbidity and mortality with consultant pharmacists was 4 billion dollars compared to 7.6 billion dollars without them. This difference translates into 3.6-billion-dollar savings ($1.6 billion in combination in treatment failure, $1 billion in new medical problem, and $1 billion in combination of treatment failure and new medical problems). Other data revealed negative therapeutic outcome: 10 to 16% (13% average) residents need no further treatment with consultant pharmacists (CP) compared with 11 to 16% (13.5% average) without them; 23 to 25% (24% average) residents needed additional drugs to regimen with CP compared with 23 to 27% (25% average) residents without them; 4 to 7% (5.5% average) cases resulted in hospitalizations with CP compared with 7 to 10% (8.5% average) without them—this translates into 3% increase at the cost of $5,415 per admission and a 2 to 4% (3% average) increase in the number of deaths with CP compared with 3 to 4 % (3.5% average) without them. Initiation of drug therapy increased to 60% and cost $6 billion after physicians visit with CP compared with $11.5 billion without them—a difference of $5.5 billion resulting in unwanted, unnecessary, or inappropriate therapy. Physicians' and pharmacists' estimates show little difference. The investigators reasonably concluded that $1.33 of healthcare resources is spent on treatment of drug-related problems for every $1 spent on drugs in nursing facility, and consultant pharmacists helped to reduce this cost by $3.6 billion.[37]

The ability of clinical pharmacists to act as independent prescribers was put to test in a long-term care facility (nursing home) in California and a study by Thompson et al. The guidelines of the California State Assembly bill 717 enacted in 1977 spell out the authority of clinical pharmacists in acting as independent prescribers. The study noted that research has shown how physicians prescribe many different types of drugs to nursing home residents without due regard to drug interactions, contraindications and adverse drug reactions. This quasi-experimental study consists of 70 experimental group patients and 82 control group patients. Two clinical pharmacists prescribed drugs to the 70 patients in the experimental group under the supervision of the facility medical director, and a family practitioner while the 82 control group patients were catered to by a private community physician, an internist. Baseline observations were made one year (February 1, 1980 to January 30, 1981) before the experiment, which started on February 1, 1981 till January 31, 1982. The pharmacists' relationship with the pharmacy was severed during the study because of the need to eliminate biases. Patients were seen and medically examined every month by the pharmacist, while the supervising physician remained aloft (no prescription and lab order or altering of pharmacist's order). He was just an administrator during the period. Baseline results showed no significant difference in age, sex, length of stay, diagnosis, hospitalization, mortality rate, discharge rate, and number of drugs between the experiment and control group in the first year of study (February 1980 to January 1981), the pre-treatment period. The study period results show no significant differences in age, sex, and diagnosis. However, there were some significant differences in average number of prescribed drugs per patient, which was 5.7 for the treatment against and 7.1 for the control group (average of 2.2 drugs difference per patient—$P < 0.05$); discharge rate to home or lower level of care, which was 8 for treatment group against 2 for control group ($P = 0.03$); hospitalization rate, which was 2 for treatment group against 8 for control group ($P = 0.06$—not significant because value P must be less than 0.05, which may be due to the small sample size); and mortality rate, which was 3 for treatment group against 10 for the control group ($P = 0.05$). All these achievements were due to drug therapy appropriateness. The savings realized from this study was $16,080 per year in drug cost (based on California average drug cost of $10 per drug); $14,400 in discharge rate to lower level (Medicaid reimbursement rate of $1,000/month in nursing home and $800/month in lower level); and $24,750 in decreased hospitalization rate (reimbursement rate of $750 per hospital day for average length of stay of 5.5 days). These savings totaled up to $55,230 for the 67 patients. The pharmacists spent one quarter of their time performing the services, and this amounted to $9,000 because pharmacists' average salary in the state in 1982 was $36,000 per year.[80]

Christensen and colleagues' study of pharmacists' interventions in Washington State Cognitive Activities and Reimbursement (CARE) project found that pharmacists are capable of reducing costs and drug-related morbidity and mortality if someone pays for it. Pharmacists in the treatment group made over 20,000 documented interventions in one year and Medicaid paid for 83% of the interventions at the rate of $4 to $6 per intervention. The project consists of 200 community pharmacies out of which 110 pharmacies were in the treatment group and 90 pharmacies were in the control group. 27% of the interventions (about 5,400) culminated in drug therapy change, and Medicaid saved about $10 to $13 for every 1,000 prescriptions dispensed.

This project was one of the two studies directed by congress through HCFA and it was designed to determine the effect of OBRA '90 legislation, which mandated pharmacists' counseling and drug use review. The study did not reveal statistical data resulting from drug-related morbidity and mortality because the interventions forestall such outcomes. It is difficult to quantify a dollar amount that would have resulted from such outcomes in terms of emergency room visits, physician/clinic visits, hospitalization, and others if the interventions had not occurred. The above Medicaid savings might appear small but avoidance of the resultant consequence is huge. The success of the program Washington State Cognitive Activities and Reimbursement paved the way for the state's Medicaid to pay for other pharmacists' cognitive services such as compliance and emergency contraception program.[27]

St. John's University College of Pharmacy, Queens, New York, sponsored two faculty officers, Drs. Brocavich and Etzel, and their students to assess the impact of pharmaceutical care on human immunodeficiency virus (HIV) inpatients at Nassau County Medical Center. Nassau County Medical Center, East Meadow, is a 500-bed teaching hospital where the two faculty members and their doctor of pharmacy students provided clinical services and interventions to infectious disease teams over 14 months (July 1993 to August 1994). Most of the HIV inpatients had developed acquired immunodeficiency syndrome (AIDS) because of disease progression and they were placed on costly multi-drug regimen with concomitant ADR, improper dosing, frequency, etc. The period was divided in 2 months rotations, each consisting of one faculty member and student who monitored each patient's organ function, concurrent disease state, allergies, laboratory/physical data, ADR, inappropriate drug usage, inadequate dosing, toxicities, frequency of administration, route of administration, drug interaction, past and present medications in combination with patient's age and gender purposely to make recommendations. The recommendations were made known to the physicians, who in most cases accepted the interventions (86%). Pharmacy made 933 interventions with a total savings of $84,476:25 for 378 patients in 14 months. This even out to $6,034 ± $3,679:45 savings per month to a hospital whose only commitment to the pharmacy was office space. The interventions consisted of 25% discontinue drug therapy (233), 22% changes in drug regimen (205), 19% changes in frequency (178), 13% changes in dosages (122), 10% laboratory data monitoring (93), 6% changes in route of administration (56), and 1% new drug therapy (9).[28]

In North Carolina, pharmacists decided to prove the worth of pharmaceutical care in improving patients' health outcome and reducing total healthcare cost to diabetic patients who were employed with the city of Asheville. Asheville permitted pharmacists to render this service to their employees and they succeeded in saving $20,000 for forty employees the first year. In addition, the forty employees' health status improved dramatically even beyond the expectation of American Diabetes Association. The American Diabetes Association's goal for hemoglobin A1c is < 7%, total cholesterol is < 200mg/dl, and low-density lipoprotein (LDL) is < 100 mg/dl. The patients' average hemoglobin A1c attenuated by 1.4% from 7.6% to 6.2%, and their total cholesterol level went down by 12 mg/dl from 210 to 198 mg/dl, while average LDL level (bad cholesterol) decreased by 20 mg/dl from 118 mg/dl to 98 mg/dl. Second-year analysis revealed greater cost savings, 78% reduction in inpatient medical cost, 30% decrease in outpatient medical cost, 62% increase in prescription drugs and 90% patient satisfaction against 59 - 70% baseline. A projected economic benefit of the program revealed initial costs of $192,000, gross savings of $287,872 per 100 people in a year, reduced absenteeism and improved productivity, decreased sick leave by 50% and reduced overall healthcare cost per patient by 28%. The project started in March 1997, and as early as 2001 about 365 employees of the city and Mission St. Joseph Health System were receiving disease state management in asthma, hyperlipidemia, diabetes, and hypertension from 32 community pharmacists. John Miall, Asheville's city director of risk management, reiterated the city's commitment to the program based on its success in reducing healthcare cost, improving patient health out come, and satisfaction.[29,30,78]

In early 2001, a study by the *Journal of the American Medical Association* (JAMA) of pediatric medication errors in hospitals revealed that the presence of clinical pharmacists in pediatric wards is 1% better than computerization of physicians' entry order in preventing errors. The study was reviewed by two physicians, who ascertained that computerization of physician entry orders would halt 93% of medication errors, while the presence of a clinical pharmacist would prevent 94% of such errors in the same ward. Combination of these two assets—computers (technology) and clinical pharmacists (adroit drug specialists)—would potentially reduce pediatric medication errors to a bare minimum of 0.5%, which is a 99.5% improvement rate. Results of the study showed that 5.7% of the errors occur in pediatric medication orders, the same as in adults, while 1.1% of the orders result in adverse drug events (ADE), three times greater than adults. Further breakdown of ADE revealed 34% incorrect dosing, 28% anti-infective medications, and 54% intravenous drugs (IV). The value of the study and its society impact was further enhanced by the deaths of a 9 months old girl in Washington Children's Hospital because of medication error in April 2001. The fragile little girl was given two doses of morphine 5mg, 2 hours apart. The surgeon wrote.5mg (point 5), which was interpreted and transcribed as 5mg by the clerk.[31]

Scott Davis studied the effectiveness of clinical pharmacists in management and treatment of adult patients with positive culture for group A, beta-hemolytic streptococcus throat infections. This was a retrospective study in which 50 control group patients received treatment from internists (physicians), physician's assistants, and nurse practitioners while 58 experimental group patients received treatment from pharmacists in Genesee Valley Group Health Association (GVGHA) Wilson Center, a health maintenance organization (HMO) of Rochester, New York. Normally, the protocol for treatment of patients in the control group is that patients see the internist, physician's assistant, or nurse practitioner (the three otherwise tagged healthcare providers); a throat culture is done; and the patient is given drugs sometimes pending results. Patients will be informed that results take 1 to 2 days and when the results are received, the provider reviews the patient's chart and prescribes medication before contacting the patient and pharmacy to follow up if positive. The treatment group's otherwise new program followed the same procedure, up to the point of receiving culture results. The result of the treatment group is sent to a pharmacy and, if positive, the pharmacist reviews the patient's chart and prescribes medication before contacting the patient to follow up. The new program was meant to save the provider's time, personnel cost, and to make things easy for patients without mitigating medical care. The results revealed that patients spent 16.7 minutes in the control group and 6.11 minutes in the treatment group ($P \leq 0.01$), a time difference of 10.5 minutes per case. Fewer patients, 21 in the experimental group return sick to the office for treatment compared with 31 patients in the control group. However, there were more re-culture visits- 10 patients in the experimental group compared to 6 patients in the control group. Re-culture visits were meant to show if the patient was free of infection or not, and patients were probably reacting to the pharmacist's role as a provider rather than dispenser (a psychological factor rather than reality). The cure rate for patients who were given oral medication for the experimental group was 73.2% (41 out of 56) and 66.7% (28 out of 42) for the control group. The overall savings for the HMO was 17 hours, 40 minutes, and this translated into $373. The pharmacists clearly showed that they produced better results in drug therapy management and cost-effectiveness than the traditional providers.[38]

Total parental nutrition is the administration of nutrition or nutrient fluid through intravenous route (parental) to patients who cannot sustain adequate oral nutrition. This nutrition therapy for ailing patients in acute care and other critical settings used to be the exclusive prerogative of other healthcare providers vis-à-vis physicians, physician assistants, nurse practitioners, nurse and others until the thought of pharmacists as therapeutic experts who can effectively managed the procedure better than others was echoed and put into practice in some institutional settings like the hospitals. The test did not only proved those that initiated the program right but also saved various institutions that practice the new procedure a tremendous amount of money. Today, TPN is under the jurisdiction of a pharmacy in almost all parts of the country and Mutchie et al.'s study is one of the studies that have been conducted on the issue so far. Mutchie et al. studied the clinical and cost-effectiveness of pharmacists' involvement in TPN monitoring at a 150-bed primary children's medical center (PCMC) in Salt Lake City, Utah. The patient paid pharmacy charges of $40 per bottle for TPN and data was collected for 12 weeks before the pharmacists' intervention. This data included the patient's age, clinical response, numbers of lab results, TPN volume, charges per day, and number of days involved. Pharmacy departments reviewed this data and convinced the administration, surgery, and neonatal departments to provide this service by monitoring clinical response, data, lab values, and made recommendations to physicians during daily rounds. The study consisted of 52 patients, 26 in the control group before the pharmacist's intervention and treatment group after the pharmacist's involvement. The results revealed that mean number of days of TPN therapy went up from 12.3 ± 9 (control group) to 14.8 ± 12 (treatment group) but the mean number of bottles and charges per day went down from 1.8 (control group—CG) to 1 (treatment group—TG) and from $72 (CG) to $50.18 (TG), a difference of $21.82/patient/day. Wastage due to outdated solutions and orders changed or discontinued after preparation of solution went down from 45 bottles (CG) at the cost of $1,800 to 6 bottles at the cost of $301:08. Clinical response for the mean age of 35 weeks old babies went up from a mean weight gain of 4gm/day for control group to 17gm/day for treatment ($P < 0.05$, student t-test) and statistics for the two groups were closely matched.[39]

Hospital costs of TPN to patients is awesome, and for some patients whose only means of survival is permanent or long-term administration of TPN, this cost can be unbearable; consequently, the pharmacy department in conjunction with hospital administration decided to go a step further in minimizing the cost by introducing home parental nutrition (HPN). Some studies have evaluated the difference between TPN and HPN and showed the cost-saving nature of HPN. One of these studies is the Brakeball et al. research that examines the HPN program at the University of Washington Hospital. The program started in 1970 with 55 patients and while in the hospital, pharmacists trained the patients who could have died from malnutrition without the services. Training included the use of a written manual and a videotape, which delineated instructions. Patients are discharged from the hospital, and with the aid of the pharmacists they started administering the HPN for 9 - 14 hours a night, thereby giving them enough time to perform normal life activities during the day. The study randomly follows the results of ten patients and came up with the following comparison. The average cost per patient was $10,071:62 per year or $48:19 per infusion per day for HPN, and $42,987:19 per year or $205:68 per infusion per day for TPN. This represents a cost savings of $157:49 per patient per day, a 76% difference. This savings translates into $32,915:14 for the 209 infusion days per year per patient and $1,810,348 per year for the 55 patients. A 76% savings in cost besides permanent institutionalization that would have crippled and reduced their quality of life means a lot to patients.[40]

Wateska et al. studied a similar program at a Cleveland clinic from March 1976 to September 1978 in Ohio. There were 17 patients in the HPN program, but the study monitored 8 patients. Physicians, nurses, and pharmacists were all involved in the training of the patients, but the pharmacists and pharmacy departments spent more time with the patients and HPN supplies than any other. The results showed an average cost per patient of $21,465 for the first year then $19,700 per year for maintenance cost or $54 per infusion day for HPN and $73,720 per year or $202 per infusion day for TPN, hospital inpatient. The savings showed 73% reduction in cost or $157,600 for the 8 patients in a year. Adachi et al. studied controlling admixture through pharmacist monitoring at St. Francis Medical Center, Lynwood, California. The study lasted from 1982 to 1983 and within the period, pharmacists review effective post-surgical prophylactic antibiotic orders after 48 hours, nursing units' IV admixtures, the refrigerators twice daily (to check for discontinued admixture), preparation of admixtures twice daily, and all 10 days or older IV antibiotic orders. The program resulted in a 39% reduction with a total cost savings of $34,674 in 1983. A minimal amount of time was said to have been spent by the pharmacists and technicians with no available data.[41,42]

Kelly et al. investigated the impact of clinical pharmacists' activities on intravenous fluid and medication administration in a 300-bed General Hospital, Kansas City, Missouri, and found a cost savings of $11.31 per patient per day. This was a randomized study involving two internal medicine units with clinical pharmacists (study group) and without pharmacists (control group). The clinical pharmacists' responsibilities were to question the necessity of IV piggyback and fluid (e.g., keep open lines); recommend equivalent alternatives such as buretrol, oral dosage, IV bolus, or IM dosage; and decrease waste arising from this administration. The study group consists of 117 patients, while the control group consists of 140 patients. The results revealed that the mean hospital stay was 7.8 days for the study group against 10.2 days for control group. The cost of IV administration without drug cost was $6,193 for study patients against $8,998 for control patients. The cost of IV piggyback was $2,464 for study group against $14,256 for control group. The cost of IV buretrol was $517 for the study group against $264 for control group. The total cost was $9,174 for the study group and $23,518 for the control group, representing a difference of $14,344. The total cost of drug administration was 32 percent for the study group against 62 percent for the control group, while non-recoupable IVPB waste was $297 for the study group and $1,166 for the control group. These costs were analyzed and reduced to cost per patient per day for IV therapy and it was $32.01 for the study group and $43.32 for the control group, representing a savings of $11.31 per patient per day.[43]

Fudge and Vlasses conducted an investigational study of third-party reimbursement for pharmacist instruction on antihemophilic factor. Hemophilia is one of the diseases that was previously thought to be managed effectively only in the hospital. Home therapy with the aid of pharmacists is now known to be as effective as hospital management. This study investigated how two pharmacists taught a patient the methodology involved in home preparation, storage, stability, and self-administration of antihemophilic factor (AHF), thereby preventing hospitalization and the resultant huge healthcare cost. The clinical pharmacists from Ohio State University Hospital designed the program at the request of the hospital in 1973 and taught the 14 year-old hemophilia patient and his parents these techniques while in the hospital. They supervised the patient in the hospital and followed him home after discharge to ensure that the child/parents mastered the procedure. The patient was asked to document all bleeding episodes and the amount of AHF used. The results showed a cost savings of $20,230 and there was a 15% increase in school attendance for the year. The success of this program led to enrollment of 23 other patients and approval of $40/patient payment for the pharmacists' services by Blue Cross of Central Ohio in October 1975.[48]

Poretz et al. studied intravenous antibiotic therapy in an outpatient setting and found a cost savings of $432,816 for 150 patients. The program was designed to reduce cost, hospital burden, physicians' workload, and free hospital beds for acutely ill patients. It was placed under direct supervision of a pharmacist, who spent half of his time on the program. Patients who needed intravenous antibiotic treatment beyond the acute phase of their illness were discharged into the program from Fairfax (VA) Hospital, a 656-bed community hospital in Washington, D.C. The 150 patients were taught normal procedures involved in home parental administration of antibiotic and the program enabled the patient to return to work or stay at home instead of the hospital. Patients mastered the procedure and demonstrated it to staff before they were released. They see their physician every two weeks or as necessary and a part-time IV nurse who spent one quarter of her time on the program was available for service. The results revealed a cost savings of $432,816 for the 150 patients or 3,048 days at a cost of $142 per day. A physician's fee of $210 ($35 per patient), pharmacist's fee of $17,500, and nurse's fee of $6,000 were part of patient's incurred charges for the home therapy.[49]

Pathak and Nold examine the cost-effectiveness of clinical pharmacy services for self-administering patients who medicate themselves with antihemophilic factor, cytarabine, calcitonin, parenteral nutrients, and injectables and analgesics at home and found a substantial savings of $833,723 for the society in two years. The pharmacy department of Ohio State University Hospitals (OSUH) trained and followed up 35 patients between September 1, 1976, and August 31, 1978. Patients' benefits were assessed in terms of hospitalization days or outpatient clinic visits saved by each patient and then converted to monetary values using the hospital average daily charges or outpatient clinic charges. Results showed that the clinical pharmacy services saved the society (taxpayer) $833,723 in two years. This translates into 46.3 hospitalization days and $11,911:30 savings per patient in a year. Other benefits of the program included savings in missed school or workdays, availability of hospital beds to other sick patients, improved quality of life, patient satisfaction, and family education that helped to reduce their anxiety.[69]

Schloemer and Zagozen conducted a two-year retrospective study on the effects of pharmacy-based pharmacokinetic consultation service for aminoglycosides in relation to hospital costs and charges. The study was performed in the 185-bed, acute-care St. Nicholas Hospital, Sheboygan, Wisconsin. The pharmacy department provided the pharmacokinetic services for aminoglycosides and theophylline. Investigators reviewed 98 patients who were on aminoglycosides with serum drug assays between April 1981 and March 1983 as study group. Pharmacokinetics properties revealed that dosing interval for aminoglycoside increases with age because of longer half-lives in an older population. For instance, it has been discovered that the mean half-lives of aminoglycosides in patients more than 30 years old is almost double that of patients less than 30 years old. This was a basic tool that the pharmacists used to arm themselves as therapeuticians or drug specialists. Physicians were in the habit of dosing aminoglycosides in all patients every eight hours before the commencement of the pharmacokinetics services by the pharmacy department because they were unaware of this crucial information about the drug's half-life. The results revealed that 41 patients (42%) had increased dosing intervals with shorter frequency (like every 12 hours), and savings ranged from $20 to $740. 44 patients (45%) received regular dosing, and 9 patients (9%) who would otherwise receive sub-therapeutic dosing with regular dosing interval were given decreased dosing intervals with longer frequency (probably every 6 hours) and the increase in drug cost ranged from $19.95 to $120, which is better than long days in a hospital or readmission for the same purpose. The net savings for the 98 patients was $6,284:55 and the drug assay cost was $9,734:20. The overall hospital costs were reduced by $563:28 for the 98 patients.[44]

Self et al. studied cost containment through medical education of early use of oral theophylline in hospitalized chronic obstructive pulmonary disease patients at the Regional Medical Center, University of Tennessee Center for the Health Sciences. Patients with acute exacerbations of COPD are treated with intravenous infusion of aminophylline and later converted to oral theophylline in hospital. The study noted other research that shows a loading dose of oral theophylline elixir followed by a maintenance dose of sustained-release theophylline tablets in two hours is as good as intravenous aminophylline in maintaining serum level at a therapeutic range of 10-20 µg/ml (trough of 5 µg/ml). This oral therapy can reduce hospital length of stay (LOS) because of early stability on oral medication. Cost comparison of these drugs at the institution shows theodur tablets and a liter of aminophylline 500mg IV fluid cost the pharmacy 2-3 cents and $1:30, respectively. The patient was charged $2:15 for the theodur tablet and $18:40 for the aminophylline drip due to personnel time and other materials like needles, pumps, etc. The aim of the study was to assess the impact of pharmacy-developed monthly education program on physicians prescribing habits and cost of theophylline therapy. The study was conducted in two phases, which are pre-ed (first two-month audit period) with no education and no clinical pharmacist on service, and post-ed (second two-month audit period) with education and no clinical pharmacist on service. Education presentation by clinical pharmacist (about 10 minutes in duration), background study, and handouts were given to physicians at the beginning of each month. Results were obtained and compared with the Mann Whitney U-test for significant difference. The hospital saved $6:56 per COPD patient while the patient or third-party payer saved $103:60 per COPD patient. The program cost $2:50 of clinical pharmacy time. There was a statistical significant difference in length of intravenous therapy between the two groups. That is to say that the education program shortened the length of therapy ($P = 0.0004$). However the LOS couldn't reach significant difference between the two groups in spite of the 3 days difference in nonsevere patients (no difference in severe patients). It was projected on the basis of this result that a total cost of $3 million and $43 million patients' charges could be saved if all hospitals were to implement the program.[45]

Levin et al. studied the effect of pharmacist's intervention on the use of serum drug assays in a 65-bed community hospital, the Good Samaritan Hospital, Baltimore, Maryland (MD). The aim of the study was to evaluate prescribers' use of serum drug assays (SDR), the impact of clinical pharmacist's education on physicians' use of SDA and drug-related patient care performance for medical audit committee. Subjective and objective criteria for each drug evaluation were based on rational indication (subtherapeutic treatment, noncompliance before admission and toxicity), rational performance (timely blood sample and achievement of steady state), and rational adjustment of dosage due to SDA results (dose and frequency of dosing). The study period experienced a greater number of admission (480 against 384 patients) but the results revealed that the number of SDAs ordered went down from 154 to 105 (digoxin, which constituted- a majority went down from 95 to 57) and number of patients affected went down from 71 to 55 ($P < 0.05$). The number of SDA without indication went down from 65 (42%) to 16 (15%) and about $2,500 cost savings was realized in patient charges during the five months period. The cost of providing the services was about $260 for the entire period (15mins/SDA). Prior to the introduction of the service, one patient whose SDA was inappropriately drawn 2 to 3 hours after digoxin dosage had a supposedly "toxic level of the drug, consequently the drug was discontinued. The patient was discharged and readmitted back to the hospital one week later for congestive heart failure (CHF). Digoxin is known to prevent or reduce hospitalization rate of CHF patients; hence, the drug (about $10/month) in this patient resulted in his readmission with concomitant wastage of healthcare resources (large sum). [46]

Elenabaas et al. investigational study at Truman Medical Center, Kansas City, Missouri (MO) revealed what it takes for a specialist to be in control of his destiny. They studied the influence of clinical pharmacist consultations on the use of drug blood level tests. It has been reported that most drug blood level tests are either done inappropriately or overused and misinterpreted because of inadequate knowledge about the test or pharmacokinetic. However, clinical pharmacists have displayed their expertise as drug specialists in this area judging by past experience. Truman Medical Center demonstrated this in January 1978 when they mandated all drug blood level tests to go through clinical pharmacists. "The policy made consultation by a clinical pharmacist a prerequisite to ordering a drug blood level test and stated that no drug level analysis would be performed without the authorization of a PharmD. The study was divided into control period (6 months, July 1977 to December 1977, prior to policy) and study period (12 months, January 1978 to January 1979, post policy). Average admissions per month during the periods were the same (634 for control group and 635 for study group) and results revealed that 908 assays in 6 months for control group against 1,083 assays in 12 months for study group were performed. This resulted in 151 ± 22 assays per month for control group and 90 ± 15 per month for study group ($P < 0.001$). A total cost saving of $12,086.61 in a year was realized. Mann-Whitney U test was used to analyze the results that took the cost of providing pharmacokinetics services into consideration. The reduction in number of assays performed was found to be 40% and this agreed with similar researches cited in the study. The study noted numerous factors such as dosage, time of dosing, quantity (size), elimination rate and sampling of time that are some of the basic principles of pharmacokinetics were often neglected by the physicians. These neglects often result in complications and misinterpretation of laboratory data; hence, education and training of most physicians by clinical pharmacists became important. Most hospitals now conduct their pharmacokinetics services through the pharmacy.[47]

Horn et al. conducted an evaluation of digoxin pharmacokinetic monitoring service in a community hospital and found improved condition of service for the hospital. The aim of the study was to evaluate the effect of pharmacokinetic service (PKS) on digoxin serum drug concentration and patient outcome in terms of LOS and toxicities. The prospective study involved 218 patients in before and after groups and with outside target range digoxin serum level. A clinical pharmacist provided the after group with PKS realizing the fact that inappropriately drawn digoxin sample (e.g., during distribution phase or before steady state) could be misleading. Results of the study showed that appropriately drawn sample was 79.3% in after group compared with 68.1% before group ($P < 0.05$, $X^2 = 5.22$). Patients in therapeutic range of 1.5-2.2ng/ml were 55% in after group (or 63.6% when physicians followed PKS dosing recommendations by clinical pharmacist) and 23.3% before group ($P \leq 0.05$, $X^2 = 3.94$). Toxicity (i.e., > 2.5ng/ml) was 10% in after group (none when PKS recommendation were followed) and 23.3% in before group. The length of stay was 11.6 days for after group and 15.3 for before group. The number of SDAs was reduced by 22% in the after group and a total cost saving of $7,920 (396 unneccesary SDAs) per year was estimated when the data/record was extrapolated to one year for the hospital. The 5 months study found 40 unnecessary SDAs with an estimated savings of $800 and the cost of providing PKS was $690 for 92 patients. The savings would have been more if the clinical pharmacist's recommendations were followed; for instance, the clinical pharmacist recommended discontinuation of digoxin in 11 asymptomatic CHF patients, 9 of which had serum level less than 0.8ng/ml (below trough level which makes treatment worthless) but was ignored.[50]

In light of the 300% increase in United States hospitals drug expenditure from $1 billion in 1972 to $3 billion in 1982 (a decade) and the more than 300% noninflationary dollars increase in University of Minnesota Hospital's antibiotic expenditures since 1982, Fletcher et al. decided to study pharmacist's interventions in improving vancomycin and tobramycin prescribing acts. The hospital had previously reviewed the chart retrospectively and found that inappropriate use of many high cost antibiotics of which vancomycin and tobramycin were the most culpable cause. A clinical pharmacist conducted the chart review, then designed education materials for vancomycin and tobramycin and proceeded to construct written information as well as oral follow up for the substitution of naficillin for vancomycin and gentamycin for tobramycin. The clinical pharmacist educated physicians and the study was conducted in two phases (phase1 --- 10/1/83 to 3/31/84 and phase 2 --- 4/1/84 to 9/30/84). Three month period before the commencement of the target drug program was control for comparison purposes. The result revealed an increase in the use of naficillin by 31% and gentamycin by 21% and a decrease in use of vancomycin by 27% and tobramycin by 12%. The total savings that resulted from the expenditures was $161, 396 compared with half full time equivalent of clinical pharmacist time spent for the success of the program (about $16,000 in 1984). The benefit /cost ratio was 10 to 1. Physicians were not mandated to follow the clinical pharmacist information consequently the effects of the program degenerated with time.[51]

Bootman et al. conducted a retrospective cohort/cost-benefit analysis study of individualized gentamycin dosage in burn patients with gram-negative septicemia and found that clinical pharmacists saved lives with pharmacokinetic services. Clinical pharmacists used pharmacokinetic services to individualize the dosage regimen for the purpose of influencing patient outcome. The study consisted of 66 patients in treatment group who received kinetics service from mid 1974 to 1976 and 39 patient in control group who did not receive kinetics service from 1972 to mid 1974 at St. Paul-Ramsey Medical Center, Minnesota, Minneapolis (MN). The results were analyzed with multivariate statistics, nonparametric and parametric tests. These results showed a positive correlation with survival when other parameters like complications, burned surface area, age and blood cultures were negative. Mortality rate for the nonkinetics group was about 30.3% more than the kinetics group and this translate to about 20 lives savings or 13% of the variance, which is 2.6 lives. However, the mean length of stay and infection were 93.2 days and 10.3 days respectively for the kinetics group and 72.3 days and 8.1 days respectively for the nonkinetics group. This 24-bed facility is one of the largest burn care center that admit 190 patients every year in Upper Midwest, US. The longer duration of stay and infection and the subsequent $24,488 increase in cost has been attributed to higher survival rate of the kinetics group over the nonkinetics group. The benefit/cost ratios for each discount rates of 1% (24.0), 6% (8.7 : 1), and 10% (4.5 : 1) were greater than 1(one) therefore the pharmacokinetics services was worthy of the expenditure.[52]

Peterson and Lake studied the role of a clinical pharmacist in reducing prophylactic antibiotic cost in cardiovascular surgery. The study was conducted in Abbott-North Western hospital, an 838-bed treatment center, Minnesota, Minneapolis. The clinical pharmacist took advantage of its numerous roles as member of pharmacy and therapeutics, infectious control antibiotic utilization review, quality assurance pharmacy management and other committees to design drug therapy options and reduce the duration of antibiotic prophylaxis from five to two days. Review of pharmacy drug purchases by the clinical pharmacist revealed that 30% of annual drug costs were antibiotics of which 57% accounted for cephalosporins purchases and cefamandole demand was extraordinary in the group. Further investigation showed that cefamandole was predominantly used for cardiovascular and orthopedic surgery prophylaxis against infection. The alternative therapy with equal efficacy and the resultant cost savings to patients, pharmacy, and hospital were delineated to the various committees. Results of the project revealed that use of cefazolin ($95/day) and cefuroxime ($66.20/day) in place of cefamandole ($155:93/day) ended in cost savings of $600,000/year to patients, $200,000/year to pharmacy and $105,000/year to the hospital in revenue Vs expenses improvement. Additional cost savings in less nursing time was $14,700/year and pharmacist time in drug preparation/distribution was $7,875/year. There were concerns about the efficacy of cefazolin (1st generation) in the coverage of staphylococcus epidermidis in comparison with cefamandole (2nd generation) a wider spectrum. However, this concern was dismissed with the inclusion of cefuroxime (2nd generation) another equally effective wide spectrum in the regimen. The efficacy of the new regimen was examined with post operative infection wound rate which showed 1.4% before the project and 1.3% after the project. This means greater efficacy in spite of the reduced duration from 5 to 2 days.[53]

Abramowitz, Nold, and Hatfield conducted a survey to ascertain the use of clinical pharmacists in reducing cefamandole, cefoxitin, and ticarcillin cost. The clinical pharmacists realized the fact that inappropriate use of hospital antibiotic accounted for 40-75% of a pharmacy budget and the above named drugs had enormous financial impact on the fiscal budget. They decided to use their drug expertise by checking for inappropriate prescriptions for the antibiotics and alternative drugs for the expensive ones. Second generation cephalosporins like cefamandole and cefoxitin have wide spectrum, require more frequent dosing, and almost double the cost of first generation cephalosporins. Antipseudomona antibiotics like ticarcillin and carbenicillin on the other hand, have similar spectrum of activities except that ticarcillin is two to four times more effective than carbenicillin and carbenicillin can overcome this deficiency by increasing the dosage. Carbenicillin is the preferred drug of choice in severely fluid-restricted patients because of sodium contents in other antipseudomonas like ticarcillin. The aim of the study was to determine the effectiveness of clinical pharmacists in recommending cefazolin ($13.14/day) as alternative therapy for cefamandole and cefozitin ($34.56-$39.44/day) and carbenicillin ($17.70/day) for ticarcillin ($41.76/day) and ascertains the subsequent financial reward at the University of Chicago hospital and clinics, Chicago, IL. The study was conducted in two phases, which are phase 1 (7/1/80-3/31/81) as control group and phase 2 (4/01/81-9/30/81) as study group. Pharmacy invoice/records were used on quarterly basis to assess the project and 8 clinical pharmacists used education program to promote the project among physicians. They encouraged the use of cefazolin and other narrow spectrum antibiotics when appropriate and other antibiotics including cefoxitin and cefamandole when culture and sensitivity results or hospital microbiology reports demanded their usage. Clinical pharmacists recommended substitutions when any antibiotic was considered inappropriate during the 90-bed segment review by each pharmacist. Results revealed that pharmacy department spent $177,310 on second-generation cephalosporin, $63,403 on first generation cephalosporin, $60,412 on ticarcillin and $10,886 on carbenicillin during phase 1. This amounted to average monthly cost $26,745 for cephalosporin and $7,922 for ticarcillin and carbenicillin and yearly cost of $233,448 for phase 1 drugs. Pharmacy purchase for phase 2 was $101,261 or $16,877 per month for cephalosporin in spite of the price increase by 7/1/81and this amounted to $118,428 savings in a year. The total cost of ticarcillin and carbenicillin in phase 2 was $28,370 or average monthly cost of $4,728 and this amounted to monthly savings of $3,194 and yearly savings of $38,382. The total savings realized from the project was $156,756 and the cost of providing clinical services was $16,000. Cefamandole and cefoxitin accounted for 59.8% antibiotic usage in phase 1 and 39.7% in phase 2. Ticarcillin usage was 77.1% in phase 1 and 16.6% in phase 2. It is worthwhile to mention that total cephalosporin dose decreased by 10% while average monthly number of patient days decrease by 4%.[54]

Knapp et al. studied the relationship between inappropriate drug prescribing and increase length of hospital stay in three General Care Hospitals in Maryland, Baltimore and found that inappropriate drug prescribing was responsible for half (50%) longer length of stay. The study consisted of retrospective review of 77 pyelonephritis medical records between January 1974 and June 1978 and the criteria used in judging appropriateness of drug were patient specificity, drug specificity, and correlation of infecting organism to drug. Investigators chose antimicrobial drugs because of wide spread inappropriate drug usage which has been documented in various studies. Results revealed that inappropriate prescribing was linked to two days or 50% longer length of stay (LOS) than appropriate prescribing. Mean LOS was 4.5 days for appropriate prescribing and 6.3 days for inappropriate prescribing (t = 3.55, P < 0.05). The result was analyzed with student's two-tailed t-test for unpaired data and found to be significant. Other variables such as age and seriousness of disease didn't make any difference, and there were some concerns that the longer duration of stay might be due to the affected physicians' desire to keep their patients longer than expected in hospital (after remission). The investigator concluded by requesting for more similar studies, and if similar results are obtained then pharmacist consultations would be necessary for improving drug therapy.[55]

Herfinda, Bernstien, and Kish studied the effect of clinical pharmacy services on prescribing in an orthopedic unit and found that clinical pharmacy services were responsible for decreased length of stay by 5.6% and decreased course of therapy per patient, number of doses, drug costs, etc. This cross-sectional study is comprised of three phases, which are 9 months of phase 1 without clinical pharmacist, 12 months of phase 2 with clinical pharmacist services, and 6 months of phase 3 after clinical pharmacist service. The study spread from July 1, 1978, to September 30, 1980, with an experimental site/clinical pharmacy services in a 500-bed university teaching hospital (University of California, San Francisco) and a control site without pharmacy services in a similar, 400-bed university teaching hospital in another California city. Clinical pharmacist provided in-service education about drugs to physicians and nurses, and took part in daily rounds, monitored patients' medication during the study phase, and documented recommendations made to physicians. Results were analyzed with chi-square test, one-way, and two-way analysis of variance (ANOVA). From phase 1 to 2, the experimental group in comparison to the control group experienced decreased length of stay by 5.6%, and decreased number of doses, course of therapy per patient, and cost of drugs including antibiotics. These decreases were statistically significant, and patients with or without implants who were on prophylactic antibiotic after drainage-tube removal had a significant reduction in duration of therapy from 106 hours in phase 1 to 35 hours in phase 2. Prescribers' overall compliance with guidelines for postoperative antibiotic prophylaxis was not significant. During the study phase, 1,196 consultations took place; 76% were unsolicited, 13% were solicited by physicians, 11% were solicited by nurses, and 47% of these consultations involved drug recommendations for specific medical condition, while 10% were dosage questions. One clinical pharmacist provided the service in the experimental site and it was difficult to find matched control site because of sufficient availability of clinical pharmacists in most sites.[56]

McKenney et al. conducted a survey on the effect of clinical pharmacy services on patients with essential hypertension and discovered that a clinical pharmacist had great impact on blood pressure control. The investigators were motivated by some concerns, which show that an estimated 85% of patients with undiagnosed, untreated, or inadequately treated hypertension and noncompliance problems arise because of adverse drug reactions, unavailable patient education programs, lack of motivation and continuity of care, prolonged waiting time, high cost of medications, and inaccessible/unavailable facilities. The investigators decided to examine the role of clinical pharmacists in meeting these needs. The study consists of 50 hypertensive patients who were randomly assigned to experimental and control groups (25 each) in Model Neighborhood Comprehensive Health program Inc., (MNCHP), Detroit, Michigan. Study patients were about 15 pounds heavier than patients in the control group and all patients' general knowledge of hypertension, dietary, and drug management were accessed with the administration of true and false questionnaires before the commencement of the program and after the last visit. Patients in both groups received medical care from two health center physicians; however, the study patients saw a clinical pharmacist every month on the basis of appointment. The clinical pharmacist rendered clinical services, which included education and many other issues, before making recommendations about therapy changes to the physician. Results showed greater knowledge of hypertension and treatment for the study group than the control group (F [1, 32] = 23.407; P < 0.01). Compliance problems in the control group remained the same before (4 patients), during (4 patients), and after (3 patients), while it improved in the study group before (6 patients), during (19 patients), and after the program (6 patients). The difference was significant (X^2 [1] = 14.487; P < 0.001). The number of control patients with normal blood pressure (BP) were before (11 out of 25), during (5 out of 24), and after the program (3 out of 21), while the study patients were before (5 out of 24), during (19 out of 24), and after the program (10 out of 24). The decrease in BP was significant in the study group compared to the control group (F [1, 46] = 21.988; P < 0.001). Most of the study patients were noncompliant and hypertensive before and after the study. The clinical pharmacist identified 59-suspected ADR because of treatment and helped to manage them through education, therapy, or dosing frequency alterations, etc. Patients complied with pharmacist's appointment most of the time (92%) and appreciated the services rendered by the clinical pharmacist.[57]

Gattis and others studied the effect of adding a clinical pharmacist to heart failure management team on reduction of heart failure events at Duke University Medical Center Institutional Review Board, Durham, North Carolina (NC), and found that such additions save lives. The study consisted of 181 heart failures and left-ventricular dysfunction (ejection fraction < 45) patients who were randomized into control and intervention groups. One clinical pharmacist provided patient education, medication evaluation, follow-up services/monitoring, and therapeutic recommendations to physicians in the intervention group, while the control group received no clinical pharmacy services. Characteristics of both groups were similar at the beginning of the study except that the intervention group patients were slightly older and a blind endpoint committee comprised of physicians evaluated the clinical events/results. During the 6 months median follow up, the results of all-cause mortality and nonfatal heart failure showed that 4 events occurred in the intervention group against 16 events in the control group (95% CI 0.07 - 0.65; P = 0.005). Patients in the intervention group received higher doses of an angiotensinogen-converting enzyme inhibitor (ACEI) than the control group (P < 0.001) and 75% of other patients who couldn't take ACEI for one reason or another were given vasodilator in the intervention group while 26% were given similar treatment in the control group during follow up (P = 0.02). Significant decrease in readmission rates was also noted in the intervention group: 29% against 42% in the control group.[58]

In light of the fact that 3 to 5% of all hospital admissions and 15 to 30% of all hospitalized patients experienced adverse drug reactions, McKenney and Wasserman decided to study the effect of advanced pharmaceutical services on the incidence of adverse drug reactions (ADR) and found that such services significantly reduced ADR. The aim of the study was to examine the impact of three levels of pharmacy services on ADR in an inpatient medical center. The three levels of pharmacy services were flock stock drug distribution system, flock stock drug distribution system with clinical pharmacy services, and unit dose drug distribution system/pharmacy technician program with clinical pharmacy services. The study period lasted thirty days at each level and a pharmacist investigator as well a nurse monitor from Boston Collaborative Drug Surveillance Program monitored the ADR with data collection. Results revealed no significant difference in the number of drugs administered during the study; however, ADR incidences dropped from 26% of 116 patients in period 1 to 16% of 112 patients in period 2 (not statistically significant, P < 0.1, chi-square analysis); toxicity and allergic reactions dropped from 11% to 6% and 4% to 1% respectively (P < 0.05, significant); and the number of patients experiencing ADR dropped from 20.7% of 77 patients in the 1st period to 15.6% of 64 patients in the 2nd period and 8.2% of 73 patients in the 3rd period (P < 0.05, chi-square analysis—statistically significant). Antimicrobials ADR dropped from 13.6% in the 1st period to 3% in the 3rd period; the length of stay in hospital decreased by 4 days from period 1 to 2 and nearly 4 days from period 2 to 3 (P < 0.01, significant). The total number of saved days from period 1 to 2 amounted to about 500 patients' days, and hospitalized patients who experienced ADR were about 50 to 80 percent more likely to stay longer than those who did not. The study buttressed the facts that with the aid of proper dosing, physicians' education, and other services, clinical pharmacists can significantly reduce incidence of ADR.[59]

Clapham et al. studied the economic consequences of two drug-use control systems in a teaching hospital by determining the impact of two pharmacy systems: pharmacist monitoring of drug therapy in patient-care area (study group) and centralized pharmacist monitoring of computerized patient profiles (control group) on length of stay (LOS), total cost per admission (TCA), and pharmacy cost per admission (DCA). The investigators' aim was to correlate appropriate pharmacotherapy with cost of care reduction, among other things. The study was performed in a 1,058-bed university teaching hospital with schools of medicine, pharmacy, dentistry, nursing, and allied health. The pharmacy department provided drug information, pharmacokinetic consultation, injectable drug program, and nutrition-support services to the entire hospital. Three pharmacy systems which are: 1. centralized unit dose cart checking (pharmacists used hospital information system [HIS] to check for accuracy and therapeutic appropriateness before filling patient's cart); 2. centralized profile monitoring (pharmacists used HIS to monitor patients' progress through their profile); and 3. patient care unit (PCU)–based monitoring (pharmacists attended rounds and used HIS to monitor patients' drug therapy) were used to examine pharmacists' impact during the study period. The study period consisted of 7 months duration from December 29, 1984, to July 20, 1985, for the control group and 5 months duration from July 22, 1985, to December 6, 1985, for the experimental or study group. Clinical pharmacists with doctor of pharmacy degrees (PharmD) provided the clinical pharmacy services. LOS data for 659 patients were examined retrospectively during the control period, while LOS, TCA, and DCA data for 496 patients were examined prospectively during the study period. The hospital admissions department had no knowledge of the study, so admission to study and control remain the same. Results revealed that the third pharmacy system (PCU) decreased the average length of stay by 1.5 days (3.8 days between 3 and 1 in the experimental period compared to control interval—$P < 0.005$), average TCA by \$1,293 ($P < 0.05$), and average DCA by \$155, while the second pharmacy system was associated with a decrease in average LOS by 0.13 days, average TCA by \$235, and average DCA by \$55.13 less than the first pharmacy system (unit dose system). The \$1,293 TCA reduction totals \$217,274 for the 168 patients in the PCU team (#3); the cost of providing the pharmacists' services was \$9,000. This represents about a \$208,000 cost savings for 168 patients admitted in the hospital. It is necessary to distinguish between control interval (retrospective review aimed at determining the effect of pharmacy in general during the study) and control group (pharmacy systems designed to differentiate areas of pharmacists greatest impact). The study, however, proves the facts that clinical pharmacists make their greatest impact when they are directly involved in patient care as providers.[60]

Stimmel et al.'s study compared the acts of prescribing for psychiatric inpatients by pharmacists and physicians and found that clinical pharmacists were better prescribers than physicians were. The California State Assembly passed bill 717, a five-year pilot project in which pharmacists are allowed to prescribe drugs under the supervision of a physician in 1977. University of Southern Californian School of Pharmacy was one of the two places where the project was executed in 1978. Pharmacists were required to pass written exams in physical assessment, pathophysiology, and clinical therapeutics before participating in the program. The study was conducted in a 40-bed health maintenance organization (HMO) mental health facility. Pharmacists where given diagnosed patients who needed treatment, and as a result they were expected to have biweekly review meetings with the supervising physicians. Two psychiatrists and three pharmacists participated in the program and were aware of the study. A panel of four clinical judges comprised of two psychiatrists and pharmacists randomly selected 60 prescriptions with a break down of 20 neuroleptic drugs, 20 anticholinergic drugs (used to treat neuroleptic-induced Parkinson's-like syndrome), and 20 antidepressants for each prescriber. A special triplicate prescription form with information about age, sex, weight, diagnosis, other drug therapy, and other diagnoses was designed for the project. These attributes or information were similar for all and the prescribers' identities were deleted from the triplicate form before evaluation. Results were analyzed with two-tailed student's t-test with $P < 0.05$, and Student-Newman-Keuls was used to compare mean scores for each prescriber. Judges mean scores were rated and found to be the same irrespective of their specialty. Data for the three categories of drugs showed the following:

Neuroleptic drugs: combined six scales showed that the pharmacists' scores were significantly better than physicians' ($P < 0.04$). The pharmacists' choice was discovered to be more appropriate without drug interactions.

Anticholinergic drugs: combined six scales showed no significant difference. Physicians' scores were better than pharmacists' in terms of drug appropriateness, while pharmacists' scores were better than physicians' in terms of directions appropriateness.

Antidepressant drugs: combined six scales showed that pharmacists' scores were significantly better than physicians' ($P < 0.003$). Pharmacists' scores were better in terms of drug necessity, positive effect on patients, appropriateness of drugs, and directions.

All drugs: combined six scales showed that the pharmacists' scores were better than the physicians' ($P < 0.001$).

The project thus vindicated pharmacists as better prescribers than physicians in treating psychiatric patients.[62]

Haig and Kiser studied the effect of pharmacists' participation on a medical team on costs, charges, and length of stay and found that such participation resulted in significant savings. The prospective study was conducted in a 774-bed community teaching hospital from February to December 1989 (11 months) and the dependent variables were LOS, total hospital charges, and total pharmacy costs and charges. The pharmacists were bachelor of science degree holders and they were not allowed to write in a patient's chart without the approval of the physician. The study consisted of 24 hours on-call control group team A (without pharmacist) and study group team B (with a pharmacist). The two teams operated independently and results were analyzed with student's t-test and chi-square. The study period was divided into four phases, which are: 1. February to June (attending physicians rotated monthly), 2. July to December (a permanent attending physician in team A), 3. February to December (the entire study period), and 4. the entire study period without LOS that is greater than 30 days. Data for 619 patients showed that study team B had significantly lower per-patient pharmacy costs ($173 against $351), pharmacy charges ($679 against $1,176), hospital charges ($6,371 against $10,236), and LOS (6.3 against 8.8 days) compared with control team in phase 1. There was no significant difference in phase 2 but phase 3 showed significantly lower per-patient pharmacy costs and charges than team A. In phase 4, team B had significantly lower per-patient pharmacy cost ($173 against $278—$P = 0.0124$), pharmacy charges ($652 against $1,020—$P = 0.0008$), hospital charges ($6,122 against $8,187—$P = 0.0013$, and LOS (5.9 against 7.2 days—$P\ 0.0036$) than control team A. Areas of greatest impact by pharmacists were drug selection, dosing, avoidance of ADR, counseling, ordering and timing of lab tests. The permanent physician in phase 2 was described as an erudite fellow with impeccable knowledge of drugs. The pharmacists made some impact during phase 2, but they were not significant.[63]

Bjornson et al. studied the effects of pharmacists on healthcare outcomes in hospitalized patients and found that pharmacists save lives and money. The one-year (–October 1990 to September 1991 for medicine and February 1991 to January 1992 for surgery) nonrandomized comparative study took place in Walter Reed Army Medical Center (WRAMC), Washington, D.C., and it was comprised of all 3,081 patients in general medicine and surgery. Data for

557 patients who were not in the study were also used. Patients were separated into five medical teams, two of which included a pharmacist and three surgery teams, one of which included a pharmacist. The dependent variables that were measured are length of stay (LOS), a measuring parameter for morbidity, drug cost per admission, and mortality. International Classification of Diseases, Ninth Revision (ICD-9-CM), was used to categorize patients, and results were analyzed with two-way analysis of variance (ANOVA), student's t-test, chi-square, descriptive and inferential statistics. The three medical teams without a pharmacist (MT) and two surgical teams without a pharmacist (ST) were the control groups, while the two medical teams with a pharmacist (MPT) and one surgical team with a pharmacist (STP) were the intervention groups. Patients transferred to intensive care units (ICU) were more from MT subgroup than MTP subgroup (8.5% against 5.9%; $X^2 = 5.8$, $P = 0.02$), and pharmacists' recommendations were 86.7% fully accepted by the MTP physicians and 82.8% fully accepted by STP physicians. Data showed significant reduction in LOS ($P = 0.032$) and drug cost per admission as Log drug cost per admission ($P = 0.048$) for intervention groups than control groups. Although there were differences in mortality rate, 21 deaths (1.75% mortality) in the intervention group compared with 46 deaths (2.45% mortality) in the control group, the statistics were not strong enough for significance ($X^2 = 1.68$, $P = 0.2$—no significant difference). The overall average cost savings resulting from the study or inclusion of a pharmacist in the team was $377 per admission, and this amounted to a $150,951 annual cost savings with a cost- benefit ratio of 6.03:1.[64]

Monson (MD) et al. studied the role of a clinical pharmacist in improving drug therapy and found that clinical pharmacists can save money as well as improve prescription-writing skills (drug therapy) and compliance. The aim of the study was to demonstrate the effect of a clinical pharmacist on physician prescribing habits, patient compliance, medical records, and documentation with chronic management of medication regimen in ambulatory setting (outpatient therapy). The study consists of 81 patients in the control group and 133 patients in the study group from a sample group of 355 patients, which was randomly selected from all clinics and followed up in a rheumatology and renal clinic. The selection of the clinics was based on complex and multiple drug regimens, while data was taken from medical records and prescription files by pharmacists (not involved in the study). Records were reviewed and examined for accuracy and completeness of physician prescriptions ordered and then compared (between rheumatology/renal clinic and pharmacy files). The control period lasted for six months without a clinical pharmacist (before), while the study period lasted for nine months after the introduction of a clinical pharmacist in the clinics. Results were analyzed for 6 months and the data showed that the control group averaged 4.6 prescriptions per patient, while the study group averaged 3.1 prescriptions per patient (P < 0.05); 60 (16%) out of 373 prescriptions dispensed to patients were not documented for the control group, while 6 (1%) out of 512 prescriptions were not documented for the study group (P < 0.001). Accuracy in terms of recording drug name, strength, dose, and directions in medical records showed that 7 (9%) of the control group patients met the criteria, while 77 (59%) of the study group patients met the criteria (P < 0.001). Prescription-duplication records showed 221 (37%) out of 594 prescriptions were duplicated for the control group (46 patients—4.8 duplicate prescriptions per patient), while 200 (28%) out of 712 prescriptions were duplicated for the study group (66 patients—3 duplicate prescriptions per patient) (P < 0.001). Compliance records showed that 15 (20%) of the control group patients and 71 (72%) of the study group patients were in compliance with all medications or 80 (33%) prescriptions for the control group against 211 (85%) prescriptions for the study group. Using 1976 data, an estimated annual savings of $31,641 resulted from $16,879 cost reduction in decreasing the number of prescriptions from 4.6 to 3.09, and $14,762 avoidance of duplication for 452 patients.[65]

Packer et al. examined the effects of pharmacists' clinical interventions on nonformulary drugs used in a 719-bed Rhode Island teaching hospital and found that the pharmacists saved the hospital money. The 1983 amendments of the social security act heralded the implementation of a prospective pricing system, and this pricing system coupled with hospital formulary that had been in existence since 1960 made the Rhode Island teaching hospital establish a governing rule for usage of nonformulary drugs. The rules required physicians to complete a "nonformulary medication request" form signed by the attending physician before nonformulary drugs could be approved and dispensed. The pharmacist was expected to influence the physicians' prescribing habits by using this system to promote effective rational drug use and decrease inventory cost through prescription checking for nonformulary drugs. Once the pharmacist cites a nonformulary drug, he is expected to contact the affected physician and possibly recommend an alternative drug in the formulary or usage of the form if the physician so desired. The four-month study (January to April 1984) was conducted with the aid of two different unit dose drug distribution systems, which are: 1. centralized unit dose pharmacy services in the 187-bed Jane Brown Memorial Building (the control group with no pharmacist in patient-care area) and 2. four decentralized pharmacy services tagged "pharmacy service units" (PSU) at the main building (the study group with clinical pharmacists providing pharmaceutical services in patient-care area). The clinical pharmacists were required to document their interventions and the time spent on it or use pharmacists' consultation log.

Results were compared, reviewed, and analyzed with student's t-test and a chi-square test. Data showed that out of 394 cases of nonformulary drug use by physicians, 388 pharmacist contacts were made (others couldn't be reached). Out of 388 contacts 230 resulted in alternative formulary drug recommendations and 149 (64.8%) of these recommendations were accepted by physician. Out of the 149 accepted recommendations, 113 (75.8%) were made by the clinical pharmacist in the study group (PSU), while the control group or centralized pharmacy made 36 (24%). Physicians' refusal to accept recommendations was 17.3% in PSU against 30.1% in centralized pharmacy. The cost savings (i.e., nonformulary-formulary drug cost) that resulted from the intervention was $2,645 or $13,573 per year. The estimated cost of providing the pharmacy services was $1,497 in a year ($993 for pharmacist's service and $504 administrative cost).[66]

Brown studied pharmacists' participation in a multidisciplinary rehabilitation team in the 340-bed Union Hospital, a community teaching hospital in Indiana, and found that such participation resulted in savings for the hospital and patients. The rehabilitation unit in the hospital is a 12-bed section with patients mostly over 60 years old on regimens consisting of several drugs for disease states. The average length of stay is four weeks or more if the debilitating conditions persist or degenerate because of other factors such as adverse drug (ADR). The multidisciplinary teams that often cater to the needs of these patients were physical therapy, psychology, nutrition, social work, nursing, and others without the pharmacists. In February 1992, the situation changed for good when a clinical pharmacist was included in the team. The role of the clinical pharmacist was to review a patient's drug regimen for appropriateness, access patient's ability to follow drug instructions, determine ADR, monitor patient's daily progress, and recommend therapy changes if need be. Patient or family's drug education starts from admission to time of discharge. The entire pharmacist's intervention was documented and reviewed every month. At the end of six months (August 1992), results showed that 83 patients received clinical pharmacy services and the pharmacist made 184 recommendations for therapeutic modification. 167 out of the 184 recommendations were accepted, with a breakdown of 19 untreated conditions, 12 improper drug selection, 27 improper drug dosage, 9 drug interactions, 56 unnecessary drugs, 16 changes in drug administration route, 27 ADR, and 1 patient's failure to receive drugs. 90% of the patients had more than 6 medications for their multiple ailments before the intervention. At the end of the six-month period, the 83 patients saved $14,990, while the hospital saved $2,700 in drug costs. The pharmacist's time spent in providing these services ranged from 8 to 10 hours in a week depending on the patient's condition and admission census.[67]

Ryan et al. studied the economic justification of the pharmacist's involvement in patient medication consultation and found that the pharmacist's involvement improved therapy and saved money. Patient compliance is a monumental issue in ensuring a patient's well-being and it is known to be influenced by two major factors, which are: 1. medication acquisition ability (traveling distance, transportation, physical well-being, finances, etc.) and 2. patient's knowledge/understanding of his disease state and treatment (medication) goals. This project was designed to examine the impact of finance, ADR, safety, and compliance with medication on patients during a medication discharge interview by a pharmacist. The study took place in a 120-bed two-surgery unit University Hospital between June 1973 and February 1974. 1000 patients participated in the program and the pharmacist spent an average of 11.2 minutes for each discharge interview. The pharmacist noticed that physicians were in the habit of prescribing expensive medication irrespective of the patient's status. The interviews revealed that many of the patients have no third-party health insurance and were not financially buoyant enough to afford the drug, so the pharmacist contacted the physician for less expensive medication or help to obtain health insurance coverage for eligible patients or write alternative formulary drugs for medical assistance program patients. Other assistance rendered by the pharmacists includes recommendation of over-the-counter medications, re-labeling of bedside medications that were to be duplicated, and clarification of illegible prescriptions. Results showed a cost savings of about $1,700 for 357 patients (35.7%); this amounted to $9:13 patient's savings per pharmacist hour of interview. Re-labeling saved $498:12 and avoided therapeutic duplication of 135 prescriptions.[68]

Meisel studied the cost-benefit analysis of clinical pharmacy services in a 250-bed community hospital, St. Joseph Hospital, St. Paul, Minnesota, and found savings of $125,648 to the hospital and patients. The hospital hired a clinical pharmacist coordinator in January 1982 and charged him with the responsibility of providing cost-effective clinical pharmacy services. The clinical pharmacist explored five major areas and results showed a cost savings of $125,648 to the hospital and patients over 3 years. The areas are: 1. direct patient care that included pharmacokinetic services, patient education, therapeutic consultations, hyperalimentation, monitoring, pain management, streptokinase team, and rehabilitation center activities participation—these services saved over $45,143 over 3 years; 2. quality assurance that included drug utilization review (e.g., better dosing resulted in cefazolin frequency changes from every 6 hours to 8 hours and acts of prescribing resulted in reduced usage of cefamandole), usage of drug serum levels, drug interactions, ADR, and medication error—these services saved $56,308; 3. drug information that included monthly publication of a drug information newsletter and provision of formal/informal drug information to staff and community. The newsletter is used to promote newer, less costly, and less toxic drugs at the expense of expensive drugs—these services resulted in a $113,471 savings over three years; 4. formulary management, which included the adoption of a closed formulary system and subsequent savings of $20,762 over 3 years; and 5. education of physicians, nurses, and pharmacy staff. The clinical pharmacy services cost $115,990 and the gross savings from executing the services is $241,638. The net cost-benefit is therefore $125,648 ($241,638 - $115,990).[70]

In 1994, Gina Upchurch, a pharmacist, established the PHARMAssist program purposely to assist senior citizens with limited incomes gain access to medication in Durham County, North Carolina. Qualified senior citizens pay $8 for up to a 100-day supply of medication with the aid of a credit card that is issued to them. Upchurch sees the patients on a routing basis (at least twice a year) to review their medication and to educate them about compliance, ADR, drugs, their disease state, and the purpose of their medication. Kristi Ward, the other clinical pharmacist, calls homebound patients at home to perform the same function. The program is said to have catered to over 800 patients' medication needs by the year 2001 and the founder won an additional $100,000 pharmaceutical care grant because of the success of the program. The annual budget is over $500,000. Senior citizens over age 65 years are the fastest-growing segment of the American society and are projected to increase from 13% in 2001 to 20% by 2030, and most of them have no healthcare insurance for medications in North Carolina as a result their enrolment in this program enabled them to obtain their medications from any pharmacy of their choice in the neighborhood. Upchurch, Catellier, and others conducted a study to examine the impact of the program on emergency room and hospital visits. Senior citizens are eligible for the program if their income is below 140% federal poverty level with no other health insurance. By June 1994, there were 394 seniors who enrolled in the program and were studied. 120 out of the 394 seniors completed 12 months in the program, while others dropped out for reasons ranging from financial ineligibility to Medicaid enrollment or death. Medication review and interviews were conducted at baseline, after 6 and 12 months. Results of the study showed that clients' knowledge of the purpose of their medication grew from 69% at baseline to 90% after 6 months and no more after 12 months (OR = 4.5, P < 0.001). Emergency room visits declined From 57% at baseline to 51% after 6 months and 39% after 12 months or 23 % reduction at 6 months (OR = 0.77, P = 0.77) and 58% reduction at 12 months (OR = 0.42, P < 0.001) after adjusting for confounding factors with logistic regression. Hospitalization rate was 48% at baseline, 46% at 6 months, and 34% at 12 months (logistic regression adjustment showed a P < 0.001, which is significant). Within the limits of self-reporting interview bias, the program was said to be successful.[72,73]

In December 2003, the Wyoming Pharmacist Association (WPA) project, officially classified as a pharmacy technical assistance program, started in Wyoming. The aims of the project were to review qualified patient's drug regime so as to avoid drug-drug interaction, assist patients in proper utilization of their medication, and help them to save money through one-on-one pharmacist's counseling. Ralph Bartholomew, pharmacy director at Admiral Beverage Health Center in Worland, Wyoming, initiated the program with Admiral Beverage's employees. The program is now sponsored by the state legislature as a joint venture of Wyoming Pharmacy Association, Wyoming Department of Health, and the University of Wyoming. Patients who are residents of Wyoming with at least two medications can enroll in the program irrespective of their income. The main service areas are Torrington, Casper, Cheyenne, and Laramie. Patients who are interested in the program are expected to call 877-246-4114 for necessary arrangements with the school of pharmacy staff via the Wyoming Department of Health. AARP helped to propagate the program throughout the state with the aid of mass campaign. Information about approved patients is sent to one of the consultant pharmacists in one of the nearest locations (given above) to the patients, and the service commenced. The patient pays a $5 co-pay and the state government pays $70 making a total of $75 for the consultation services. The pharmacist communicates with the patient and physician about the services. The program started with a budget of $100,000 and later received an additional $300,000. As of May 13, 2004, 350 people called WPA, 335 packets were mailed to them, and 100 cases were completed. The program has been applauded by the state legislators, physicians, patients, and pharmacists who are now reimbursed for cognitive services instead of product-oriented services. John Vandel, dean of the school of pharmacy, University of Wyoming, noted that physicians have no time to spend with their patients on medication regimen, so they are happy with the program. The program is said to have saved Admiral Beverage employees hundreds of dollars on prescriptions drugs per month. One employee saved $400 per month because his medication bill went down from $525 to $125 per month as per Ralph Bartholomew, the originator of the program. These achievements were used as testimonies by Bartholomew and John Arross, former Wyoming Pharmacy Association president, to convince Wyoming legislators to approve the program (WPA) as a statewide project after hearing.[82]

Lai and Sorkin studied a cost-benefit analysis of pharmaceutical care in Maryland's Medicaid population from a budgetary perspective and found that pharmaceutical care saved Medicaid $89,287.76. In view of the dramatic increase in Medicaid expenditure from $12 billion in 1975 to $126 billion in 1993, the University of Maryland Center on drug and public policy decided to enter into agreement with the Maryland Department of Health and Mental Hygiene to render pharmaceutical care services program (PCSP) to Medicaid recipients. The aim of the study was to determine the economic impact of pharmaceutical care on Medicaid patients in four Baltimore hospitals, primary care outpatient clinics, Maryland or how appropriate drug use, cost-effectiveness of physician prescribing habits, and avoidance of hospitalization resulting from ADR can save money instead of restrictive formulary/placing unnecessary economic burden on the less fortunate. The quasi-experimental pre- and post-test design consists of a control group selected from equally matched Medicaid patients one year (April 1, 1992, to March 31, 1993) before the commencement of PCSP and an intervention group selected from 1,036 Medicaid patients who received pharmaceutical care from two clinical pharmacists (with a PharmD) one year after PCSP began. 473 intervention group patients were finally selected for the study after scrutiny. Maryland Medicaid awarded $200,000 to the PCSP program in a year and this resulted in $84,362.93 prorated cost for the 437 patients. Results were analyzed with sensitivity analysis and it revealed the total Medicaid cost for the control group pre-intervention was $1,642,787.88, while post intervention was $1,851,315.54. In the PCSP group, pre-intervention was $1,456,223.84, while the post intervention was $1,491,100.81. The difference between the two groups yielded a direct benefit of $173,650.69 minus the cost of the program ($84,362.63), giving a net present value (NPV1) of $89,287.76 or $204.32 per patient for the first year. The net present value at a 4% discount rate was calculated to be $724,203.70 per 437 patients or $1,657.20 per patient in 10 years' time. It was projected that if the service was extended to all Maryland Medicaid non-institutionalized adult patients, the state would save up to $22 million from the program in the preceding year.[76]

One of the most daring researches about clinical pharmacy services is Bond et al.'s study of the interrelationships among mortality rate, drug costs, total cost of care, and length of stay in United States hospitals. The investigators used a 1992 database of American Hospital Association's (AHA) Abridged Guide to the Healthcare Field (3,444 hospitals), National Clinical Pharmacy Services (NCPS—1,599 hospitals), and Healthcare Finance Administration (4,822 hospitals) mortality data. Multiple regression analysis was used to evaluate the severity of illness, relationships, and associations. The study population is comprised of data for 1,029 hospitals matched for mortality, 1,024 hospitals matched for length of stay, 1,016 hospitals matched for total cost of care, and 934 hospitals matched for drug cost. These four healthcare outcomes were measured against various pharmacy variables but one variable, which is the number of clinical pharmacists per occupied bed in the hospitals, was correlated with positive outcome in all four categories. The clinical pharmacy services were basically pharmacokinetic consultations, therapeutic monitoring, drug-protocol management, adverse drug reaction (ADR) monitoring, drug counseling, drug history during admission, and participation in total parental nutrition (TPN) team, medical rounds, and cardiopulmonary resuscitation (CPR) team. Results revealed the following:

Mortality: Death rate declined from 113/1,000 to 64/1,000 admissions (43% decrease) as the number of clinical pharmacists increased from the tenth percentile (0.34/100 occupied beds) to the ninetieth percentile (3.23/100 occupied beds). This decrease amounted to 395 deaths per hospital with an admission rate of 8,061.39 ± 6,721.89 per year or 1.09 deaths/day/hospital. The 1992 mean pharmacist salary in hospital was $43,791 ± $12,206; reduced to the tenth and ninetieth percentiles, the mean salary became $320. Consequently, every $320 spent on pharmacist salary averts a single death in the hospital and mortality (death) rate is an excellent measurement of health outcome or quality of care. Clinical pharmacists have the greatest impact on mortality rate; however, dispensing pharmacists and technicians helped to enhance the service.

Length of stay (LOS): Three pharmacy variables correlate with a decrease in LOS and they are: drug protocol management by pharmacist, which was associated with decrease 432.76 patients-days per hospital or 152,998.80 patient days per 354 hospitals or 442,572.80 patient days per 1,024 hospitals (1% of all patient days). The cost of providing the pharmacist services in 1992 was $1,650 or $3.81/patient day saved (slope—1.30, P = 0.008). This amounted to a savings of $244.88 in LOS for every $1 spent on the pharmacist (C/B = 1; 244.88). Pharmacists' expertise in drugs helped to prevent inappropriate prescriptions and decreased ADR, which are known to increase LOS. Pharmacist participation in medical rounds resulted in a 164.82 patient-day reduction per hospital or a 25,178.46 patient-day reduction in 153 hospitals or a 168,514.65 patient-day reduction in 1,024 hospitals (0.3% of all patient days). The cost of providing the service was $31,652/year or $192.04 per patient day saved. This amounted to a savings of $4.86 in LOS for every $1 spent on a pharmacist (C/B 1:4.86; slope—1.71, P < 0.001).

The number of clinical pharmacists per occupied bed: The mean LOS decreased from 10.17 to 5.39 days/patient as the number of clinical pharmacist increased from the tenth percentile to the ninetieth percentile (i.e., from 0.34 to 3.23/100 occupied beds). This amounted to a 47% decrease in LOS or decrease of 4.78 days per patient.

Total cost of care: The death rate decreased from 105/1,000 to 68/1,000 as the total costs increased from the tenth percentile ($287,205/occupied bed/year) to the ninetieth percentile ($495,305/occupied bed/year). This amounted to 35% decrease or 298 deaths per hospital with an admission rate of 8,061.39 ± 6,721.89 in a year or 0.82 deaths reduction/day/hospital (slope—5846720642, R2 14.9%, $P < 0.0001$).

Drug cost: The death rate decreased from 91/1,000 to 72/1,000 admissions as drug costs increased from the tenth percentile ($4,623/occupied bed/year) to the ninetieth percentile ($19,628/occupied bed/year). This amounted to a 21% decrease or 153 deaths reduction per hospital with an admission rate of 8,061.39 ± 672.89 in a year or 0.42 deaths/day/hospital (slope—38609852, R2 8.2%, $P < 0.0001$).

The investigators concluded by recommending increased role or number of clinical pharmacists for patient care while decreasing the functions or number of pharmacists in dispensing and administrative cadre. They used the results of the study to warn against unnecessary decrease in cost, which might harm patients by decreasing quality of care. "Clinical pharmacist was the best indicator of improved patient care outcomes and reduced cost."[71]

Bond and Raehl of the Texas Technical University Health Sciences Center, School of Pharmacy, studied data from the National Clinical Pharmacy Services and Medicare databases and found consistent patterns in aggregate analyses as well as specific diseases. The data showed the following results:

---That the total cost of hospital care in U.S. can be reduced by five billion dollars with the addition of 1 to 3 clinical pharmacists per 100 hospital beds. This reduction was correlated with the provision of six specific clinical pharmacy services such as $5.6 million per hospital from drug information services and $8 million per hospital from medical-rounds participation.

--- 43% reduction in the number of patient deaths (average of 1.09 averted deaths per day) in hospitals with the highest level of clinical pharmacist staffing compared with lowest level of clinical pharmacists' staffing.

--- In warfarin management services, hospitals without pharmacist/warfarin provided services incurred 2,786 more deaths, $234 million more patients' charges, 316,589 more patient days, 429 more patients suffering from bleeding complications, and 8,991 more whole blood units used for transfusion because of bleeding complications.

--- In heparin management services, hospitals without pharmacists/heparin-provided services incurred 4,664 more deaths, $651 million more Medicare charges, 494,855 more patient days, 145 more patients suffering from bleeding complications, and 9,784 more whole blood units used for transfusion because of bleeding complications.[81]

OTHER STUDIES

Other studies include: Haltom et al., an eleven-year review of 305 articles of pharmacy literature, documenting the value and acceptance of clinical pharmacy (*Drug Intelligence and Clinical Pharmacy* 20 [1986]: 33-34); Schumock et al., an eight-year (1988-1995) economic evaluation of 104 articles of clinical pharmacy service (*Pharmacotherapy* 16[6] [1996]: 1188-1208); Abramowitz et al. ($91,071 to $202,815 cost-savings study of controlling moxalactam and cefotaxime use with a target drug program (*Hospital Pharmacy* 18 [1983]: 416-20); Bollish et al. 81% improvement in Obtained SLs or Pharmacokinetics services study of establishing an aminoglycoside pharmacokinetic monitoring service in a community hospital (*American Journal of Hospital Pharmacy* 38 [1981]: 73-76); Alexander et al. $40,000 annual cost savings from inappropriate therapy study of therapeutic use of albumin(*Journal of the American Medical Association* 241 [1979]: 2528-29); Alexander et al., $85,000 projected annual cost savings from monitoring and education of MDs on appropriate use of albumin (therapeutic use of albumin) (*Journal of the American Medical Association* 247 [1982]: 831-34); Hatoum et al. $221,056 annual cost savings study of patient care: contributions of clinical pharmacists in four ambulatory care clinics (*Hospital Pharmacy* 27 [1992]: 203-206, 208-209); Britton et al. $55,715 one-year cost-savings study (43.6% cost/patients/day) of cost containment through restriction of cephalosporins (*American Journal of Hospital Pharmacy* 38 [1981]: 696-99); Katz et al., $33,196 annual cost-savings study of savings achieved through cephalosporin surveillance (*American Journal of Hospital Pharmacy* 35 [1978]: 1521-23); Suzuki et al. $22,295.72 annual cost-savings study of the cost benefit of pharmacists' concurrent monitoring of cefazolin prescribing (*American Journal of Hospital Pharmacy* 40 [1983]: 1187-91); Guernsey et al. over $77,000 annual cost avoidance from inappropriate use of STCs study of utilization review of theophylline assays: sampling patterns and use (*Drug Intelligence and Clinical Pharmacy* 18 [1984]: 906-12); Klotz et al. $39,459 annual cost savings study of improved pharmacy services through pharmacist participation in medical rounds (*American Journal of Hospital Pharmacy* 33 [1976]: 349-51); Slaughter et al. $60,000 annual cost avoidance waste (49% irrational indications assays) study of appropriateness of the use of serum digoxin and digitoxin assays (*American Journal of Hospital Pharmacy* 35 [1978]: 1376-79); Schweigert et al. study of hospital pharmacy as a source of drug information for physicians (38% of drug inquiries) and nurses (46% of drug inquiries) (*American Journal of Hospital Pharmacy* 39 [1982]: 74-77); Elenbaas et al. study of the clinical pharmacist in emergency medicine, which showed that 87% of MDs feel that CPs (clinical pharmacists) are capable of offering primary care (*American Journal of Hospital Pharmacy* 34 [1977]: 843-46); Greenlaw study of evaluation of a computerized drug-interaction screening system (51% elimination of drug interaction) (*American Journal of Hospital Pharmacy* 38 [1981]: 517-21); Ivey et al. study of the $41,028 annual cost savings achieved through use of less-concentrated amino acid solution (*American Journal of Hospital Pharmacy* 36 (1979): 57-59); Roberts et al. study of the $23,844 annual cost savings from a pharmacy program to reduce parental nutrition costs (*American Journal of Hospital Pharmacy* 38 [1981]: 1519-20); Lash, $446,013 third-party cost savings from the study of financing hospitals and clinical pharmacy services (*Hospital Pharmacy* 15 [1980]: 78-88); Munzenberger et al. study of cost-impact analysis of selected clinical pharmacy functions in three hospitals (*American Journal of Hospital Pharmacy* 31 [1974]: 947-53); Dick et al. study of cost-effectiveness comparison of a pharmacist using three methods for identifying possible drug-related problems (*Drug Intelligence and Clinical Pharmacy* 9 [1975]: 257-62); Thompson study of cost-analysis of comprehensive consultant pharmacist services in the skilled nursing facility (*California Pharmacy* 26 [1978]: 22-24); Chrischilles et al. study of cost-benefit analysis of clinical pharmacy services in three Iowa family practice offices (*Journal of Clinical Hospital Pharmacy* 21 [1985]: 742-47); Covinsky et al. study of the impact of the docent clinical pharmacist on treatment of streptococcal pneumonia (*Drug Intelligence and Clinical Pharmacy* 16 [1982]: 587-91); Saklad et al. study of clinical pharmacists' impact on prescribing in an acute adult psychiatric facility (*Drug Intelligence and Clinical Pharmacy* 18 [1984]: 632-34); Self et al. study of medical education provided by a clinical pharmacist: impact on the use and cost of cortiscosteroid therapy in chronic obstructive pulmonary disease (*Drug Intelligence and Clinical Pharmacy* 18 [1984]: 241-44); Phillips et al. study of the determination of total cost-effectiveness of drug therapy (*American Journal of Hospital Pharmacy* 44 [1987]: 67); and many others.

The availability of this preponderance of evidence/studies has convinced many in the literary world, medical community, and some patients/consumers of the greatness and destination of pharmacy while others remain ignorant or skeptical simply because they refuse to acknowledge the evidence or pretend not to see it. In the medical community, physicians' school of thought and opinion about pharmacy varies from the indifferent attitude group to the great opposition group.

Indifferent attitude group: The majority of the traditional medical doctors fall into this category because they developed this indifferent attitude about pharmacy/pharmacists. They secretly admired clinical pharmacists' dexterity about drugs and acknowledge them as drug experts/therapeuticians. They seek their assistance from time to time about drug information and therapeutic judgment but showed great reservation/restraint when it comes to professional freedom/liberty for pharmacy/clinical pharmacists. Publicly some of them are prepared to do anything humanly possible to silence the clinical pharmacists, conceal facts about their studies, or pretend not to see the studies at all. Some physicians (a small number) in this category are the vocal minority of indifferent attitudes. They are contented with the present status of the pharmacist and will do anything humanly possible to preserve it. The views of these vocal minorities permeate the mainstream even against the wishes of some, and it is readily visible in the argument of the American College of Physicians-American Society of Internal Medicine (ACP-ASIM)'s paper on the scope of pharmacists' practice. The paper was a direct response to the 1999 Institute of Medicine study on medication errors. One of the most powerful statements from the paper is

"ACP-ASIM believes prescriptive privileges and initiation of drug therapy should remain under physician authority because of lack of pharmacist experience, the difference in educational training, and lack of supporting evidence."

One can conveniently analyze this statement by starting with lack of pharmacists' experience and supporting evidence. These are two issues that tend to trivialize the overwhelming evidence and preponderance studies cited above and in other places about clinical pharmacists' activities and achievement in the medical world. This view about experience and evidence relies on either ignorance of facts or the fact that the authors are trying to shy away from the truth by pretending not to recognize the studies. It is obvious that this statement did not take into consideration studies that showed that prescriptions written by clinical pharmacists are better than those written by physicians. The difference in educational training would have been more meaningful if it had specifically addressed the issue of pharmacy curriculum that presently does not teach or encourage the act of prescribing anywhere in the country or world (that is, nowhere in pharmacy curriculum, be it in the classroom, internship, residence, or fellowship is the act of prescribing taught, because such a move would be unlawful—state and federal laws ban pharmacists from prescribing). Even then one would have expected a moderation of views and thoughts in such a way that encouraged schools of pharmacy to change their curriculum by incorporating prescriptive acts that would empower the profession to aid other branches of medicine in minimizing medication errors and improving patients' therapeutic outcome. This statement, which appears to be driven by ego, selfishness, and lack of patients' interests, is one of the characteristics of the present status that encourages robbing Peter to pay Paul. These thoughts ought to be discouraged because clinical pharmacists, as acknowledged by some physicians in the above studies, have established themselves as formidable prescribers, skillful therapeuticians, drug experts, and therapeutic consultants in spite of the odds against them. Study upon study has vindicated them despite the fact that they are not taught the act of prescribing in school. Heaven and Earth know that the sky is the limit if and when schools of pharmacy decide to incorporate acts of prescribing in their curriculum. Schools of pharmacy presently teach their students how to check prescriptions, police prescribing habits of others, and everything about drugs (including dosages, frequency, effective combination of drugs, etc.—all schools might not do it the same way and it might not be everything about drugs in some schools, but nothing is supposed to be off the table about drugs in all schools of pharmacy). Many will argue that in order to be effective prescription monitors, one needs to know the act of prescribing, but the truth is that there is a difference between how to prescribe drugs and how to check for irregularities in prescriptions or prescriptions' appropriateness.

The usage of difference in educational training in the above statement can readily be correlated with difference in profession training/curriculum, a phenomenon that permeated all branches of medicine and buttresses the need for specialty. Thus, surgery curriculum is different from dentistry, internal medicine, general practitioner, ophthalmology, and others in order to prove their expertise. If there is no difference in training, one will be tempted to ask what makes a surgeon a surgeon, or a dentist a dentist, or an optometrist an optometrist, or a cardiologist a cardiologist. Be that as it may, like every other branch of medicine, pharmacy would have to run a curriculum that differentiated it from others by emphasizing its core curriculum about drugs, the basic rudimentary values of drug knowledge/treatment, and others on the students/graduates. Judging by the present-day curriculum, pharmacy is not an exception to the rule of professionalism in comparison to others such as engineering, dentistry, accountant, veterinary medicine, and others. Pharmacy course content and the number of years spent in school training rank high and even higher than some other professions that control their destiny. As a matter of fact, some branches of medicine such as dentists, optometrists, and veterinary medical doctors spent the same number of years in school training as the pharmacists and they become autonomous medical practitioners without residency requirements, if that is the major crucifixion. The question then is why is pharmacy treated differently like a child in his own area of jurisdiction? If residency is the bone of contention, the aim is to use it to augment and strengthen pharmacy, be it the addition of one to two years or more, and not to use it as a detriment in weakening the profession. All schools of pharmacy now have residency programs for interested graduates, and some graduates especially those just graduating from school are taking advantage of it. At any rate, ACP-ASIM's statement is a realization of the degree of pharmacy importance and the indispensable role the profession is beginning to play in the medical field. "The mere issuance of this statement goes a long way to show the degree of perturbation that confronts the medical world about clinical pharmacists/drug expert and contemporary day issues/reality." Realizing that they were fighting a losing battle, sometime in early 2002 the ACP-ASIM modified its views about pharmacy by endorsing the following: 1. immunizations, 2. physician education about drug interactions and cost, and 3. patient education about medications and drug safety as an extended scope of practice for pharmacists. Dr. Gans, the APhA executive vice president, in his review of the document on "opinions and insights" in *Pharmacy Today*, noted that ACP-ASIM's position was too myopic and defiant in the acknowledgement of pharmacists' success especially in nursing homes for 30 years and some projects like the Asheville and IMPACT. He argued that the healthcare system will be centered on patients/consumers and those who can provide them with low-cost high-quality service instead of physicians/hospitals that are the bone of contention in physicians' view. He marveled at the astonishment of having AphA write the scope of practice for physicians the same way the latter wants to control pharmacists' scope of practices.[77]

Unlike the previous, 1999 position/paper, the ACP-ASIM cited some research studies that justified pharmacists' years of education, residency, fellowship training, and work experience as drug/therapeutic experts. Dr. Gans's opinions and insights appear to have missed a vital key point about the ACP-ASIM's statement and that is "drug information for all branches of medicine." The ACP-ASIM's published position/paper cleverly excluded this vital point because such a move would have negated physicians' kingship position over pharmacists in relation to drug treatment. That is to say, such a statement would provide the public cogent reason to question physicians' authority and the reason why they must prevail over pharmacists about drug treatment. The facts remain that the second point, which is "physician education about drug interactions and cost" ought to be physicians' education about drug, which is the same as drug information, drug interactions, and costs. No matter what the ACP-ASIM does to divert attention from the main issue by trivializing pharmacy/pharmacists' awesome contributions to health care system to mere physician education about drug interaction and cost, nothing can take away the fact that all drug information centers in pharmacy, schools of pharmacy, hospitals, nursing homes, and other places are run by clinical pharmacists. These drug information centers and the clinical pharmacists provide enormous drug information and guidance to physicians and other medical personnel across the country today. However, the issuance of this statement is a sign of good omen to come to pharmacy; if not for any other reason, at least they have acknowledged research studies and pharmacy's crucial role in the medical field. This is something they denied in the past. In light of the above endorsement, anybody has the right to query physicians' supremacy over pharmacists if the former is to rely on the latter for education about drug interaction and cost or it is all right for the latter to educate the former about drug interactions and cost.

Supporters' group: In between the indifferent attitude and great opposition group of physicians are few traditional medical doctors, many of whom are recent graduates who support pharmacy fervently and are prepared to do anything for pharmacy's professional freedom. These recent graduates went to medical schools with a curriculum that emphasized specialty and interdisciplinary cooperation within the medical field in the interest of patients. Like the physicians with an indifferent attitude, they acknowledge the drug expertise of clinical pharmacists and are willing to take the recognition a step further by supporting pharmacy liberation or autonomy. Some of these supporters are cited in the various studies about clinical pharmacists' impact on healthcare system. They are not shy to seek clinical pharmacists' assistance in terms of drug knowledge and therapeutic judgment because they know that this is their area of jurisdiction or specialty. They see the clinical pharmacists as colleagues and coequals rather than subservient professionals.

Great opposition group: These are the traditional medical doctors who vehemently oppose pharmacy's autonomy. The majority of them graduated from an old medical school curriculum, the curriculum that emphasizes conglomeration of all branches of medicine (cardiology, optometry, ophthalmology, dentistry, pediatric, internal medicine, surgery, etc.) into one, thus making medical doctors jacks of all trades, masters of none. This set of physicians is at times considered the "old bridge"; they know how to describe the pharmacist in their own world as "a drug clerk, who is by no means different from a law school bookseller or librarian." To them, the pharmacist is a pharmacist irrespective of doctor of pharmacy degree or clinical experience. They don't want to hear anything about clinical pharmacists; they are in the old world and would prefer to take the whole world back to those days in spite of today's medical advancement through specialization. Needless to say that these doctors' perception of a pharmacist as a zombie of the medical field is enough to justify their reasoning that pharmacy/pharmacists cannot be used as a good source of drug information. They would rather sink in an ocean of drug information or die than seek the assistance of a pharmacist. Others in this category are those whose feelings of inadequacy create an uncertain world for themselves because of clinical pharmacists. They liken all their woes and failures to the emergence of clinical pharmacists. Left alone, they would prefer to remain in the old world as the only existing autocratic king with unquestionable absolute power in the medical field. They forgot about the fact that the existence of ophthalmologists, dentists, podiatrists, cardiologists, and others has not stopped the general practitioners from attending to patients' eye problems, tooth/mouth problems, children's problems, and others. Few conservative fellows among these physicians would love to go to the extreme with their views instead of modifying them, but they are in most cases surprised to see that their action is tantamount to threading a dangerous dinosaur's pathway or heading towards the dustbin of history. A typical example is the 1997 scenario at a 500-bed New York medical center where pharmacists under the leadership of Dr. Joe (PhamD) developed treatment protocols, therapeutic interchange, disease state management systems, pharmacoeconomic therapeutic evaluation, intravenous (IV) to oral (PO) therapeutic modification, and other methods in order to ensure cost-effective drug therapy/management. Unfortunately, these changes did not go down well with Dr. Gerald, one of the traditional medical doctors who have been with the medical center for several years. He was basically mad about the fact that he was being forced out of practice because of younger and less costly medical staff. He claims that pharmacy reports are used as an excuse for the excommunication attempts; consequently, he personally appealed to Dr. Joe to remove his patients from the preceding pharmacy report so that he would have enough time to rectify his prescribing habits.[75]

TREATMENT IS TO PHARMACY AS TO WHAT DIAGNOSIS IS TO OTHER BRANCHES OF MEDICINE

If general practitioners with profound didactic class work about diagnosis can go into residence and practice to master drug knowledge and treatment, what makes anyone think that pharmacists with profound didactic class work about drug knowledge and treatment cannot master diagnosis during residence and practice?

It is important to note that at the end of the day, it is not how far we train our medical personnel that matters but how well they impact the patients. We might train our medical personnel to be rocket scientists, but if the patients find greater comfort, relief, and cures with uneducated herbalists, that is where they are going to seek treatment.

REFERENCES

1. Pauley, T., R. Marcrom, and R. Randolph R. Physical assessment in the community pharmacy. *American Pharmaceutical Association NS 35 (1995):* 40-49.

2. Ojo, P., and L. Lai. Provider's cost and patient's benefit from pharmacists' accessibility to a minority community. Ft Lauderdale, Fla.: Nova Southeastern Univ., 1999, 1-16.

3. Braden, L. L. Compensation for cognitive services in the community pharmacy. American Pharmacy. NS 35 (1995): 58-65.

4. Penna, P. M. Managed care and the community pharmacists. American Pharmacy. NS 35 (1995): 54-60.

5. Friebele, E. Veteran pharmacists learn to provide clinical care. Journal of American Pharmaceutical Association NS 36 (1996): 580.

6. Pharmacy updates. Florida Pharmacy Today (September 1998): 25-27.

7. Carter, B. L., D. J. Barnette, E. Chrischilles, et al. Evaluation of hypertensive patients after care provided by community pharmacists in rural setting. Pharmacother 17 (1997): 1275-84.

8. O'Neil, C. K., and T. I. Poirer. *Impact of patient knowledge, patient-pharmacist relationship, and drug perceptions on adverse drug therapy outcomes. Pharmacother* 18(2) (1998): 333–40.

9. Pharmacy updates. *Florida Pharmacy Today (October 1999): 30.*

10. *Manning, A. Hospital druggists fix many errors, dosing mistakes could be fatal. USA Today* (1996) (from *New York Health System Pharmacist Journal).*

11. MS Pharmacy Association. The need for pharmacists' care. National Data Corp. (1995): 1.

12. Otto, A. Errors decrease when pharmacists make rounds through ICUS. Pharmacy Today 5(8) (1999): 1.

13. Christensen, D. B. Collaborative practice agreements further evidence of acceptance and success. Journal of American Pharmaceutical Association 41 (2001): 15-16.

14. Sommers, S. D., N. Chaiyakunapruk, J. S. Gardner, and J. Winkler. The emergency contraception collaborative prescribing in Washington State. Journal of American Pharmaceutical Association 41 (2001): 60-66.

15. Posey, M.L., Expanding pharmacy's horizon: VA's pharmacotherapy innovations. Journal of American Pharmaceutical Association NS 37 (1997): 379-382.

16. Allen, K., M. Snider, T. Pauley, and T. H. Self. Asthma management initiated by community pharmacists improves outcomes: Two case reports. Journal of American Pharmaceutical Association NS 37 (1997): 440-42.

17. Munroe, W. P., K. Kunz, C. Dalmady-Isreal, L. Potter, and W. H. Schonfeld. Economic evaluation of pharmacist involvement in disease management in a community pharmacy setting. Clinical Therapeutics (1997) 113-123.

18. Smith, C. P., and D. B. Christensen. Identification and clarification of drug therapy problems by Indian health services pharmacists. Annals of Pharmacotherapy 30 (1996): 119-23.

19. Keeney, E. M. Pharmacists, technicians can enhance hematology/oncology services. Pharmacy Today 3(3) (1997): 1 and 11.

20. Bluml, B. M., J. M. McKenney, M. J. Cziraky, and R. K. Elswick Jr. Interim report from project impact: Hyperlipidemia. Journal of American Pharmaceutical Association 38 (1998): 529-34.

21. Epstein, Debbie. Making an IMPACT: a ground breaking new study clearly demonstrates the value of a pharmacist-administered cholesterol management program. Retail Pharmacy News (September 1998): 1, 34-35.

22. English, T. Patients, pharmacists reflect on impact of foundation project. Pharmacy Today. 4 (1998): 1, 15.

23. Solomon, D. K., T. S. Portner, G. E. Bass et al. Clinical and economic outcomes in the hypertension and COPD arms of a multicenter outcome study. Journal of American Pharmaceutical Association 38 (1998): 574-85.

24. Njoku, O. Pharmacy-based immunization programs get noticed. Pharmacy Today 5(8) (1999): 10.

25. Posey, M. L. Medicare prescription drug benefit: An opportunity for Pharmacy. Pharmacy Today 5(8) (1999): 4.

26. Park, J. J, P. Kelly, B. L. Carter, and P. P. Burgess. Comprehensive pharmaceutical care in the chain setting. Journal of American Pharmaceutical Association NS 36(7) (1996): 443-51.

27. Posey, M. L. Medicaid payments for cognitive services: Washington State pharmacists' responds; report on Journal of the American Pharmaceutical Association study. Pharmacy Today (October 1999): 6 and 9.

28. Brocavich, J. M., and J. V. Etzel. Clinical and economic impact of pharmacy faculty and students on an inpatient population infected with the human immunodeficiency virus. The New York Health—System Pharmacist (April 1996): 8-10.

29. Jackson, M. We can improve patient outcomes. Florida Pharmacy Today June 65(6) (2001): 7-8.

30. Bunting, B. A., J. P. Miall Jr., D. G. Garrett et al. Providing pharmaceutical care issues, initiatives, and insights. Pharmacy Times Supplement (March 2000): 15-27.

31. Posey, M. L. Pediatric medication errors in hospital: Pharmacists' efforts important. Pharmacy Today 7(6) (2000): 5.

32. English, T. What's wrong with the healthcare system? Part 2: IOM report calls for major reforms. Recent case studies indicate pharmacists may be ahead of curve. Pharmacy Today 7(4) (2001): 1, 3, 31.

33. Dillon, C. L., J. R. Lopez, and C. M. Leyba. oxazepam cost—savings conversion. Hospital Pharmacy 36 (2001): 639–44.

34. Bond, C. A., (PharmD), and R. Monson (MD). Sustained improvement in drug documentation, compliance, and disease control: A four-year analysis of an ambulatory care model. *Archives of Internal Medicine* 144 (1984): 1159-1162.

35. Gray, D. R., S. M. Garabedian-Ruffalo, and S. D. Chretien. Cost justification of a clinical pharmacist-managed anticoagulation clinic. *Drug Intelligence and Clinical Pharmacy* 19 (1985): 575-80.

36. Powers, D. A. Antimicrobial surveillance in a VAMC teaching hospital— Resulting cost avoidance. Drug Intelligence and Clinical Pharmacy 20 (1986): 803-805.

37. Bootman, J. L., D. L. Harrison, and E. Cox. *The healthcare cost of drug-related morbidity and mortality in nursing facilities. Archives of Internal Medicine* 157 (1997): 2089-96.

38. Davis, Scott. *Evaluation of pharmacist's management of streptococcal throat infections in a health maintenance organization. American Journal of Hospital Pharmacy* 35 (1978): 561-566.

39. Mutchie, K. D., K. A. Smith, M. W. Mackay et al. *Pharmacist monitoring of parental nutrition: Clinical and cost-effectiveness. American Journal of Hospital Pharmacy* 36 (1979): 785-787.

40. Brakebill, J. I., R. A. Robb, M. F. Ivey et al. Pharmacy department costs and patient charges associated with a home parental nutrition program. American Journal of Hospital Pharmacy 40 (1983): 260-63.

41. Watesk, L. P., L. L. Sattler, and E. Steiger. *Cost of a home parenteral nutrition program. Journal of the American Medical Association* 244 (1980): 2303-04.

42. Adachi, W. D., A. Y. Endo, and J. Y. Tanaka. Controlling admixture waste through pharmacist monitoring. American Journal of Hospital Pharmacy 41 (1984): 883.

43. Kelly, K. L., J. O. Covinsky, K. Fender, and J. L. Bauman. *The impact of clinical pharmacist activity on intravenous fluid and medication administration. Drug Intelligence and Clinical Pharmacy* 14 (1980): 516-520.

44. Schloemer, J. H., and J. J. Zagozen. Cost analysis of an aminoglycoside pharmcokinetic-dosing program. *American Journal of Hospital Pharmacy* 41 (1984): 2347-51.

45. Self, T. H., R. F. Ellis, H. L. Davis, and M. D. Lee. Early use of oral theophylline in hospitalized chronic obstructive pulmonary disease patients: Cost containment through medical education. *Drug Intelligence and Clinical Pharmacy* 19 (1985): 749-53.

46. Levin, B., S. S. Cohen, and P. H. Birmingham. Effect of pharmacists' intervention on the use of serum drug assays. *American Journal of Hospital Pharmacy* 1981: 38: 845-51.

47. Elenbaas, R. M., V. M. Payne, and J. L. Bauman. Influence of clinical pharmacist consultations on the use of drug blood-level tests. *American Journal of Hospital Pharmacy* 37 (1980): 61-64.

48. Fudge, R. P., and P. H. Vlasses. *Third*-party reimbursement for pharmacist instruction about antihemophilic factor. *American Journal of Hospital Pharmacy* 34 (1977): 831-34.

49. Poretz, D. M., L. J. Eron, and Goldenberg et al. Intravenous antibiotic therapy in an outpatient setting. *Journal of the American Medical Association* 248 (1982): 336-339.

50. Horn, J. R., D. B. Christensen, and P. A. de Balaquiere. Evaluation of a digoxin pharmacokinetic monitoring service in a community hospital. *Drug Intelligence and Clinical Pharmacy* 19 (1985): 45-52.

51. Fletcher, C. V., R. M. Giese, and J. H. Rodman. Pharmacist interventions to improve prescribing of vancomycin and tobramycin. *American Journal of Hospital Pharmacy* 43 (1986): 2198-2201.

52. Bootman, J. L., A. I. Wertheimer, D. Zaske, and Rowland. Individualizing gentamycin dosage regimen in Burns patients with gram-negative septicemia: A cost-benefit analysis. *Journal of Pharmaceutical Sciences* 68(3) (1979): 267-72.

53. Peterson, C. D., and K. D. Lake. Reducing prophylactic antibiotic costs in cardiovascular surgery: The role of the clinical pharmacist. *Drug Intelligence and Clinical Pharmacy* 19 (1985): 134-37.

54. Abramowitz, P. W., E. G. Nold, and S. M. Hatfield. Use of clinical pharmacists to reduce cefamandole, cefoxitin, and ticarcillin costs. American Journal of Hospital Pharmacy 39 (1982): 1176-80.

55. Knapp, D. E., D. A. Knapp, M. K. Speedie et al. *Relationship of inappropriate drug prescribing to increase length of hospital stay. American Journal of Hospital Pharmacy* 36 (1979): 1334-37.

56. Herfindal, E. T., L. R. Bernstein, and D. T. Kishi. *Effect of clinical pharmacy services on prescribing on an orthopedic unit. American Journal of Hospital Pharmacy* 40 (1983): 1945-51.

57. McKenney, J. M., J. M. Slining, R. H. Henderson et al. *The effect of clinical pharmacy services on patients with essential hypertension. Circulation* 48 (1973): 1104-11.

58. Gattis, W. A., V. Hasselblad, D. J. Whellan, and C. M. O'Connor. *Reduction in heart failure events by addition of a clinical pharmacist to the heart failure management team. Archives of Internal Medicine* 159 (1999): 1939-45.

59. McKenney, J. M., and A. J. Wasserman. Effect of advanced pharmaceutical services on the incidence of adverse drug reactions. American Journal of Hospital Pharmacy 36 (1979): 1691-97.

60. Clapham, C. E., C. D. Hepler, T. P. Reinders, M. E. Lehman, and L. Pseko. *Economic consequences of two drug-use control systems in a teaching hospital. American Journal of Hospital Pharmacy* 45 (1988): 2329-40.

61. Mayer Olivia. Travis Watts: Teacher and clinician. Community Pharmacy. Nov/Dec 2001: 14 - 16.

62. Stimmel G. L., W. F. McGhan, M. Z Wincor et al., *Comparison of pharmacist and physician prescribing for psychiatric inpatients. American Journal of Hospital Pharmacy* 39 (1982): 1483-86.

63. Haig, G. M., and L. A. Kiser. *Effects of pharmacist participation on a medical team on costs, charges, and length of stay. American Journal of Hospital Pharmacy* 48 (1991): 1457-62.

64. Bjornson, D., W. O. Hiner, R. P. Potyk et al. *Effect of pharmacist on healthcare outcomes in hospitalized patients.* American Journal of Hospital Pharmacy 50 (1993): 1875-84.

65. Monson, R., C. A. Bond, and A. Schuna. *Role of the clinical pharmacist in improving drug therapy.* Archive of Internal Medicine 141 (1981): 1441-44.

66. Packer, L. A., C. D. Mahoney, D. S. Rich, and P. J. Louis. *Effect of pharmacists' clinical interventions of on nonformulary drug use.* American Journal of Hospital Pharmacy 43 (1986): 1461-66

67. Brown, W. J. *Pharmacist participation on a multidisciplinary rehabilitation team.* American Journal of Hospital Pharmacy 51 (1994): 91-92.

68. Ryan, P. B., C. A. Johnson, and R. P. Rapp. *Economic justification of pharmacist involvement in patient medication consultation.* American Journal of Hospital Pharmacy 32 (1975): 389-92.

69. Pathak D. S., and E. G. Nold. *Cost*-effectiveness of clinical pharmaceutical services: A follow - up report. *American Journal of Hospital Pharmacy* 36 (1979): 1527-29.

70. Meisel, S. *Cost*-benefit analysis of clinical pharmacy services in a community hospital. *Hospital Pharmacy* 20 (1985): 904-906.

71. Bond, C. A., C. L. Raehl, and T. Franke. *Interrelationship among mortality rates, drug costs, total cost of care, and length of stay in United States Hospitals: Summary and recommendations for clinical pharmacy services and staffing.* Pharmacotherapy 21(2) (2001): 129-41.

72. Price, Suzanne. Pharmacist wins $100,000 grant for senior pharmaceutical care program. Pharmacy Today 7(8) (2001): 9, 27.

73. Catellier, D. J., E. A. Conlisk, C. M. Vitt, K. S. Levin, M. P. Menon, and G. A. Upchurch. *A community-based pharmaceutical care program for the elderly reduces emergency room and hospital use.* North Carolina Medical Journal (2000): 1-7.

74. English, T. *Increased pharmacist/physician collaboration urged by ACP-ASIM.* Pharmacy Today 7(1) (2001): 3.

75. Katz, S., and R. Digregorio. Pharmacoethics: Withholding prescribing data from a utilization committee. *The New York Health-System Pharmacist.* 16 (1997): 7-8.

76. Lai, L. L., and A. L. Sorkin. Cost-benefit analysis of pharmaceutical care in a Medicaid population—From a budgetary perspective. *Journal of Managed Care Pharmacy* 4 (1998): 303-308

77. Gans, J. A. Pharmacists' scope of practice: Critiquing the physicians' view. Pharmacy Today 8(2) (February 2002): 14.

78. Miall John Jr. The Ashville project: A successful model to emulate - Advance practice institute: Diabetes AphA publication. March 2002.

79. Williams, J. S., M. Straight, T. Hoang, and T. Phan. Survey: Florida retail pharmacists' feelings on administering vaccines to pediatric and adult patients. *Florida Pharmacy Today* 12 (July 2002).

80. Thompson, J. F., W. F. McGhan, R. L. Ruffalo et al. Clinical pharmacists prescribing drug therapy in a geriatric setting: Outcome of a trial. *Journal of the American Society for Geriatric* 32(2) (1984): 154-59.

81. Posey, M. L. Lemons to lemonade: Making the most of consultants' visits to hospitals. *Pharmacy Today 10(11) (November 2004): 1, 18, 23.*

82. Berry, Derek. Wyoming PharmAssist: A revolution for the profession. Pharmacy Today 10(6) (June 2004): 1, 36.

83. Physicians and pharmacists team up. Generic Rx Product Report - Pharmacy Times supplement (Fall 2003): 1,15.

84. Cannistra, Justine. Pharmacists reduce preventable adverse drug events. Pharmacy Today. November 2003: 11.

85. Cannistra, Justine. North Carolina CPPs can now prescribe controlled substances. Pharmacy Today. November 2003: 22.

CHAPTER NINE

MEDICAL PROFESSION, HANDWRITING, AND ERRORS

Science and technology have shaped the world and changed humanity for good. Some of the greatest impact of science and technology is in medicine, and e-prescribing has emerged as the latest development. E-prescribing is a prescriber computer order entry (PCOE), a computerized form of writing prescriptions and sending it to the pharmacy through the Internet or printing the computerized prescription for patients to take to the pharmacy. The aim of e-prescribing is to eliminate handwriting, the consequences of illegible writing, and the subsequent adverse effects on the society. As good as it sounds, e-prescribing is in its infancy and even when it becomes widely available, will it be possible to eliminate illegible writings in the world? The answer is no, because of the following: Worldwide availability of technology, computers, and/or Internet services in medicine is low, financial resources for the implementation of such projects in many parts of the world is a great problem, electricity/good telecommunications systems that are a vital part of e-prescribing is a problem in some parts of the world, and last but not the least, the same pressure that complicates handwriting is likely to complicate e-prescribing for medical practitioners. For instance, a physician using PCOE selected occlusal-HP (salicyclic acid solution 17%) instead of ocuflox (ofloxacin solution 0.3%) with "use as directed" direction for a patient's pinkeye and sent the order to the pharmacy for dispensing. The patient's counseling by the pharmacist revealed that the medication was intended for eye instead of wart (hard skin lesion) removal, so necessary steps were taken to correct the error and prevent the mistake. The patient could have been blinded with the occlusal-HP instead of ameliorating the condition.[11]

Worldwide opinion of medical practitioners and handwriting seems universal and unfavorable. Perhaps the last place any medical practitioner would love to be judged about handwriting is public court of opinion, and a lot has been said about the issue. Some argue that the medical practitioners' writings are comparable to third-graders or elementary school children's writing, while a few others go further to say that if these writing styles were displayed at a certain level in kindergarten, the teacher would have probably identified the problem, worked on it, and called the parents for assistance. How is it that a professional that goes through some of the most intense educational training that humanity has to offer or one of the greatest professions in the history of mankind ends up with this kind of bad reputation in the most basic fundamental/rudimentary educational training? Is there any place where these writing styles are taught in medical schools if the problem is universal? The answer is no.

Handwriting is taught at an early stage in life and it develops over time through practice. Although handwriting is not taught at advanced education stages in life including medical schools, the practice is alive and individualized. Volumes of work, academic assignments, class work, and others build up pressure on students or anybody, and in an attempt to manage the situation properly the affected person develops a coping mechanism. Built-up pressure creates volcanic eruptions under the ground and the subsequent explosion on the surface of the Earth. Bad handwriting is a coping mechanism used to diffuse pressure and prevent explosion such as mutation in the spirit of Charles Darwin's theory of evolution by natural selection. Few medical practitioners cannot even read their handwriting at times because their mood at the time of writing is different from their mood as at the time they are called upon to interpret it. Bad handwriting starts with shorthand forms of writing notes during lectures and classes. The more shorthand forms of writing you see in students' notes, the greater the pressure on the affected student. Some perfect their shorthand forms of writing to the point where it becomes a norm for them in every situation even where there are no pressures. Few practitioners in this category specialize in writing for themselves. They constantly put themselves in the position of the writer as well as the reader. They think that everybody that reads their handwriting possesses supernatural intelligence or a doctor of philosophy in psychology/writing to read their mind and decipher the handwriting whenever they come across it. The irony of it all is that these practitioners double their task/job each time they write for public consumption, because they are constantly called upon to spend more precious time interpreting their handwriting for the readers.

Shortly after graduating from medical school, some practitioners go into practice and discover that the volume of work is not different from what they encountered in school; consequently, they retain the writing skills they developed in school. At various times they mix shorthand forms of writing with normal forms or write some few letters and use their pen to stretch out the remaining letters of the word in zigzag fashion or a scribbled manner or in the form of a line till the end with a period. Very few practitioners may want to use the gesture as a cover-up for spelling deficiencies like every other human being. At times these writings have nothing to do with pressure but a mere show-off or bragging attitude. However, some are able to purge themselves of these writing skills after graduating from medical school. These sets of practitioners have good perception of the public and the society. They are conscious of their writings because they know it is better to be safe than to be sorry. They acknowledge the fact that no matter how sophisticated a reader is, good writing enhances effective communications, saves time, avoids medication error, prevents therapeutic delay, makes things easier, and promotes understanding between the writer and the reader without unnecessary destructive interference. Moreover, they know that their writing can be read and diagnosed by the worst reader or the least educated person in the society.

Many will argue that medical school training is not an excuse, neither is it an exception to other professional/formal school training, because lawyers, engineers, schoolteachers, and many others go through similar school pressure. In as much as one would not like to jump to fallacy of haste generalizations about professional pressure and formal school training, it is worthwhile to say that pressure in various medical schools, law schools, engineering schools, and others varies. This is not enough reason to defend bad writing, because no matter what happens, no human writing is worthy of a human life and other consequences it unleashes on the society. Pressure causes volcanic eruptions and bad handwriting. The best way to deal with pressure and prevent it from exploding is to reduce it by any means necessary. Human writings' toll in the medical community involves all and sundry. In January 1996, a conference on hospital medication errors was held in Boston and the aim of the conference was "how to prevent errors from occurring." The conference was a direct result of Betsy Lehman's tragic story. Betsy Lehman, a 39 year-old lady at the time of her death in December 1994, was a health columnist at the *Boston Globe*. She was given four times the dose of her chemotherapy to fight breast cancer at the famous Dana-Farber Cancer Institute.[1] She developed a swollen body, abnormal EKGs, and blood tests that were ignored and treated as part of normal adverse reaction in a clinical trial or experimental treatment. She eventually died as a result of the toxicity and the mistake wasn't detected until two months after she passed away.

Stephen Fried, the author of *Bitter Pills* and husband of Diane, a patient who was floxed by Floxin in 1992 and never regained her normal self, was in the conference. Mr. Fried had gone to the conference with the hope of learning more about prescribers' inadequate drug knowledge and communication problems with patients, something he believed were the key factors in Diane's irreversible condition for a trivial illness. However, he was disappointed to note that the conference focused merely on hospital system errors rather than general problems that would have included his wife's condition. The conference was sponsored by the Institute for Healthcare Improvement (a nonprofit organization) and hosted by Dr. Lucian Leape, a pediatric surgeon. Dr. Leape enumerated his United States statistics, which showed that 1.3 millions Americans suffer various forms of injuries because of treatment in the hospital in a year. He went further to highlight the fact that 180,000 Americans out of this number died every year, 69% of the errors are preventable and 20% of the errors are attributable to medication errors, or 7% of all patients in the hospital encounter serious medical errors (i.e., without those that are injury free). Breakdown of medication errors showed 39% are due to prescribing, 38% to administrative, 12% to transcription, and 11% to dispensing. He drew a direct analogy with other spheres of human endeavor in the U.S. and discovered that hospital errors alone in the medical field (without nursing home, community clinics and pharmacies, and others) are comparable to three jumbo-jet crashes per two days, 84 unsafe landings per day, 16,000 lost parcels of mail per hour by the postal service, and 32 bank check errors per hour by the bank. He noted that unlike the medical practitioners, airline pilots died with their passengers (a probable reason for apathy) and the system dwells on whom to blame rather that what went wrong. In a hypothetical situation, he assumed that a doctor probably makes errors 1% of the time and the pharmacist and nurse make error 0.1% of the time because they are more careful about drugs than doctors are. He later introduced Michael Cohen, a pharmacist and "a single voice in the wilderness" of medication error.[1]

Michael Cohen developed the habit of collecting reports of medication and device errors in early 1970s as a young pharmacist with Temple University Hospital, Philadelphia, and later founded a nonprofit organization known as the Institute for Safe Medication Practices (ISMP) in 1989. The medication error reporting section of the organization was later relinquished to United States Pharmacopoeia (USP) in late 1990s. Though he had no statistics because most of the collected errors over the years were anonymously reported to him, Cohen informed the audience that the errors were mostly due to unreadable doctor's orders, confusing product labels, or improper IV connections. Pharmacists and nurses who were at the receiving end of medication errors' blame made most of the reports to Cohen to justify their innocence to a large extent. In *Bitter Pills*—appendix "The Antidotes," Mr. Fried highlighted nine points on "how to make your doctor write smarter prescriptions." One of the nine points stressed the fact that the patients need to "ask what each prescription is for," and a section of it says, "If you can't read something on the prescription, ask what it says—doctors' handwriting is notoriously illegible."[1]

"Doctors' handwriting is notoriously illegible" is a general comment about all doctors and not just some. Unfortunately, this comment is not a personal view that can be dismissed with ignominy but a worldwide opinion. At what point will the practitioners who are mostly guilty of this ominous act that has tinted and stigmatized the whole medical community say enough is enough, it is time to put our house in order by calling a spade a spade, and do the right thing by writing legibly for public consumption? It is difficult to quantify how many lives have been lost as well as the resultant economic consequences of dangerous bad handwriting on a worldwide scale. In 1995, the Supreme Court of Alabama affirmed a jury verdict in which the plaintiff was awarded $100,000 compensatory damages and $150,000 punitive damages making a total of $250,000 against a corporate pharmacy. In the lawsuit tagged *Harco Drugs Inc. v Holloway*, the plaintiff alleged that the pharmacy had insufficient institutional controls over how prescriptions were filled. The corporate pharmacist had incorrectly filled the plaintiff's prescription for tamoxifen with tambocor (flecainide acetate), a cardiac arrhymic medication for breast cancer medication, because of illegible handwriting. During the hearing, another pharmacist, who works for the corporate pharmacy and who was present when the plaintiff came back to question the prescription that was misfiled, claimed that the prescription was illegible and as a result he would have committed the same error at a busy time. However, the Court heard that the pharmacist acknowledged the practitioner as an oncologist and the medication as a heart disease drug. The court's bone of contention was the prescription's illegibility and the highly unusual nature for the prescriber, an oncologist, to prescribe dangerous heart medication. These two issues were sufficient enough to raise a red flag for the pharmacist; consequently, the Court believed that the corporate pharmacy that is responsible for its employees' actions under the vicarious liability principle acted in a reckless manner, disregarding the safety of others. The monetary reward according to the court was to compensate for the irreparable physical injury/damage as provided by the law (second-best solution). The authors of the article argued that this case and the law here are interpreted to mean that pharmacists must look at the therapeutic implication of unclear order especially patient's condition and practitioner's area of jurisdiction before filling the prescription.[2]

This case readily brings into play the issue of collective responsibility for pharmacists. Pharmacy is perhaps the only profession in the world where people can be held responsible for others' mistakes instead of their sole mistakes. Normally people are held responsible for their own actions. If an order is unclear and it is glaring to all and sundry, no matter where it is tendered, that the order is unclear one would have expected the finality of the case to rest there and then on the culprit. Anytime the Court uses the collective responsibility principle to drag a case like this and take away the onus duty from the culprit to alibi, no one knows the kind of message the Court is trying to send. Is the public right to infer from such judgment that the pharmacist is the medical doctor's superior or supervisor as far as therapeutic use of drugs is concerned, hence they are supposed to make better judgments (as a mind reader) when an order is not clear or an inferior/subordinate who is nobody but a dispenser in the medication-use process and in that capacity as a dispenser, he is supposed to function as a monitor? It is ironic to see that the Court that once considered the pharmacist as a drug clerk whose only function is to sell drugs with no drug knowledge, now thinks that the pharmacist can act as a therapeutic judge. In order to play this role effectively the pharmacist has to be recognized as the master of his fate and controller of his destiny (an independent practitioner) rather than a monitor. As a dispenser, what time does the pharmacist have to audit all drugs in a prescription, decide the therapeutic nature, dosage, frequency, duration, drug interaction from profile, side effects, practitioner's specialty, drugs within and outside practitioner's specialty, make numerous futile phone calls to verify prescriptions, and others in a busy store of 300 to 500 prescription drugs per day? Moreover, practitioners have need to prescribe drugs in and outside their specialty and some are generally unkind whenever pharmacists call to question the use of drugs. Besides the practitioner, some patients are easily irritated when the pharmacist questions their diagnosis in an attempt to investigate rational use of drugs. Thus, these phrases are not unfamiliar to any pharmacist:

> Prescriber—my role is to prescribe and your role is to dispense, so you don't question me about how I treat my patients.

> Patients—the main job has been done; your role is to give me the drug as a dispenser. You don't question me about diagnosis because that is between me and the doctor.

In another scenario, the court awarded $2.5 million in compensatory damages against a chain pharmacy in North Carolina. As nebulous as the case sounded, the court heard that the physician intended to prescribe prednisone 80mg daily for a renal-failure patient and the pharmacist interpreted the direction as 80mg four times daily making a total of 320mg daily. The pharmacist defended herself by claiming that her concern about the dosage made her call and verify the prescription. She said that a lady answered the phone, put her on hold, and returned later to confirm the dosage as 320mg per day. However, the head of the clinic asserted a different view by maintaining that the clinic was closed on Saturday, the day the pharmacist allegedly made the phone call to verify the prescription. The patient filled the prescription the first time and refilled it again two weeks later in the same chain pharmacy but at a different location and with a different pharmacist. The end result was that the patient ended up in the emergency room with oral thrush, and later lung bacterial infection, aspergillosis, brain fungal infection with various operations in the hospital, permanent kidney failure, and dialysis. The patient sued the physician for negligently writing the prescription and the chain pharmacy for negligently dispensing the drug. Ironically the clinic and the physician settled with the patient for $10,000 before trial, while the chain pharmacy bore the brunt of the case through jury verdict. The chain pharmacy wanted to share the award with the clinic, but the court refused, claiming that the case against the clinic and the physician was weak because the pharmacist couldn't convince the court about the phone call. An expert, a pharmacist from another state, testified that the dosage was too high irrespective of where the prescription was filled.[3] Here is another case where a pharmacist is held solely responsible for a prescriber's writing problem and the culprit is let off the hook by the Court because of pharmacist collective responsibility.

Around April 2001, the *Washington Post* highlighted the tragic death of a 9-month-old baby because of a handwriting problem. The pediatrician prescribed ".5mg" (point 5mg) morphine for the baby's pain after surgery, and it was to be administered intravenously (IV). The unit secretary transcribed this dosage as 5mg instead of ".5mg" into the medication administration record (MAR) and it was administered by an experienced nurse. The baby received two doses two hours apart, after which he developed cardiac arrest and breathing cessation. This was the second episode in less than a year involving the same drug, dosage, mistake, and problem but with a different practitioner. The ISMP (Institute for Safe Medication Practices) issue of *Safety Briefs* on November 15, 2000, highlighted the problem and drew attention to it as one of the first medication safety issues to be published by ISMP 25 years ago. The publication as at then dealt with usage of a decimal dose without a leading zero (i.e., 0.5mg instead of ".5mg," as in this case).[4]

Illegible prescription orders and hospitals' inability to act was such a great concern to an administrator that he decided to write Dr. Darryl Rich of the Joint Commission on Accreditation of Healthcare Organizations (JACHO) a letter inquiring about JACHO standards with regards to the issue. In the letter, he noted that an investigation conducted about illegible orders as part of medication use evaluation (MUE) in the hospital revealed that few practitioners were responsible for 80% of the illegible orders. These practitioners resisted every attempt to correct and educate them about the issue; consequently, the pharmacists resorted to a guessing game because they gave up the ideal of calling to verify illegible order. The pharmacists complain that they have no time to verify illegible orders and the hospital couldn't do anything because of pharmacists' nationwide shortage and the hospital's inability to deal with culprit practitioners. Dr. Rich, the associate director of Surveyor Development and Management, Division of Accreditation operations at JACHO, in response highlighted the various JACHO standards, which include:

- The use of MUE as part of a hospital's privileging and credentialing program in physicians' renewal. Violation of this is a type 1 recommendation for the hospital (MS. 8. 1.2).
- The use of JACHO order, which states that a medication order must have "degree of accuracy, completeness, and discrimination necessary for their intended use" (IM. 3). This order is in place in the absence of MUE.
- The use of JACHO order, which requires hospital medical record review for "presence, timeliness, legibility, and authentication" and "action is taken to improve the quality and timeliness of documentation that impacts patient care" (IM. 7. 10).
- The use of JACHO order, which requires that "accurate, timely, and legible completion of patient's medication records," be used to assess physician's privileging and credentialing program not only in aggregate terms but specific in comparison of particular physician to norm (MS. 8. 2. 3).
- The use of JACHO order, which requires pharmacists to review all medication orders and clarify illegible order with prescriber (TX. 3. 5. 2).

Dr. Rich, who coincidentally is a clinical pharmacist, informed the administrator that clarifying an illegible order is an important part of pharmacists' job and most pharmacists will respond to correction if treated like an "adult." Any pharmacists who fail to perform their job are subject to disciplinary action by the hospital and board of pharmacy.[5] The existence of these orders is an indication that any institutions or hospital will be cited and fined by JACHO for violations. Dr. Neil Davis, the editor-in-chief of *Hospital Pharmacy*, addressed the issue in his editorial article and noted that acceptance of this "long-standing, serious health hazard" is not only a national disgrace (medical records cannot be read because of bad writing) but an indication that patients' safety comes last because of tradition and health professionals' inability to change the system. He called on each institution to select a committee that would accumulate data, assess the damage, identify culprits, explain the effects of bad writing to culprit, what to do in order to rectify the problem, and the consequences of noncompliance. He equally suggested that a personal visit to a culprit is necessary to show the extent of damage and gravity of offense. Culprits can be advised to print if necessary, spend more time to write clearly, use assistance (other staff) in writing orders then and countersign immediately, and/or use committee-approved preprinted prescription orders.[6]

Prescription writing problems in the medical field have become such a perplexing issue that *Pharmacy Today* and *Pharmacy Times* pharmacy news magazines now devote a page or column in every publication to address the problem. The December 2002 issue of *Pharmacy Times* highlights two prescription blanks that were written for a patient (sample I and II). One of the prescription blanks, sample I, has eight medications and not a single one of them was legible. The pharmacist spent two days trying to verify the prescription, and at a dead end he was able to reach the nurse who requested a faxed copy of the prescriptions. Ironically, the second prescription blank contains only one medication, which was equally unreadable.[8] Initially, the pharmacist thought that the prescriber was trying to conserve prescription blanks for economic reasons or from a desire to squeeze everything in one blank or whatever reason; hence, eight medications were written on one blank. However, the sight of the second blank with just one medication raised a lot of inexplicable questions—a puzzle. The January 2003 issue of *Pharmacy Times* highlights another two prescriptions in which Don Raymond, a pharmacist from Montana, tried in vain with the patient to make out three drugs in a single blank (sample III). The pharmacist later called the doctor and left a message to unravel the mystery after wasting so much time trying to read the prescription. The doctor from another state, Wyoming, responded four days later to clarify the drugs. Dr. Harper-Velazquez, a clinical pharmacist from Maryland, called to clarify the second prescription hard copy (sample IV), and the doctor called back later to decipher the four drugs on it. The March 2003 issue of *Pharmacy Times* showed how pharmacist M. Chantz Eyring of Walgreens #2708, Farmington, New Mexico, used his job experience in combination with the technician, Charlene Waldron, to match the prescriber's writings from the patient's profile and previous prescriptions written by the same prescriber (sample V). The patient left the pharmacy before anyone could ask her anything about the prescription; however, she confirmed the investigation before the drug was dispensed to her during counseling. In sample VI, pharmacist Mark Pass of Lawrence Pharmacy, Gainesville,

Georgia, had to call the nurse for clarification before he was able to figure out the beginning and end of the prescription hard copy.

In sample VII, pharmacist Joby Nellickel of Walgreens, Bronx, New York, is used to getting this kind of prescription from this prescriber, who is equally bombarded by other pharmacists for the same reason. The moment the pharmacist got the prescriber on the line, he gave all the necessary information about the prescription only by mere mention of the patient's name. The pharmacist, Dilesh of Patel of Hillcrest Pharmacy, Pennsauken, New Jersey, was able to decipher the drug in sample VIII. Pharmacist Nicholle Binek and her colleagues in Target Pharmacy, Moorhead, Minnesota, together with the patient were unable to decipher the prescription on sample IX, so they waited till the next day to clarify the order with the prescriber. Sample X did not end as peacefully as others because the pharmacist, Chaim Kurz of Echo Drugs, Flushing, New York, thought he could decipher the prescription but ended up with the wrong deduction. The patient was probably counseled about the fact that the medication was used for headache and this made the patient call the prescriber about the medication error. He demanded to know why he was given medication for headache, so the prescriber called the pharmacy to correct the prescription. The pharmacist said sample X is a typical example of the reason why prescriptions should be typed. In sample XI, pharmacist Sherry Southern of Huff Drug, Hazard, Kentucky, commented about the fact that the prescriber must have had a real bad day to scribble medication like that on a hard copy. She claimed that illegible writing pattern is a normal thing for this prescriber, but this was so bad that she couldn't make out anything from the order about the drug. Pharmacist Kimberly Bickford of Albertsons Pharmacy, Mansfield, Texas, and her technician in sample XII recognized the fact that few drugs come in 7.5mg doses and the scribble on the blank did not look like one of them. The pharmacist equally knew her patient's profile and regimen and this did not look like one of them, so she called to verify the prescription. And many others; in the summer of 2003, concerned about medical error resulting from handwriting made Florida State legislators and the governor to pass into law a bill requesting all healthcare prescribers to either write/print legibly or type all prescriptions. The Bill S2084 was signed into law by the governor of the state.[7,10] Governor Phil Bredesen of Tennessee state, on March 29, 2005 signed a similar bill S.B 470 into law. The law requested any written orders from podiatrists, dentists, physicians, surgeons, nurse practitioners, optometrists, osteopaths, or physician assistants (the recognized health care providers) "must be legibly handwritten or typed so that (they are) comprehensible by the pharmacist who fills the prescription."

In law, we say "justice delayed is justice denied." The same phenomenon can be applied to the medical field in terms of treatment modalities; hence, one can reasonably say that therapy delayed is therapy denied, and this condition can spill over a lot of problems in the medical field. A seriously ill patient without medications for two days because of clarity can end up in the emergency room, thereby doubling medical cost, complicating patient's health problem because a stitch in time saves nine, negating all previous work of healthcare practitioners, making matters worse for patients in terms of returning back to normal activities/work, and complicating issues for patients' relatives, caregivers, dependents, healthcare practitioners, and others affected by patient's ill health.

THERAPY DELAYED IS THERAPY DENIED

—— Dr. P. Ojo

Dr. Rich joked about the fact that every time he presents doctors' handwriting as a major topic in a symposium, there is an immediate amusement (laughter) by the audience. As perplexing as the amusement, it is not only peculiar to his audience but a universal phenomenon. Not a single pharmacist in the world would deny how many times they have been questioned by the patients about their ability to read doctors' handwriting. Though pharmacists are denied their rightful place in medical community, it is fair to say that as trained therapeuticians, they are able to use their expertise to draw inference from most of the writings. Dr. Rich's comment about pharmacists' behavior when treated like an "adult" could be analyzed in several ways. Either by omission or commission such comment could be inferred to suggest that pharmacists are treated like children one way or the other by the authorities in the discharge of their duty. This comment could have been treated with ignominy if it was made by an outsider, but with the comment coming from a deep insider who has been part and parcel of pharmacy, there is a clear indication that he has either personally experienced this problem or has observed others go through the problem. It is fair to say that each time an adult is treated like a child, there is something wrong, and as far as pharmacy is concerned everything is correlated with its bondage with other branches of medicine. Every branch of medicine is independent; thus, they treat each other as equals. If one practitioner happens to call another practitioner, be it the same specialty or a different specialty, for any reason including handwriting clarification everybody in the vicinity can easily feel the tension, ovation, and high degree of response. The moment the name pharmacy is mentioned the equation changes and so does the tension, ovation, and degree of response, as if to say the groaning child is around the corner again. What can you do for or with him? If you can't chastise or pet him to stop groaning, you can ignore him or do something to stop the groaning. Little wonder why people can put pharmacists on hold and forget about them in the hospital. This is besides other frustrating problems such as: the doctor is not in this unit or around, endless calls to track a practitioner, if you do not know who wrote the prescription we can't help you, we can't trace a practitioner with a license or DEA number, can you make anything out of the signature? and others. Pharmacists are human beings and as humans they are sensitive to their second-class-status treatment in the medical community; hence, many will stop at nothing in trying to retrieve their personal dignity, image, and self-worthiness. In economics, we say scarcity determines value; thus, anything that is common on Earth demands less value and commands less respect. One of the ways pharmacists can retrieve their respect is to minimize calls for handwriting verification to other practitioners' office. The assertion of the fact that a pharmacist can face disciplinary action if he fails to call and verify illegible orders for something he did not do while doctors, the culprit of the illegible order, will receive pats on the back is another way one can trace pharmacists' treatment as a child.

Pharmacy is a Branch of Medicine and not an Errand Boy of Medicine.

Pharmacists' second-class status in the medical community is uncalled for. As noted earlier, if any branch of medicine deserves specialty and liberation, the poison we pump into our body in the name of drugs ought to be the first priority/option, but unfortunately, it has become the last if anyone is paying attention to the plight of pharmacy. Bad writings in most cases are the resultant consequences of pressure, and the best way to deal with pressure is to reduce it. An independent pharmacy profession, like every other branch of medicine, will use its expertise, intellect, and technical know-how acquired through years of school training and practice to enrich and supplement other branches of medicine and enhance medical practice all over the world. An autonomous pharmacy that is devoid of any unnecessary interference is not a profession that will antagonize other branches of medicine or stop other branches from performing their job; rather, it is an opportunity for the professional to exercise his right of self-determination as master of his fate and controller of his destiny. Much of the pressure experienced during medical school training and professional practice will subside with autonomous pharmacy. Assisting pharmacy to stand on its feet is a challenge to the entire medical community because professional bondage is not a thing of the past but an impediment on the wheel of progress. Pharmacy or doctor of pharmacy graduates, fellows, residents, interns, and students that go on rounds like other branches of medicine will use their knowledge to reduce morbidity and mortality resulting from adverse drug reactions/drug problems, enhance drug delivery systems, improve quality of life for patients, increase therapeutic outcomes with drugs, reduce escalating healthcare costs, and boost healthcare systems for all and sundry.

Hospital administrators have acknowledged the crucial role of pharmacists/pharmacy in overall healthcare provision especially the reduction of a hospital's risk. This was revealed in a survey conducted by *Drug Topics* and *Hospital Pharmacy* report. These administrators rate hospitals' risk reduction as the most important role played by pharmacy in six areas.[9] Pharmacists' role in hospital risk reduction goes a long way to show their effectiveness in minimizing and preventing errors. An independent pharmacy profession will enhance this role and promote an interdisciplinary relationship with other branches of medicine.

I

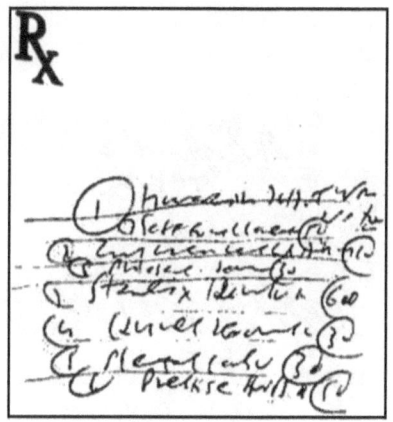

II

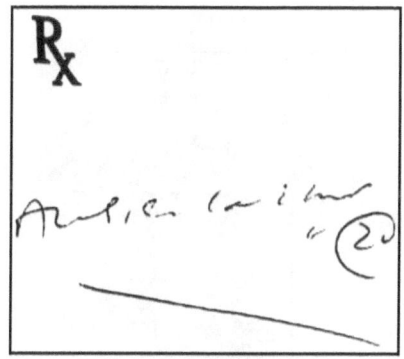

III

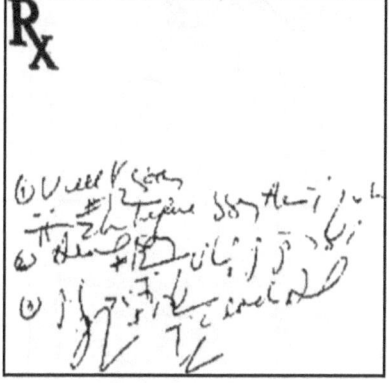

IV

V

VI

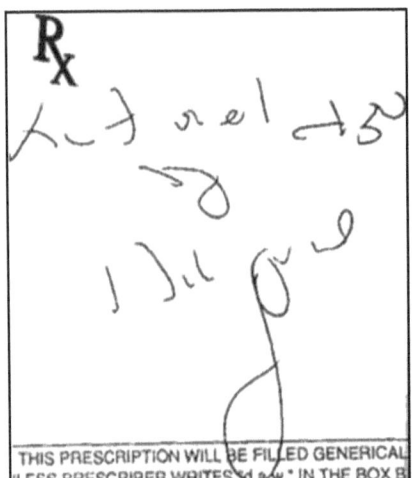

VII

VIII

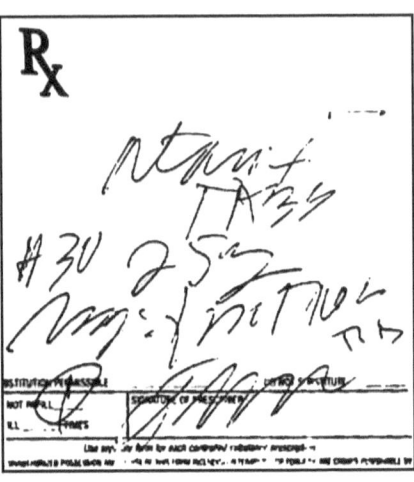

IX

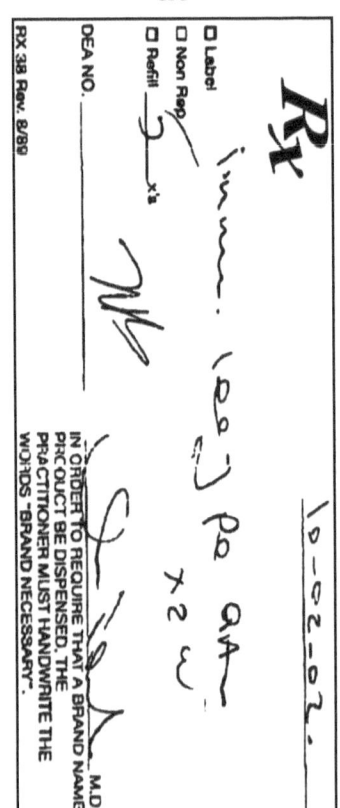

X

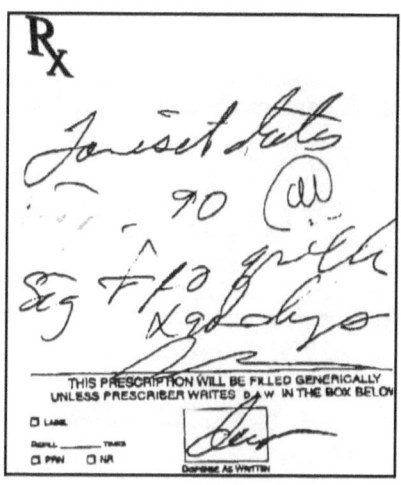

XI

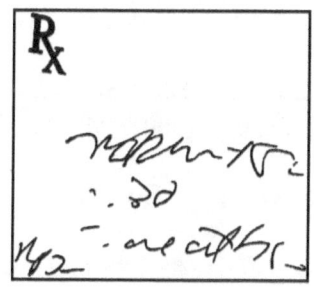

XII

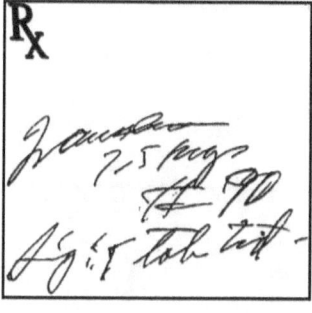

REFERENCES

1. Fried, S. *Bitter pills*. A Bantam Book, 1998, 309-*312, 391*.

2. Brushwood, D. B., and K. Mullan. *Corporate pharmacy's responsibility for a dispensing error. American Journal of Health-System Pharmacy* 53 (1996): 668-70.

3. Simonsmeier, L. M. The dosage was too high no matter where the Rx was filled. Pharmacy Times 62 (December 2002).

4. *Error leads to child's death. Letter in Institute for Safe Medication Practices*, May 2, 2001. Cited in *Florida Pharmacy Today.* (June 2001): 8-*10*.

5. Rich, D. S. *Ask the Joint Commission (illegible prescription handwriting, blanket medication order, "range" medication orders, automatic stop orders). Hospital Pharmacy* 36(7) (2001): 786-*89*.

6. Davis, N. M. *The Joint Commission doesn't think that illegible handwriting is a joke. Hospital Pharmacy* 36(6) (2001): 585-*86*.

7. Can you read these Rxs? *Pharmacy Times* 56 (January 2003).

8. Can you read these Rxs? *Pharmacy Times 50 (December 2002).*

9. Vecchione, A. Hospital administrators laud pharmacists for their role. Drug Topics 45 (April 2001).

10. Jackson, M. *Legislative update. Florida Pharmacy Today* (June/July 2003):
8-*10*.

11. Error alert. Pharmacy Today 10(11) (November 2004): 20-21.

CHAPTER TEN

EPILOGUE

In summary, the creation of pharmacy in Baghdad in the 9th century AD unknowingly brought specialization to medicine and set a milestone in the history of mankind. Unfortunately, this creation became much like a human conception (pregnancy) that did not result in the birth of a child for eleven centuries. Human history is riddled with topsy-turvy happenings, oppression, captivity, deprivation, bondage, trials, tribulations, wars, and victories. Part of this human history is women's struggle against men's domination; Copernicus and Galileo against church doctrines; the Israelites' struggle for freedom; African National Congress, Mandela, Steve Biko, and others against South African apartheid regime; the American War of Independence against the United Kingdom; and many others. Pharmacy has a lot in common with these human struggles even though others can now count their blessing while pharmacy remains in bondage, and good news about the profession's liberation has yet to be written in the *Guinness Book of World Records*. Medicine is equally an interesting part of this human struggle/history.

At the beginning, medicine was inseparable because man learned the art of harnessing anything in his environment to heal his ailment alongside gathering and hunting during the Stone Age. Over the ages, medicine went through series of reformations and transformations. Some of these reformations and transformations are, notably, the Hippocratic doctrine and Flexner panel report. Hippocrates (c. 460-377 BC) struggled to retrieve medicine from superstitious belief and place it on a scientific base with clinical observation and rationalized study of the human body with its functions during the fifth century BC. A lot of effort helped to materialize Hippocrates's principles but the practice of medicine was without standards and forms for many years until the beginning of the twentieth century. That is to say, the *modus operandi* of medicine was very much based on an apprenticeship mode of training. The inadequacy of the apprenticeship mode of training, in some cases without formal college education, led to a huge public outcry especially in United States of America (USA), and this public outcry resulted in the creation of Flexner panel around 1908. The Flexner panel examined the *modus operandi* of medical schools in U.S. and Canada and published its report in 1910. Flexner panel concentrated it efforts on allopathic medicine and declared others null and void. The report led to drastic reformation of medical schools. Some of the implemented policies included the proscription of osteopathic medicine, chiropractics, homeopathic medicine, and acupuncture; declaration of pharmacy as a non-profession; abandonment of the apprenticeship mode of training, to be replaced by internship/residences; closure of two thirds of the existing medical schools; and production of clinicians and specialists.

Pharmacy is a Branch of Medicine and Not an Errand Boy of Medicine.

Specialists opened a new phase in medical history and much of it rests on various branches of medicine. As noted above, medicine was inseparable at the beginning because it existed as a whole entity, but specialists catalyzed the existence of various branches of medicine as separate entities. In the U.S., the introduction of Medicare in 1965 and military settings (the army) helped to fuel the development of these branches/specialties in medicine. There are many branches of medicine but at the tail end of the 20th century, the U.S. has about 24 recognized boards of medical specialties according to the American Board of Medical Specialty directory. It is important to note that these 24 boards of medical specialties do not include dentistry, optometry, and veterinary medicine. The establishment of these boards in the U.S. started with ophthalmology in 1917; otolaryngology in 1924; obstetrics and gynecology in 1930; dermatology in 1932; pediatrics in 1933; psychiatry and neurology, orthopedic surgery, and radiology in 1934; urology and colon and rectal surgery in 1935; pathology and internal medicine in 1936; surgery in 1937; anesthesiology and plastic surgery in 1941; physical medicine and rehabilitation in 1947; preventive medicine in 1948; thoracic surgery in 1950; family practice in 1969; allergy and immunology and nuclear medicine in 1971; emergency medicine in 1979; and genetics in 1980. Implementation of Flexner's report resulted in the genesis of these specialties. By and large, in spite of the setback, pharmacy can precisely look at these branches of medicine and say, "Before Abraham there were men." A brief review of pharmacy showed that pharmacy played a pivotal role in medicine as a whole entity, because at the beginning all that mattered was anything that treated human ailments. At this stage pharmacy was synonymous with medicine; thus, one can reasonably say that pharmacy was medicine and medicine was pharmacy.

Anything in the form of active ingredients from plants and other resources was used to treat human ailments, and these things at one point or another were considered drugs. Everything about drugs is pharmacy and everything about pharmacy is drugs. People used drugs during the Paleolithic or Neolithic period around 600,000 to 10,000 BC. Shaman, the earliest known witch doctor or priest, used drugs to heal his patients around 30,000 BC. The four earliest great human civilizations, namely Egyptian, Mesopotamian, Greek, and Roman empires used and advanced drug treatment for the benefit of mankind. Egyptians compounded drugs and used various dosage forms in delivery it to the body. Asu, the experienced healers of Mesopotamia, advanced various dosage forms such as enemas, ointments, suppositories, and tablets in the treatment of patients. In the Greek Empire, the humoral theory of Hippocrates aided Dioscorides in writing the first book about drugs, an encyclopedia of drug caption *Materia Medica*. Galen and his followers opposed the Hippocratic principle, blended superstition and magic spells with drugs in treating patients. Generally, the use of drugs declined in the Roman Empire because of the activities in the monasteries (monks). The monks believed in spiritual healing because they wanted to emulate Jesus Christ's life activities.

The Islamic religion came into being in the 7th century AD. Mohammed, an orphaned child, introduced the religion and encouraged his followers to respect, learn, translate, and advance the writings of the previous great civilizations. Islamic scholars consequently learned from the great works of Hippocrates and Dioscorides of the Greek Empire and Galen of the Roman Empire. They translated these great works into Arabic and sought to transform medicine to great heights. They rejected the notion that the bitter a pill is or the fouler tasting a concoction is the better it is. Advancement in the medical field led to better dosage formulation, which precisely is more fragrant and more palatable drugs and other attractive forms of medication. As the desire to prepare more sophisticated medicine, improve existing ones, and invent new drugs increased so did the desire to have specialists within the medical field take care of this phenomenon. One of the Islamic scholars, physicians, and first ever known pharmacist to rise to the occasion was Dr. Rhaze (AD 860-932). Dr. Rhaze created pharmacy out of basic necessities for specialty and the need to advance the new profession. The new specialists (pharmacists-physicians) became dexterous in the acts of manufacturing, counseling about drug usage, compounding, and dispensing of drugs to patients with or without prescriptions from their colleagues, other physicians. Pharmacy thrived in various Arab cities then spread to Europe. After the fall of the Roman Empire, the monks that once abhorred drug treatment began to encourage pharmaceutical growth. Monasteries grew their own herb gardens for pharmaceutical use. Two monasteries, which are the learning centers founded in 10th century AD by Cassiodarus at Salerno, Italy, and Toledo, Spain, played a great role in the spread of pharmacy to Western Europe. Although the Islamic learning center in Fez, Morocco, founded AD 859, is considered the first university in the history of mankind, Western scholars credit the monastery learning center in Salerno, Italy, as the first university in Europe and at times the world. University learning centers spread around the world in Fez, Morocco—AD 859; Al-Azhar, Egypt—AD 990; Bologna, Italy—11th century; Paris, France—AD 1150; Oxford, Britain—AD 1167; Salerno, Italy—AD 1180; Cambridge, Britain—AD 1248; Timbuktu, Mali—AD 1320; Sankore, Padua, and Prague—AD 1347; and others. Pharmacy was very much part of these universities' learning culture. Donnolo, a Jewish scholar and physician, made good use of his Salerno influence and Arab data in producing the first drug formulary book, *Antidotory*, in the 10th century.

The invention of movable-type printing in 1436 by Johannes Gutenberg (1397-1468) helped chemists, botanists, and physicians to print their investigative works on plants for medicinal purposes. Valerius Cordus was one of the medical scientists who used such gesture in publishing his work *Dispensatorium*, the first recognized pharmacopoeia used in compounding drugs, in Nuremberg, Germany, in 1546. The Renaissance period in Europe is marked by great voices like Paracelsus, the father of toxicology — all are poison, known for his heresy and reactionary views of traditional medicine. The practice of pharmacy took a different turn with the advent of apothecaries in Europe. Apothecaries were recognized medical practitioners who rendered medical services to the poor, downtrodden, underserved, less privileged, and less fortunate members of the society, who couldn't afford the high medical fees of university-trained physicians in most parts of Europe during the 17th and 18th centuries. By the 19th century the apothecaries had elevated their status through university education and scientific research to become the equals of university-trained physicians. They left behind the job of selling drugs to druggists and chemists. This was the state of affairs in which pharmacy was imported to some British colonies including United States of America. Records showed that some American apothecaries like Brown and Talbot operated like their British counterparts. Restriction of apothecaries as general practitioners to a mere dispensing function started in America in the early 19th century, and the modalities for training physicians gradually changed from preceptorships to hospital-clinical experience with a major focus on prescription-writing skills. Apothecaries became dispensers and the compounding of drugs was left as part of their functions. The first medical college in the country, the Medical College of Philadelphia, was established in 1765 and the desire to curtail medical school curriculum from embracing pharmacy school curriculum led to the formation of Philadelphia College of Apothecaries (later Pharmacy) in 1821. In 1820, the United States Pharmacopoeia (USP) was approved as a standard for physicians' prescription-writing skills and pharmacist/apothecary's desire to compound drugs accurately. The apothecaries together with some druggists and chemists teamed up to form the American Pharmaceutical Association in 1852 in Philadelphia.

Industrial Revolution brought an end to apothecaries and resulted in a new era of count and pour for the pharmacists. Pharmaceutical industries took over drug manufacturing from the apothecary, perfected the act, and engaged in large-scale production of drugs. Pharmacists filled their shops with these drugs and dispensed them with written prescription from prescribers. Pharmacists' education has gone through many hurdles, with vocational courses and three-year programs at the beginning in U.S. In 1928, the American Association of the Colleges of Pharmacy (AACP) adopted the four-year bachelor of science/pharmacy degree program as the entry level for pharmacists. This was later upgraded to five years in 1960. The five-year program was a compromise for those who, on one hand, felt pharmacists needed a six-year doctorate program in order to match the status of other branches of medicine, gain public confidence, and raise the practicing standards of pharmacy; while on the other hand were others such as the employers and National Association of Retail Druggists (NARD) who felt such a gesture was unnecessary because there was no market for doctorate program and nobody needed six years of educational training for a profession that restricted one's performance to count and pour or throw pills from one bottle to another. The latter group equally claimed that there would be unnecessary increase in labor costs and a scarcity of pharmacists because students would generally prefer to add one additional year for better remuneration in other branches of medicine instead of pharmacy. The views of the latter group were supported by an earlier code of ethics adopted by the American Pharmaceutical Association (AphA) in 1922. This code of ethics prevented pharmacists from discussing the therapeutic effects of drugs with patients and it was repealed in 1969 more than four decades later.

The era of count and pour brought great disservice to pharmacy profession, as many people couldn't draw direct relationships between pharmacists' remuneration, educational training/requirements, and services. This issue became much more evident every time people compared pharmacy to other professions such as engineering, teaching, journalism, nursing, and others that require greater output of knowledge, more professional services/demand, but less educational training (four years in most cases). Though certain pharmacists are pleased with the status of count and pour, other progressive, optimistic, and forward-looking pharmacists felt the imperative need to advance the profession in a clinical direction because technological advancements endeared the availability of robots, automation, and computerized systems that threatened to take away count and pour system from the pharmacists. The yearnings of the progressive pharmacists coupled with the demands of pharmacists' educators brought the issue of six-year doctor of pharmacy degree programs, a program that started in 1950 at the University of California, San Francisco back as hot topic. Three decades after the adoption of the five-year degree program, the American Association of the Colleges of Pharmacy (AACP) was once again facing a dilemma and the reality of time. However, this time there was no escape in the adoption of the six-year doctor of pharmacy degree program as entry level for pharmacists. The AACP and the American Council on Pharmaceutical Education in 1989 sent a letter of intent to all schools of pharmacy to adopt the six-year program as entry level and the program was eventually approved in 1992 with an implementation date set for 2005.

In 1933, the election of Franklin Roosevelt as president of the United States of America ushered in a new era of social reform through which the Social Security Act was enacted in 1935. The Social Security Act protects against unemployment, and offers retirement benefits and health insurance for everybody who deserves it. Medicare, health insurance for the elderly paid for through payroll tax deductions and Medicaid, health insurance for the poor sponsored by the federal and state governments was enacted later in 1965 as part of the Social Security Amendment Act. These social reforms, especially Medicare and Medicaid, changed healthcare system in America for good and it resulted in soaring healthcare products, services, and increased drug usage. Increased demand for healthcare products, services, and drug usage resulted in price gouging that escalated way out of proportion, serious adverse drug reactions that precipitated high morbidity and mortality rates as well as increased hospital admission, and other problems. Statistics revealed that healthcare's fraction of the gross national product rose from 5.2% in 1960 to 13.9% in 1993 and 14.4% by the year 2001; the medical fraction of the consumer price index (CPI) rose by 7.3% when other goods and services rose by 2.8% annually; prescription drugs, on the other hand, rose from $2.7 billion in 1960 to $12 billion in 1980, $103.9 billion in 1999, and $121.8 billion in 2000. Pharmacy is the only profession in the world where professionals can spend five to six years in educational training and at graduation the young aspiring graduates/professionals are told to forget everything they learned in school and face reality of life by way of professional-service demands. The harsh reality is that they cannot write anything about patients, drug therapy, and therapeutic outcome. Teachers with four years of educational training write lesson notes and teach their students, engineers with four or five years of school training draw plans and execute their projects, architects with four years of school training draw building plans and see the end results, and lawyers with four to six years of educational training design their clients' cases and go to the court to marshal out their plans and other professional services.

Gradually, people begin to comprehend the plight of a pharmacist in the medical field—overeducated, underutilized, and marginalized professionals—while billions of dollars are spent on drugs and drug therapy without specialists. Ironically, many other aspects of medicine including life and non-life-threatening issues have specialists caring for them. The first gesture in this realization process came from the United States Congress when the Omnibus Budget Reconciliation Act (OBRA) of 1990 was passed. OBRA '90 mandated pharmacists to perform drug-utilization review (DUR) and counsel patients before dispensing drugs. Though clinical pharmacy was already in existence before OBRA '90, it was the first legal backing for pharmacists to have a direct impact on patients' healthcare. Counseling was a limited form of practice for pharmacists because it did not guarantee professional autonomy/freedom but aided pharmaceutical care. Clinical pharmacy started in 1930s when some pharmacists went into a hospital for post-baccalaureate internship training program. Clinical pharmacy then began to grow with Mr. White of Virginia transforming his traditional pharmacy amid criticism into an office practice setting in 1960, and the University of California, San Francisco, establishing a clinical practice in 1966 in a monumental 9th floor project that eventually changed hospital pharmacy for good. Around 1975, the American Council on Pharmaceutical Education (ACPE) and the federal government used the clinical pharmacy experience at the University of California, San Francisco, to force schools of pharmacy to include clinical pharmacy in their education programs. Consequently, clinical pharmacy became the criteria for pharmacy education reimbursement, and the availability of hospital pharmacy became a criteria for Medicare reimbursement.

Hepler and Strand's landmark research brought pharmaceutical care into being in the early 1990s and pharmaceutical care became the rallying point for pharmacists in modern history. Pharmaceutical care confronted problems similar to what counseling and clinical pharmacy did and the most crucial part of these problems was pharmacy autonomy. Other issues such as excess workload, pharmacy layout, inadequate privacy and financial rewards for counseling, clinical pharmacists' (PharmD) services against first-degree-holder pharmacists affected pharmaceutical care services. One of the most vital ingredients that propelled pharmacy to greater heights through counseling, pharmaceutical care, and clinical pharmacy services is the introduction of the doctor of pharmacy degree (PharmD) program. Initially many wonder if pharmacy as a profession deserves six- to seven-year doctorate program for dispensing function only, but as time goes on many issues that endeared pharmacy as a medical specialty rather than an errand boy of medicine began to unravel themselves and buttress the need for doctor of pharmacy degree.

Some of these issues include: the message of Paracelsus (1493-1541), the father of toxicology, that claims that all substances including chemicals/drugs are poisons and the only thing that differentiates poison from remedy is the right dose. This fact becomes much more evident when one realizes that drugs, like every other thing in life, have their own pattern; for example, pharmacokinetic properties (absorption, distribution, metabolism, and excretion—ADME), and once inside the body they have no master. Contemporary problems deserve contemporary solutions, and these days in age when technological advancement is the order of the day, longevity/extended life spans coupled with chronic illness are common factors. Chronic illness brings with it multiple drug usage and it is not unusual to find an elderly patient these days on a daily regimen of 20 or more drugs in the management of their disease states. If we have specialists taking care of all spheres of life including cars and non-life-threatening cases such as massage, dermatology, dentistry, and others, doesn't it make sense to have specialists taking care of the poisons (drugs) we pump into our bodies every day? It is worthwhile to remember that the poisons we pump into our bodies as remedies for any ailment at dawn can send us to our grave at dusk. Multiple drug usage has a concomitant effect on the body besides the intended indication. The most crucial concomitant effects of drugs in the body are adverse drug reaction (ADR).

Numerous studies have revealed the devastating effects of ADR on the nation's healthcare system. Some of these studies include: Drs. Bootman and Johnson's 1995 study that showed how ambulatory care patients spend over $76 billion every year on drug-related illness; a 1994 meta-analysis prospective study by Lazarous et al. that showed that ADR is responsible for 106,000 deaths annually (making ADR anywhere between 4th - [by conservative estimates] and 6th-[by liberal estimates] leading cause of deaths—a stable statistic for 3 decades) and 2,216,000 hospitalizations (making ADR responsible for 6.7% hospitalization of patients); a 1995 National Ambulatory Medical Care Survey that showed that 2 million patients visited physicians' offices because of ADR—an estimated 7.7 visits per 1,000 persons, with a breakdown of physicians (e.g., internists, family, and general practitioners) accounting for 55.98%, specialists such as pediatricians and dermatologists accounting for 15.96%, nurses alone accounting for 29.6% and physician assistants alone accounting for 16.6% of medication-related visits; a 1992 Fink study that showed that $76.56 billion was spent on drug-related morbidity and mortality when $75 billion was spent on prescription drugs alone the same year; a Berg et al. noncompliance study that showed that patients' noncompliance cost businesses $50 billion, hospital admissions $25 billion, nursing home admissions $5 billion, and pharmacy $8 billion; a 1990 World Health Organization (WHO) report that showed that ADR cost the U.S. 1.6 million hospitalizations and 160,000 deaths; and others.

In 1952, two years after the initiation of a doctor of pharmacy program by the University of California, Dr. Harry Gold, a physician, requested for a specialty within the medical field that specializes in pharmacology and clinical medicine. These specialists were to be classified as clinical pharmacologists. Pharmaceutical industries, some medical schools, and physicians lauded the idea but the American Medical Association (AMA) and other physicians groups opposed it strongly. Clinical pharmacology eventually died a premature death and was replaced with clinical pharmacy. It is strange to note that the same AMA and other physicians groups that supported other specialties of medicine including surgery and anesthetics find it difficult to support a therapeutic pharmacology/clinical medicine specialty. In the first place, why was anesthetics created as a specialty? Was it that the surgeons and other physicians were not smart enough to handle anesthetics during surgery and other situations or because of the intricacy involved in drug therapy? Ironically, anesthetics is an infinitesimal part of drug therapy/pharmacy that does not even constitute up to 1% (one percent) of some pharmacy textbooks or paraphernalia. As noted in an early chapter, the only reason why anesthetics was created as a specialty was because the surgeons unanimously demanded for it.

Dr. Raymond Woosley was so moved by the safety record of the Netherlands as the world's safest drug nation and the degree of ADR's devastating impact on the American society, as well as healthcare professionals' and public apathy about drug knowledge, that he decided to suggest the establishment of the Center for Education and Research in Therapeutics (CERT) in the 1970s and again in the 1990s. Dr. Flockhart supported the idea and planned to implement it with Dr. Ray through government funding. The Federal Drug Administration (FDA) commended the idea but lamented the lack of funds to execute it. Dr. David Burkholder, a clinical pharmacist, established the first known academic drug information center at the University of Kentucky Medical Center, Lexington, shortly after graduating from the first class of the doctor of pharmacy degree program at the University of Michigan in 1962. As a pioneer of a drug information center, Dr. David's center was renowned for disseminating quality drug information to all medical personnel including physicians, medical students, and nurses. In the absence of government funding, colleges of pharmacy and some hospital pharmacies waded in to fill the vacuum by spreading drug information centers created by Dr. Burkholder across the country. Today, these drug information centers are renowned for their activities and for translating Drs. Woosley and Flockhart's dream into reality.

These and other issues buttress the need for drug or therapeutic specialists, and no one in the medical field stands in a better position to grab the bull by the horns and drag it to the altar than the pharmacist. In order for the pharmacist to serve his originally intended role or as therapeutician/drug specialist, he needs to arm himself with the doctor of pharmacy degree and effective drug knowledge. Currently the profession is far from its intended role/position in the medical field, yet overwhelming evidence supports the profession as the indisputable therapeutic/drug specialty within medical field. Two pieces of outstanding evidence substantiate the profession's claim above and they are schools of pharmacy curriculum in comparison to other branches of medicine and the numerous studies that showed the tremendous impact of clinical pharmacists/pharmacists on our healthcare system. Statistical analysis of data collected from various schools, as enumerated in chapters 5 and 6, showed that in the United States of America the following situation prevails:

—Physician assistants operate in various categories across the nation in physicians' office. Most states have little or no restriction on their prescribing authority. In Florida, for example, physician assistants can prescribe over 617 prescriptions drugs, while the pharmacists can only dream of less than 50 drugs in the same category. In terms of course content as basic qualification for the prescriptive authority, the physician assistants are exposed to an estimated one pharmacy or drug-treatment course out of every 14 courses in one academic year (maximum of two courses, and that is if 28 courses are offered in the only year devoted to classroom work out of the two-year program) before rotation and there is no residence requirement. The clinical pharmacists (regular pharmacists), on the other hand, are exposed to an estimated 7 (8 for regular pharmacists) pharmacy or drug-treatment courses out of every 10 courses, making a total estimate of 42 courses in three years (32 courses for regular pharmacists in two years) before rotations.

—A certified nurse practitioner or midwife operates in and outside a physician's office. Certified nurse practitioners have similar or greater prescribing authority than physician assistants in most states. Few of them operate independently with a physician's name as the figurehead in some of their prescriptions' hardcopy and none in some others. Their sole claim for this prescribing authority is an estimated 1 (one) pharmacy or drug-treatment course out of every 25 courses in two years (2 years program after the first degree) without a residency requirement (1 out of every 50 courses for regular nurse—4 years program for the first degree). There is low probability of taking more than 25 courses in two years. The clinical pharmacists on the other hand take an estimated 7 out of every 10 courses, making a total estimate of 42 courses in three years, yet they cannot dream of the crumbs that fall from the prescribing table of CNP. Little wonder why prescriptions are thrown at patients like candy bars or prescriptions written by nurses and PAs account for 46.2% (29.6% for nurses and 16.65% for PAs) of physicians' office visit because of ADR as per a 1995 medical care survey.

—Psychologists with no drug knowledge or drug courses in their curriculum have been granted prescriptive authority in few states, while others such as social workers in hospitals, physician's office managers/secretaries, etc., without any pharmacy or drug-treatment courses in school, but on the basis of years of experience in a physician's office/hospital, are next on the prescriptive line of authority list. The pharmacists with their years of school training in drug treatment watch amazingly.

—The dentists can write any prescription for the pharmacist to dispense and their justification for this lies in an estimated one pharmacy or drug-treatment course out of every 33 courses in three years (maximum of 3 courses in 3 years and that is if the school offers 33 courses in a year before rotation) without a residence requirement. They spend the same number of years in school training as the clinical pharmacists, who take an estimated 7 pharmacy or drug-treatment courses out of every 10 courses (maximum of 42 in 3 years before rotation).

—The veterinary medical doctor can prescribe any medication for the pharmacist to dispense to animals. The veterinary medical doctor's prescribing authority lies in the acquisition of an estimated one pharmacy or drug-treatment course out of every 13 courses in three years (maximum of 6 courses in 3 years and that is if the school offers 26 courses in a year before rotation) during school training, and this is without any residence requirement. Like the dentists, they spend the same number of years in school as the pharmacists, who take an estimated 7 pharmacy or drug-treatment courses out of every 10 courses (maximum of 42 in 3 years before rotation).

—The optometrists can write prescriptions for a lot of drugs unimaginable to the pharmacists, and their justification for this lies in the acquisition of an estimated one pharmacy or drug-treatment course out of every of 17 courses in three years (maximum of 4 courses in 3 years and that is if the school offers 22 courses in a year before rotation) during school training and this is without any residency requirement. Like the dentists and veterinary medical doctors, optometrists spend the same number of years in school training as the clinical pharmacists.

—All branches of medicine including various specialty, traditional, and osteopathic medical doctors have unlimited prescribing authority. They can prescribe anything for the pharmacists to dispense and their justification for this lies in the acquisition of an estimated one pharmacy or drug-treatment course out of every 17 courses in two years (maximum of 4 courses in two years and that is if the school offers 34 courses per year) during school training before rotation and residency. The clinical pharmacists, on the other hand, acquire an estimated 7 pharmacy or drug-treatment courses out every 10 courses (maximum of 42 courses in three years and that is if the school offers 20 courses per year) during school training before rotation but without a residency requirement (residency is optional for graduates). They have little or no prescriptive authority.

The world study of the same curriculum at Ile-Ife/Benin City, Nigeria, in Africa; Beijing, China, and Japan in Asia; Sydney in Australia; London, UK in Europe; and Rio de Janeiro, Brazil, in South America showed a trend similar to the United States of America in North America with little or no variation. The study found that in sharp contrast to the number of pharmacy or drug-treatment courses available to these professionals during school training, traditional medical doctors and osteopathic practitioners with specialties such as allergy and immunology, anesthesiology, dermatology, emergency medicine, family practice, internal medicine, genetics, neurology, nuclear medicine, obstetrics and gynecology, ophthalmology/otolaryngology, pathology, pediatrics, physical medicine and rehabilitation, psychiatry, preventive medicine, radiology, surgery, and urology and veterinary medicine (without residency), acquire an estimated 8 diagnosis-related courses out of every 10 courses. The physician assistants are exposed to the same estimated 8 out of every 10 courses in just a one-year academic program before rotation and without residency, while the certified nurse practitioners are exposed to an estimated 7 out of every 10 diagnosis and nurse-related courses. The dentists are exposed to approximately 9 out of every 10 diagnosis and dental-related courses. The optometrists are exposed to an estimated 8 out of every 10 diagnosis and optometry-related courses, while the clinical pharmacists, on the other hand, are exposed to estimated 2 out of every 10 diagnosis-related courses. The world and United States's statistics are similar in this regard, and the data confirmed the fact that other branches of medicine are trained diagnosticians, dentists, and optometrists, while the clinical pharmacists/pharmacists are trained therapeuticians/drug specialists.

Numerous studies have shown the activities of clinical pharmacists to be life and money-saving for humanity. Some of these studies include: the July 1999 *Journal of the American Medical Association* publication that reported a clinical controlled study in which Dr. Leape (MD) drew national attention to the fact that pharmacists' (Dr. Lyman, clinical pharmacist with a PharmD in this study) participation in therapeutic decisions can identify and prevent many potential errors in drug therapy, and a total savings of $270,000 per year was realized; in December 1995, the National Data Corporation reported a cost savings of $752,391 per year in Nebraska because of 878 pharmacist interventions; a Veteran Affairs health care center in Northern California report showed an estimated cost-savings advantage of $139,380 to $216,800 between April and August 1996 because of clinical pharmacists' interventions, which involved initiation, monitoring, continuity, and modification of therapy as well as ordering of laboratory reports to correlate pharmacotherapy as an independent prescriber; a Munroe et al. study that showed a Blue Cross/Blue Shield (BCBS) cost savings of $143.95 to $293.39 per patient per month because of pharmacists' interventions; a Waddell et al. study that showed 7 months cost-savings of $24,000 at Walter Reed Army Medical Center, Washington, D.C.; the popular two-year hyperlipidemia project IMPACT (Improve Persistence and Compliance with Therapy), which started in January 1996 and in December 1997 persistence rate was 84%, compliance rate was 84.3% and 44.3 to 62.5% patients achieved National Cholesterol Education Program (NCEP) lipid goals compared to less than 40% compliance rate and 18% congestive heart failure patients at cholesterol target/goal with traditional medical doctors; a Park et al. hypertension study that showed how pharmacists' interventions raised blood pressure control from 17.4% (baseline) to 52.2% ($P < 0.02$) in four months (NHANES—National Health and Nutrition Examination Survey—revealed that 24% of hypertensive patients on physician-prescribed medications have their blood pressure under control); a St. John's University College of Pharmacy–sponsored project that showed 14 months cost savings of $84,476.25 for 378 patients at Nassau County Medical Center, East Meadow, because of pharmacists' interventions; a Yale-New Haven Hospital study that showed how pharmacist involvement in asthma care saved $172,397 per 50 high risk patients in a year, reduced emergency room visits by 64% and hospital admissions by 63%, while correct use of inhalers went up from 25 to 90%; a Thompson et al. study that showed how clinical pharmacists can act as independent prescribers and save a California nursing home about $55,230 per 67 patients in a year; a Wateska et al. study that showed a 73% cost reduction or savings of $157,600 per 8 TPN patients at a Cleveland clinic in a year; a Poretz et al. study that revealed a cost savings of $432,816 for 150 outpatients on intravenous antibiotic therapy; a Fletcher et al. study that revealed a cost savings of $161,396; a Peterson and Lake study that revealed a cost savings of $600,000 per year to patients, $200,000 per year to pharmacies, and $105,000 per year to the hospital by using less-expensive antibiotics to achieve the same goal as the expensive one; a Gattis et al. study that showed a decrease in the mortality rate and nonfatal heart failure incidents for heart failure and left ventricular dysfunction patients, from 16 in the control group to 4 in the intervention group, and a decrease in readmission rates from 42% to 29%; a Stimmel et al. study that showed that prescriptions written by clinical pharmacists is better than those written by physicians in terms of three classes of drugs for psychiatric patients; a Pathak and Nold study that showed a cost savings of $833,723 in two years; and a Bond et al. study that showed, among other things, how the involvement of a clinical pharmacist with just $320 spent on the salary averts one death in the hospital every time.

All these achievements are with due regard to the fact that nowhere in pharmacy school curriculum is the act of prescribing taught or encouraged, because such a move would be tantamount to violation of the law. As per contemporary school curriculum, pharmacists are only taught how to monitor therapy; consequently, it is easy to visualize the fact that the sky would be the limit for liberated pharmacy.

"Pharmacy Is in Bondage with Other Branches of Medicine."

A drug specialist/expert survey in U.S. showed that public view of pharmacists as drug specialists/experts is beginning to materialize in spite of the odds. The world's public opinion seems to agree to a large extent with United States's public opinion about pharmacists as drug specialists/experts. The liberation of pharmacy as an independent profession like other branches of medicine will enhance pharmacists' status as trained therapeuticians or drug specialists/experts and reduce the tension in the medical community. This tension in the form of patients' needs/demands, inadequate practitioners in many areas, and lack of drug specialists/therapeuticians in the medical community and others has resulted in bad handwriting, inadequate monitoring, short-lived/inadequate attention for patients, unpoliced adverse drug reaction, and unmonitored drug interaction resulting from inadequate knowledge and others. Pharmacists as trained therapeuticians need to be the master of their fate and controller of their destiny like other professionals or specialists in the medical field.

In spite of the activities of clinical pharmacists in the United States, regular pharmacists in China, rural areas, most developing countries, and other places around the world function as independent practitioners rendering medical services to those in desperate need of it. In light of these, pharmacy is crying loud and clear to the great lady of New York Harbor—the Statue of Liberty—the American president, American congressmen and -women, Americans, goodwill people of the world, all those who know the implications and ramifications of bondage/oppression, and all citizens of the world, to liberate him from the yoke of oppression, and professional bondage. Bondage is not a joke; all those who have experienced it know what it means, and that is why the great democracies of the world such as the United States of America disdain it, and it can be argued that

—No to human bondage is no to professional bondage.
—No to human subservience is no to professional subservience.
—No to human captivity is no to professional captivity.
—No to human oppression is no to professional oppression.
—No to human deprivation is no to professional deprivation.
—No to human aberration is no to professional aberration.
—No to dehumanization is no to de-professionalization.

Once again, the United States of America—home of the brave and land of the free—spreads its tentacles beyond human freedom to other spheres of human endeavors—pharmacy's professional liberation/freedom. America is at another milestone and threshold in the history of mankind—setting historical records straight and vindicating the just, thereby liberating one of the greatest professions in the history of mankind for the benefit of this and future generations.

APPENDIX

The issues discussed in this section may or may not be related to the subject matter of the book; however, they are considered important and crucial to the world in a bid to make it a better place to live in by all and sundry. Some of these issues, especially the reflection of retrogressive forces in third world countries such as Nigeria, are meant to create better societies around the world. These forces are not only drawing back the hands of the clock in terms of human development and technologically advancement but unleashing a series of untold hardships on their people because of selfishness and greed. All it takes is to have less than 1% of the population/wrong people in power. Some people will question the relevance of the pope John Paul II using his position to bring the plight of his people in Poland to the world's attention or the relevance of Dali Lama using his position to bring the plight of his people in Tibet to the world's attention. By so doing, the world learned a lot and greater forces are brought on the evil retrogressive forces. The whole world now talks about surviving Indian democracy, the largest democracy in the world, because the right ingredient for the survival of democracy (e.g., government official cars, law and order, accountability, good media, checks and balances, ridding the government of corruption/bad elements such as the corporate crooks in U.S., etc) is in place.

If India was as rich as Nigeria or Saudi Arabia, it is easy to see that we would have been looking at another Japan in the making. These days we are worried in America because of the number of U.S. jobs shipped to India, and that is because the society has what it takes to attract foreigners by putting democracy on the right track. China's communism has a similar gesture that makes the society look like a social-capitalist nation in spite of the leaders' preaching, which runs contrary to the people's wish and desire for true democracy. India and China have a lot in common with most third world countries, vis-à-vis the prevalence of abject poverty among the vast majority of the people and other issues. There is nothing black and white in human ills or retrogressive forces because evil knows no one. Human beings are human beings anywhere you go in the world, and any society that is not able to purge itself of human ills cannot see the light of the day. It is in light of this that the investigator reflects below with some pabulum on his unique experience as highlighted in chapter 6.

INVESTIGATOR'S UNIQUE EXPERIENCE

The investigator's unique experience has a lot to do with the fact that the University of Ife (now Obafemi Awolowo University), Ile-Ife, Nigeria, was an eye-opener for him, and presently the deplorable situation of the school and other issues in the country deserve the world's attention. (Nigeria is like a cancer patient who is dying of his ailment but prefers to hide his disease from those who can possibly help to ameliorate the situation or cure him.) Besides high academic excellence and educational standards, the University of Ife in its glorious days was blessed not only in terms of grandiose buildings and a fanciful campus, but also with functionary offices with basic necessities. In January 2001, when the investigator visited the campus because of the world study, he was astonished to see the degree of degeneracy that had besieged the university and its offices, and this is reminiscent of almost everything in the country. Any sane human being that saw the University of Ife in its glorious days would lament and cry the beloved country, Nigeria, at the sight of the faculty of health sciences (medicine) dean's office. Things have gotten so bad that at the request of the investigator, faculty officers could not produce any current catalogue (handbook) because of the economic predicament of the nation and the university. He was given the only available copy, which dated back to 1988-90. At the faculty of pharmacy, he had to pay for photocopies of the only available faculty-corrected copy of the catalogue (handbook), which dated back to 1987-90.

The world's study has to start from somewhere; at any rate, some will query the choice and uniqueness of the University of Ife (Great Ife as it is commonly referred to by the students) if not for personal aggrandizement and selfishness. The investigator was born and brought up in a rather hopeless, feudalized society where hereditary is the bane of the society. People do not only see hereditary properties as a matter of life and death resulting in a bitter family acrimony and deaths, in some cases for as little as a mud house; but people's aspirations especially young children were pretty much tied to the apron springs of their parents' status, achievement, and influence in the society. That is to say, the type of schools you attended, social interaction, and other issues were closely linked to who your parents were. The investigator's great-grandmother was thoroughly schooled by the system, which she passed on to other generations by crooning in the ears of the younger ones the values and greatness of the family/system through oral history. She wasn't educated, but to her last day on the surface of this Earth, she could tell story upon story without loosing a fragment of it to all little children that came across her way. She emphasized the greatness of the family by virtue of her being a descendent of the second in command to the royal family (granddaughter of Ezomo of the

Benin Empire) and her marital status to a descendant of the royal family as per Benin legend (Oloton of the Benin Empire). She also preached the essence of dignity in poverty by reminding us that she might be poor with nothing to inherit when she died but no one would come to us to say she owed him or her anything, even the slightest penny. She always said that a good name is better than riches.

She maintained the fact that there is dignity in poverty if only you can house and feed your family without debt or begging for alms. These two values, "hereditary and poverty," resonated constantly and played a tremendous role in the investigator's life all through secondary/high school. He had often wondered if there was an escape from these two phenomena that weighed heavily on the society even with education. At any rate, he has seen the importance of education and what a difference it makes in people's life. He cherished the egalitarian societies such as the Ibo society of Nigeria (equality and not the greed), the Kikuyu society of Kenya, and others where children grow with the ideals that life is not a bed of roses but what you make of it. Irrespective of their parents' status, wealth, and position, children in these societies learn surviving skills and how to explore their talents from an early age rather than resign their fate and condemn their life's ambition at the mercy of hereditary bondage, waiting and praying in some cases for their parents' death in order to inherit the properties or position. Quite too often, children that inherit their parents' properties or position without laboring for it do not know the value. They end up like the prodigal son, squandermania and wretchedness before the end of the day (back to square one or zero).

The investigator's admission to the University of Ife by late 1979 changed his views about "hereditary and poverty," and forever radicalized his approach to life issues. People can be born in a hereditary society and not be condemned by hereditary bondage or their parents' riches, status, position, and wealth. The investigator's first year on the campus coincided with the rise to power of Wole Olaoye as student union president and Femi Falana as public-relations officer. He experienced for the first time the true meaning of democracy and not the sham democracy that existed in the society, where people can kill anybody including their opponents and they will say nothing is going to happen and nothing will surely happen; people can rig elections in the name of power and tell you nothing is going to happen and nothing will surely happen; people can use their money to buy votes or give people dinner and everybody will mortgage their conscience for a little gesture that will cost them millions of dollars (hundred or thousandfold of the initial expenditure through embezzlement and corruption); and people see the government treasury (government money is nobody's money) as an inexhaustible bar of money/wealth so when you have the opportunity, dupe and loot as much as you can—fortunately for this set of people and unfortunately for the nation (present and future generation), politics offers a good avenue to achieve their aim of get-rich-quick mania. If and when these people discover that they are not capable of achieving their aim directly by becoming the president, governor, or other political elected position, they will look around and identify whom they can use as a puppet to achieve their aim.

Years upon years after independence, Nigeria has graduated into a nation that does not only eulogizes riches and power but also makes laws and orders to be obeyed by the poor in defense of the rich, powerful, and traditional rulers. Power, riches, and traditional rulers' positions are the easiest way to be above the law. People do not see the essence of the lawyers because justice is at the mercy of riches, power, and traditional rulers' positions. Traditional rulers' positions in most cases are hereditary and are not accessible to all and sundry, while power and riches, on the other hand, are at the mercy of anyone who can grab and use them for their own selfish purposes. The sham leaders created societies with direct links between riches/power and goodness. Consequently, if you are rich and powerful everybody identifies you as a good man from a good family even if you have armed robbers working for you all over the place or you looted the bank treasury or burnt down the government building to cover your guilt/loot of government treasury, etc. These issues coupled with the preaching of religious leaders such as Reverend Idahosa that it is a sin to be poor (we are not talking about spiritual poverty here but materialistic or monetary poverty; what an irony and a sharp contrast to the teachings of the Bible—it is a sin to be poor; where do you expect a night guard or security officer with a merger salary and who is an ardent member of your church to get the money to match the status of rich people in your church?). Under these conditions, it wasn't difficult for the vast majority of the people to lose sight of their vision and sense of direction all in the name of get-rich-quick mania. People's yearnings and aspirations become how to live above the laws and orders of the land through riches (the easiest way to acquire both positions—riches and power). Consequently, a lecturer in a university can resign his productive role as a lecturer to become a redundant traditional ruler because that is a role that serves him best, with people worshipping him, paying him homage, and eulogizing his power and riches.

This is the type of society with a sham democracy that brought Alahaji Shehu Shagari to power as president of the most populous black nation on the surface of this Earth. Bakinzuwo, a stack illiterate who couldn't differentiate between mineral resources and mineral soda (a common name for sodas like Coke) or a running mate and someone running after him, became governor of a state and thus introduced Bakinzuwocracy in the midst of numerous educated people. People did not see the danger in vesting the future of millions of human lives in the hands of an ignorant man who did not know what he was doing in the highest position of the state, because everything was normal to them. They were laughing and joking about the awesome display of ignorance, while the state was sinking. Alahaji Shehu Shagari is a man who in a true democratic society would not have succeeded in winning a local government election but was able to bulldoze himself to the highest position of the land because people knew they could easily use him to achieve their aim.

During his inept, malfeasant, maladministrated, corrupt, and inefficient administration that is worse than the type that characterized New York City before the election of La Guardia as mayor and the subsequent cleanup in the 1930s, Nigeria as a nation started degenerating. Shagari set the necessary machinery in motion for a downward trend and created a nation where people now think of retrogressiveness rather than progress as way of life. Thus, it is not difficult for any sane or right-thinking human being who knew Nigeria from independence to identify the fact that Nigeria of 1980 is better than Nigeria of 1990, Nigeria of 1990 is better than Nigeria of 2000, and Nigeria of 2000 will be better than Nigeria of 2010. Most of the infrastructure such as railways, seaports, drainage systems, good roads, streetlights, traffic lights, industries, good schools (contemporary universities are like '70s colleges or high schools in terms of infrastructures; same is true of elementary schools in places of high schools; however the quality of education remains the same because that has to do with direct dealing with human beings—at any rate it is fair to say that it is affected by availability of equipment in some place), airports, etc., have been destroyed and replaced with nothing. It is not unusual to see school children carrying chairs on their heads to schools in some localities. We grew up in Benin with airplanes flying over our heads; these days children have to be in dreamland to see airplanes flying over their heads. The sight of a present-day, isolated landing field in place of the functional Benin Airport of the 1970s is enough to bring tears to sane eyes. This is the capital of a state with a population of about 7 million people, yet the people want to develop, attract foreign investors, and move along with the rest of the world. How are you going to develop and attract foreign investors with an isolated landing field? Secret cults like the Ogboni Society of Nigeria and other destructive forces that are reminiscent of the old archaic societies are all back in full force and operate like no man's business.

When you see people crowded in junky cars and molue buses in Lagos, you wonder what has gone wrong with our reasoning faculty. We cannot even plan effectively for our people or maintain the things we inherited from colonial power—what a shame. A loaf of bread that cost 1 or 2 naira in the 1980s is now about 200 to 300 naira, and ordinary water is a luxury in some places.

Ikpoba River Dam, which started when I was in elementary school in the '70s, is yet to be commissioned and up till today Benin City, a state capital, has no potable drinking water provided by the government. Security is at an all-time low level with people barricading their houses like jails. Motorcycles (Okada Air) in Benin City and other places in the country have now become a popular means of public transportation, an abomination in the 1970s or 1980s—what a shame. In the midst of it all, these people have not lost their faith and good sense of humor—suffering and smiling as per Fela Anikulakpo Kuti. One of the generals, Banbagida, that presided over the country's worst time in history helped to catalyze Shagari's degeneracy machinery and created a favorable atmosphere for his twin brother in destruction, Abacha the dons, to ascend to power and put the finishing touches to the degeneracy. Banbagida, a civilian in uniform, thought he was the Diego Maradona of Nigerian politics only to get to power and discovered that he is a physician that could not heal thyself. Despite other things, including using a huge amount of government money to entice, bribe, and buy people over to his side, Dele Giwa's mysterious death with a letter bomb because of investigative journalism or the nullification of the Abiola election results that paved way for Abacha the dons to ascend to power, he came into office at the time the local currency was about two naira to one U.S. dollar, and as of the time he was leaving, it was more than eighty (between Eighty and one hundred) naira to one dollar. Banbagida is said to have used some of his ill-gotten wealth to buy himself a big, luxurious private jet and asked his in-law to donate it to him as a birthday gift. Ceteris peribus, if we literally accept that it was a true donation (almost everybody knows it is not), we can compare a similar gesture in American politics. As rich as U.S., any president that accepts a car donation talkless of an airplane while in office has a lot of explanation for the public or citizens especially if he is running for second term in office — that is accountability, law and order or using public opinion to guide your conscience while in the highest position of the land. Stunned and flabbergasted by the awesome display of enormous/grandiose wealth on Obasanjo's farm, visiting ex-president Julius Nyerere of Tanzanian, East Africa is said to have asked speechless then-ex-president Obasanjo if he had made his farm's money from his first term in office as president.

In Nigeria, if you going into public or government office as a hundred or thousandaire and leave as a millionaire or billionaire, people hail or sing praise of you out of sheer ignorance. If anyone goes to the same position and comes out same way or poorer or slightly richer, people show no mercy in condemning him because they are quick to label him as a mogul or moron, however patriotic he may have been. They compare people's achievements in terms of their personal investment irrespective of their status or positions held. They don't know that government's money is their money and corruption/

embezzlement robs them of the benefits of such money. Moreover, a president that duped his country thousands of dollars has no moral justification whatsoever to query another that duped his country millions or billions of dollars. Obasanjo's second term in office as president may or may not be a blessing, but generally speaking his first time in office was more of a blessing to the country (the 1970s—Nigeria's good days or the only decade of progress) because his regime was an offshoot of General Murtala Mohammed, a man who tried to wipe out corruption and thus put the country on the right track to greatness but was assassinated by the evil retrogressive forces or enemies of progress. Some people say that Obasanjo invested his money in the country unlike others such as Abacha the dons or the Dikkos, even Banbagida. There is no excuse for corruption and embezzlement. However good the gesture may be in the eyes of these fellows, the wrong message has been sent to millions of people who saw him as a role model, and the nation is bound to reap the trickle-down effects of such bad leadership qualities especially at a crucial time in the nation's development. Thus, if you ask people to manage a place like the airport or a school, they are much more interested in how much personal investment (e.g., if one man acquired 5 houses from managing the place, another [possibly the successor] must acquire up to 7 or 10 houses as sign of improvement) they can acquire by defrauding the place rather than looking at the goodness or future or societal benefits of the place.

After many years in power as a dictator, Banbagida now wants to come back and perform his political jinx, something he couldn't achieve as a dictator but hopes to do so as a politician, and Nigeria being what it is for now (blindfolded and incapable of learning from the past, and Banbagida with his endless tricks/enormous amount of stolen money to bribe and manipulate people), people will not be surprised to see him back in power with all his reminiscent acts. Nigeria's downward trend is bound to continue until something drastic occurs to revolutionize the nation in terms of people's thinking, attitudes, hopes, yearnings, and aspirations. Nigeria has become a big toothless bulldog on a straight road of destruction heading for a doom. No amount of political correctness can put things right on this road except a total reversal or 180-degree turnaround. The only decade of progress that Nigeria as a country after independence and the bitter civil war of the 1960s can proudly talk of is the 1970s. What is this? Colonialism or racism or slavery or imperialism. As a matter of fact, the condition is so bad now that if you conducted a poll in some areas about the return of colonialism, people would readily second the idea because they are yearning for serious resolution. All it takes is to have wrong people in power (less than 1%) and mislead/misdirect the masses or the rest of the country. These people (less than 1%) had the golden opportunity of selling their ideology to the masses of the nation right from birth and sociologists say when you raise a child in a den of snakes or lions, the child learns to behave like snakes or lions when he or she grows up. Most of these people are the wayward men who introduced public spraying of money (public insanity) to African culture in the 1950s and '60s and forever tarnished African public ceremonies in the eye of the world or world community. No sane human being who worked hard for his monthly or weekly salary will go to any public ceremony and in a matter of some seconds spray the money on anybody because of instantaneous praises. These men have no regard for money because they did not work for the money they stole or embezzled from their respective offices and their brains work in a negative direction, so this is one of the by-products of that negativity. There were no good laws to curtail the excesses of these men; as result they spread their waywardness to the rest of the society. How can a society that believed in public spraying of money (public insanity) evolve in the modern-day world when the phenomenon itself encourages corruption and unscrupulous activities? For instance, two principals of two schools (one corrupt and the other a dutiful, patriotic citizen) go to a public ceremony and the corrupt one starts spraying his ill-gotten wealth (money). All of a sudden, musicians as well as other people start singing praises of him. The dutiful, patriotic citizen is humiliated and he needs no soothsayer to prophesize to him that he is in trouble with his family (wife, children, and others), who witnessed everything, because they are going to demand to know if both of them are doing the same job. With this kind of pressure coming from various places and no incentives for being patriotic, gradually the good patriotic citizen begins to change his way to incorporate the corrupt practices of the corrupt principal, and that is how you mess up the society. These are human ills that have nothing to do with the color of one's skin, and it is pathetic. The irony of it all is that when things are fallen, people fold their hands or sits hand akimbo and watch amazingly with a lackadaisical attitude as if to say what is my business in it? It is the government, and when the problem comes everybody cries woe.

Wole Olaoye was a student as well as columnist in one of the nation's magazines or newspapers. He used his writings in his columns to decry the ills of the society, especially the sham politicians who specialized in looting the nation's treasury and womanizing. During the student union election, the opponent saw this as a weakness and decided to capitalize on it especially among the female students in female hostels. The news spread and the majority of the students were outraged. They said this will never happen but kept their peace and equanimity until the speech night, which is election eve (a day before the election). On speech night, all aspirants, especially presidential aspirants, face a mammoth crowd of the student body to talk about their manifestos (plans) and be challenged with a barrage of questions from selected campus journalists. Besides speech night, there were other forums such as the press night that is designed to drill all aspirants before the students. Wole out-flashed his opponent in all forums including speech night. The investigator, yet to be completely socialized into campus life the first semester in the school, was in one of the cafeterias reading (a food service center that is commonly converted into reading place by students after food service) at night when he suddenly noticed a stream of students pouring into the cafeteria after speech night, with palms fronds and broken tree branches, chanting, "Wole Wole o Wole Wole—Wole for president, Wole Wole." At first he was astonished. Further inquiring with various students revealed all that had taken place, so he had no option but to join the mammoth crowd of supporters of Wole after speech night.

Wole was just like every other student, probably from a poor family with lots of stories to tell about hereditary and poverty. He won the election gallantly and set out to organize the most effective administration ever witnessed by students in the campus. Femi Falana, now a nationally recognized attorney, also won as the public-relations officer position. Besides students' self-help project that started building dormitory to ease overcrowding of students in the main hostels and other issues, during his administration a few words from the president was enough to galvanize students into action against the ills of the society by mobilizing students for peaceful protest. Ife students became very active politically, registering about 11 protests against the inept Shagari's regime at federal, state, and local levels. It was easy for Ife students and all well-meaning Nigerians to visualize that Nigeria was heading for a doom, which is the result of today's Nigerian society, and greater catastrophe in the future if nothing is done to reverse the course. Ife students were so active against the societal ills that they would sacrifice the goose that laid the golden egg by risking their lives, forsaking lectures/courses, and mobilizing school/commercial buses sponsored by the student union to convey students to Lagos from Ile-Ife, a journey of about 450 miles. They protested the federal government's unwarranted action at the federal capital, Lagos, all to ensure a prosperous future for all Nigerians.

The effectiveness of Great Ife students in propagating the nation's true course was so much that a renowned lecturer, an erudite scholar, political activist, and an indomitable lion by the name of the late Professor Ayodele Awojobi decided to leave his school, the University of Lagos, to deliver his powerful, famous lecture "Austerity Measure: Where Has Our Oil Money Gone" at the University of Ife, Ile-Ife. Well-meaning Nigerians, such as Professor Awojobi, Ife students, and even Shagari's political opponent, Chief Obafemi Awolowo, warned the nation seriously of the dangerous path it was treading. Yet Shagari and his cohorts, who were never satisfied with their loot of the nation's treasury, always had answers for everything to cover their guilt in the midst of the ailing faces of the masses. "The nation is in perfect shape," "The economy is healthy and sound (a few months later the Austerity measure was introduced)," "People are not yet eating from the dustbins," "Some must die so that others can live," and many others. In a true democratic society such as the type that existed in Great Ife campus, there is hell no way Shagari, a grade-two-teacher certificate holder, could have matched the greatness of his opponent, a renowned scholar and lawyer, in discussing the nation's issues, vision, and direction before the masses. Barrister Awolowo is at times described with mixed feelings as the Thomas Jefferson of Nigeria that never materialized. Yes, he was corrupt to a certain extent with the acquisition of the inexplicable Marroko Beach properties and others, but not the match of Alahaji Shehu Shagari and his cohorts such as the Dikkos. It was easy to visualize Awolowo's vision and the direction for the nation rather than the visionless and directionless Shagari. People had no problem identifying with Shagari because their personal gains in terms of looting the nation's treasury were not only paramount to them but greater that the nation's interest and the interest of generations yet unborn. There were instances where Shagari couldn't stand the mammoth crowd of people and his cohorts assured him not to worry because they would deliver the election at all cost, come rain or sun.

Money politics (excessive expenditures) and special interest groups were almost an abomination in Great Ife campus politics; in short, you would be doing yourself a great disfavor while favoring your opponent's election bid if you were associated with these two evils in politics. Before the end of Shagari's regime by the military junta, one of his cohorts, Omoboriowo, rigged himself to power as a governor of a state and he couldn't even stay in the state to rule. He had to rule the state from the federal capital, Lagos, under the umbrella of Shagari's federal authority. (If you win a free and fair election, you will love to be among the people that elected you because their enthusiasm alone is enough to silence the opposition and protect you; the reverse is the case when you rigged the election.) Some of his supporters were lynched to death and there were spontaneous riots all over the state because people took the law into their own hands to seek justice and get him at all costs. Shagari supported him fervently by mobilizing federal forces (military and police) to calm the state and keep him in power while he remained safe in the federal capital. Though not in support of military government, if the military junta had not stepped in, the federal forces would have succeeded in calming the state using the power that be to suit selected leaders through divide and rule tactics—and before anybody is aware of anything, the national ruling party would be the order of the day in the state. This is how a sham democracy works and the reason why most third world countries find it difficult to practice true democracy.

Little wonder why Nigeria is how it is today, with all its great potentialities that once endeared him as a hot contender of the United Nation's Security Council-member as the only black nation. Nigeria, the most populous blacks nation on the surface of this Earth, has become a nation of squandermanias. A nation where people readily lose sight of their vision, ambition, direction, conscience, ethics, and morality, all in search of money and the wealth, is not there, neither are they getting the money (so in the long run they lose everything including money, soul, conscience, morality, ethics, vision, and direction). A nation that keeps rotating in a vicious circle repeating catalogue of past mistakes, all because of old layers who looted the treasury very time they were in office. Instead of building a just society for all and sundry including themselves, these reactionaries looted the treasury with the notion that they could guarantee a decent life for themselves, their family, and descendants yet unborn. Unfortunately for them, they discovered that the chaos that they created and masterminded out of greed, selfishness, and covetousness engulfed the society and all their loot. The so-called monumental loot they thought would guarantee a decent life for their descendents could not even last their lifetime; consequently, they had to wangle their way back to office and repeat the same scenario with the aid of government control media, and the almost good-for-nothing government apparatus such as the police force. They have successfully programmed the nation to be blindfolded to its past mistakes and misdeeds. Nigeria is now the laughingstock of the world and a good source of blacks' ridicule anywhere in the world—what a colossal waste of human and natural resources—somebody needs to wake up the sleeping giant of Africa.

Around mid-1981, Wole's one-year tenure in office was over and one of his lieutenants had become the president even though people were still clamoring for continuation of his regime. News had spread to the campus that a student was murdered and the decapitated body was found close to the marketplace. There were different rumors surrounding the death and one of the most popular was that the death was connected to ritual killing. Ritual killing (in the 20th century?) spread so fast like wildfire in winter or the harmattan (dry) season bush (woods). The spillover of students' political consciousness from Wole's regime was still very much alive; hence, Great Ife students left no stone unturned and rose to the occasion. A peaceful protest was planned for June 7, 1981; some radical students had planned to burn down the Oni of Ife's palace (king's palace) but the student union wasn't going for that because the vast majority of the students were peaceful. The police were notified and they gave their blessing to the peaceful protest. However, at the middle of the protest in

Ile-Ife, the police that had given their blessing to the peaceful protest opened fire shooting directly at innocent, defenseless, and armless students. At the end of the day, four more students lay dead, and June 7 massacre (as coined by the students) quickly became world news. Numerous news reporters, political activists, well-meaning lecturers, and others besieged the campus to calm the students down. Students were outraged, many were clamoring for justice for the five dead souls, while a few others requested to turn the university's chemical laboratory into a weapons factory for revenge. The good voices eventually prevailed after careful thoughts that further violence would escalate issues, worsen the problem, and result in more students' death. No matter what, students could never match government-backed forces (military and police). Some of the lecturers and political activists promised to take up the issue at the national level and get justice for the students. This is an integral story of the investigator and the University of Ife in those days, a university in Africa, not Europe or the U.S., where students were in the forefront denouncing the Vietnam War and other issues. As a matter of fact, if you are someone that cherishes, acknowledges, and appreciates radicalism as an effective means of social change and you went through the University of Ife in those days without imbibing the act, know that for the rest of your life you can never be a radical. It is not out of place to say that you pass through the University of Ife without the university passing through you no matter the degree of your academic excellence. The University of Ife is the first place where I discovered that no matter who you are, as long as you are a citizen of this world, you have an impact or say-so in the running of affairs of your society. In the eyes of those responsible for Nigeria's backwardness and those who have turned the great nation into a nation of beggars, the investigator will always remain an Ife student until the society changes for good.

PABULUM FOR THE WHOLE WORLD

*** By the very nature of man, the solution for human problems does not lie in the extremism of capitalism or socialism but in between. Human beings are human beings anywhere you go in the world; extremism of socialism kills competition (essential ingredient for human survival/existence), creates laziness, the idea of people taking things or other people for granted, and eventually the system collapses. Extremism of capitalism is the opposite of socialism: the rich getting richer and the poor getting poorer. Unfortunately, the rich cannot live in isolation without the poor or else the wealth loses its value and it becomes meaningless. Moreover, the bulk of the wealth is derived from the poor. If the poor are going to be allowed to serve to death in the midst of abundance of the rich and some of the heartless rich are going to pretend as if they don't see anything, then there will be an increased wave of robbery, prostitution, crime, senseless killing (the rich boost with wealth while the poor boost with death because they have nothing to lose, and that is one of the few things they have in common with the rich), other human vices, and eventually the system collapses.

*** By the very nature of man, the solution for human problems lies in the socio-capitalist system and the *modus operandi* for operating such a system on a percentage basis (e.g., 20/80% or 30/70% or 35/65% or 40/60% or 50/50%) depends on the prevailing circumstances in any human society. The operation of a two-party systems in a polarized democratic society can help to balance these two extremes (socialism and capitalism) in a healthy manner. (When the ruling party is going too far to the left or right, the other is swept to power to restore normalcy and sanity, as it is practiced in U.S.—alternatively both parties can incorporate both extremes by remaining in the center and the matter of ideology or identifying with people's yearnings and aspirations becomes the *modus operandi* for winning election.)

*** If we need to know the truth about homosexuality, we might need to study the relationship between homosexuality and civilization/wealth/wealthy society/publicity. In some cases, the richer a man is the more he allows his mind to wander about impossibilities and unrealistic life issues because he is not preoccupied with the basic necessities of life or the more he tends to query the authority and existence of God. I am not homophobic, but if we do not know how to set boundaries for our civilization, freedom, and liberty, God will set them for us. Celibacy (Catholic) is, of course, an exceptional case where man made law against nature becomes the rule for many, while some celibates allowed nature to take it due course in a normal or aberrated fashion. There is no doubt that such studies will definitely vindicate God, justice, biblical sayings such as it will be easier for a camel to pass through the eye of a needle…, and morality, and prove that there is nothing hereditary in lifestyle choices. One of the most unfortunate things in human history is the correlation of homosexuality with racism. As a black man, if I had a choice I wouldn't subscribe to anything different from the way God created me, and racism is a matter of creation and not a matter of choice. Homosexuality is a human behavioral issue that borders on lifestyle choices like prostitution, alcoholism, drug addiction, drinking habits, singing habits, stealing habits, kleptomania, eating habits, womanizing, workalcohlism, and many other good and bad behaviors. Addiction to any of these behaviors (e.g., alcoholism or drugs) can result in the victim thinking of hereditary factors as a means of justifying his action. It is not unreasonable to say that if we look around the world, we will find some pseudo-scientists that can use hereditary factors to buttress such actions, if funded adequately. The more a taboo or an abomination becomes acceptable as a norm in any society, the greater the societal practice of it, the more aberrant the society becomes, and the greater they alienate themselves from God. Let no one be deceived: there is hell no way any human being on the surface of this Earth can produce offspring (baby) without the opposite sex. Artificial insemination or cloning also needs opposite-sex cells (chromosomes) for adequate reproduction. Cloning is a product of an animal, which is a product of a sexual relationship. A cloned product of a sexual relationship has problems sustaining adequate life now; will it be possible for the cloning of cloned products to stand the test of time and sustain adequate life about 500 years from today? That is a subject of scientific evolution and a puzzle for future generations to answer.

*** The powers of the laws and judiciary manifest their greatness and reign supreme whenever it takes its judiciously blindfolded toll on the rich, powerful, and so-called "born greats" in the society. Any time, it becomes meek in the eyes of these people while it takes a harsh tone with poor, defenseless citizens, it merely betrays its weakness, and this is a recipe for a catastrophic demise of any society, however great it may be. I don't care about the greatness of any leader, king or queen; anytime the court adjourns its sittings to take evidence for adducing proceedings in the leader's place or the king/queen's palace, the law loses its value. Consequently, the power of the laws and the judiciary are not only questionable but render its machinery and integrity worthless because it can no longer guarantee equality before the law and the blindfoldedness of its judgment.

*** The time has come when humanity and indeed all traditional rulers from the British monarchy in Europe to the least African king and Asian king in Japan should come to the self-realization that monarchy has outlived it usefulness in the world. Any attempt to encourage this outdated phenomenon (pharaohs have descendents in our contemporary society) is not only tantamount to retrogressiveness but encouraging parasitism of the world's economy. Humanity created the phrase "born great" and will also discard the ideal when the time comes. Besides the unhealthy rivalry between the old and the young with the latter silently praying for quick exit of the former in order to catalyze his or her ascension to power/throne, it is worthwhile to note that the essence of life, which is struggle for survival, striving for better status, and competition stands defeated to any human being who at birth knows the end result of his or her life. The easiest way to lose success is to think that you have succeeded, and right from birth the "born greats" think that they have succeeded in life. The great men of America, the forefathers of America's independence, democracy, freedom, liberty, and happiness, fought gallantly till the last drop of their blood to set humanity free of hereditary bondage. Here we are today, almost two and half centuries later, glamorizing royalty and monarchs, and these forefathers are spinning in their graves wondering what has gone wrong with the American dream and ideology they fought for. It is important to realize how much disservice we pay to them every second or minute we spend glamorizing royalty and monarchs. Remember some of the words of our great men: "We hold these truths to be self-evident, that all men are created equal" We all came through the same process and will leave through the same process.

*** We are fast approaching the age when family name adoption and leadership will no longer be automatic and incumbent upon the man as a result of marriage but a democratic process for the couple like every other political entity in life, because there can't be two captains in a boat (it will wreck). The couple's democratic process, whether for life, a decade, a year, or a percentage basis (e.g., 50/50, 75/25), will very much become part of the wedding vows and possibly be a great resolution for most marital problems/high divorce rate in the interest of the family, children, future generations, modern society, civilization, and democracy. Home administration is the genesis of a democratic society and home leadership can't be run differently from the nation's leadership. A divided home with single parent doesn't argue well for/with children, civilization, liberty, freedom, and survival of true democracy. In fighting against women's oppression by men, the civilized world must be very careful so as not to turn the oppressed into the oppressor, because we are already feeling the ripple effect of this issue that placed men in a disadvantageous position whether in the UK, the U.S., etc.

*** Africa is a partner in the world's peace, progress, technological advancement, and economic development and not a liability, as some would make us believe. The United States of America single-handedly rebuilt Western Europe after The Second World War's devastation, Japan after the Hiroshima and Nagasaki atomic bomb catastrophe, Israel after the Jewish Holocaust/persecution, and now Iraq and Afghanistan. The U.S. can equally do a lot to help rebuild one of the black nations and thus produce a role model for others. It is important to know that all the human tragedies above put together did not last half a century, and slavery with its devastating economic woes lasted for centuries. The U.S. did the right thing in developing these places because it needed partners on the world's stage, and Africa is a viable partner too. The U.S. or the world cannot continue to wait until disaster strikes Africa before it acts; they can help Africa to help itself.

*** The United States of America and South Africa are a microcosm of the global village, the world's conscience, and a better world to come. The U.S. holds the key to that destination; thus, the blacks in South Africa will be very responsive to the prevailing circumstances in America, and if it is possible for America to have a democratically elected black president then it will be possible for South Africa to have a democratically elected white president, and a true message will be sent across the globe that any human being can aspire to any height in any country, including the presidency of the nation, without prejudice, race, or creed provided the person identifies himself with the people's yearnings and aspirations.

*** The easiest way to make a mockery of democracy and use it as rubber stamp for despotism in a polarized society is to have a system of more than two political parties.

***If you cannot follow others, you cannot lead others; similarly, if you cannot obey law and order, you cannot make law and order.

*** The human accent: a wonderful human attribute and one of the basic qualifications for human beings. All human beings have it. The fact that you are not sensitive to your accent signifies nothing but a home environment or how easily you adopt another place as a home environment. When America or any other country's president speaks and a hearer cannot identify his accent/voice after a repeated performance, there is something wrong with either the hearer or (rarely) the speaker. The same people that claimed that Arnold Schwarzenegger couldn't speak English voted him to power as governor of California in the United States, the sixth largest economy in the world.

*** The essence of parenthood is being authoritative, knowing when to be strict and loving or tough and permissive, and how to control your emotions in dealing with children. Permissive (tolerant) and authoritarian (harsh) parents know little or nothing about love and the value of life; they specialize in constructing a broad, smooth path for their children to go into the street. So what kind of parent are you?

*** In most cases, besides children born to drug addicts, who are in danger of behavioral problems, you show me one hyperactive or attention-deficit child and I will show a parent(s) who has been reckless with the child's discipline right from day one.
["It is easier to give Ritalin (a drug for hyperactivity/attention deficit disorder) than parenting." - Dr. Robert Pihl, PhD, Professor of Psychology/Psychiatry, McGill University, Montreal, Quebec, Canada]

*** If what we do for ourselves dies with us and what we do for others remains as monuments to immortalize our name, then we must learn how to do good. However, people must beware of goodness because it is not all that glitters that is gold, and there are hypocrites everywhere around the world.

*** If you are one of those that believe the fact that certain people are born great while others like yourself are born slaves/peasants that is your funeral. Hold no man culpable for your misfortune, because you are the architect.

*** Do you know that according to health psychologists, over 1,000 people die everyday in U.S. alone because of smoking? So please think about your life and ask if you actually love yourself each time you light a cigarette to smoke.

*** Lie! Lie! Lie! Human lies. No human being on the surface of this Earth is above lying, be it the request for (just) a minute when five minutes is actually needed for a task or the denial under oath of a murder by an assassin. However, the basic foundation for societal evolution and progress is truth. Any society that is not built on truth is doomed to a catastrophic demise. Tell me the truth so that we can start building the society from here, and it is important that you know that we can only deal with degrees of honesty.

***Environment is a key factor in every human life; anyone that underestimates it underestimates himself. If you take care of your environment, the environment will in turn take care of you and you will be in total control of everything and your enemies will want to live with you. If you fail to take care of your environment, your environment will not fail to take care of you but will do so in a negative manner; thus, you will be at the mercy of all mishaps and natural disasters and your children will be the first to desert you.

PABULUM FOR THE ENTIRE BLACK WORLD

*** Is the black man actually cursed or this is more of a human problem of which one race has been able to put his house in order and the other is just wandering up and down pondering where to start and continue the great work of his ancestors? Yes, slavery was a human shame that devastated the black world but we cannot continue to use slavery as an excuse for everything. Human daily struggle between evil and good will always result in the prevalence of one over the other. When evil prevails and engulfs goodness and the society sits hands akimbo, watching amazingly with a lackadaisical attitude, then the society is doomed for a catastrophic end. If goodness prevails, on the other hand, then success is bountiful.

*** Many lovers of Africa felt somehow elated to hear how Europe underdeveloped Africa. How heartsick will they be to hear how Africans underdeveloped Africa? If there are brains in the world, there are brains in Africa; if there are geniuses in the world, there are geniuses in Africa; if there are mediocres and dons in the world, there are mediocres and dons in Africa. The problem with most African nations is that the mediocres in conjunction with the dons have colluded to lead them astray while the brains and geniuses are relegated to the background. Africa is blessed with many human and natural resources to annex for the benefit of mankind; hence, the great future generations of Africa cannot afford to let the continent down like we did.

*** The people to develop Africa are in the villages and until the present generation of blacks, especially those in and from the continent, are prepared to face reality, call a spade a spade, and put our house in order, there is nothing to prevent the world from liking our generation to the era when Europe barbarians invaded and ravaged the European continent, destroying the civilization and all that existed before them because of selfishness. ("I belong to the wasteful generation." —Wole Soyinka, Nobel laureate)

*** Without a major breakthrough that endears black representation in the form a membership in the United Nation Security Council, not just in terms of sympathy but worthiness, then the present generation of blacks has nothing remarkable to justify our existence and the greatness of our ancestors especially in Egypt, the Ghana Empire,

Mali, Songhai, Zulu, etc. Contemporary blacks, be it from the era of Toussaint-Louverture's slave revolution that precipitated Haiti's (previously including the Dominican Republic) independence as the only black nation in Western Hemisphere in 1791 till the occurrence of the major breakthrough, have nothing to say about the greatness of the past and indeed future generation of blacks.

*** Words of mouth are not enough to express one's gratitude to the black brothers and sisters of the United States of America for the role so far played in the post-slavery emancipation of blacks all over the world. Without the blacks in America it is easy to visualize the fact that today's progress would have been half a century or more backwards. The so-far incomplete good reputation that blacks enjoy all over the world today owes a lot to the blacks in the U.S. The blacks in America owe it not only to themselves but also to their ancestors and indeed future generations of blacks to assist one black nation to stand on its feet and be a role model for others to follow.

*** Besides the various human tragedies that resulted in the loss of many innocent souls in places like Germany (Jewish Holocaust), Kosovo, Ethiopia, Somalia, Rwanda(Hutu/Tushi genocide), and others, Nigeria and Jean Bertrand Aristide (Haitian president—what a disgrace and disservice to the memory of Louverture) are the two greatest twentieth-century embarrassments to the entire black world.

*** Our enemies or the enemies of our nation, Nigeria, are those in high and low places that seek the nation divided permanently so that they can remain in offices as president, governors, ministers, permanent secretaries etc., the ten per centers — corrupt officers that seek bribery or 10 percent for every awarded contracts and those that make the nation look big for nothing before international circle
    — January 15, 1966 ----- Major Kaduna Nzeogwu

*** The idea of a global village is a reality and not an illusion or Hollywood fiction; let us strive to make the world a better place to live in. Black nations like Mali, the Ashante Empire, the Benin Empire, the Zulu kingdom, and others excelled even during slavery, so we have no excuse for the present-day woes. It is a shame that in spite of numerous blacks' successes in business all over the world, we cannot produce a formidable black nation. The issue of racial equality and the idea of people seeing themselves as human beings instead of blacks and whites will continue to plague humanity until black nations exalt themselves and one becomes a role model for others.

*** In the early 1960s, Kwamen Nkrumah called on African nations to seek "the kingdom of political freedom first and every other thing will follow." Today, I call on all African nations and third world countries to seek the kingdom of law and order first and every other thing will follow. Thus, if any society or nation is going to stand by, hands akimbo, and watch while one man rises to power, loots the government treasury, asks everybody to shut up, or barricades himself with gangs of hoodlums, criminals, and armed robbers as a necessary weapon in terrorizing people so as to rule in fear—it is the laws of the land that permit the atrocities and those laws remain at stake until the ills of the society are cured.

WORDS OF WISDOM FOR ALL

The turbulent and topsy-turvy nature of the world we live in makes it difficult for many people to succeed or achieve their aim/goal in life. However, those who want to overcome their obstacles in life can equip themselves with these four pieces of wisdom by four great people. With these words of wisdom among others, success is likely to be yours provided you know what to do at the right time, place, and moment.

"No one can make you feel inferior without your consent."
—Eleanor Roosevelt

"Life struggle is not about being the strongest or weakest person. No sooner than later we discovered that the act of winning belongs to the man or woman who does not only think of winning, but acts like a winner. The greatness of a man is not defined by his number of successes, but by the number of rises and falls (how often he rises, falls, and breaks to pieces then picks up the pieces, patches them together, and rises again)." —Obafemi Awolowo

"Class struggle: the good ones triumph, the bad ones are eliminated, but the best always remain in the race." —Russell Saundra

"Only if you have been to the deepest valley will you appreciate the magnificence of being on top of the mountain." —Richard Nixon

(In a nutshell, life is not a bed of roses nor is it an ideal experience for the so-called "born great." May your road be rough and bumpy so that you will know how to manipulate it.)

INDEX

A
Abacha 566, 567
Aba Riot 2
Aberdeen 470
Abiola 2, 133, 566
abomination 3, 168, 566, 570, 574
abortion clinic 119
Abramowitz 494, 511, 523
absorption 10, 119, 138, 139, 184, 552
academic doctors 166
academic reputation 205
academic researchers 422
accidents xiii, 147, 159, 162
accountant 11, 103, 196, 514
acetylation 140
acetylators 140
ACP-ASIM 513, 515, 524
Acupuncture 378, 379
acupuncture 22, 39, 378, 379, 380, 546
acute care nurse practitioner 344
Adachi 487, 521
Adams, David 55
adherence 91, 152, 161, 165, 180, 184, 377, 386, 454
ADR 13, 16, 18, 19, 89, 141, 142, 147, 148, 150, 151, 152, 158, 172, 177, 188, 189, 192, 193, 194, 195, 196, 465, 467, 471, 480, 483, 497, 498, 504, 505, 506, 508, 509, 552, 553, 555
adverse drug events 146, 184, 468, 484, 525
adverse drug reaction ix, xv, 10, 13, 14, 15, 16, 49, 89, 141, 147, 149, 160, 172, 179, 180, 199, 201, 380, 447, 467, 481, 497, 498, 509, 523, 540, 550, 552, 558
advertising 12
Africa 1, 3, 66, 133, 179, 183, 187, 359, 360, 375, 376, 378, 380, 392, 408, 439, 441, 450, 451, 556, 572, 576, 579, 615
African National Congress 3, 545
African Public Ceremonies 568
agricultural science 368
Agriculture Bureau of Chemist 121
agriculturists 103
AIDS 13, 81, 483
ailments 12, 15, 16, 22, 39, 44, 47, 50, 51, 55, 57, 58, 67, 79, 85, 86, 87, 88, 90, 91, 93, 107, 108, 138, 331, 333, 355, 455, 464, 504, 546
Akershus 184
Al-Azhar 548
Alberta province 186
albumin 139, 511
alchemist 92
alcoholism 142, 574
alcohol dehydrogenase 140
Alexandria Hospital 144
all-cause mortality 498
allergist 9
allergy and immunology 48, 331, 451, 453, 546, 556
Almshouse 98
alternative medicine 39
Alvarez, Eric 168
amalgam war 52
Amboy, Perth 97
ambulatory care xiii, 146, 149, 151, 361, 466, 472, 511, 521, 552

American Association of Colleges of Pharmacy 8, 21, 125
American Board of Anesthesiology 40, 50
American Board of Radiology 73
American Board of Surgery 40, 50, 73, 74
American Dermatological Association 53
American Hospital Association statistics 480
American Indian community 447
aminophylline 490
amphotericin B 109
analysis of variance 496, 502
analytical chemistry 93, 94
anatomy 53, 64, 76, 88, 90, 98, 362, 414
ancestors 579, 580
Andorra 112
Anesthesiologists 40, 452
anesthesiology xiv, 40, 44, 48, 50, 80, 85, 88, 331, 546, 556
anesthetics 40, 42, 43, 44, 50, 109, 452, 553
Anikulakpo Kuti, Fela 566
Animalium 76
annual cost savings 502, 511
annual savings 447, 473, 503
ANOVA 496, 502
Anthony Leeuwenhoek 65
antibiosis 107
antibiotic 17, 20, 107, 108, 121, 154, 156, 159, 161, 447, 461, 487, 488, 492, 494, 496, 522, 557
antibiotic resistance 20
anticholinergic drugs 500
anticoagulation 150, 174, 177, 447, 467, 470, 473, 521

anticoagulation management service 447, 470
antidepressants 109, 140, 153, 447, 500
Antidotary 91
antifreeze 121
antigen-antibody 49
antihemophilic factor 488, 489, 522
antimicrobial surveillance 474
antiquity period 88
anuria 121
Aparasu 151, 199
Apartheid 3
apothecary 12, 37, 93, 95, 96, 97, 102, 103, 549
apprenticeship 7, 8, 9, 64, 67, 77, 95, 96, 98, 99, 178, 334, 354, 545
Arab 89, 90, 547
archaic pharmacist 117
architect 9, 11, 167, 171, 578
Aristide, Jean Bertrand 580
Aristotelian physics 2
Aristotle 76
armed robbers 564, 581
army 4, 48, 49, 71, 102, 546
arrhythmia 16, 42
Arross, John 507
art 51, 82, 334, 422, 445, 446, 545
Asheville 18, 116, 448, 461, 483, 515
Asia 66, 359, 360, 377, 378, 381, 386, 390, 391, 408, 439, 450, 451, 556
Asipu 87
aspirin 109, 161
Association 7, 19, 23, 24, 37, 40, 48, 50, 53, 55, 56, 59, 60, 61, 62, 66, 67, 71, 72, 73, 75, 76, 78, 79, 80, 81, 83, 100, 104,

107, 118, 124, 144, 146, 172, 179, 181, 183, 185, 199, 447, 448, 460, 461, 466, 468, 478, 484, 507, 508, 511, 518, 519, 520, 521, 522, 549, 550, 553, 556
association 53, 105, 119
asteroid 408
asthma 16, 19, 49, 144, 150, 174, 448, 464, 467, 476, 477, 478, 484, 557
Asu 87, 547
Athanasius 91
Athens 480
atoxyl 108
attending physician 144, 501, 503
attorneys 119, 453
Aurelius, Marcus 89
Austerity measure 570
Australia xi, xviii, 66, 112, 183, 184, 187, 359, 360, 378, 392, 396, 406, 407, 423, 438, 439, 440, 441, 450, 451, 453, 556
Austria 112
automation 110, 550
autopsy 68, 184, 452
Avignon 93, 94
avoidance of ADR 501
Awolow, Obafemi 360, 443, 455, 562, 569, 582
Ayodele Awojobi 569

B

Babylonians 87
baccalaureate degree 7, 96, 192, 272, 281
bachelor of dentistry 413
bachelor of optometry 443
bachelor of pharmacy 407
bachelor of science 8, 104, 177, 267, 273, 275, 277, 279, 300, 313, 315, 316, 342, 344, 348, 349, 377, 378, 417, 470, 501, 549
bachelor of veterinary science 415
bacitracin 108
Bacon, Rogers 65
Bacteria resistance 153
Baghdad 7, 22, 90, 446, 545
Bakinzuwo 564
Bakinzuwocracy 564
Bakr, Abu 89
balance sheets 11
Baltimore 53, 58, 83, 208, 336, 358, 490, 495, 508
Baltimore hospitals 508
Banbagida 566, 567
bankers 12
barbers 52, 94
Barcelona 94, 96
barefoot doctors 180
Barrett, Collen 2
Bartholomew, Ralph 507
Bartolomea 69
baseline data 472
basic necessities of life 573
Bellevue Hospital 98
Benedict of Nursia 91
benefit/risk ratio 160
Benin City xviii, 443, 450, 451, 454, 556, 566, 615
Benin Empire 563, 580
benzodiazepines 109, 141, 472
Berg 152, 200, 553
Bergner 479
Berlin 52, 72, 77, 95
Bernstein 523
Berryville 123
Betsy Lehman 529
Bidell Airy, George 66
Biko, Steve 3, 545
bill 124, 146, 150, 174, 202, 448, 469, 500, 507, 536

bill 717 500
binding affinities 142
biochemistry 43, 414
Biologics Control Act 121
biology 69, 107, 166, 334, 360, 368, 387, 407, 409, 410, 414
biopsychosocial model 14
bipolar disorder 119
Birmingham 419, 444, 522
Bitter pills 200, 544
Blackstone, William 54
block 58, 213, 413
blood brain barriers 139
blood cholesterol meters 464
blood pressure meters 463
blood sugar meters 464
Blue Cross of Central Ohio 488
Bologna 92, 548
bombs 445
Bond 98
Bootman xvi, 16, 146, 148, 149, 172, 199, 342, 447, 460, 480, 493, 521, 522, 552
Boston 18, 68, 72, 79, 97, 98, 100, 498, 529
bovine pleuropneumonia 78
bradycardia 42
Brakeball 486
Brazil xi, xviii, 66, 187, 360, 424, 427, 430, 438, 441, 442, 450, 451, 453, 556
Brazilians 450, 455
Breu, Joseph 23
Briceland 468
British Empire 1, 392
British Medical Journal 123
British monarch 575
Brocavich 483, 520
Brown, Bartholomew 96
Brunei 112
bubonic plague 175

Buddha 72
Budget Reconciliation Act 113, 146, 152, 551
Bureau of Animal Industry 78
Burkholder, David 122, 167, 172, 553
business executives 12
Butler, Tait 79

C

cadaver 98
California nursing facility 18
California State Assembly bill 481
Canada 2, 7, 38, 77, 111, 112, 185, 186, 187, 202, 546, 577
cancer xiii, 16, 17, 43, 58, 73, 75, 143, 146, 147, 148, 421, 529, 531, 562
capitalism 573
Capitol Hill 24, 25, 26
carbamazepine 119, 140
carbenicillin 494
Carbrita 184
cardiologist 9, 45, 138, 514
cardiology 6, 23, 80, 516
cardiovascular surgery 381, 494, 522
CARE 285, 482
career advisers 191
Carnegie Foundation 7, 38, 85, 205
caseworkers 20
Casper 507
Cassian, John 91
Cassiodorus 91
catalog 62, 221, 228, 229, 235, 237, 239, 241, 243, 252, 255, 257, 266, 267, 300, 311, 335, 357, 358, 359
catastrophic coverage 151
Catellier 506, 524
Caucasians 140

Caventous, Joseph 93
cefamandole 494, 505, 523
cefazolin 474, 494, 495, 505, 511
cefoxitin 474, 494, 523
cefuroxime 494
Celsus, Caius 50
Centers for Disease Control and Prevention 153
center of health sciences 424
centralized profile monitoring 499
centralized unit dose cart 499
Central Hospital 184
cephalosporin 108, 495, 511
certified nurse practitioner xii, xv, 20, 155, 173, 237, 272, 335, 342, 344, 345, 347, 353, 376, 378, 392, 407, 422, 424, 440, 441, 554, 556
chain 105, 106, 164, 165, 467, 475, 520, 532
chaos 88, 571
Charcot, Jean-Martin 59
Charity Hospital 98
Charles Darwin 88, 528
Charles Dickens 77
Charles Walton 172
Chemists xviii
chemotherapy 107, 374, 529
Cheyenne 507
chi-square 473, 480, 496, 498, 501, 502, 504
Chicago 61, 69, 76, 144, 466, 475, 495
Chile 112
China xi, xix, 65, 180, 184, 203, 360, 377, 378, 380, 386, 450, 451, 453, 454, 556, 558, 561
Chinese pharmaceutical processing 378
Chinese pharmacology 378, 379, 380

chiropractics 22, 546
chiropractic medicine 39
chiropractors 12, 44
chirurgical faculty 52
chloramphenicol 108
cholestech LDX blood analyzer 478
Christendom 89
chronic illness 86, 116, 143, 157, 552
church 1, 2, 4, 6, 88, 90, 91, 94, 110, 545, 564
cipro 108
civil war 567
Class struggle 582
clay 86
clergy 12, 94, 464
clergymen 12
clinical analysis 187, 424, 433, 435
clinical director 333
clinical medicine 62, 172, 380, 384, 553
clinical pharmacists xi, xii, xiii, xiv, xv, xvi, xix, 13, 14, 15, 16, 18, 40, 44, 80, 116, 117, 120, 125, 163, 166, 171, 175, 181, 188, 190, 193, 197, 330, 347, 351, 352, 353, 355, 375, 380, 407, 422, 441, 447, 448, 450, 451, 452, 463, 466, 467, 469, 470, 472, 473, 474, 475, 481, 484, 485, 487, 488, 491, 493, 494, 496, 497, 499, 500, 502, 503, 508, 509, 510, 511, 513, 515, 516, 523, 551, 554, 555, 556, 558
clinical pharmacist practitioners 469
clinical pharmacologists 158, 172, 553
clinical pharmacology xiv, 43, 80, 134, 158, 160, 172, 200, 422

clinical pharmacy ix, x, xii, 18, 103, 110, 113, 122, 123, 124, 125, 134, 160, 163, 171, 178, 179, 180, 181, 183, 185, 188, 190, 196, 200, 352, 375, 377, 402, 421, 422, 423, 424, 446, 448, 450, 454, 461, 463, 470, 471, 489, 490, 496, 497, 498, 499, 504, 505, 508, 510, 511, 523, 524, 551, 553
clinical phase 331, 332, 333, 336, 337, 338, 339, 341, 342, 348, 349, 350, 352, 415
Clinical rotations 195
clinics 64, 173, 174, 395, 471, 473, 476, 495, 502, 508, 511, 530
cloning 15, 574
CNN/USA Today/Gallup poll 12
CNN/USA Today Gallup poll 464
cocaine 42
Coggeshall, George 100
Cohen, Lita 159
Cohen, Michael 530
Cohen, William 149
Colcord, Samuel 100
Colegio 94
colistin 108
Coll, Rena 177
collective responsibility xiii, 155, 156, 531, 533
college de pharmacie 94
college of dental medicine 427
College of Philadelphia xviii, 95, 98
college teachers 12, 464
colonialism 567
colonial era 98
combined six scales 447, 500, 501
communism 561
community ADRs 148
community pharmacy 104, 106, 164, 174, 182, 461, 518, 519

community teaching hospital 501, 504
company executives xv, 446
comparative analysis xi, 439
complaints 55, 115, 161, 164, 171, 194
complex and multiple drug regimen 502
compliance 8, 13, 20, 105, 125, 143, 150, 152, 192, 193, 195, 196, 333, 465, 471, 472, 475, 477, 479, 483, 496, 502, 505, 506, 521, 557
compounding 7, 12, 90, 91, 92, 94, 95, 99, 100, 103, 106, 122, 137, 194, 547, 548, 615
compounding of drugs 99, 548
computerization 110, 484
computer industry 163, 192, 206
concomitant 89, 184, 354, 454, 467, 483, 491, 552
Confucius 72
congestive heart failure 464, 467, 479, 491, 557
Congress 49, 70, 78, 121, 122, 480, 551
congressmen 12, 558
conjugation 140
Constantine 89, 91
Constantinople 89
consultation 12, 15, 118, 150, 157, 161, 180, 464, 465, 468, 489, 491, 496, 499, 503, 505, 507, 509, 522, 524
consumer model of care 14
contemporary pharmacists 118, 166, 174, 179
continuing education 56, 70
contraindication 161
control group 17, 18, 149, 184, 447, 468, 471, 472, 473, 475, 476,

477, 481, 482, 485, 486, 487, 491, 493, 495, 496, 497, 498, 499, 501, 502, 503, 508, 558
control regions 183
Cook, Stephanie 479
Copernicus and Galileo versus the Church 2
coping mechanism 528
Cordus, Valerius 92, 548
Cornwallis 4
corruption 561, 563, 566, 568
cost-benefit analysis 195, 464, 473, 493, 505, 507, 512, 522
cost-benefit analysis study 473, 493
Costa Rica 112
cost benefits 16, 177
cost effective 16, 115, 120
cost effectiveness 16, 115
cost minimization 16, 195
cost utilization 16, 177, 195
counseling 18, 114, 116, 119, 135, 137, 150, 152, 155, 161, 162, 163, 174, 180, 465, 467, 468, 470, 478, 483, 501, 507, 509, 527, 535, 547, 551
Coverage Act 113, 150
cram schools 104, 105
creatinine clearance 141
Crile 72
Crookes, William 66
Crusades 90
Cuba 112
culture 87, 89, 91, 96, 108, 140, 180, 407, 485, 495, 548, 568
Cuomo, Thomas 446
cure rate 464, 485
curriculum xi, xviii, 7, 8, 43, 44, 61, 62, 63, 66, 68, 70, 77, 98, 100, 124, 167, 176, 177, 179, 181, 187, 205, 207, 272, 330, 333, 355, 357, 376, 387, 391, 395, 396, 419, 439, 441, 448, 513, 514, 516, 548, 554, 555, 556, 558

D

Dali Lama 561
Dalton, John 66
Damascus 90
Dana, Charles 55
Dana-Farber Cancer Institute 529
Dark Ages 2, 65, 88
data analysis 111, 211, 235, 287, 300, 332, 348, 351, 376, 438
David versus Goliath 1, 3
Davis, Neil 534
Davis, Scott 485
DEA xv, 470, 539
decentralized pharmacy 124, 503
decision analysis techniques 480
degree abbreviations 197
degree titles 197
democracy 4, 82, 561, 563, 564, 570, 575, 576
democratic society 37, 565, 570, 573, 576
Denmark 112, 185
dentist xii, xv, xvi, xix, 9, 10, 11, 12, 14, 22, 45, 52, 67, 80, 117, 167, 168, 178, 191, 333, 334, 336, 337, 353, 356, 376, 378, 382, 388, 391, 392, 396, 406, 423, 439, 440, 441, 451, 452, 453, 455, 464, 514, 517, 536, 555, 556
dentistry xii, xiv, 9, 23, 48, 51, 52, 55, 62, 63, 66, 78, 80, 81, 135, 138, 166, 168, 197, 205, 237, 335, 336, 337, 339, 340, 348, 353, 363, 376, 377, 388, 390, 391, 396, 402, 406, 413, 414,

415, 417, 423, 424, 427, 440, 450, 499, 514, 516, 546, 552
Departibus Animalium 76
Department of Health and Human Services 190
depression 106, 121, 153, 157, 201, 332, 464, 467
dermatologist 9, 11, 53
dermatology xii, xiv, 13, 23, 44, 48, 53, 80, 138, 215, 331, 360, 380, 407, 546, 552, 556
descriptive univariate analysis 450
despotism 577
Detroit 69, 468, 497
Devaldes 65
diabetic 18, 19, 55, 58, 142, 154, 177, 183, 193, 194, 448, 483
diagnosis xii, xvi, 7, 8, 9, 10, 22, 39, 44, 49, 51, 53, 55, 57, 58, 59, 60, 69, 70, 71, 72, 73, 74, 75, 76, 86, 113, 114, 117, 147, 155, 157, 177, 195, 197, 198, 209, 210, 211, 212, 213, 214, 215, 216, 217, 218, 219, 220, 221, 222, 223, 224, 225, 226, 227, 228, 229, 230, 231, 232, 233, 234, 235, 236, 237, 238, 239, 240, 241, 242, 243, 244, 245, 246, 247, 248, 249, 250, 251, 252, 253, 254, 255, 256, 257, 258, 259, 260, 261, 262, 263, 264, 265, 266, 267, 268, 269, 270, 271, 272, 273, 274, 275, 276, 277, 278, 279, 280, 281, 282, 283, 284, 285, 286, 287, 288, 289, 291, 292, 293, 295, 296, 297, 298, 299, 300, 301, 302, 303, 304, 305, 306, 307, 308, 309, 310, 311, 312, 313, 314, 315, 316, 317, 318, 329, 331, 332, 335, 336, 337, 338, 339, 340, 341, 342, 343, 344, 345, 347, 348, 349, 350, 351, 352, 353, 355, 361, 362, 363, 364, 365, 366, 367, 368, 369, 370, 371, 372, 373, 374, 375, 377, 379, 381, 382, 383, 384, 386, 387, 388, 389, 390, 391, 395, 397, 398, 399, 400, 401, 402, 403, 404, 405, 406, 407, 410, 411, 412, 414, 415, 416, 417, 418, 419, 420, 421, 422, 423, 425, 426, 427, 428, 429, 430, 431, 432, 433, 434, 435, 436, 437, 438, 439, 440, 441, 442, 463, 482, 500, 517, 532, 556
diagnosis specialist 8, 195
diagnostician 8, 342, 354
diastolic blood pressure 475, 476
didactic classwork 195, 351, 352
dietician 150, 480
digitalized thermometers 464
Dikkos 567, 570
Diocletian 89
Dioscorides 87, 90, 91, 547
diphenhydramine 109
diphtheria vaccine 121
Dipiro 43, 172
discovery process 157
Discussion 451
disease state 66, 115, 150, 193, 448, 454, 463, 465, 466, 467, 471, 477, 478, 483, 484, 504, 505, 506, 517, 552
disease state management 448, 454, 463, 465, 466, 477, 478, 484, 517
Dispensatorium 92, 548
dispensers 118, 137, 385, 463, 548
dispensing error 20, 544
dissolution 139

distillation 93
distribution 10, 42, 138, 139, 141, 184, 450, 472, 492, 494, 498, 552
divide and rule 570
division of labor 335
DNA 58, 140, 416
doctor of optometry 68
doctor of pharmacy degree 402, 422, 424, 470, 499, 516, 550, 551, 553, 554
doctor of philosophy 402, 528
documentation 65, 73, 86, 115, 116, 151, 180, 196, 381, 454, 465, 472, 478, 502, 521, 534
Dominica 112
Donnolo 91, 548
Down Syndrome 58
doxycycline 108
dress code 164, 165
drug-related morbidity and mortality 13, 16, 17, 19, 113, 146, 148, 152, 203, 342, 353, 460, 480, 482, 521, 553
drug clerk 516, 532
drug cost 146, 461, 482, 487, 490, 494, 496, 502, 504, 508, 510, 524
drug experts xi, xiv, xix, 44, 86, 125, 162, 446, 448, 450, 470, 513, 514
Drug Information Center 123, 160
drug interactions 10, 86, 115, 139, 143, 150, 161, 162, 180, 181, 200, 380, 481, 500, 504, 505, 515
drug knowledge xv, 8, 9, 10, 23, 40, 41, 43, 99, 104, 106, 152, 160, 170, 175, 176, 177, 178, 193, 195, 337, 422, 448, 449, 452, 463, 467, 514, 516, 517, 529, 532, 553, 554, 555
drug mechanism of action 42, 142
drug problems x, xiv, 16, 115, 125, 145, 158, 163, 178, 185, 189, 470, 480, 540
drug protocol management 509
drug regimen 13, 14, 18, 21, 141, 143, 184, 193, 471, 480, 483, 504
drug research 152, 160
drug safety program 150, 160
drug selection 16, 192, 501, 504
drug specialist xi, xvi, xviii, 8, 10, 13, 15, 20, 21, 23, 37, 117, 142, 143, 145, 163, 170, 173, 176, 178, 190, 195, 197, 380, 448, 449, 452, 455, 456, 478, 484, 489, 491, 554, 556, 558
Drug Topics 23, 460, 540, 544
drug treatment ix, xiii, xiv, xv, xvi, 8, 9, 14, 22, 39, 40, 41, 42, 44, 73, 85, 143, 150, 195, 209, 210, 211, 212, 213, 214, 215, 216, 217, 218, 219, 220, 221, 222, 223, 224, 225, 226, 227, 228, 229, 230, 231, 232, 233, 234, 235, 236, 237, 238, 239, 240, 241, 242, 243, 244, 245, 246, 247, 248, 249, 250, 251, 252, 253, 254, 255, 256, 257, 258, 259, 260, 261, 262, 263, 264, 265, 266, 267, 268, 269, 270, 271, 272, 273, 274, 275, 276, 277, 278, 279, 280, 281, 282, 283, 284, 285, 286, 287, 288, 289, 291, 292, 293, 295, 296, 297, 298, 299, 300, 301, 302, 303, 304, 305, 306, 307, 308, 309, 310, 311, 312, 313, 314, 315, 316, 317, 318, 329, 332,

333, 334, 336, 337, 338, 339, 340, 341, 342, 344, 347, 348, 349, 350, 351, 352, 353, 354, 361, 362, 363, 364, 365, 366, 367, 368, 369, 370, 371, 372, 373, 374, 375, 376, 380, 381, 382, 383, 384, 386, 387, 388, 389, 390, 391, 392, 395, 397, 398, 399, 400, 401, 402, 403, 404, 405, 406, 409, 410, 411, 412, 414, 415, 416, 417, 418, 419, 420, 421, 422, 423, 425, 426, 427, 428, 429, 430, 431, 432, 433, 434, 435, 436, 437, 438, 439, 440, 441, 463, 515, 547, 555
drug use control 17
Duggar 108
duplicate therapy 146, 186
duplication 180, 473, 503, 505
Durham 38, 123, 497, 506
Durham-Humphrey amendment 123
Durham-Humphrey Amendment Act 38

E

E-prescribing 527
écoles préparatoires 96
école de plein exercice 96
economic barriers 20
education ix, xvii, 5, 6, 7, 47, 49, 52, 56, 61, 68, 77, 92, 94, 95, 100, 103, 104, 111, 115, 117, 122, 125, 143, 150, 153, 160, 164, 170, 173, 179, 180, 181, 186, 190, 197, 203, 206, 243, 334, 355, 377, 378, 381, 392, 407, 424, 461, 465, 474, 475, 477, 489, 490, 491, 492, 493, 495, 496, 497, 499, 504, 506, 511, 515, 522, 528, 546, 548, 549, 551, 563, 565
education of physicians 92, 506
Edward, Jackson 64
effectiveness 118, 119, 141, 142, 150, 195, 461, 466, 472, 473, 478, 485, 486, 489, 495, 508, 512, 521, 524, 540, 569
Egypt 65, 86, 88, 89, 92, 378, 408, 548, 579
Ehrlich, Paul 107
electrical engineer 167
electricity xvi, 527
electroencephalogram 157
Eli Lilly 158
emergency medicine 48, 53, 54, 81, 156, 214, 331, 512, 546, 556
emergency room 13, 116, 146, 148, 151, 152, 156, 159, 189, 464, 471, 475, 476, 477, 480, 483, 506, 524, 533, 537, 557
emergency room visits 13, 116, 148, 151, 152, 189, 464, 471, 475, 476, 477, 480, 483, 557
Emerson, Joann 150
Emery, Alan 58
empiricism 107
endocrinology 57, 60, 70, 80, 216
enema 86
engineer xvi, 10, 11, 12, 103, 165, 196, 333, 334, 355, 529, 550
engineering xvi, 9, 195, 206, 334, 353, 421, 514, 529, 549
England 52, 54, 65, 81, 93, 94, 112, 202
Engle, Janet 144
epizootics 78, 79
errand boy of medicine xii, xiv, xix, 164, 170, 552
erythromycin 108, 153, 161, 173
especiadors 93

essence of life 575
essential hypertension 184, 497, 523
esthetics 52
ether 50, 98
Ethiopia 87, 580
ethnicity 140, 142, 199
ethylene glycol 121
Etzel 483, 520
Europe 52, 53, 59, 66, 79, 88, 89, 90, 91, 93, 94, 97, 123, 133, 185, 359, 378, 408, 409, 422, 423, 424, 439, 440, 441, 450, 451, 547, 548, 556, 572, 575, 576, 579
excretion 138, 184, 552
experimental group 18, 447, 481, 485, 496
experts xiv, 14, 15, 119, 162, 445, 448, 455, 480, 485, 515, 558
expert panel 480
Externship 254, 305, 309, 314, 316, 374
Ezomo xviii, 562

F
Falana, Femi 563, 569
family name 575
family nurse practitioner 177, 344
family practice 44, 48, 55, 56, 80, 81, 168, 174, 216, 330, 331, 512, 546, 556
Fatal ADR 147
father of toxicology 92, 138, 548, 552
Fauchard 51
fellowship 191, 195, 513, 515
fen-phen 154
feudalized society 562
Fez 92, 548
Fink 152, 199, 552

Finland 112
first branch of medicine xiii, xiv, 6, 38, 138
first impression 114, 164, 165
Fishbein, Morris 56
Fleming, Alexander 108
Flexner, Abraham 5, 7, 38, 85
Flockhart, David 158, 159, 172, 553
Florence 94
Florey 108
Florida administrative codes 176
Florida congressman 167
Florida Department of Health 173, 201
Florida Pharmacy Association 120, 168, 188, 446
Florida Pharmacy Today 120, 135, 168, 200, 201, 460, 461, 518, 520, 525, 544
Florida Society of Health System Pharmacists 167
Florida State legislator 536
floxin 108
Fluid 264, 410
food ix, 4, 10, 20, 76, 78, 86, 115, 118, 120, 121, 125, 139, 143, 195, 263, 380, 471, 569
Forand 110
forefathers of Americas independence 575
foreign pharmacy graduates 191
forensic medicine 361
formulary management 506
Fortune 2
foundation year 419
fourth largest continent 424
Fox study 21
France xi, xviii, 19, 51, 52, 59, 65, 69, 77, 93, 94, 95, 96, 97, 112, 408, 548

Francke, Don 172
Franklin, Benjamin 66
Frank Krusen 70, 82
Fraunhofer, Joseph 66
freedom xiii, 3, 23, 38, 47, 116, 168, 347, 513, 516, 545, 551, 559, 574, 575, 576, 581
free drug 139
free nitrates period 143
free sample 156, 159
Freund 72
Friedrich 93
future generation 86, 170, 190, 408, 559, 564, 574, 576, 579, 580

G
G6PD 140
Galen 88, 90, 91, 92, 547
Galetta 157
Gallup poll 12, 158, 447, 453, 464
Gamgee 79
GAMSAT 392
Gangeness 174, 201
Gans 152, 515, 525
Garabedian-Ruffalo 473, 521
Garcão 184, 203
Gariepy 202
Gates, Bill 171, 206
Generali 148, 201
general anesthetic 42, 139, 176
general certificate of education 360
general health problems 464
general practice 22, 55, 56, 59, 85, 407
general practitioner 11, 15, 22, 44, 45, 48, 55, 56, 79, 94, 96, 99, 100, 117, 138, 142, 151, 178, 330, 380, 476, 514, 517, 548, 552

Genesee Valley Group Health Association 485
genetics 48, 57, 58, 81, 82, 85, 331, 451, 452, 453, 455, 546, 556
genetic abnormality 157
genetic composition 452
geniuses 579
Georgia 68, 114, 480, 536
Gerald 517
Gerard 91
Germany 52, 65, 69, 72, 77, 78, 92, 95, 96, 107, 112, 408, 548, 580
Ghana 392, 579
Giwa, Dele 566
glycosylated hemoglobin 19, 183, 448
Gocht 72
Gold, Harry 172, 553
Goliath 3
Golodner, Linda 149
Goodman and Gilman 43
Good Morning America 2, 154
Good Samaritan Hospital 490
Good Samaritan law 54
government xviii, 1, 4, 5, 15, 37, 44, 54, 87, 88, 100, 110, 111, 122, 125, 149, 160, 162, 163, 174, 180, 185, 334, 359, 381, 465, 480, 507, 550, 551, 553, 561, 563, 564, 565, 566, 568, 569, 570, 571, 572, 581
government control media 571
government treasury 563, 564, 581
Grabadin 92
Grabenstein, John 479
graduate certificate in clinical pharmacy 405
graduate programs 49, 179, 183, 187, 396, 402
graveyard dosing 192
great opposition group 512, 516

Greece 87, 112, 185
Greek 65, 76, 87, 88, 89, 91, 378, 408, 547
griseofulvin 109
Gross Domestic Product xiii
guilds 65, 94
Gutenberg 51, 92
Gutenberg, Johannes 92, 548

H
habitable continents x, 359, 439, 449
Hadrian 89
halothane 109
Hammond 59
Handwriting 528
Hansten, Phillip 161
harmattan 571
Harris, Chapin 52
Harvey Cushing Society 75
Hatfield 494, 523
Hayden, Horace 53
Hazen, Al 65
HCFA 483
healthcare cost 15, 19, 110, 113, 146, 149, 150, 172, 175, 178, 180, 188, 189, 194, 196, 447, 460, 465, 480, 483, 488, 521, 540
Healthcare delivery 134, 461
Healthcare Finance Administration 508
healthcare providers 448, 454, 467, 469, 475, 479, 485
health insurance 110, 113, 150, 190, 505, 506, 550
Health Maintenance Organization 113, 186
health psychologists 578
health screenings 465

heart disease xiii, 17, 146, 147, 148, 447, 470, 479, 531
hematologists 57
hematology 70, 80, 107, 227, 362, 478, 519
hematuria 474
Hemophilia 488
hemorrhage 473
Henry, Patrick 4
Henry Ford Hospital 468
Hepler x, 17, 19, 113, 114, 134, 146, 172, 188, 201, 523, 551
herb 85, 90, 91, 547
herbal products 22, 447
hereditary 49, 562, 563, 564, 569, 574, 575
Hiddemen, Joan 159
high school diploma 197, 272, 300
Hippocrates 47, 58, 72, 76, 87, 90, 91, 445, 545, 547
Hiroshima 576
Hispanics 450, 451, 453, 455
HIV 13, 230, 483
HMO 12, 113, 186, 191, 465, 466, 485, 500
HMO managers 12
Hoechst 152, 158
Holland 65, 112
Hollywood fiction 580
homeless fellow 138
homeopathic preparations 22
home leadership 576
home of the brave 559
Home therapy 488
Hong Kong 112
hormone replacement therapy 467
Horner, Franklin 154
hospitalization 13, 18, 141, 146, 147, 149, 151, 152, 180, 195, 447, 464, 465, 467, 471, 473,

475, 477, 480, 482, 483, 488, 489, 491, 508, 552
hospitalization days 489
hospitals 13, 15, 16, 20, 48, 49, 54, 78, 90, 95, 97, 98, 99, 116, 124, 125, 148, 156, 160, 173, 174, 179, 181, 189, 196, 395, 396, 421, 447, 453, 461, 484, 486, 490, 492, 508, 509, 510, 512, 515, 525, 533, 540, 555
hospital admission xiii, 16, 19, 146, 148, 151, 152, 477, 498, 499, 550, 553, 557
hospital charges 501
hospital pharmacy 102, 110, 123, 124, 181, 511, 551
human accent 577
Human evolution and advancement 13
human genome 57, 58
human ills 561, 568
human immunodeficiency virus 483, 520
human tragedies 576, 580
Humoral theory 107
Hutu 580
hydrochlorothiazide 109, 141
hydrocortisone 109, 173
hydrolysis 140
hyperlipidemia 19, 174, 177, 448, 478, 484, 557
hypertension 16, 19, 58, 177, 184, 448, 464, 467, 478, 484, 497, 520, 557
hypnotics 22, 43, 109
hypotension 42

I

Ibn-Imran 90
Ibo society 563
Idahosa 564
Ife students 569, 571
illegible writing 527, 536
Illinois Supreme Court 118
imipramine 109
immune system disorders 49
immunizations 467, 515
immunohistochemistry 69
imperialism 567
inappropriate prescribing 495
inappropriate prescription 480, 494, 509
inappropriate regimen 20
incantations 86, 87
increased rate of hospitalization 13, 16
independent pharmacy 467, 540
Indian democracy 561
Indian health services 519
indifferent attitude group 512
industrialization 103
inferiority complex 330
infusion day 487
Innocent III 91
insurance 12, 14, 15, 110, 113, 146, 173, 354, 380, 466, 477, 505, 506, 550
insurance coverage 380, 505
insurance salesmen 12
intensive care unit 15, 19, 147, 468, 502
interdisciplinary cooperation 117, 516
interdisciplinary courses 334
internal medicine 13, 44, 48, 55, 57, 166, 174, 216, 331, 360, 362, 380, 487, 514, 516, 546, 556
international baccalaureate 381
Internet prescription service 120
internist 9, 18, 57, 80, 138, 447, 482, 485

internship 7, 8, 9, 41, 55, 57, 122, 124, 194, 195, 214, 216, 218, 224, 246, 297, 318, 333, 349, 387, 388, 392, 395, 397, 406, 423, 424, 427, 439, 441, 513, 546, 551
intern year 407
intervention regions 183
intravenous 17, 447, 484, 485, 487, 488, 490, 517, 521, 557
investigational study 488, 491
Iranian dynasty 89
Iraq 22, 408, 576
irrational therapy 186
Islamic 7, 65, 74, 89, 90, 547
isoniazid 109, 140, 176
Israelites 4, 545
Italy 65, 68, 91, 112, 548
Ithaca 79
IV bolus 487
IV buretrol 488
IV piggyback 487

J

Jackson, James 98
Jackson, John 59
JAMA 17, 56, 121, 146, 147, 149, 161, 200, 484
JAMB 360, 366
James, William 72
Jansens 65
Japan xi, 66, 108, 111, 112, 180, 203, 381, 382, 385, 386, 390, 391, 556, 561, 575, 576
Jefferson, Thomas 4, 570
Jennings, Robert 77
Jerome 91
Jesus Christ 91, 445, 547
Johnson, Abigail 2
Johnson, Tim 150
Johnston, John 97

joint admission matriculation board 360
journalists 12, 569
Journal of American Medical Association 17, 121
Journal of the American Pharmaceutical Association 16, 83, 135, 199, 200, 201, 202, 203, 520
judiciary 5, 575
Jung, Andrea 2
jungle, the 121
junior residency 333

K

kanamycin 108
Kansas City 154, 487, 491
Kassam 186, 203
Katen, Karen 2
Kazmierczak, Les 466
Kefauver-Harris 124
Kelly 17, 487, 520, 521
Kenosha 475
Kesler 176
Kesley, Frances 123
Kessler xiv, 158
Khadija 89
Kikuyu society 563
Kimble, Kodak 172
King 4, 68, 82, 95, 98, 413, 444
King Jr., Martin Luther 23, 188
King Saul 4
Kish 496
Klaproth, Martin 93
Knapp 17, 173, 174, 201, 495, 523
Knowlton 149, 199
Koch, Robert 79
Kosovo 580
Kristen 158

L

L. T., Post 65
Lagos 565, 569, 570
LaGuardia 144
LaGuardia Marriott Hotel 144
land of the free 559
Laramie 507
largest continent 377, 408
largest country 187, 377, 424
largest democracy 386, 561
law x, xiii, xvi, 5, 6, 7, 9, 10, 11, 54, 63, 77, 78, 79, 81, 97, 110, 113, 116, 118, 120, 124, 151, 162, 167, 171, 175, 178, 195, 200, 205, 206, 281, 335, 354, 422, 469, 516, 529, 531, 536, 558, 561, 564, 566, 570, 574, 575, 577, 581
Law, James 79
laws of the land 453, 581
law of comparative advantage 335
Lazarous 147, 552
Lazarus, Shelly 2
LBVAMC 473
Leape, Lucia 468
least knowledgeable healthcare practitioner about drugs 449
left ventricular dysfunction 557
legislators 173, 507
legislature 5, 507
Lemgo City 95
length of stay xvi, 17, 149, 461, 474, 482, 490, 492, 493, 495, 496, 498, 499, 501, 502, 504, 508, 523, 524
lens 65
leukocytes 107
licensure 104, 380
lidocaine 42
lifestyle changes 14, 466, 479
life expectancy xiv, 14, 111, 112
life span 111, 143, 465, 552
Life struggle 582
Likert scale 449
limitations 10, 92, 142, 188, 194, 336, 338, 340, 341, 343, 347, 349, 351, 353, 376, 391, 392, 406, 423, 455, 469
Lincoln, Abraham 54
linguistic barrier 360
Lister, Joseph 79, 99
Little Axe 447
liver enzymes 140
local anesthetic 42
local currency 566
London 52, 59, 92, 94, 96, 409, 413, 444, 450, 451, 453, 454, 556
long-term care 13, 120, 148, 152, 172, 471, 480, 481
long-term care facilities 13, 120, 480
longevity 111, 143, 552
Louisiana 97, 98
Lyman, Christopher 468
Lyman, Ray 63
Lyndon Johnson 111
Lynwood 487
Lyons 77, 96

M

machine 72, 193
macrolide 108
magic 71, 86, 87, 108, 547
magic bullet 108
Mali 92, 548, 580
Malone, Daniel 193
Malta 112
managed care 146, 149, 161, 173, 189, 191, 200
Mandela, Nelson 1, 3, 6, 545
manic depression 157

manifestos 568
Maori and Pacific program admission scheme 407
Maradona, Diego 566
market 93, 103, 104, 109, 117, 118, 120, 121, 123, 153, 158, 163, 171, 188, 190, 191, 201, 350, 549
Market forces 191
Marseilles 93, 95
Martin of Tours 91
Maryland 52, 134, 208, 331, 332, 357, 358, 490, 495, 507, 535
Maryland Medicaid 508
Massachusetts 50, 96, 98, 99, 100, 468
Massachusetts General Hospital 50, 98, 468
massacre 572
master of pharmacy 402, 404
Master of Science 8, 281, 282, 284, 287, 288
Materia Medica 87, 547
Mayer 460, 470, 523
McCarthy 6, 134, 461
McCauley 51, 81, 135
McGee, Alice 159
McGrath, Judy 2
McKenney and Harrisons study 16
mean hospital stay 487
mean weight 486
Mecca 89
mechanism of action 158, 172, 446
Medicaid 15, 111, 112, 113, 134, 150, 174, 201, 465, 466, 479, 482, 506, 507, 520, 525, 550
medical assistance program 505
medical board of New South Wales 392
Medical College of Philadelphia 100, 548
medical cost 19, 448, 484, 537
medical doctors xii, xiii, xv, xvi, xix, 1, 9, 10, 12, 13, 14, 21, 37, 39, 66, 67, 79, 80, 125, 144, 166, 167, 168, 169, 170, 178, 183, 190, 191, 195, 197, 331, 332, 334, 340, 354, 355, 360, 375, 380, 384, 390, 391, 392, 406, 413, 423, 438, 439, 440, 441, 464, 471, 476, 513, 514, 516, 555, 556, 557
medical malpractice 54
medical paraphernalia 169
medical rounds 509, 511
medical school xiv, xviii, 5, 6, 7, 8, 9, 10, 38, 39, 41, 53, 55, 58, 60, 62, 63, 64, 66, 67, 70, 77, 79, 80, 97, 98, 100, 143, 145, 158, 168, 172, 177, 178, 196, 206, 207, 262, 331, 332, 333, 340, 341, 357, 359, 360, 363, 366, 368, 376, 378, 381, 385, 387, 389, 390, 392, 396, 413, 419, 422, 424, 439, 442, 516, 528, 529, 540, 546, 548, 553
medical team 468, 501, 502, 523
Medicare 15, 48, 49, 110, 111, 112, 113, 125, 134, 150, 202, 466, 467, 480, 510, 520, 546, 550, 551
Medicare Catastrophic 113
medication-dispensing 193
medication administration record 533
medication error 469, 484, 505, 513, 514, 520, 529, 530, 536
medication experts 158, 447
medicinal chemistry 43, 107, 124
medieval period 90, 93
mediocres 579
Memphis 474

Mendel 57
mental analysis 19, 113
Merck 478
meta-analysis 147, 199, 552
metabolism 10, 57, 138, 140, 142, 184, 472, 552
meteorologist 11, 162
methotrexate 109
methylation 140
metoprolol 109
Mexico 77, 112
Miall, John 484
Michigan 62, 497
microbiologists 107, 334
microbiology 43, 334, 353, 362, 495
microcosm 359, 576
microscope 65, 69
midwifery 44, 289, 291, 335, 344, 345, 348
millennium 48, 81, 111, 188, 189, 190
Mills, Wilbur 110
Ministry of Health 181
Minneapolis 469, 493, 494
Minnesota 68, 70, 73, 174, 177, 465, 469, 479, 492, 493, 494, 505, 536
Minnesota Board of Pharmacy 465
Minnesota Pharmacy Association 465
miracles xiv, 14, 52, 446
missiles 445
Missouri 56, 68, 150, 154, 291, 487, 491
mockery of democracy 577
module 213, 421
Mohammed 89, 547, 567
Moissan, Henri 93
Monasteries 90, 91, 547
monitoring of efficacy 180, 454

Monks 91
Monroe, Marilyn 171
Montana 291, 348, 349, 351, 352, 469, 535
Montpellier 93, 94, 96
moon xix, 408
Moore, Ann 2
Morgan, John 97, 98, 102
Morley, Peter 164
morphine 93, 109, 484, 533
mortality xiii, 13, 17, 89, 146, 148, 149, 152, 172, 177, 189, 192, 194, 196, 200, 447, 461, 479, 480, 482, 483, 502, 508, 509, 524, 540, 550, 557
most knowledgeable healthcare practitioner about drugs 449, 451
moxibustion 379, 380, 454
Mulcahy, Anne 2
multidisciplinary team 504
multiple chronic conditions 150
multiple prescription drugs 150
Multiple regression analysis 508
Mutchie 486, 521
Mylan pharmaceutical company 472
myocardial infarction 16

N

Nagasaki 576
nalidixic acid 108
Nanjing hospitals 181
National Cholesterol Education Program 479, 557
National Health and Nutrition Examination Survey 476, 557
Nebraska 469, 470, 557
negative therapeutic outcomes 480
Neolithic 86, 547
neomycin 108

nephrology 57, 70, 80
Nerva 89
Netherlands 112, 160, 185, 553
neuroleptic drugs 140, 500
neurologist 9, 45
neurotoxin 121
news media 159
Newton, Isaac 65, 171
New drug 107
New Jersey 81, 96, 97, 461, 536
New Mexico 20, 178, 207, 535
New Orleans 76, 98
New South Wales Dental Board 397
New York City Society of Hospital Pharmacists 144
New York State 7, 59, 81, 104, 134
New York Times 5
New Zealand 19, 407
NHANES 476, 557
niche x, 117, 164, 463
Nigeria ix, xi, xviii, 2, 66, 179, 372, 442, 443, 450, 451, 453, 454, 556, 561, 562, 563, 564, 565, 566, 567, 569, 570, 571, 572, 580, 615
19th Amendment 2
Nixon, Richard 113, 582
Nkrumah, Kwamen 581
Nold, E.G. 447, 461, 489, 494, 523, 524, 558
Non-Western origin of the profession 22
nonadherence 183
noncompliance 16, 20, 145, 147, 152, 186, 193, 465, 477, 491, 497, 535, 553
nonformulary drug 503, 524
Nooyi, Indra 2
Nordbyhagen 184

North America 4, 66, 73, 290, 359, 376, 378, 380, 408, 439, 440, 451, 470, 556
North Carolina 18, 116, 174, 202, 448, 469, 479, 483, 497, 506, 524, 525, 532
Norway 184, 185
Nova Southeastern University xi, xviii, 15, 135, 208, 336, 337, 338, 341, 350, 357, 615
NSAID 141, 152
nuclear medicine 48, 85, 88, 331, 556
nuclear physicists 6
nuclear reactor 445
null hypotheses 449, 452
Nuremberg City 92
nurses xv, 12, 18, 20, 99, 123, 125, 150, 151, 160, 281, 343, 344, 376, 446, 455, 465, 467, 468, 471, 473, 487, 496, 506, 512, 530, 552, 553, 555
nurse midwifery 348
nurse practitioner 11, 150, 155, 173, 175, 176, 177, 178, 281, 344, 345, 347, 442, 467, 470, 471, 485, 536, 554
nursing homes xvi, 13, 116, 148, 150, 467, 515
nursing home medical director and administrator 480
Nyere, Julius 566

O

Obasanjo 566, 567
obstetric/gynecology 13
obstetrics and gynecology 48, 214, 216, 331, 407, 546, 556
of physician entry orders 484
Ohio 16, 68, 105, 208, 338, 339, 479, 487, 488, 489

ointments 87, 547
Oklahoma 447, 470
Olaoye, Wole 563, 568
old bridge 516
old civilizations 378
old layers 571
old medical school curriculum 516
old world 516
Oloton xviii, 563
Oman 112
Omnibus 113, 146, 152, 551
omniflox 108, 158, 159
Omoboriowo 570
oncology 13, 57, 60, 70, 73, 80, 214, 216, 218, 227, 407, 478, 519
Oni of Ife 571
ophthalmologist 9, 15, 44, 63, 64, 68, 157, 330, 451
ophthalmology 13, 23, 44, 48, 61, 62, 64, 66, 166, 197, 213, 214, 215, 330, 331, 360, 514, 516, 546, 556
oppressed group 170
optics 62, 65, 66
optometrist xv, 9, 11, 15, 44, 62, 68, 167, 330, 333, 338, 353, 354, 406, 514
Optometrists 68
optometry xi, xiv, 9, 23, 48, 61, 62, 63, 64, 66, 67, 80, 83, 138, 166, 205, 237, 246, 247, 248, 249, 250, 251, 252, 253, 254, 329, 330, 335, 337, 338, 339, 348, 353, 400, 401, 402, 417, 418, 419, 423, 450, 516, 546, 556
Opus Magnus 65
Organon 76
organ transplants 49
orthopedic 48, 213, 453, 494, 496, 523, 546

Orthopedic surgery 74
orthopedic unit 496, 523
osteopathy 39, 166
osteoporosis 140, 467
otolaryngology 48, 60, 61, 215, 331, 452, 546, 556
outdated solution 486
outpatients 16, 151, 447, 474, 557
over-the-counter medications 109, 115, 152, 464, 505
overuse 153, 186
oxazepam cost-savings conversion 471
oxidation 140
oxytetracycline 108

P

Pabis 18
pabulum 561
Padua 92, 548
Paine, Thomas 4
pain management 51, 59, 505
Paleolithic 86, 547
palm computer 18
pamaquin 108
papyrus 76, 86
parametric test 493
Pare, Ambroise 51
parent-child 14, 281, 344
parent-child model 14
parental nutrition 125, 485, 486, 512, 521
Paris xi, xviii, 52, 91, 94, 96, 548
Park-Davis 109
Parker, Paul 172
Parks, Rosa 5, 6
Pasteur, Louis 79, 107
Pathak 447, 461, 489, 524, 558
pathologist 9, 451, 452, 453

pathology 48, 53, 64, 65, 66, 68, 76, 85, 98, 330, 331, 362, 407, 414, 546, 556
pathophysiology 43, 500
patient-care area 499, 503
patient care unit 17, 499
patient education 470, 497, 498, 505, 515
patriotic citizen 568
PCOE 527
peaceful protest 24, 569, 571
peak flow meters 476, 477
peasants 577
pediatricians 44, 151, 178, 355, 451, 453, 455, 552
pediatrics 48, 55, 57, 70, 80, 82, 166, 174, 177, 214, 216, 331, 360, 380, 407, 546, 556
peer review 119
Pelletier, Joseph 93
penal colony 392
penicillin 108, 141, 153
Pennsylvania Hospital 98, 102
period 18, 63, 86, 87, 88, 90, 121, 141, 183, 186, 361, 413, 475, 482, 483, 487, 490, 491, 493, 498, 499, 501, 502, 504, 529, 547, 548
peripheral neuropathy 123
persistence 152, 479, 557
Peterson and Lake study 557
pharmaceutical care x, xii, 12, 13, 16, 18, 19, 110, 114, 116, 117, 122, 134, 137, 150, 162, 163, 179, 180, 184, 185, 186, 199, 201, 202, 203, 312, 313, 448, 461, 463, 465, 466, 469, 475, 480, 483, 506, 507, 520, 524, 525, 551
pharmaceutical companies pressure 153

pharmaceutical industries 37, 103, 106, 107, 137, 150, 191
pharmaceutical statistics 43
pharmacien 95
Pharmacist x, xii, xiv, xv, xvi, xix, 5, 6, 10, 11, 13, 17, 18, 19, 21, 44, 45, 83, 90, 95, 103, 105, 106, 110, 114, 115, 117, 118, 119, 120, 123, 144, 150, 154, 155, 164, 167, 168, 169, 170, 172, 174, 177, 182, 185, 186, 188, 189, 190, 196, 198, 200, 201, 202, 330, 342, 350, 353, 354, 376, 380, 381, 392, 405, 406, 423, 439, 446, 447, 448, 450, 451, 453, 454, 456, 457, 458, 459, 460, 463, 464, 465, 466, 467, 468, 470, 472, 473, 476, 477, 479, 480, 482, 484, 485, 486, 487, 488, 490, 491, 492, 494, 495, 496, 497, 498, 499, 501, 502, 503, 504, 505, 506, 507, 509, 510, 511, 513, 516, 518, 519, 520, 521, 522, 523, 524, 525, 527, 530, 531, 532, 534, 535, 536, 539, 547, 549, 551, 553, 554, 555, 556
pharmacodynamics 10, 86, 125, 138, 142, 200, 333
pharmacoeconomics 16, 43, 135, 297, 310, 405
pharmacognosy 96, 124, 374, 375
pharmacokinetics 15, 43, 86, 125, 138, 142, 184, 200, 489, 492, 493
pharmacokinetics services 125, 489, 492, 493
pharmacology 62, 66, 80, 107, 124, 158, 172, 177, 421, 422, 553
pharmacotherapy 461, 468, 471, 499, 519, 557

pharmacy-developed monthly education program 490
pharmacy autonomy 116, 117, 118, 120, 163, 180, 551
pharmacy calculations 43
pharmacy charges 486, 501
pharmacy cost per admission 499
pharmacy officials 37
pharmacy organizations 23, 38, 39
pharmacy service units 503
pharmacy technician 118, 120, 124, 197, 465, 498
Pharmacy Times 135, 461, 520, 525, 535, 544
Pharmacy Today 135, 178, 199, 200, 201, 202, 203, 460, 515, 519, 520, 524, 525, 535, 544
PHARMAssist program 506
PharmD x, 8, 104, 105, 118, 120, 122, 125, 137, 144, 162, 163, 166, 167, 168, 170, 174, 175, 179, 188, 189, 191, 197, 292, 294, 295, 298, 300, 301, 303, 306, 308, 311, 348, 377
phase I 360, 363, 376
phase II 360, 363, 376
phase III 360, 363
phase P 360, 363
phenytoin 109, 139, 176
Philadelphia College of Apothecaries 100, 549
philanthropists 110
Philistine 3
Phillips, Stacy 159
physical assessments 115
physical medicine 48, 70, 71, 82, 85, 331, 451, 546, 556
physical medicine and rehabilitation 48, 82, 331, 451, 546, 556
physical pharmacy 43
physical sciences 124, 300

physical therapist 480
physician xv, 7, 9, 11, 14, 20, 38, 54, 55, 56, 64, 69, 70, 73, 80, 88, 91, 92, 97, 98, 102, 114, 116, 119, 145, 148, 150, 151, 152, 154, 155, 167, 171, 172, 173, 174, 175, 176, 178, 184, 190, 207, 237, 267, 330, 335, 341, 342, 347, 353, 376, 378, 392, 407, 422, 424, 440, 441, 452, 453, 456, 459, 460, 465, 467, 470, 471, 480, 482, 483, 485, 488, 497, 500, 501, 502, 503, 505, 507, 508, 513, 515, 523, 524, 527, 532, 534, 536, 548, 552, 553, 554, 555, 556, 557, 566
physician assistants xv, 20, 150, 151, 155, 173, 175, 176, 178, 207, 341, 347, 376, 378, 392, 407, 422, 424, 440, 441, 467, 470, 471, 485, 536, 552, 554, 556
physician visits 148, 152, 480
physics 65, 66, 73, 95, 124, 334, 353, 360, 368, 387, 409
physiology 53, 61, 62, 64, 66, 69, 76, 88, 98, 141, 196, 414
Pihl, Robert 577
pilots 6, 530
pioneers 48, 53, 70, 71, 355
Pius, Antonius 89
plastic surgery 15, 48, 73, 75, 177, 546
pneumoccal pneumonia 17
pneumonia 16, 147, 153, 202, 480, 512
podiatry xiv, 23, 80
Poirier 185, 202
poisons xii, xiv, 9, 92, 138, 552
Poison Squad 121

policemen 12
political activists 572
Polo, Marco 65
polymorphism 142
polymyxin B sulfate 109
polypharmacy 143
poor collection of data 467
Pope 91
Pope Alexander III 91
Poretz 447, 461, 488, 522, 557
Portugal 184, 185, 203, 408
Portuguese xviii, 424, 450
positron emission tomography 59, 452
postmortem 184
poultry 77
powerhouse 408
powers of the laws and judiciary 574
practitioners xii, xiii, xv, xvi, xix, 12, 15, 20, 22, 39, 41, 47, 48, 49, 51, 53, 56, 64, 68, 71, 77, 79, 89, 93, 97, 103, 107, 116, 117, 118, 142, 154, 157, 163, 168, 170, 171, 173, 174, 175, 177, 178, 180, 187, 191, 192, 193, 194, 201, 330, 347, 355, 396, 407, 446, 451, 452, 454, 455, 465, 467, 469, 472, 473, 474, 514, 527, 528, 530, 531, 532, 533, 537, 539, 548, 556, 558
Prague 92, 548
pre-clinical 41, 331, 332, 333, 336, 337, 338, 339, 340, 341, 348, 349, 350, 351, 352, 375, 376, 391, 392, 406, 409, 413, 415, 422, 423, 438, 439, 440, 441
pre-clinical didactic class work 41
preceptor 9, 98, 99
pregnancy tests 464

prescriber computer order entry 527
prescribing xvi, 6, 18, 19, 20, 23, 37, 38, 137, 141, 145, 150, 158, 173, 175, 176, 178, 187, 194, 347, 376, 447, 448, 460, 471, 472, 490, 492, 495, 496, 500, 502, 503, 505, 508, 511, 513, 517, 519, 522, 523, 525, 527, 530, 554, 555, 558
prescriptions xii, xv, xvi, 12, 13, 19, 37, 90, 95, 97, 106, 109, 148, 152, 153, 154, 155, 161, 162, 167, 186, 188, 198, 342, 392, 423, 441, 447, 466, 467, 468, 469, 473, 477, 482, 500, 502, 505, 507, 513, 527, 530, 531, 532, 535, 536, 547, 554, 555, 558
prescription blank 535
press night 569
preventable errors 147
preventive medicine 48, 71, 331, 454, 546, 556
primary care providers 173, 201
privacy 117, 180, 381, 454, 551
private consultation areas 478
private jet 566
Procter Jr., William 100, 135
prodigal son 563
professionalism 100, 103, 227, 514
professional autonomy xii, 163, 551
professional course 192
professional phase 209, 211, 212, 214, 216, 218, 221, 223, 224, 226, 228, 229, 231, 233, 235, 237, 239, 241, 243, 246, 249, 252, 255, 257, 260, 263, 266, 267, 269, 271, 272, 273, 275, 277, 279, 282, 284, 287, 288, 289, 292, 295, 298, 300, 301,

303, 306, 308, 311, 313, 315, 316
professional slavery 540, 559
profiles 123, 124, 499
prontosil 108
prophet 168
propofol 42
prospective study 492, 501, 552
prostheses 52
prosthetic replacement 51
protein binding 42
protesters 25
prothrombin tests 464
prothrombin time ratio 473
Prussia 52, 95
psychiatrist 12, 45, 48, 178, 451, 472, 500
psychiatry and neurology 48, 546
psychologists 20, 178
Ptolemy theory 2
publicity 573
public court of opinion 527
public insanity 568
public institutions 205
public opinion xi, xv, 448, 455, 558, 566
public perception 453
public spraying of money 568
Puerto Rico 172, 331
pulmonary disease xiii, 147, 447, 461, 475, 490, 512, 522
pulmonologist 80
pulmonology 70, 80
puppet 564
Pure Food and Drug Act 121
pyelonephritis 17, 495

Q

quality assurance 494, 505
quality of health 112
quasi-experimental study 481

Quebec 185, 577
Queens 483
questionnaire xviii, 194, 449
quinine 93, 108
quinolones 108, 139

R

rabies vaccine 107
racism 567, 574
radiology xiv, 48, 72, 73, 80, 85, 166, 215, 331, 361, 407, 546, 556
radionuclides 59, 452
Raymond, Don 535
reactionaries 571
receptors 142, 196
recommendation 114, 492, 505, 534
reduced absenteeism 19, 448, 484
refractionists 63, 65, 68
refusal to dispense 186
regimen 11, 19, 20, 119, 143, 152, 153, 185, 188, 193, 194, 196, 467, 474, 480, 483, 493, 494, 502, 507, 522, 536, 552
regimen changes 467
Registered nurse 272
remuneration 104, 174, 188, 190, 191, 272, 549
Renaissance 68, 92, 93, 548
renewal fee 175
rennin 140
residence xii, 7, 8, 9, 10, 21, 41, 52, 105, 118, 124, 167, 173, 175, 333, 339, 353, 354, 513, 517, 554, 555
resident physician 97, 98
results 12, 17, 18, 99, 115, 137, 147, 148, 157, 161, 183, 184, 186, 188, 195, 332, 347, 375, 390, 391, 424, 447, 450, 451, 452,

453, 457, 466, 467, 469, 472, 475, 478, 482, 485, 486, 487, 488, 489, 491, 493, 495, 496, 498, 501, 502, 504, 505, 510, 551, 566
retrogressive forces 561, 567
Rhazes 7
rheumatology xiv, 57, 80, 472, 502
rheumatology and renal clinic 472, 502
Rhode Island teaching hospital 503
Rich, Darryl 533
Richmond 478
Rinderpest 77, 79
Rising, Waite 172
rising cost of health care 15, 16
Ritalin 577
robotic approach 106
rob Peter to pay Paul 21
Rochester 75, 177, 485
rockets 334, 445
Roentgen, Wilhelm 72
Romans 65
Roman Catholic Church 90
Roman Empire 88, 89, 90, 91, 547
Roosevelt, Eleanor 582
Roosevelt, Franklin 550
Rosemount 465
Ross, Mike 150
rotations x, xvi, 41, 57, 118, 194, 195, 216, 220, 221, 225, 226, 238, 248, 251, 254, 256, 257, 263, 267, 269, 270, 272, 292, 293, 295, 297, 303, 313, 314, 318, 332, 334, 336, 337, 338, 342, 349, 350, 351, 352, 354, 362, 367, 381, 382, 383, 386, 387, 388, 389, 392, 395, 397, 399, 406, 412, 413, 415, 417, 422, 423, 427, 437, 438, 439, 440, 483, 554

Roussel, Hoechst Marion 152
rudimentary educational training 528
Rudolf Virchow 69
rural dwellers 174
Russia 52, 408
Rwanda 580

S

S4 drugs 400, 406
Salerno 91, 548
salt 139, 191, 206
Salt Lake City 149, 486
salvarsan 108
Samitha, Sushrutha 73
Sankore 92, 548
San Diego 23
San Marino 112
Saudi Arabia 561
Sawyer, Diane 161
Scheele, Wilhelm 93
schools of pharmacy xi, xvi, xviii, 7, 8, 43, 96, 104, 120, 122, 124, 125, 160, 162, 164, 172, 178, 179, 183, 185, 187, 189, 191, 194, 196, 350, 359, 448, 513, 515, 550, 551, 554
school absenteeism 477
school days 464
Schwarzenegger, Arnold 577
scientific method 7, 39
scope of pharmacists practice 513
Sebuncuoglu, Serafeddin 50
second-generation cephalosporin 495
second largest continent 360
second smallest habitable continent 408
secretaries 20, 555
Seinfeld, Jerry x, 5, 167

Seinfeld/Robot practicing pharmacist 20
Self 447, 460, 461, 490, 512, 519, 522
senate 146
senators 12
senior residency 333
sepsis 16, 99
serum drug assays 489, 490, 522
Shagari, Shehu 564, 570
Shaman 86, 547
sham leaders 564
sham politicians 568
Sheboygan 489
Shefcheck 155, 172, 175, 201
Shippen Jr., William 98
shorthand forms of writing 528
shuttle 445
Sicily 89
sick leave 19, 448, 484
sign-on bonus 190
Singapore 112
single proton emission computer tomography 59
sinusitis 154
slave 37, 55, 580
slavery 148, 168, 545, 558, 559, 567, 576, 579, 580
sleeping giant of Africa 571
Slovenia 112
smallest habitable continent 392
Smalley 152
smart label 193
Smith 168, 183, 470, 519, 521
smoking 5, 142, 467, 578
smoking cessation 467
Snell 65
SOAP format 115
socialism 180, 573
Social Security Act 110, 150, 550

social security disability beneficiary 477
social worker 150, 165, 196, 476, 555
societal ills 569
socio-capitalist 573
sociological barriers 20
Socrates 72
software 192
soldiers 48, 49
Somalia 580
soothsayer 190, 568
South America 66, 187, 359, 378, 424, 438, 439, 441, 450, 451, 556
South Dakota 150, 470
spacer device 476
Spain 89, 90, 91, 96, 112, 360, 408, 548
Spalitto, Anthony 154
Spanish 168, 193, 408
specialist 11, 56, 64, 82, 116, 139, 142, 162, 190, 354, 380, 396, 407, 452, 491
spectacles 61, 65, 68
speech night 568
Srnka Quentin 152
St. Joseph Hospital 505
St. Louis 81, 120, 291, 351, 358
St. Nicholas Hospital 489
St. Paul 469, 493, 505
St. Philips Hospital 98
stage III hypertension 476
state governors 12
state health departments 396
State University 83, 105, 208, 332, 338, 339, 357, 479, 488, 489
Statio 92
Stephen Fried 156, 157, 529
Stimmel 447, 460, 500, 523, 558
stock brokers 12

store 106, 123, 155, 164, 193, 466, 532
Strand x, 19, 113, 114, 134, 146, 163, 164, 172, 551
streptomycin 108
stroke xiii, 147, 148, 194
study group 17, 472, 476, 487, 489, 491, 495, 497, 499, 501, 502, 503
sub-therapeutic treatment 20
subtherapeutic dosing 153
sulfanilamide 121
Sumerians 87
summer 536
Sumon, Sakolchai 179
superiority complex 330
superstitions 88
supporters 3, 516, 569, 570
suppositories 87, 547
Supreme Court of Alabama 531
suramin 108
surgeon 6, 9, 22, 40, 41, 42, 44, 48, 50, 51, 52, 60, 73, 75, 92, 94, 96, 97, 98, 177, 197, 396, 450, 451, 452, 453, 484, 514, 530, 536, 553
surgery 6, 22, 40, 41, 42, 44, 45, 48, 49, 50, 51, 52, 55, 60, 64, 66, 72, 73, 74, 75, 78, 80, 81, 85, 88, 90, 91, 93, 166, 174, 177, 197, 213, 214, 216, 256, 331, 355, 361, 362, 380, 388, 407, 422, 450, 452, 479, 486, 494, 501, 505, 514, 516, 533, 546, 553, 556
surgical team 502
surrogate physicians 155
Sweden 111, 112
Swiss 92
syphilis 53, 56
systolic blood pressure 475, 476

T
tabes dorsalis 59
tablets 87, 490, 547
taboo 574
Talbot, Robert 96
talking pill bottle 193
Talley and Laventuriers study 16
tambocor 531
tamoxifen 140, 531
Taylorville 466
teacher 10, 76, 79, 167, 333, 528, 570
Tegata campus 381
television advertisements 152
Tennessee xviii, 119, 121, 474, 490, 536
tetracycline 108
Thailand 179
Thailand Ministry of Health 179
thalidomide 123
thallium 121
Theophrastus 87, 92
therapeutic xi, xii, xiv, xvi, xix, 20, 23, 37, 70, 73, 86, 89, 92, 106, 108, 114, 115, 116, 117, 119, 125, 138, 141, 142, 147, 150, 153, 162, 169, 170, 171, 175, 176, 177, 180, 184, 187, 195, 196, 197, 198, 330, 375, 380, 400, 421, 422, 446, 447, 448, 468, 471, 473, 480, 485, 489, 490, 492, 498, 499, 504, 505, 509, 511, 513, 514, 515, 516, 517, 529, 531, 532, 540, 549, 550, 553, 554, 556
therapeutician xii, xiv, xvi, xix, 8, 10, 15, 23, 37, 40, 44, 116, 117, 143, 145, 150, 170, 175, 176, 178, 187, 190, 195, 196, 197, 375, 380, 451, 463, 489, 513, 514, 539, 554, 556, 558

therapeutic judge 532
therapeutic outcome 70, 115, 150, 169, 380, 446, 448, 469, 480, 514, 540, 550
therapeutic physician xi, xii, xiv, xvi, xix, 23, 37, 117, 125, 143, 170, 176, 187, 196, 197, 198, 330, 375
therapeutic range 447, 473, 490, 492
therapy xiii, xiv, 10, 13, 14, 16, 17, 19, 42, 49, 70, 109, 114, 115, 116, 117, 125, 138, 139, 142, 143, 146, 147, 150, 152, 158, 159, 160, 161, 167, 171, 172, 175, 177, 178, 180, 186, 188, 192, 193, 194, 195, 196, 197, 199, 200, 201, 421, 447, 461, 467, 468, 470, 471, 473, 475, 476, 477, 478, 480, 482, 483, 485, 488, 490, 494, 495, 496, 497, 499, 500, 502, 504, 505, 511, 513, 517, 518, 519, 522, 524, 525, 537, 538, 550, 551, 553, 557, 558
three big powers 408
thromboembolism 473
Ticarcillin 495
Timbuktu 92, 548
timing of lab tests 501
Toni, Bernardo 68
tooth extraction 51, 67
Torrington 507
Total cost of care 510
total cost per admission 17, 499
total parental nutrition 509
Tower of Babel 408
toxicity 16, 17, 20, 42, 92, 138, 139, 140, 142, 154, 179, 192, 477, 491, 498, 529

traditional Chinese medicine 180, 377, 379
traditional medicine 92, 181, 360, 378, 386, 454, 548
traditional rulers 564, 575
Trajan 89
transfusion 510, 511
transportation 76, 78, 79, 173, 505, 566
treatment x, xv, 7, 8, 9, 14, 15, 20, 22, 37, 39, 44, 45, 48, 49, 51, 53, 55, 56, 57, 58, 59, 60, 63, 65, 66, 70, 71, 72, 73, 74, 75, 76, 80, 85, 86, 88, 92, 93, 113, 115, 116, 143, 145, 148, 157, 169, 170, 177, 180, 183, 184, 186, 192, 193, 194, 195, 197, 331, 332, 334, 336, 337, 338, 340, 341, 343, 345, 347, 350, 351, 352, 354, 376, 379, 385, 391, 392, 400, 406, 407, 417, 421, 422, 423, 438, 439, 440, 441, 446, 450, 453, 454, 463, 471, 473, 475, 476, 477, 481, 482, 485, 486, 488, 491, 492, 493, 494, 497, 498, 500, 505, 512, 514, 515, 517, 529, 530, 536, 539, 547, 554, 555, 556
treatment failure 148, 481
treatment group 186, 471, 473, 475, 482, 485, 486, 493
treatment protocols 517
Tromp 185
Truman, Harry 110
Trunet 19
Tuina 378, 379
Tushi 580
two great races 360
typan red 108
typist 167
Tyson, Mike 171

U

Umar 89
Umezawa 108
unit-dose system 17
United Kingdom 58, 66, 69, 98, 112, 113, 185, 409, 413, 415, 417, 419, 421, 422, 423, 441, 450, 545
United Nations Security Council 571
United States xii, xviii, xix, 4, 6, 7, 38, 41, 47, 52, 55, 66, 78, 96, 99, 110, 112, 179, 185, 199, 201, 202, 360, 380, 392, 408, 424, 441, 449, 453, 455, 458, 461, 508, 524, 530, 546, 548, 550, 551, 554, 556, 558, 559, 576, 577, 580, 615
United States Hospitals 524
unit dose drug distribution system 498, 503
Universitas Aromatariorum 94
University of Arizona 146
University of London 96, 413, 415, 444
University of Michigan 104, 122, 172, 553
University of Wyoming 507
unnecessary prescriptions 153
Upchurch, Gina 506
Upjohn 109
Upper Midwest 493
urgent care 13
urology 48, 85, 88, 331, 546, 556
Utah 486
Uthman 89

V

vaccinations 186, 479
Valencia 94
VANCHCS 471
vancomycin 15, 108, 153, 492, 522
Vandals 90
Vandel, John 507
venerology 360
verapamil 109
Verhoeff 64
Vermont 54
Verona 94
Veterans Affairs Medical Center 193
Veteran Administration 116, 467, 471
Veteran Administration Medical Centers 116
veterinarian 9, 11, 12, 77, 78, 79, 83, 167, 451, 455
veterinary medicine xi, xviii, 9, 48, 76, 77, 78, 79, 80, 83, 237, 335, 339, 340, 348, 353, 424, 450, 514, 546, 556
vicarious liability principle 531
Virginia 123, 144, 477, 551
vitamins 22
vocational courses 104, 549
volunteer 110, 121
Von Haller, Albrecht 59
Von Helmholtz, Hermann 66
Von Hohenhein, Philippus Aureolus Theophrastus Bombastus 138
Vullemin, Led 107

W

Waddell, James 478
Waksman 107, 108
Ward, Kristi 506
warfarin 109, 139, 447, 474, 510
Warren, John 98
Washington, George 4
Washington Post 124, 533
Washington State 469, 482, 519, 520

Wateska 487, 557
Watson 58
Watts, Travis 447, 460, 470, 523
weather 11, 162
weight management 467
Weistein 108
West Africa school certificate 360
White, Andrew 79
White, Eugene 123, 172
Whitman, Meg 2
Wigand 5, 6
Wiley, Harvey 121
Williams, John Whitridge 60, 82
William I 52, 95
window of opportunity 114
Winfrey, Oprah 2, 159
Winter 243, 244, 245, 246, 247, 248, 249, 250, 251, 252, 253, 254, 263, 264, 265, 268, 269, 292, 293
Wisconsin 208, 339, 341, 342, 475, 479, 489
Woertz, Pat 2
womanizing 568, 574
womb of medicine 7, 40, 85, 89
women versus men 1
wonder drug 109, 121, 156
woods 571

Woofendale, Robert 52
Woosley, Raymond 159, 553
words of wisdom 164, 582
working poor 113
work days 464
Worland 507
World Health Organization 147, 152, 553
World War II 48, 49, 78, 81, 108
Worrall, Cathy 177
Wyoming Department of Health 507

Y

Yale-New Haven Hospital 477, 557
Yanofsky 58
Yodian 180
Yoh 447, 460

Z

Zahnarzt 52
Zahnbrecher 52
zidovudine 109
zombie 157, 516

About the Author

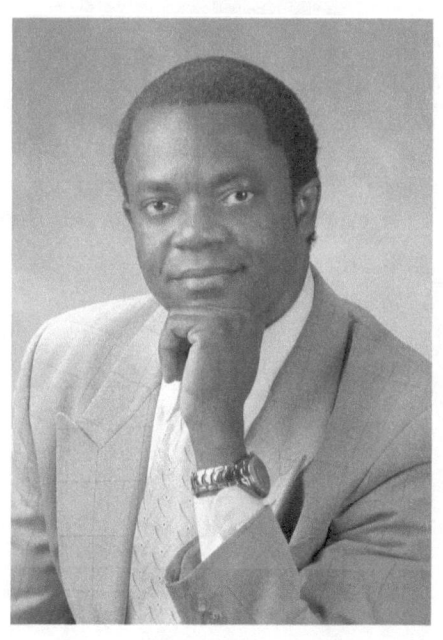

Dr. Patrick Ojo was born and brought up in Benin City, Nigeria, Africa. He attended Benin Baptist Model Primary School, Evboneka Grammar School (high school), and Eghosa Grammar School briefly for one year before proceeding to University of Ife, Ile-Ife, for a degree in chemistry. He taught briefly at Government Girl's College Ngelzarma, Borno State, as Assistant Head of the Science Department, and Oghada Grammar School, Edo State, as Head of the Science Department before migrating to the United States in 1988. While in the U.S., he worked with New York City Department of Homeless Services as a caseworker; at the same time he attended New York City Technical College (to complete pre-pharmacy school requirements) and Long Island University, College of Pharmacy, Brooklyn, New York, for his first degree in pharmacy. He became a U.S. citizen in 1996. In 1997 he moved to Florida State for a professional pharmacy practice. He later enrolled in Nova Southeastern University, Fort Lauderdale, Florida, for a Doctor of Pharmacy degree, and he graduated in 1999. He has practiced professional pharmacy in various settings: community (Winn-Dixie Pharmacy), hospital (North Shore Hospital, Miami, etc.), closed (compounding prescription pharmacy), in a correctional facility (prison pharmacy), and/or institutional pharmacy.

www.ingramcontent.com/pod-product-compliance
Lightning Source LLC
LaVergne TN
LVHW091526060526
838200LV00036B/500